FOUNDATIONS OF
HEALTH SCIENCE

Allyn and Bacon, Inc.
Boston, London, Sydney, Toronto

FOUNDATIONS OF HEALTH SCIENCE

third edition

Barbara Osborn Henkel

Professor of Health Education

Chairperson, Department of
    Health and Safety Studies
California State University at
    Los Angeles

Richard K. Means

Professor of Health Education
Auburn University

James M. Sawrey

Professor of Psychology
Academic Vice-President
Austin Peay State University
Clarksville, Tennessee

Jack Smolensky

Professor of Health Education
San Jose State University

Library of Congress Cataloging in Publication Data

Main entry under title:

Foundations of health science.

    Bibliography: p.
    Includes index.
    1. Hygiene.   I. Henkel, Barbara Osborn, 1921–
RA776.F775   1977   613   76–52905
ISBN 0–205–05739–X

contents

Contents

preface

The 1970s may be one of the most important decades of the century relative to changes in health care. Are you prepared to cope with it? The attainment and maintenance of effective levels of wellness (health, if you choose) is now accepted as a right in the United States, as well as in a number of other nations. The system of medical care in the United States is being increasingly criticized, sometimes rightfully, sometimes wrongfully. Our provisions for health and medical care are geared to therapy, some of which is exotic and so expensive that it is not available to many. Even if money were to be made available for such care, there is not the manpower to provide it.

Some of the knotty problems currently facing us, the layman as well as the professional, include these questions: How should health care be provided? Who should provide it? What should health care comprise? When should it cease? and should responsibilities for maintaining health and wellness extend beyond self to society?

Subsidization by government for health care is increasing, but how much can we afford to pay, and what should be included? Is it reasonable to underwrite the cost of dental care, vision and hearing, and psychological treatment? Should personal medical records be maintained in a central file under our social security number, for example? This could promote efficiency, but it could also curtail privacy.

Since the availability of care is unevenly distributed, should primary care providers, such as physicians, be forced to practice for a specified time in rural or ghetto areas? How much responsibility can be delegated to an extender, such as the physician's assistant? Exactly what is the role of the nurse-practitioner? How should health professionals be controlled—by peer or consumer review under the auspices of government or of private organizations? Should professionals be required to participate in a continuing education program for relicensure?

Since orientation toward therapy rather than prevention seems short-sighted, why don't the medical community and the underwriters of care such as insurance companies provide for preventive care for the majority? Too many times the consumer asks for a preventive medical examination but does not obtain an adequate one or cannot get it paid for by his or her insurance plan. How is "adequate" determined? Should the exotic treatments be made available to all?

If a choice is to be made, who makes it? For example, in kidney failure, a transplant may be recommended. Such transplants have the best chance of surviving when the kidney is obtained from a close relative. If you were a father of several young children, would you give up one kidney to *one* of these children? It might jeopardize your health and therefore your potential for caring for your family. How much of the family income should go for the care of a chronically, maybe terminally, ill relative? How far should we go to keep a severely defective baby alive when the life expectancy may be but a few years, or the quality of life may be at a very low level? Let us say that a relative is in a deep coma and has suffered extensive brain damage. This person cannot live without artificial aid such as a respirator. How long would you want him to live? Who is going to disconnect the respirator (pull the plug)—you, the nurse, or the physician? Is this murder? What about abortion, is that murder? If abortion is not murder, why the furor about doing research on the products of abortion? If a woman has the right to control what happens to her body, then why should her male partner be required to give consent to an abortion procedure or to sterilization? Does the State have a right to curtail what she does? These issues involve moral decisions, but health knowledge can aid in arriving at a decision.

Should our responsibilities for maintaining health extend beyond personal needs to the needs of society? Is it right for us to refuse a vaccination and thus threaten others? Does our right to privacy (not naming a venereal disease contact, for example) take precedence over the rights of those to whom we might have transmitted disease? As long as we do not ostensibly harm others, should we be permitted to abuse dangerous substances, such as vitamins, aspirin compounds, sleeping pills, alcohol, and narcotics, by using large amounts?

Are you, as an accountable adult, prepared to participate in making decisions about some of these questions? Prevention seems to be the key concept. As health professionals slowly move to an increasingly preventive orientation in providing health care, are you prepared to assume responsibility for maintaining health and improving wellness levels of yourself and your family? The purpose of this text is to help adults to value

the concept of prevention and to practice preventive behavior. They
should:

1. Make intelligent and knowledgeable decisions about health matters
   and problems
2. Know what constitutes wellness and levels of good health
3. Use desirable health practices that promote optimal health levels
4. Improve levels of health by understanding how the body functions
5. Select competent health advisors
6. Utilize the resources in the community to solve health problems
7. Identify deviations from normal to obtain necessary health care
8. Critically evaluate health information and services
9. Identify and counteract some of the hazards of sedentary life
10. Cope with problems that grow out of crowded living conditions
11. Analyze the health implications inherent in a life span increased by
    medical and public-health advances
12. Support government and private programs that promote health locally,
    nationally, and internationally.

We have done several things in this book to make it more valuable
to the reader. One was to integrate descriptions of anatomy and physiology
with discussions of specific health problems. Some years ago health textbooks were like anatomy and physiology texts. Readers would get bogged
down in details about muscles, bones, nerves, and systems of the body.
Health educators gradually stopped using this approach and concentrated
on explaining what to do, but they gave minimal emphasis to the *why* of
doing. We have tried to incorporate the *why* with the *how*.

Today's adult is confronted wtih a myriad of complex and perplexing
health problems, decisions, and responsibilities that must be handled
during an era marked by rapid scientific and technological advances, as
well as by changing social conditions. What is appropriate behavior this
week might change next week. In the fields of health science and medicine, though, there are yet many unknowns. Health practitioners must still
rely on their past experience, intuition, and personal judgment in deciding
what to do. No one has all the answers. Reputable practitioners and
scientists may hold diametrically opposite points of view. In this book, we
have tried to maintain a middle-of-the-road position based on what is
widely accepted by authorities in various fields. However, in hope of being
provocative, we have included reprints of articles that present a different
point of view, or at least approach our point of view from a different angle.

A number of college students have contributed anecdotal descriptions of various health problems encountered by themselves or their

friends. These anecdotes are interspersed throughout the chapters. It is hoped that these will exemplify the very real problems that face us as well as make the textual material more interesting.

Illustrations are included to emphasize a particular aspect or clarify a concept. A number of tables are placed in the appendix, as are the glossary, the bibliography, and suggested readings from selected sources. This placement enables use of these items without detracting from the textual material.

The arrangement of the chapters allows for flexibility in keeping with specific needs and interests of the readers. One chapter does not necessarily build on previous ones. The content was selected on the basis of immediate and future needs, health interests, attitudes, knowledge, and practices of college students and young adults as revealed by studies, surveys, and our own experience in the fields of psychology, medical science, health and physical education, and public and community health.

We hope that this third edition proves a valuable adjunct to the college instructor in his efforts to increase levels of health knowledge, create attitudes favorable to desirable health practices, and motivate young adults to improve their health behavior. We hope also that this book will provide a foundation that will be of value to the reader in making decisions about health behavior in this rapidly changing world.

Barbara Osborn Henkel
Richard K. Means
James M. Sawrey
Jack Smolensky

FOUNDATIONS OF HEALTH SCIENCE

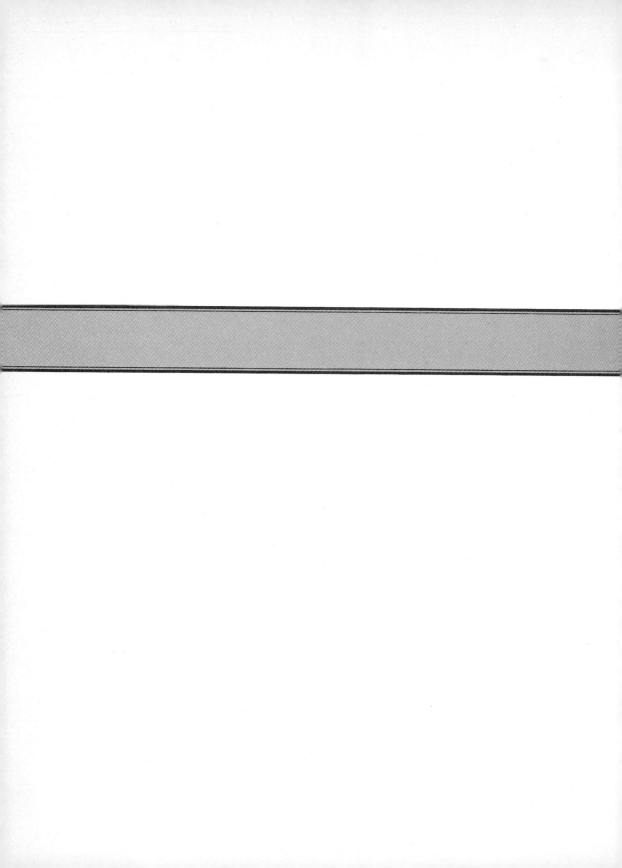

HEALTH CONCEPTS

chapter one

We live in a time of spectacular change, in a world beset with confusion, fear, and frustration. Political, social, technological, economic, and scientific developments pose complex questions and problems.

Together with circumstances that threaten existence itself, there are unlimited potentialities today for a fullness of life heretofore impossible. The giant strides made in science and medicine in recent years offer promise of a far safer and healthier world for the decades ahead. Although many perplexing personal and community health problems remain to be solved, scientists in numerous fields are steadily advancing the boundaries of knowledge, removing more and more obstacles to man's mastery of health and life.

Health is but one of the factors college students must consider in meeting their obligations. It is one of the most important, however, for it has a direct influence on all others. Sound health practices are the foundation of individual effectiveness—physical, social, academic, mental, and emotional. But when we are well, concern for our health is a remote consideration in relation to more pressing needs and desires. Although opportunities for healthful living surpass those of any previous generation, young adults don't always take advantage of them. Because of changing attitudes and the availability of services, a student is likely to seek medical

1

care for obvious physical and mental health problems; however, the same student may not practice behavior that could prevent health problems, especially when such behavior interferes with other interests.

Many factors influence the well-being of college students. There is great competition for their time and energy. Many students are working part or full time, and many are on limited budgets. Crowded living conditions and off-campus living create problems.

There are problems of safety and of increasing amounts of leisure time—outgrowths of automation. College students are part of an extremely mobile population that, because of new and faster modes of travel and closer relations between nations, is becoming increasingly cosmopolitan.

College students are engaged in a struggle for independence from parental control and adult supervision in general. At the same time they appreciate guidance that presents alternatives while allowing freedom of choice and action. Students are also engaged in a struggle for status, which involves a strong desire to conform to college modes of dress, behavior, diet, rest, and sleep. During the college years, a tendency toward sedentary habits of living frequently begins to assert itself.

Finally, college students are nearing the time when they will have to handle family responsibility, parenthood, and other adult problems. In a relatively short time many will assume leadership roles as citizens, civic leaders, and policy makers in their communities.[1]

Figure 1.1 provides a summary of some of the factors influencing sound health and effective college living. Understanding how the self interacts with the social environment is an integral aspect of the modern concept of health and life.

The sciences contributing to health comprise a variety of fields that are broad in scope and complex in action. In general, there is a good deal of misunderstanding and misconception concerning the relationships between these fields and the nature of health itself. Research reveals that the health knowledge, attitudes, and practices of the general population are inadequate to meet modern pressures and demands effectively. We are bombarded with health information via radio, television, newspapers, magazines, and other media, but while much of that information is authentic and scientifically accurate, some shades the truth or is deliberately misleading.

HEALTH IN THEORY AND PRACTICE

The word *health* was derived from the Anglo-Saxon word *haelth*, which meant the condition of being safe and sound, or whole. Until the

FOUNDATIONS OF HEALTH SCIENCE

Figure 1.1 Today's College Student. The modern college student is confronted with numerous problems relating to adjustment.

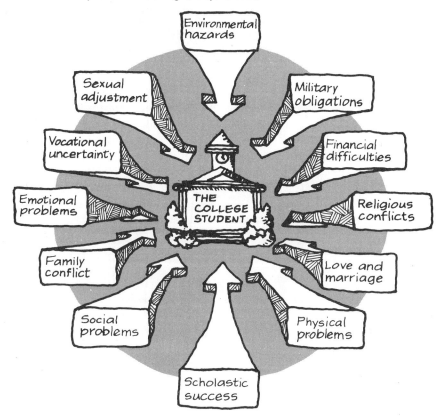

twentieth century, health was visualized in a negative way, as freedom from disease, defect, or disability. Some people confused being able to stay in a vertical position with being in good health: as long as one could stand and walk, he was not ill. "Everything will be all right as soon as he is on his feet." This idea is still held by some.

Today, health has various meanings for different people. To the professional athlete it often carries a far different connotation than it does to the student, teacher, bus driver, or businessman, because health is not easily or wholly measurable, and it comprises different components. Modern thought measures health in terms of an optimum state of living effectiveness. Health is construed as a vital process that involves the whole person and his unique pattern of living. This idea is apparent in the widely accepted definition developed by the World Health Organization. Fifty-four member nations endorsed the following statement in 1948 at the first World Health Assembly: "Health is a state of complete physical, mental

Figure 1.2 Modern Man's Health Potential. The range and levels of health and illness, extending from zero health (death) at one end of a continuum to optimal health at the other end. (Source: Howard S. Hoyman, "Our Modern Concept of Health," *The Journal of School Health*, 32:254, September, 1962. Copyright 1962, American School Health Association, Kent, Ohio 44240.)

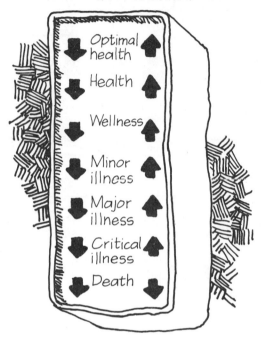

and social well-being, not merely the absence of disease or infirmity."[2] The components of health (physical, mental, and social well-being) are interactive. Alteration of any one, for either better or worse, will be reflected in the other two.

Another definition of health is proposed by Hoyman, who asserts that "Health is optimal personal fitness for full, fruitful, creative living."[3] He also points out the wide range and various levels of health and illness. These can be illustrated on a continuum that ranges from death, at one end, to optimal health, at the other end. (See Figure 1.2.)

It is more difficult to make the distinctions between the levels of good to optimal health than between the levels of illness. Beginning at the lower end of the scale, we identify the levels by the following characteristics: *Critical illness* implies grave sickness approaching death; *major illness* is an incipient, subclinical, or manifest disease or disability of a serious, incapacitating nature; *minor illness* indicates a milder sickness or ailment.

Wellness suggests degrees, or levels, of health—a state of being well that ranges from a suboptimal level of barely being well to high-level wellness, or *optimal health,* which is the realization of one's full potentialities.

Optimal health is seldom attained and rarely maintained. This is evident from the most casual observation of the practices of others or an analysis of one's own behavior. Many college students, for example, knowingly sacrifice appropriate habits of healthful living when confronted by the variable pressures of life on a modern campus. Sound health is gained not merely by *knowing* but by *doing* as well.

Good health is not often perceived as a goal in itself, except perhaps by the hypochondriac. Those who do not perceive it as a goal in itself may be only vaguely aware of its immediate effect. Until injury or illness strikes, few give more than a passing thought to the importance of good health, despite the fact that it is a means of attaining goals and a requisite for success in almost every field of endeavor.

Health is a changing, dynamic quality of life. What we should do today may be inappropriate tomorrow. The application of research findings to improving dietary practices, perfecting organ transplants, and preventing and controlling disease illustrates how scientific progress influences well-being.

THE HUMAN BODY

The human body is one of the wonders of nature. In good health, it enables us to attain the fullest enjoyment of life. In distress or illness, it possesses an amazing ability to adapt and recuperate. The marvels of the human organism are captured in these words of Shakespeare:

> What a piece of work is a man! How noble in reason! how infinite in faculties! in form and moving how express and admirable! in action how like an angel! in apprehension how like a god! the beauty of the world, the paragon of animals.

Care of this marvelous mechanism must be based on a knowledge and appreciation of how it works. This understanding provides the foundation for health decisions and is part of the armamentaria that protects against the quack with his array of false advice and worthless nostrums.

The study of the human body has frequently been compared to the assembling of different parts of a picture puzzle. We might begin to put a puzzle together at any point—the bottom, middle, or sides. What the picture might be does not become apparent, however, until a considerable number of pieces are in place. So it is with an analysis of the structure and function of the human organism. The different systems and organs can be described somewhat independently and in no particular order. But all are closely interrelated and intricately dependent upon one another for harmonious functioning.

INTERRELATIONSHIPS OF THE BODY

It has long been recognized that one's health is dependent not only upon a sound physical state but also on emotional and mental well-being. As far back as the Graeco-Roman period of history, Juvenal asserted, *"mens sana in corpore sana"* ("a sound mind in a sound body"). And John Locke, founder of modern psychology, borrowed from that ancient saying when he stated:

> A Sound mind in a Sound Body is a short, but full description of a happy State in this World. He that has these two, has little more to wish for; and he that wants either of them will be but little the better for anything else. Men's happiness or Misery is most part of their own making. He, whose Mind directs not wisely, will never take the right Way; and he, whose Body is crazy and feeble, will never be able to advance in it.

The Mind and the Body

It is increasingly apparent that the mind and the body are inseparable. In fact, the medical profession recognizes this phenomenon as the field of psychosomatic medicine. *Psychosomatic,* a term compounded from the Greek words *psyche* ("mind") and *soma* ("body"), exemplifies the idea that certain physical aberrations may have a psychological or emotional origin.

There are numerous everyday examples of the interrelationship between the mind and the body. It is known that anger, fear, pain, and other strong emotions affect bodily efficiency and may retard digestion or even cause nausea, headache, or other symptoms of physical distress. News of the death of a loved one may cause fainting, trembling, or some other physical reaction. Being involved in, or viewing the aftermath of, a serious accident may precipitate emotional responses that result in physical reactions. These and similar experiences frequently alter the normal functioning of various systems and organs of the body.

Just as the emotions affect the physical state, the condition of the body greatly determines the serenity of the mind. Exhausting physical work, especially when performed under stress or tension, does much to influence ensuing social behavior. Some people become cross or sullen when hungry or tired. Nearly everyone is familiar with the effects of a severe toothache, headache, earache, or backache on the emotional state.

Psychogenic Disorders

Severe emotional shock, traumatic experiences, or situations involving persistent stress and conflict may produce serious and permanent effects. They may cause mental illness, as well as a variety of physical symptoms. These are described in Chapters 6 and 7. Since serious repercussions may occur years after the actual emotional experience, the patient and the physician may not recognize the connection between a disease and its psychic cause.

According to reliable authorities, a great many persons who seek medical advice and care do so because of past or present emotional problems, some of which are deep-seated. It is frequently stated by physicians that one-half of the ailments they treat are complicated by psychogenic factors.

FACTORS THAT HELP TO DETERMINE HEALTH

A number of closely interrelated factors play a vital part in the development and maintenance of sound health. Many of these influences are readily apparent—heredity, nutrition, rest, sleep, exercise, disease, fatigue, and accidents. Other factors are less obvious but nevertheless significant. These include the effect on well-being of aging, excesses of certain noxious substances, abnormal growth and development patterns, family instability, noise and vibration, and various glandular deficiencies. Research in the biological and behavioral sciences is beginning to provide answers regarding how some of these factors relate to well-being.

HEALTH VALUES AND VALUING

Considerable attention in recent years has been devoted to the ways in which values affect health behavior and to the process by which individuals clarify personal values about health. Dalis and Strasser defined a value as:

. . . a characteristic or attribute of some general realm of living which is considered desirable by an individual.[4]

With respect to health, numerous value judgments influence the way one thinks and behaves. These focus on those areas of human concern that are controversial—marijuana use, venereal disease, smoking, fluoridation of water supplies, sexuality, and others.

Three aspects and seven criteria have been identified by Raths, Harmon, and Simon as significant in the valuing process. To determine a value, they assert, the individual must go through the process depicted in Figure 1.3.

Smith and Ojemann proposed the following four-step model for making personal decisions about health.

> Step One—Examine what motivating forces seem to be operating in a given situation. What feelings are [you] trying to satisfy through the behavior under consideration?
> Step Two—Devise and examine the probable intermediate and remote effects of possible alternative ways of satisfying these motivations.
> Step Three—Apply [your] personal standard to the proposed course of actions to determine if the effects of the action and the standard are compatible.
> Step Four—Decide either for or against the selected behavior at this point in time.[5]

How one reacts in a given situation is strongly related to one's basic needs and values. The promotion and maintenance of optimal health must involve the development of a personal value system. It is helpful from time to time to reexamine our own values in order to live more realistically and successfully. In order to reappraise our values realistically, we must know the consequences of different behaviors. This text defines those consequences.

Figure 1.3 The Values Clarification Process. Adapted from Louis Raths, Merrill Harmon, and Sidney Simon, *Values and Teaching* (Columbus, Ohio: Charles E. Merrill Publishing Co., 1966).

CHOOSING:	(1) freely
	(2) from alternatives
	(3) after careful consideration of the consequences of each alternative
PRIZING:	(4) cherishing, being happy with the choice
	(5) willing to affirm the choice publicly
ACTING:	(6) doing something with the choice
	(7) repeatedly, in some pattern of life

FOUNDATIONS OF HEALTH SCIENCE

COLLEGE HEALTH PROGRAM

College health programs are available to aid students. Some are comprehensive; others are minimal, providing services that supplement and complement those of the family physician. The student health center functions much like any other clinic. Its procedures are designed to appraise, protect, maintain, and promote health. Appraisals for abnormalities include vision and hearing tests, laboratory analyses of blood and urine, X rays, lung function evaluations, and checks for cancer (including gynecological examinations). The health center personnel frequently treat minor ailments, dispense medications for such illnesses, and care for injuries. More and more programs include family planning services and counseling about sexual concerns and problems. The staff will help students find appropriate assistance in the community when it is needed. The identification and correction of remediable defects and the provision of services for handicapped students are also aspects of college health programs. Proper follow-up, guidance and counseling, and planning of individual programs for those with special problems are essential.

Counseling and guidance programs include such services as aptitude and interest testing and appraisal, vocational exploration and advisement, and academic-program planning. The counseling staff helps students who request aid in making the numerous decisions with which they are confronted. Clinical psychologists or psychiatrists should be available to work with the few students who have serious personality disturbances or are mentally ill. Prolonged psychotherapy is rarely provided by colleges and universities, but those in need of it are helped to find treatment.

Counseling and guidance services meet the problems arising out of emotional and social relationships. Following are a few of the decisions that must be made by college students, as well as all other young adults:

1. What profession or vocation to choose
2. Whether or not to stay in school
3. What academic programs or classes to take
4. How to maintain good family relationships while establishing one's independence
5. How to solve problems within the family stemming from physical or emotional illness, including alcoholism
6. How much emotional and economic assistance to expect from the family
7. Whether or not to live at home, live alone, share facilities, or live in a group setting such as a sorority or fraternity
8. Whether or not to work

9. How to get along in an academic setting: how to study, what to expect from college personnel, and how to relate to college faculty and staff
10. What to do about conflicting points of view regarding religion, political philosophy, and value systems
11. How to choose friends and get along with peers
12. How to establish and determine man-woman relationships
13. Whether or not to marry or establish a "home"
14. What to do about incapacitating emotional problems.

HEALTH INSTRUCTION

Since health is a state of being, it cannot be taught. But how to achieve this state of being can be taught. As an applied science, health education draws its body of knowledge from a number of scientific fields. These include the biological sciences, such as anatomy, physiology, and microbiology; the physical sciences, comprising chemistry and physics; the behavioral sciences, including sociology and psychology; and such disciplines as medicine, pharmacology, dentistry, and public health. To sift from each of these fields those aspects that pertain to healthful living necessitates critical and continuous evaluation and a constant alertness to new developments. In this book, the elements of healthful living are organized into groups of related problems to aid you in making decisions and assuming responsibility for the health of yourself, your family, and your community.

Physical, mental, and social well-being, the three components of health, must be in balance. (See Figure 1.4.) They are so interrelated that a change in one effects a change in the others. Discussions of health in this book presume this relationship. Physical, mental, and social well-being are discussed separately only for the purpose of clarification.

The need for health education has become increasingly apparent. The long range benefits were described as follows:

> The ultimate value of health education cannot be measured by ordinary standards or in ordinary periods of time. One bit of health information properly applied may save a life now or forty years from now. That single life may be so valuable to society that this health education learning may be of greater value than any other bit of learning that the individual may have experienced.[6]

PROBLEMS AFFECTING WELL-BEING

Table 1.1 contrasts the top ten causes of mortality (death rate) in 1900 and today. Today, diseases of the cardiovascular-renal system are in first

Figure 1.4 The Unity of Health. The modern concept of health reflects the total unity of man—the physical, mental, and social dimensions of living.

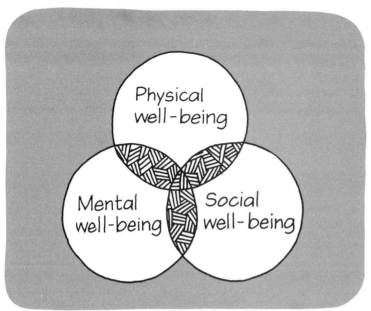

place. Also among the top ten are conditions such as accidents, suicide, and cirrhosis (related to alcohol abuse in many instances), which have psychosomatic components.

In 1900, five communicable diseases were among the top ten, while

Table 1.1 Leading Causes of Death in the United States

1900	Rank	Today
Tuberculosis	1	Major cardiovascular diseases
Pneumonia and influenza	2	Cancer
Enteritis, gastritis, colitis	3	Accidents
Diseases of the heart	4	Influenza and pneumonia
Stroke or apoplexy	5	Diabetes mellitus
Kidney diseases	6	Cirrhosis of the liver
Accidents	7	Suicide
Cancer	8	Bronchitis, emphysema, and asthma
Diseases of early infancy	9	Homicide
Diphtheria	10	Congenital anomalies

Adapted from data from the National Vital Statistics Division, National Center for Health Statistics, 1976, and from "Current Mortality Reports of the Metropolitan Life Insurance Company," *Statistical Bulletin,* 57:11, February, 1976.

only two attain this questionable distinction today. Progress in the control and prevention of the infectious diseases has largely accounted for this profound change. Better means of detection, diagnosis, and reporting of the incidence of noncommunicable or chronic-degenerative diseases has undoubtedly contributed to their statistical rise. Technological and mechanical advances have had an impact on mortality, especially in the case of accidents.

A limited amount of data reflects health needs and problems specifically related to the college-age group. Such data reveal conditions that are considerably different from problems of the total population. The following statistics and trends have been reported in recent literature.

1. A study at Cornell University revealed that 96 percent of the students required medical care during from one to eight semesters of their academic careers.
2. Accidents are the leading cause of death for ages one through forty-four; they cause more than half of all deaths for the age group fifteen to twenty-four.
3. An estimated 16 percent of all new admissions to state mental hospitals are patients between sixteen and twenty-nine years of age.
4. The number of delinquency cases in juvenile courts has risen steadily each year since 1948.
5. Persons less than twenty years old account for an estimated 22 percent of all cases of infectious venereal diseases.
6. One-fourth of the population under age twenty-one have defective vision.
7. Approximately 10 percent of the school-age population have speech defects or disorders.

A 1973 study of students in a community college in San Francisco indicated a higher prevalence of health problems than was formerly suspected.[7] The researchers found that 20 percent of the enrolled students had some chronic problem on file with the Student Health Service. Morbidity rates were highest for such health problems as conditions requiring major surgery, asthma, major orthopedic problems, hepatitis, mononucleosis, nervous breakdown, heart trouble, tuberculosis, epilepsy, diabetes, and the sexually transmitted diseases. A number of other health problems were reported in the study, without reference to incidence. These included weight problems, drug problems, pregnancy and abortion, sexual problems, suicide, family planning, and severe emotional crises.

A critical look at the leading causes of death for ages fifteen to twenty-four in the United States, presented in Table 1.2, reveals some interesting health implications for college students. Even the most casual perusal of

FOUNDATIONS OF HEALTH SCIENCE

Table 1.2   Rates of Leading Causes of Death in the United States, by Sex, for Ages 15 to 24 Years

Cause	Death Rate per 100,000 Population	
	Male	Female
Accidents	109.5	28.0
Homicide	20.7	6.1
Suicide	17.0	4.3
Cancer	9.1	5.9
Heart disease	3.5	2.3
Pneumonia and influenza	2.4	1.6
Stroke	1.4	1.4
Diabetes	.5	.5
Cirrhosis of liver	.4	.3

Statistical Abstract of the United States, 1975. Washington, D.C.: Superintendent of Documents, U.S. Government Printing Office, 1976.

the data is distressing. Three of the four leading causes of mortality in this age group have distinct psychogenic components. Homicide and suicide rates particularly illustrate the need for increasing attention to emotional problems.

IN CONCLUSION

Health progress in the twentieth century has been spectacular. It has materially raised the expectancy of life and better living to a previously undreamed of degree. Through the Peace Corps, UNESCO, the World Health Organization, and similar agencies and programs, prospects have been made bright for peoples throughout the world.

By following sound principles of healthful living and by using the scientific resources designed to protect and promote health, the individual of today will live longer and more healthfully than ever before.

It is desirable to ponder one question concerning the future of man's well-being. Will modern technology and science ultimately provide the utopia that has been sought through the ages? Has the scientific world reached the threshold of the very thing that sent Ponce de León on his quest some four centuries ago? Perhaps an answer lies in the provocative words of Dubos:

While it may be comforting to imagine a life free of stress and strains in a carefree world, this will remain an idle dream. Man cannot hope to find another Paradise on earth, because paradise is a static concept while human life is a dynamic process. . . . The earth is not a resting place. Man has elected to fight, not necessarily for himself but for a process of emotional, intellectual, and ethical growth that goes on forever. To grow in the midst of dangers is the fate of the human race, because it is the law of the spirit.[8]

In the following article, René Dubos succinctly describes the "fights" facing us.

Notes

1. Adapted from Report of the National Conference on College Health Education. *A Forward Look in College Health Education* (Washington, D.C.: American Alliance for Health, Physical Education and Recreation, 1956), pp. 9–10.

2. *Constitution of the World Health Organization* (Geneva, Switzerland: World Health Organization, 1946), p. 3.

3. Howard S. Hoyman, "Our Modern Concept of Health," *Journal of School Health,* 32:253, September, 1962.

4. Gus T. Dalis and Ben B. Strasser, "The Starting Point for Values Education," *School Health Review,* 5:3, January-February, 1974.

5. Lester V. Smith and Ralph H. Ojemann, "A Decision-Making Model," *School Health Review,* 5:7–9, January-February, 1974.

6. Commission on Philosophy, Division of Health Education, American Alliance for Health, Physical Education, and Recreation, "A Point of View for School Health Education," *Journal of Health, Physical Education, and Recreation,* 33:26, November, 1962.

7. Judith Carey and E. Lance Rogers, "Health Status and Health Knowledge of the Student in the Changing Community College," *American Journal of Public Health,* 63:126–33, February, 1973.

8. René Dubos, *Mirage of Health—Utopias, Progress, and Biological Change* (New York: Harper & Brothers, 1959), pp. 235–236.

HUMAN ECOLOGY

René Dubos

Nowadays there is a tendency to believe that modern medicine consists exclusively of a few sensational recent discoveries—miracle drugs, spectacular techniques, sophisticated immunization methods. This tendency is dangerous, for it deflects attention from another aspect of modern medicine which is just as remarkable and perhaps of greater practical importance. If the health of the public has improved in many regions during recent decades, the improvement is due not only to certain specialized medical procedures, but also—and probably to a greater extent—to a better understanding of the effects of

From WHO Chronicle, Vol. 23, No. 11, published by the World Health Organization, 1969.
René Dubos is professor of pathology and microbiology and a well-known ecologist.

man's environment and way of life on his physiological and mental state. Our health is better than that of our ancestors to the extent that our lives are more in accord with what I would choose to call biological wisdom. The scientific expression of that biological wisdom is human ecology, i.e., knowledge of the relationships between man and the innumerable factors of his environment.

It would be easy and pleasant for me to devote this entire lecture to an inventory of the progress of modern medical science. But I feel that it will be more productive to consider in what respects that science is inadequate, particularly when it comes to coping with the new ecological crisis that at the present time is threatening almost every country in the world.

The word "environment" has in

our day acquired an ever more tragic connotation, both in primitive agrarian societies and in industrial urban societies. It connotes, for example, malnutrition and infection in most of the poor countries, chemical pollution and mechanization of life in all the prosperous countries. The ecological crisis is everywhere so menacing and takes such varied forms that the term "human ecology" has come to be used only for certain situations that might lead to biological or mental disaster. Yet human ecology embraces far more than this tragic view of the relationships between man and his environment. Ecology teaches us that all the physical, biological, and social forces acting upon man impart a direction to his development and thus mold his nature. The body and the mind are constantly being modified, and hence shaped, by the stimuli that induce formative reactions. It is to be hoped that a time will come when human ecology will be able to pay greater attention to the positive and beneficial effects of the environment than to its pathogenic effects.

The social mechanisms whereby society tries to create a more or less artificial environment better adapted to man's needs and desires constitute an extremely important aspect of human ecology which I shall not attempt to discuss here. The other aspect of human ecology consists of the biological processes whereby the organism as a whole tries to adapt itself to environmental forces. The importance of these adaptive phenomena for health has frequently been demonstrated in the course of history. I shall mention a few examples of this.

In the narrative of his travels, Christopher Columbus speaks with admiration of the magnificent physical condition of the natives he discovered in Central America. In the eighteenth century, Cook, Bougainville, and the other navigators who ranged over the Pacific also wondered at the excellent health of the island populations of Oceania. Many other explorers were similarly impressed on their first contact with the Indians, the Africans, and later, the Eskimos. The legend of the noble savage, healthy and happy, thus has its origin in the descriptions published by the explorers who observed certain native populations when they were still undeveloped and almost completely isolated from the rest of the world.

There was certainly a lot of false romanticism in the illusion that the noble savage was free from disease and social restrictions because he lived in a state of nature. But, all the same, this romantic and oversimplified view of man's estate has been partly justified by the studies in physical and social anthropology conducted on what contemporary anthropologists call man the hunter. These studies were recently the subject of a symposium under that title, in the course of which descriptions were given of the characteristics of populations that live without agriculture and even without tools, except for a few primitive objects they employ to derive their sustenance from wild plants and animals. It appears that this way of life, though so close to nature and therefore lacking any medical assistance, is compatible with a good state of health. But I like to emphasize the fact that primitive populations undergo rapid physical and mental deterioration as soon as they come into close contact with the

FOUNDATIONS OF HEALTH SCIENCE

modern world, and thus lose their ancestral manners and customs. The noble savage who seemed so healthy and happy in the eighteenth century had often become a human wreck by the nineteenth.

The epidemiological facts suggest that the good health of primitive peoples, like that of wild animals, is a manifestation of a biological equilibrium between the living creature and its environment. This equilibrium persists as long as the conditions of human ecology remain stable, but is broken as soon as the conditions change. The enormous problems of malnutrition, alcoholism, and infectious disease, which caused such a rapid physical deterioration among the primitive populations in the seventeenth, eighteenth, and nineteenth centuries, recurred in all the Western countries at the outset of the Industrial Revolution, when their working classes, originating largely from agricultural regions, underwent massive and sudden exposure to conditions of life that were then new to them.

NO TIME FOR ADAPTATION

Adaptation to industrial society is now far advanced in the prosperous countries, but this is only a temporary phase. New problems are arising from the fact that the second Industrial Revolution is causing sudden and far-reaching changes in the physical environment and in everyday living, thus creating a new and as yet unstable ecological situation. The changes naturally bring their own specific dangers, which undoubtedly underlie what we nowadays call the diseases of civilization.

Indeed, we might say that in our day, human ecology is undergoing an almost universal crisis because man is not yet adapted, and probably never will become adapted, either to the biological impoverishment of the very poor countries or to certain environmental influences that the second Industrial Revolution has introduced into the rich countries. It might be supposed that man, since he still has the same genetic make-up as in the past, could once again use the biological mechanisms that enabled him in the Stone Age to colonize a large part of the globe, and so could adapt himself to the conditions of physiological impoverishment or industrial intoxication of present-day life. But this is neither certain nor even probable, because the present changes are of a kind almost without precedent in human history.

Until now, changes in the pattern of living have generally been so slow that it took several generations before they affected all classes of society. This slowness enabled the entire range of adaptive forces to be brought into play: physiological and even anatomical characteristics, as well as mental reactions and particularly social organization, little by little changed. Nowadays, on the contrary, everything changes so quickly that the processes of biological and social adaptation do not have time to come into play. Whether from the biological or the social point of view, the father's experience is now of practically no value to the son.

It is also a known fact that the human faculty of adaptation, great as it is, is not unlimited. It is quite possible that the stresses of present-day living are taking it near its extreme limits.

In the course of his evolution, man has constantly been exposed to inclement weather, fatigue, periodic famine, and infection. To survive these dangers, he has had to develop in his genetic code hereditary mechanisms that have facilitated certain processes of adaptation. But man now has to face dangers of another kind, without any precedent in the biological past of the human species. He probably does not possess adaptive mechanisms for all the new situations to which he is exposed. Moreover, the evolution of biological mechanisms is far too slow to keep up with the accelerated pace of technological and social change in the modern world.

It is certain, for example, that there is no possible means of adaptation to nutritional deficiencies that persist for long periods. Many children in their growth phase succumb to them. If they survive, they cannot satisfactorily realize the potentialities of their genetic endowment; they are condemned for the rest of their lives to anatomical, physiological, and mental atrophy. A population continuously subjected to nutritional deficiency can only degenerate.

Industrial technology has introduced into modern life a range of substances and situations that man has never known in his biological past. It is probable that he will never be able to adapt himself to the toxic effects of chemical pollution and of certain synthetic products; to the physiological and mental difficulties caused by lack of physical effort; to the mechanization of life; and to the presence of a wide variety of artificial stimulants. We should probably add to this list the disturbances to natural body rhythms arising from the almost complete divorce of modern life from cosmic cycles.

There are no grounds for the fear that all deviations from the natural order that result from technological change will be dangerous to health. Far from it. It remains true, however, that the more a population is exposed to modern technology the more it appears to be subject to certain forms of chronic and degenerative disease—conditions called for precisely that reason the diseases of civilization. Premature death caused by these diseases is not due to the lack of medical care. In the USA, for example, scientists and especially physicians have, paradoxically, a shorter life expectancy than other groups, although they belong to an economically privileged class. Certain demographic studies show that the life expectancy beyond the age of 35 may have decreased somewhat during the last few years in the big cities of the USA.

MAN'S AMAZING TOLERANCE

Everyday life seems to give the lie to the anxieties expressed in the previous pages, since modern man appears to be just as adaptable as Stone Age man. An extraordinary number of people have survived the terrible ordeals of modern war and the concentration camps. Throughout the world it is the most crowded and polluted cities, those in which life is at its most ruthless, that attract most people, and it is their population that is increasing at the greatest rate. Men and women are working all the time in the midst of the infernal noise of machines and telephones, in an atmosphere polluted with chemical fumes and tobacco smoke.

This remarkable tolerance of man toward conditions so different from those in which he has evolved has given rise to the myth that, through technological and social progress, he can modify his way of life and his environment indefinitely and without risk. That is simply not true. As I stated earlier, modern man can only adapt himself insofar as the mechanisms of adaptation are potentially present in his genetic code. Furthermore, it is certain that in many cases the apparent ease with which man adapts himself biologically, socially, and culturally to new or unfavorable conditions constitutes, paradoxically, a threat to individual well-being and even to the future of the human race.

This paradox arises from the fact that the word "adaptation" cannot be applied unreservedly to the adjustments that enable human beings to survive and function under modern conditions. Indeed, in man, sociocultural forces distort the effects of the kind of adaptive mechanisms that operate in the animal kingdom.

For the biologists, the expression "Darwinian adaptation" implies harmony between a species and a given environment, a harmony that enables it to multiply and, at the appropriate moment, to invade new territory. In the terms of this definition, man would appear to be remarkably well adapted to the conditions of life that exist both in high industrialized societies and in developing countries, since the world's population is continuing to increase and to occupy an ever greater proportion of the land surface of the globe. However, what would constitute a biological success for another species is a serious social threat to the human species. The dangers arising from the increase in world population show clearly that the Darwinian concept of adaptation cannot be used if the well-being of humanity is taken as a criterion of its biological success.

For the physiologist, a reaction to environmental stress is adaptive when it neutralizes the disturbing effects of such stress on the body and mind. In general, physiological and psychological adaptive responses are a factor tending towards the well-being of the organism at the time when they occur. In man, however, they may in the long term have detrimental effects. Man is capable of acquiring some degree of tolerance toward environmental pollution, excessive stimuli, a harassing social life in a competitive atmosphere, a rhythm completely foreign to natural biological cycles, and all the other consequences of his living in the world of cities and technology. This tolerance enables him to resist successfully exposure to influences which, at the outset, are unpleasant or traumatic. However, in many cases such tolerance is only acquired through a set of organic and mental processes that risk giving rise to degenerative manifestations.

THE THREAT OF IMPOVERISHED HUMANITY

Man can also learn to put up with the ugliness of the environment in which he lives, with its smoky skies and polluted streams. He can live without the scent of flowers, the song of birds, the life-enhancing spectacle of nature, and the other biological stimuli of the physical world. The suppression of a number of the pleasurable aspects of life and the stimuli that have conditioned his biological and mental evolution may have no manifest deleterious effect on his physical appearance or on his efficiency as a cog in the economic or technological machine, but there is a risk that, in the long run, it may impoverish his life and lead to the gradual loss of the qualities we associate with the idea of a human being.

Air, water, soil, fire, and the natural rhythms and diversity of living species are important not only as chemical combinations, physical forces, or biological phenomena but also because it is under their influence that human life has been fashioned. They have created in man deep-rooted needs that will not change in any near future. The pathetic weekend exodus toward the countryside or the beaches, the fireplaces that are still built in overheated urban apartments, the sentimental attachments formed for animals or even plants all bear witness to the survival deep down in man of biological and emotional urges acquired in the course of his evolution, of which he cannot rid himself.

Like the giant Antaeus in the Greek legend, man loses his strength as soon as he loses contact with the earth.

Human ecology therefore requires a scientific and intellectual attitude differing from that which would be adequate in general biology and even in the other biomedical sciences, because it has to deal with the indirect and long-term effects ex-ercised by the environment and way of life, even if those factors have no apparent immediate influence. It would be easy to illustrate the importance of those indirect and long-term effects by discussing, for example, the part played by the abundance or scarcity of food, the various forms of chemical and microbial pollution, the effects of noise or other stimuli, the density of and especially the rapid changes in the population; in brief, all of the environmental forces that act on man in every social class and in every country. Here, however, I shall confine myself to pointing out that the most important effects of the environment and way of life are often difficult to recognize because they only show themselves indirectly and after a lapse of time.

The early stages of life are of exceptional importance because to a large extent they determine what the adult will become. The young organism never forgets anything. All the factors that act upon it therefore contribute to the psychosomatic formation of the individual. The younger the person, the more malleable he is and the more easily affected by environmental influences. Hence the importance of the first stages of life, including those within the womb. These long-term and indirect manifestations of the environment are still poorly understood, but it is fortunately possible and even easy to study them experimentally since in animals, as in man, prenatal conditions have a profound and often irreversible effect, bearing on the anatomical features of the adult as well as on metabolism and behavior. Animal experiments will therefore make it possible to see what is not easily seen in man, to understand what is not obvious to our minds and, consequently, to take action with a view to alleviating certain untoward or even disastrous consequences of the influences to which man is exposed at the beginning of his life.

Of course the environment continues unceasingly to transform the organism. However, the first years of life have effects so profound and irreversible that they are the most important part of human ecology. I am emphasizing this fact because it seems to me that it should influence the general policy of WHO and encourage scientists to devote more effort to the problems of childhood. It is beyond doubt that the establishment of an atmosphere favorable to the biological and mental development of the child is the most economical way of improving world health.

A better understanding of the effect of environment at the beginning of life on growth and development gives a deeper sense to the definition of health made famous by the preamble to the WHO Constitution: "Health is a state of complete physical, mental and social well-being and not merely an absence of disease or infirmity." This "positive health" advocated by WHO implies that a person should be able to express as completely as possible the potentialities of his genetic heritage. That heritage, however, can only find true expression to the extent that the environment transforms genetic potentialities into phenotypic realities. It is in this way that human ecology might finally become identified, as I expressed the hope that it could at the beginning of this lecture, with the positive and beneficial effects of the environment.

The word "health" in the sense that I have chosen to give it describes not a state but a potentiality—the ability of an individual or a social group to modify himself or itself continually not only in order to function better in the present but also to prepare for the future. Ideal health will, however, always remain a mirage, because everything in our life will continue to change. The doctor and the public health expert are in the same position as the gardener or farmer faced with insects, molds, and weeds. Their work is never done. Man quickly grows tired of conditions of life that had originally seemed attractive. Individually and collectively he will look for adventure, and this forces him to live under constantly new conditions, with all the unforeseen occurrences and threats to health involved in change.

There is no question, however, of turning back. A society that does not move forward quickly deteriorates. Indeed, it cannot even survive in a world where everything is in a state of flux. Civilizations can only succeed and survive by exploring the unknown and accepting the risks involved in plunging ahead into the future. Technology would soon cease to develop if a certificate of absolute safety were required for every technical innovation and every new product.

It is therefore inevitable that economic and social progress should always be accompanied by hazards to health, whatever the advances made by medicine and hygiene.

This fact gives the doctor and the hygienist a still more important social role than they have at the present moment. It consists in recognizing as swiftly as possible, and even in anticipating, the medical problems that will arise increasingly as a result of the accelerated rate of technological and economic innovation. For this purpose it is becoming urgent to set up what might be called listening posts to record the first signs of pathological disorders that might threaten to spread to society as a whole. For example, the effects of atmospheric pollution, changes in food habits, the almost universal and constant use of new drugs, and automation in industry and in every aspect of life are still unforeseeable but could doubtless be detected before health disasters become widespread. It is a matter of satisfaction that this social responsibility is already recognized in certain sectors of the public service. Thus, thorough studies of the biological effects of ionizing radiation have been undertaken with a view to developing in advance practical methods of protection against the probable consequences of the industrial use of radiation. There would be no point in quoting here studies of the same kind already undertaken by WHO on the effect of drugs and insecticides. This far-sighted attitude will have to be generally adopted. In the future the development of technological innovations should always include parallel scientific studies on the long-term effects of these innovations on human ecology.

As Jacques Parisot wrote, "To cure is good but to prevent is better." Humanity will only be able to avoid the hazards of the future by extending its scientific knowledge and showing greater social conscience.

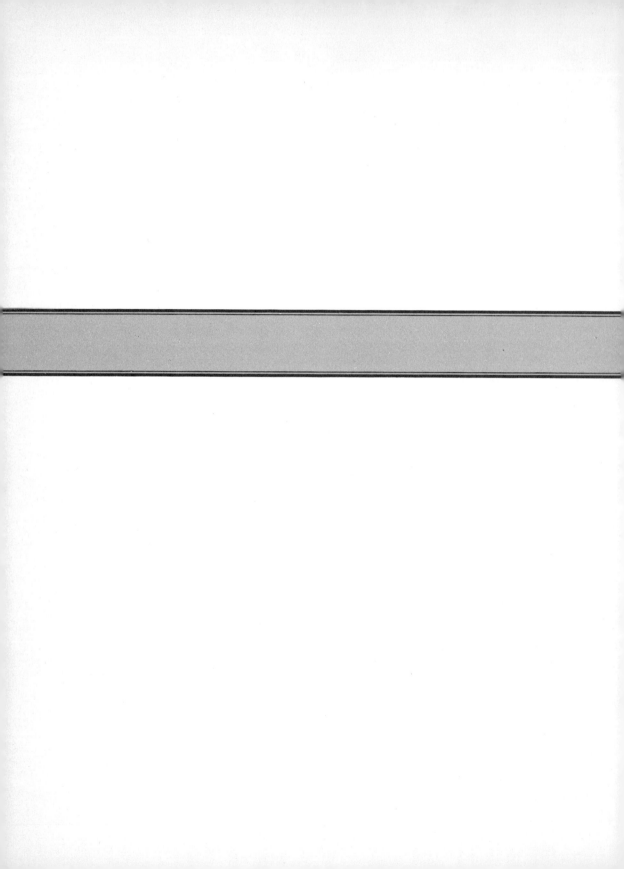

HEALTH INFORMATION: PRODUCTS AND SERVICES

chapter two

The American consumer and his purchasing practices have undergone a considerable transformation. A shrinking work week and an accompanying increase in personal income have resulted in more free time and greater spending power to enjoy it. Children and teenagers have become major consumers, and everyone exercises considerable individuality in buying. In past generations, the selection of products and services was relatively limited, but today's manufacturers, noting the needs and demands of the new consumer market, are producing a multitude of innovations, such as the do-it-yourself hobbies and activities. Billions of dollars are spent each year on reading material, sports, club activities, movies, social events, recordings, television, advanced education, recreation, travel, and other pursuits. These, in turn, have stimulated alterations in dress, eating habits, patterns of family living, and economic values. Today's consumer is confronted with a wide choice that necessitates careful analysis and decision-making. Never before have people been confronted with such an array of health products, specialized medical advisors, and sources of information pertaining to health. This vast choice of products, services, and information, complicated by high-powered advertising and pressure selling, has grown at an unprecedented rate in recent years. The direct and indirect effects on well-being of the use, wise or unwise, of these many resources are profound. Therefore, programs of consumer health education are necessary for everyone—the young, the working adult, and the aged; the sick and the well; the rich and the poor.

QUACKERY AND FRAUDULENT HEALTH PRACTICE

In nearly every aspect of health, and for every kind of human misery, there exist quackery and fraudulent health practices. The modern consumer is highly susceptible to the food, drug, and cosmetic racketeers who promise new or renewed health. The actual bill for fake medical treatments, health nostrums, and dietary preparations is reported to be well in excess of one billion dollars annually.

The Quack

A *quack* is a fake or incompetent medical practitioner who pretends to possess knowledge about the treatment of disease and illness. Some are licensed and some merely pretend to be licensed. *Quackery* is the practice of medicine by such a person. This limited dictionary definition is commonly broadened today to include all who are inadequately trained or offer false information.

Cameron, in his booklet *The Cancer Quacks,* identifies three kinds of fake medical practitioners. The first of these are the "dumb quacks," who know not, but know not they know not. They are usually uneducated persons who understand little about medical practice. "Deluded quacks" often have some education but limited knowledge of scientific research methods. Thus, their treatment is ordinarily based on faulty observation and equally faulty reasoning. "Dishonest quacks" are by far the commonest type. They know not and know they know not. Therefore, they trade on the forlorn hopelessness of the ill. Such persons are without scruples and moral sense. They are in the business for one reason only—to make a killing, which they often do in several ways.[1] In any case, the quack's patients lose precious time in obtaining treatment that could save their lives.

Certain characteristics distinguish quacks from qualified physicians. The quacks' operational procedures and claims are intended to create and maintain a steady market. Their practices may be distinguished by one or more of the following:

1. Use of scare methods to arouse fears of personal ill-health
2. Dominating motive of making money

3. Extensive advertising, often based on testimonials and case histories
4. Claim of persecution by other physicians or "medical trusts"
5. Disrespect of surgery, X ray, immunization, or certain drugs
6. Guarantee of a quick or definite cure that is usually not founded on scientific fact
7. Diagnosis and treatment based on a single theory, such as a special or secret machine or formula
8. Refusal to consult with reputable physicians
9. Proclaimed association with the Diety or some divine inspiration

Nostrums and Drugs

Nostrums are special remedies or treatments sold only by the quack. These products are frequently hailed as surefire methods of treatment guaranteed to cure many or all diseases and ailments. Such a product may bear the name of the quack or a reputable-sounding name of a research or scientific organization. Nostrums are sometimes advertised as "health tonics," "magic potions," or "miracle substances."

The nostrum is distinctly different from proprietary and standard drugs or compounds. Proprietary compounds are patented products manufactured by reputable pharmaceutical companies. They are used by competent physicians in supplement to standard drugs defined in the *United States Pharmacopeia* or *The National Formulary* of the American Pharmaceutical Association. The formulas for many common drug products are given in these pharmacopeias. Any drug that bears the symbol "U.S.P." or "N.F." meets specifications or standards established for the product.

Remedies through the Ages

Quackery probably began with the first ailment of man. Certainly the forerunners of some modern beliefs and customs pertaining to the art of healing had their origin as far back as the primitive period. Banishment of illness was originally based largely upon belief in magical power and supernatural forces. Sickness, injury, and pain were treated by attempts of the medicine man or tribal prophet to drive demons from the body.

Evidence indicates that quackery existed in many of the ancient nations, whose people had a profound belief in magic and a firm faith in the healing powers of the gods. One of the oldest nostrums, still in use today, is a drug called *hiera picra,* which is cathartic. The concoction was extensively used, supposedly to cure a variety of ailments, by Arabic, Greek,

Roman, English, and American physicians, as well as by quacks who overestimated its powers. Some quacks attempted to imitate its ingredients.

Whole books and numerous articles have been written about the gullibility of the consumer and the success of quackery throughout time. The words of P. T. Barnum, "There's a sucker born every minute," have a true and ominous ring.

Modern Areas of Quackery

The following brief statements illustrate some of the classic nostrums that have been peddled for millions of dollars in more recent years. Some of these are described in detail in the references cited in the Bibliography.

Figure 2.1 Advertisement of an Indian Physician in Boston. Note the statements claiming the cleansing of the blood of all disease. Today, professional ethics of reputable health advisors prohibit such advertising.

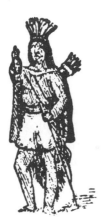

R. GREEN, M.D.
INDIAN PHYSICIAN,
No. 38 BROMFIELD STREET,
BOSTON,

Has, with his INDIAN REMEDIES, treated with complete success more than 50,000 cases of CHRONIC DISEASES His practice is attended with complete triumph in cases of CANCER, SCROFULA, and all CHRONIC DISEASES.

The discovery of a plaster that will draw out CANCERS, with all their roots, without injury to the surrounding parts, and a remedy like the INDIAN PANACEA, which will cleanse the blood of all humors, are triumphs in medical science never before achieved.

His medicines are all VEGETABLE, and act in harmony with the laws of life; and so perfectly do they cleanse the blood of all disease, that out of several thousand cases of CANCER and SCROFULA which he has cured, not a case can be found where the disease has ever troubled them afterwards.

Consultations, personally or by letter, upon all diseases, free of charge. Circulars with full reference, sent by mail free.

Eksip. A combination of magnesium carbonate, ordinary talcum, and starch, that was supposed to cure diabetes and making dieting unnecessary in weight control.

Perkins patent tractor. A device, made of two three-inch-long rods of brass and iron, that was supposed to be applied to the head to draw pain and disease from the body.

Electro bracelet. An ordinary bracelet with minute copper tubing, worn to treat muscle pain, contusions, sprains, arthritis, and rheumatism.

Cherry's salve. A concoction of lead salt, fatty oil, and camphor that was claimed to cure blood poisoning, ulcers, and pneumonia by drawing out the poison and corruption.

Magic spike. A device that supposedly contained radioactive power that produced emanations capable of curing cancer, diabetes, leukemia, and arthritis.

Vibrator chair. An electrically operated chair claimed to have therapeutic value in the treatment and cure of impure blood, arthritis, heart trouble, circulatory diseases, and cancer.

Cook describes the story of Yang, a Shanghai patent medicine merchant who made a fortune selling a son-producing tonic to expectant mothers:

> In China of old, boy babies were much more valuable than girl babies; so naturally there was a fine potential market for Yang's Son-Producing Elixir for Pregnant Ladies. The tonic actually was nothing more than a bottle of spring water with a dash of flavoring. But Yang guaranteed unconditionally that expectant women who drank it in the recommended dosage would give birth to boys. The lady customers figured it must be good stuff, because Yang offered a money-back guarantee. . . .
>
> Half of Yang's customers were delighted. They gave birth to boy babies. To these mothers, Yang's tonic was a magnificent preparation, and Yang was a national hero. All these happy women gave him enthusiastic testimonials which he used as scientific evidence in advertising Yang's Son-Producing Elixir to other pregnant ladies.[2]

Although all areas of health concern are potentially susceptible to quackery, fraudulent health practices have been directed most strongly to a special few. Generally the diseases most difficult to diagnose and treat and the human desire to improve one's personal appearance have been most widely exploited by the charlatan. Diseases whose causes are unknown are particularly exploitable by the quack and his nostrums.

Arthritis and rheumatism cures. By the time they are 60 years of age, more than 90 percent of the population in the United States suffer from arthritis and rheumatism, for which there is no cure. Only the symptoms of these diseases can be effectively treated. In their search for temporary relief from pain, the victims are often easy preys for the quack. Arthritis sufferers spend millions of dollars each year for misrepresented drugs, devices, and treatments.

Leading the list of cure-alls for these diseases are the therapeutic devices. Copper bracelets, vibrators, colored lights, and various radioactive materials foster the financial success of the incompetent practitioner while they delay the victim's obtaining proper medical attention. Numerous drug

Figure 2.2 Arthritis Quackery. A new principle that "reversed the death process into a life process" was claimed for this $30 "oxydoner." The sufferer simply attached the metal disk to his ankle and put the cylinder into a bucket of cold water to cure his arthritis. The colder the water, the faster the arthritis would disappear, according to the accompanying circular. Actually, reports the Arthritis Foundation, this gadget is completely useless. (Courtesy of the Arthritis Foundation.)

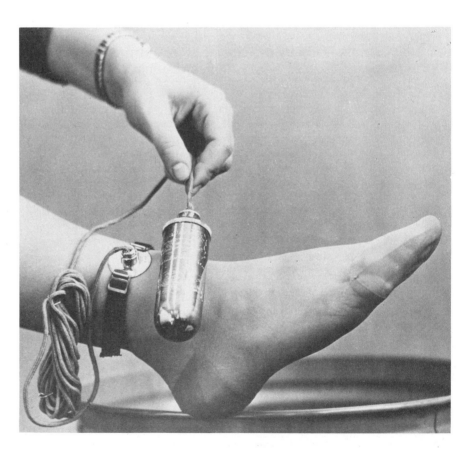

FOUNDATIONS OF HEALTH SCIENCE

preparations and chemical substances have also been offered as sure relief from arthritis.

A detailed description of the exploitation of the often agonizing aches and pains of the arthritic is provided in *The Arthritis Hoax*.[3] Some of the fraudulent remedies that have been used include the Atomotrone, which consisted of a kitchen cabinet, a sun lamp, panes of colored glass, and two fruit jars and sold for $300; Thiede's Stretch-to-Health Head Harness, which was especially designed to cure osteoarthritis victims; the Zerret Applicator, which supposedly expanded all the atoms of the body for only $50; and "immune milk" for arthritis at $1.70 a quart. (Some of these are still being used.) Many extravagant claims have also been made for pokeberries, O-Jib-Wa Bitters, Tri-Wonda, alfalfa, sea water concentrates and other "wonder" foods and drugs.

Cancer cures. One of the most tragic of the common types of fraudulent medical practice depends on the desperation of cancer victims. Because only certain types of cancer can be cured (and those types must be detected early), because the public greatly fears the disease, and because its causes are not yet known, the promises of the quack often inspire hope in the patient.

Drug cures for cancer were peddled long before scientists proved that chemotherapy was valuable. Radium capsules, pastes, medicines, poultices, enzymes, caustics, salves, ointments, and numerous other worthless pills and preparations offered "sure cures" to those inflicted. Many such concoctions supposedly "drew out the roots of cancer."

The use of krebiozen is strongly criticized by the Food and Drug Administration, medical authorities, and scientists who say it has no value in curing cancer. However, there are those who say that denying them "use of this product" is interfering with their personal freedom of choice. Numbers of people are traveling to other countries to obtain krebiozen. It is available illegally in the United States.

Another cancer "treatment" was purveyed by a couple who opened a "clinic" in the basement of a church in a large eastern industrial city. The details of this case are almost unbelievable.

> The man of the team was formerly a tire salesman, and the woman, before expertizing cancer, managed a cafeteria. Their secret "medicine," which must be swallowed on the premises, was smuggled out by a newspaper reporter who posed as a patient in order to get at the fantastic facts about the enterprise. On careful analysis by laboratory scientists, the medicine proved to contain water, vinegar, fly specks, and insect wings.[4]

Probably the most famous case was that involving the Hoxsey Cancer Clinic, which claimed to cure internal malignancy with a mixture of various powders, barks, roots, and other substances. Scores of individual testimonials were published over the years by the clinic, although no cancer cures were scientifically substantiated. The treatment, handed down from grandfather to father to son, was dispersed through several outlets. One clinic was established in 1936 in Dallas, Texas, followed by another in Portage, Pennsylvania. It was not until 1960 that these operations were officially ended by federal court action.

Other disease cures. Numerous other cures for chronic and degenerative diseases are promoted by quacks. Some of these nostrums and treatments are for leukemia, cardiovascular disease, sinus disorders, ulcers, diabetes mellitus, goiter, kidney diseases, anemia, epilepsy, liver diseases, and allergies.

One of the strangest operations in the modern era of quackery took place shortly after World War II in the backyard of a modest home in Long Beach, California. Here "Doctor" Beebe established his "health yard," consisting of overhead wires that, he claimed, miraculously transmitted healing cosmic rays. Although there was no charge for space beneath the contraption, thousands of people purchased activated grain and water for the cure of anything from tired blood to arthritis. By the time the city council was able to force him to leave for the health and safety of surrounding homes (not because of fraud), this nonmedical man had amassed a fortune.

The charlatan also preys on victims suffering from the simplest to the most serious communicable diseases. Among conditions that are frequently susceptible to the wiles and wares of the quack are venereal disease and the respiratory related ailments, such as the common cold, influenza, tonsillitis, tuberculosis, and bronchitis.

Fraudulent therapeutic devices. One of the most lucrative schemes in the field of quackery involves the sale, use, or home leasing of devices believed to diagnose and treat disease. These fraudulent machines and instruments may be elaborately designed to appear like reputable devices. Since use of these machines and instruments delays the obtaining of competent medical attention, the result is often permanent damage or fatality.

The therapeutic-device-oriented quack strongly depends upon strength of impression and smooth talk. He usually promises new health or improved vigor through the use of his machine. Frequently the device is promoted by claims that it works by using the mystical powers of magnetism, radio waves, electricity, colored lights, atomic energy, cosmic rays, or other unknown forces and unexplained phenomena. One such machine actually found a corpse to be in first-rate health.

An example of a useless but unfortunately popular gadget was the orgone accumulator, described below.

About the size of a bathtub, it consists of a wooden box lined with zinc, and it is supposed to draw into it a kind of "cosmic energy" called orgone, which is claimed to be very good for cancer, sexual impotence, and anything else you have and don't want. The patient sits in the tub, or "orgone accumulator" as it is advertised, where he allegedly absorbs the energizing, disease-combatting, youth-preserving power of the universe.[5]

While many worthless devices have been successfully condemned through court proceedings, there are still an amazing number of highly scientific-sounding contraptions in use, some by quacks themselves, others by patients at home. A few typical machines are the electric Plasmatic Therapy Device, for the fake treatment of over forty diseases and conditions; the Theraphone instrument, which is said to produce healing sound waves in various frequencies; Holder's Electronic-Oscillating Condensator, which is said to locate toxic conditions in the body; the Neurolinometer, which is supposed to measure nerve interferences and diagnose any abnormal bodily function; and the Oscilloclast and the Oscillotron, whose short-wave transmissions supposedly provide beneficial treatment for over 180 diseases and ailments.[6]

Cosmetic quackery. The American consumer, either young or old, is ever alert for new products that will erase wrinkles, eliminate blemishes, restore beauty, and improve personal appearance. In response to an ever-increasing demand, cosmetic preparations flood the market, bearing claims that they remove unsightly skin problems, nourish body tissue, or promote new loveliness. These external lotions, ointments, creams, and salves come in numerous forms and a wide range of prices. The ingredients, commonly advertised as beneficial, often include hormones, vitamins, fish or animal oils, enzymes, and other special lubricants. Aside from softening and partially cleansing the skin, such products are of little value. Some, such as antibiotic and hormone salves, are harmful.

The gullibility of the consumer is illustrated by the millions of dollars that are spent each year on such questionable products and services as weight increasers, bust developers, mole and bunion removers, eyelash growers, and dimple makers. The sale of eyeglass prescriptions by mail and baldness preparations that "feed the hair roots like a plant" further emphasize this point.

According to the Food, Drug, and Cosmetic Act, cosmetics are defined as articles, including components of such articles, intended to be rubbed, poured, sprinkled, or sprayed on, introduced into, or otherwise applied to the human body or any part thereof for cleansing, beautifying, promoting attractiveness, or altering the appearance.

Cosmetic preparations, properly applied, can enhance personal appearance, but "miracle" cosmetics are one of the oldest forms of quackery. The desire for youthful attractiveness is a potent motivator in the United

States, and many people are willing to spend a great deal of money for products that promise what they cannot perform. There is no way to nourish the skin by creams or lotions or falsely labeled "skin foods" applied from the outside. False and misleading names are applied to many cosmetic products. No known substance or combination of substances can live up to the promises suggested in any of the following names: contour cream, crow's-foot cream, deep pore cleaner, eye wrinkle cream, scalp food, skin conditioner, skin firm, skin tonic, eyelash grower, and wrinkle eradicator.

Considering the millions of daily applications of innumerable cosmetics, the incidence of skin rashes and other irritations from their use is very low, says the American Medical Association. Nevertheless, sufficient numbers of cases of dermatitis directly traceable to the use of cosmetic products come to the attention of the dermatologist and the manufacturer to warrant continued search for safer products. Some of the skin problems that might be traceable to cosmetics are dry, scaly, itchy skin; red, swollen eyelids; rash on the neck and ears; pigmented spots on exposed areas such as the cheek; and skin problems around the fingernails. Compounds that are powerful enough to bleach or cause peeling are potentially dangerous.

Cosmetics containing hormones do not rejuvenate the skin and remove wrinkles. They may be dangerous, in fact. Experimental data on the use of sex steroids in cosmetics indicate that some hormones, both active and inactive biologically, cause slight histological thickening of the epidermis of aged skin. Dermal changes are questionable, and there may be clinical effects. In the amounts that can be safely incorporated into cosmetic preparations, topically applied estrogens and progesterone have no effect on human sebaceous glands and oil secretion.

Other areas of quackery. Many frauds are perpetrated on the public in other areas of human misery and despair, such as alcoholism, deafness, eye conditions, dental problems, hernia, foot abnormalities, hemorrhoids, hair problems, weight problems, and the tobacco habit. Older persons, who are prone to these and other health disabilities and who represent an increasingly larger part of the population, are a special target group for the fraudulent health practitioner.

The field of dentistry also includes charlatans, who fleece the public with fraudulent schemes related to conditions of the teeth and the supporting structures of the mouth. Mail order dental plates and home dental kits are among the most ridiculous.

The Educational Division of the National Better Business Bureau, in the booklet entitled *Facts You Should Know about Health Quackery,* advised that products should not be sold to the public or purchased by individuals (1) if they are dangerous to health or life when used without proper supervision, (2) if they are worthless for the purposes for which they are offered, and (3) if they are offered for conditions for which they alone do not constitute competent treatment, when unwise self-treatment may permit the conditions to progress so far that damage cannot be repaired.[7]

APPRAISING HEALTH INFORMATION

The American consumer is bombarded with a multitude of factual and pseudoscientific information pertaining to health. This information, much of it colored by advertising, fills the airways of radio and television, per-

Figure 2.3 Del Rey Masso Therapy Unit. Seized from the offices of a California chiropractor in 1966, this device produces a weak galvanic current that can be used to stimulate voluntary muscle tissue. Upon questioning, however, the practitioner freely admitted that he was using this therapy unit for treatment of many serious diseases. (Courtesy of the American Cancer Society, Long Beach and State of California Health Department.)

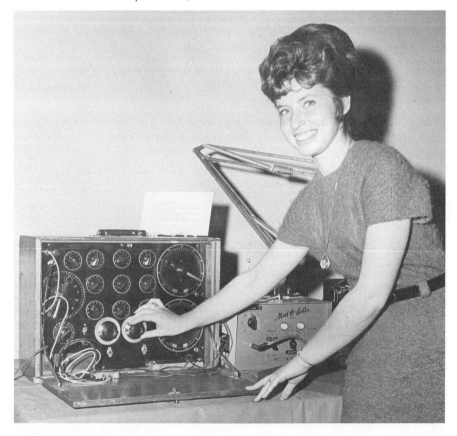

vades the pages of newspapers and magazines, and decorates billboards throughout the nation.

Criteria for Intelligent Evaluation

Information of all types should be scientifically appraised. Only through a sound application of fundamental criteria and an unbiased evaluation of all impinging factors can one be sure of the authenticity of what has been communicated. Certainly particular care should be taken concerning information that is to serve as a basis for the selection and use of products and services influencing health.

Rudyard Kipling, in his *Just So Stories,* cleverly identified the interrogatives of evaluation when he said:

> I keep six honest serving-men
> (They taught me all I knew);
> Their names are What and Why and When
> And How and Where and Who.

The following list contains more specific ways by which one can assess the value and reliability of health information.

Author. Do the individuals or organizations offering the information possess a good reputation in the health sciences? Are they qualified? What is their educational background and experience?

Intent. What is the predominant purpose of the information or material? Is it opinionated? Has it been written to promote the sale of a particular product or service?

Content. Is the information presented reliable, scientific, realistic, unbiased, and unprejudiced? Has the topic been comprehensively treated to assure adequate coverage of the major issue or question? Does it demonstrate sound reasoning and philosophy?

Organization. Has the material been logically and progressively developed? Are there important omissions or apparent gaps in the data? Are they easily understood? Has proper substantiation of supporting information been made through documentation?

Timeliness. Is the information up to date? Would more recent research influence the content? Does the information reflect current and acceptable thought?

Sources of Health Information

With such an abundance of available information pertaining to health, not all of it is equally reliable. It is as important to be able to identify questionable sources of health information as it is to be aware of those that are most valuable and accurate.

Erroneous beliefs and superstitions. The average American is relinquishing the mystical beliefs and superstitions of the past in favor of more scientific attitudes. The number of persons duped each year by fraudulent practices is evidence, however, that there is resistance to abandoning old notions. Tradition and cultural influence have undoubtedly contributed to the persistence of certain misconceptions about health. Although false, the following beliefs are still prevalent.

Boils are caused by bad blood.

Toads cause warts.

A cat will suck the breath out of an infant.

Certain communicable diseases are caused by the night air.

Whiskey is a good antidote for snakebite.

Disease and illness are a punishment for sin.

Birthmarks on a child are caused by experiences of the mother during pregnancy.

Butter is good for a burn.

Copper bracelets or rings will relieve arthritis.

Vitamins should be taken for energy.

Certain foods have special healing properties.

A bowel movement should occur daily.

Swallowing grape or watermelon seeds will cause appendicitis.

Seawater has certain minerals that will cure cancer.

Commercial sources. Health information found in the advertising and other materials disseminated by commercial and business organizations, ranges from most reliable to unreliable. Most reliable is the valuable, authentic information available from such groups as life insurance companies, councils supported by food manufacturing concerns, and pharmaceutical firms. These companies have developed many excellent materials for use in schools and colleges as well as for the general public.

Some commercial groups are unreliable when they use the health motive as a front to sell their products. The information emanating from such sources is often distorted. Claims and promises sometimes border on fraudulent practice through the exploitation of special health values of a product or misrepresentation of its benefits. Several books supporting such claims have become best-sellers, illustrating the gullibility of the American public.

Nearly 26.5 billion dollars were spent in the year 1974 for advertising.

Figure 2.4 Health Foods and Reducing Preparations. Safflower oil capsules "for use as directed with the CDC 'Calories Don't Count' weight control program" were taken off the market because the book included false claims regarding weight reduction and heart disease. (Courtesy of Food and Drug Administration, U.S. Department of Health, Education and Welfare.)

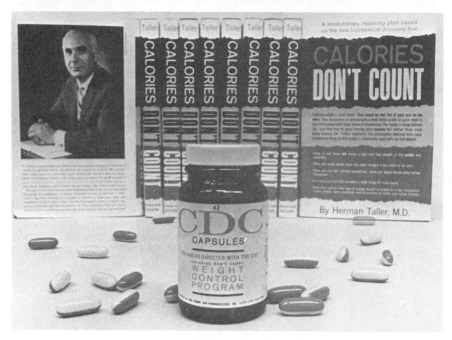

The pleas and promises of the advertiser are everywhere: in whatever one reads, wherever one rides or walks, in whatever one hears, and in virtually every life situation.

The commercially spoken and printed word reaches all consumers in numerous ways many times each day, unfortunately often from the health salesman, cultist, herb-doctor, quack, faddist, and health huckster. In the horse-and-buggy days of medicine, dissemination of knowledge was by word of mouth and therefore was limited to a few people at a time. Today a message can reach millions instantaneously, so false information has greater impact than it did in the past.

Disraeli once remarked, "There are three kinds of lies: lies, damned lies, and statistics." An examination of claims for certain typical products is enlightening concerning statistical information related to health. You might hear or see such claims as the following hypothetical statements:

Users of "Toothachers," amazing new dentifrice, report 30 percent fewer cavities.

FOUNDATIONS OF HEALTH SCIENCE

Figure 2.5 Advertising—Estimated Expenditures by Medium: 1960–1974.

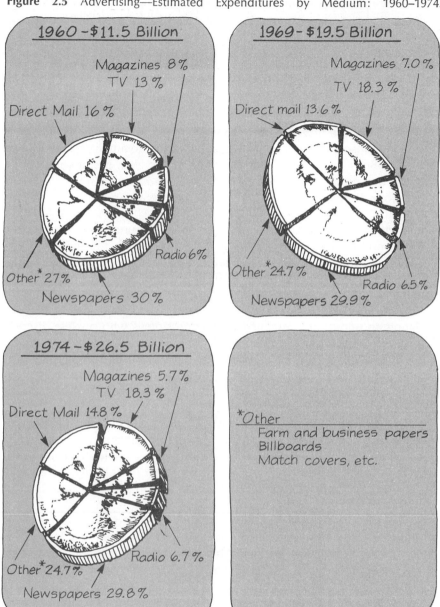

1960 – $11.5 Billion

Magazines 8%
TV 13%
Direct Mail 16%
Radio 6%
Other* 27%
Newspapers 30%

1969 – $19.5 Billion

Magazines 7.0%
TV 18.3%
Direct mail 13.6%
Other* 24.7%
Radio 6.5%
Newspapers 29.9%

1974 – $26.5 Billion

Magazines 5.7%
TV 18.3%
Direct Mail 14.8%
Radio 6.7%
Other* 24.7%
Newspapers 29.8%

*Other
Farm and business papers
Billboards
Match covers, etc.

(Source: *Statistical Abstract of the United States, 1975.* Washington, D.C.: U.S. Government Printing Office, 1976, p. 791.)

Three out of five eminent doctors smoke "Coughies" cigarettes.

"Cohist" clears up common cold discomfort and distress in just twenty-four hours.

We guarantee new loveliness for tired hair with "Tint Glow."

"Gurgle" mouthwash, with chlorohexophosphate, halts unpleasant breath in just five seconds.

Modern science has made fantastic discoveries and has unequivocally proved their value in combatting some of man's most pressing problems. This makes unsophisticated consumers susceptible to anything that appears scientific. But a brief analysis of the listed statements, permits interesting observations about such statistics and claims.

Before disposing of your present toothpaste and running out to purchase a tube of "Toothachers," it might be well to check the reliability of its manufacturer's claim. A close examination might uncover that only ten cases composed the experimental group upon which the evidence was based. It may have taken the investigators a dozen tries, but sooner or later, by chance, the proper test group displayed the necessary reduction in dental caries. A true statistic?

The manufacturers of "Coughies" used the age-old gimmick of associating an undesirable practice with professionals who possess discriminating intelligence. In this case, however, it is unrealistic to assume that doctors, regardless of their prominence, have the inside dope on which cigarette is least harmful. How many groups of five were surveyed to find one in which three doctors smoked this brand? The best response to this and similar proclamations is, "So what!"

The marvelous new drug "Cohist" might well fulfill just what it claims —but so do many other things. Nothing is of special value in either curing or ameliorating cold symptoms. The choice words of Henry G. Felsen provide the clincher in this case. Although no medical authority, he astutely observed that "Proper treatment will cure a cold in seven days, but left to itself a cold will hang on for a week."

The advertisers of "Tint Glow" skillfully exploited three vague terms to entice even the most discriminating consumer: "guarantee," "new loveliness," and "tired hair." They may be analyzed by the questions, "What kind of guarantee does one really have?" "How can 'new loveliness' be measured?" and "What is 'tired hair'?" Perhaps the underexposed and microscopically small black-and-white "before" picture, as contrasted with the vibrant "after" photograph produced in full color, had something to do with the statement's allure.

Two prominent deceptions are illustrated by the mouthwash statement. First, the advertisement made careful reference to the highly scientific-sounding substance chlorohexophosphate. (This term was coined for this discussion. Who knows whether it is plain water, perfume, sulfuric acid, or a nonsense word?) It is also gratifying to realize that the product will stop unpleasant breath in just five seconds, just as the advertisers claim. They do not add that so does candy or that "even your friends might not tell you" the results ten seconds later.[8]

Credentials and testimonials. Health information provided by the quack, health salesman, cultist, or huckster should obviously undergo careful scrutiny, but how does one know who they are? These people rely largely upon creating an emotional atmosphere and on having a reassuring and pleasing personality. They often have a long list of impressive credentials, records of past successes, and elaborate testimonials. A testimonial is a statement made by an individual or a group attesting to the value or benefits of a particular product or service. It may be given by a faithful follower, sometimes in good faith, or it may be fabricated or paid for. Regardless of the source, testimonials serve as the backbone of nostrum and quack advertising and should be considered unreliable.

Testimonials are considered to have no scientific authenticity. Most professional organizations, such as the American Medical Association, consider them unethical and discourage their members from issuing or supporting them. A number of court actions and specific studies have indicated the lack of value of such statements. A United States Post Office Department investigation, for example, revealed that 75 percent of the individuals providing current testimonials were actually dead. Some of these persons, in fact, had died from the very diseases of which they were reportedly cured.

Reliable sources of health information. Governmental and private agencies that provide protection against fraud and dangerous or useless products are probably the most reliable sources of health information. The national offices of these agencies answer inquiries regarding consumer health problems. Most of these organizations publish or distribute extensive materials that are helpful references for further information.

The family physician, the college Student Health Service, or a health education instructor should be able to provide reliable information. Within the community, advice and assistance can usually be obtained from the local or county health department, the county medical society, or one of the numerous voluntary health agencies.

EVALUATING HEALTH PRODUCTS

The health products market is extensive, ever changing, and constantly expanding. It includes highly specialized items that do particular things and more general items that purportedly remedy all problems of mind and body. Health products are eaten, drunk, inhaled, sniffed, sprayed, rubbed, or put on in any number of ways. They may be purchased in almost any quantity and in a variety of colors, shapes, and sizes. Depending upon individual desires or taste, they may be found bottled, canned, boxed, tubed, dehydrated, or frozen.

Selecting reliable and safe health products is important for the consumer in terms of both health and economy. The choice is usually complicated by the existence of numerous brands, packages of all shapes and sizes, and a wide range of prices. It behooves the buyer to know exactly what he is getting for the money he spends. The discriminating consumer will not be fooled by misleading advertising, low cost, or colorful and elaborate trimmings in selecting health products. The following criteria are helpful purchasing guides:

1. Be aware of acceptable standards of quality and the values of the products to be purchased in order to have a basis for comparison.
2. Follow the advice of a qualified physician in the selection of drugs and chemotherapeutic agents.
3. Learn the exact contents or ingredients of the article being purchased by carefully reading the label, and compare different brands.
4. Utilize the research findings of testing and rating services and consumer organizations.
5. Avoid products and devices that claim to cure all diseases or to be a surefire method of treatment for specific health problems.
6. Purchase products that bear a seal of acceptance or that carry government approval.
7. Be skeptical of products and devices that are promoted by high-pressure advertising, propaganda techniques, testimonials, or other dubious procedures.
8. Buy health products on the basis of need, from reputable dealers, and in the quantity recommended for the particular problem at hand.

SELECTING HEALTH SERVICES

The modern consumer is faced with many important decisions regarding the selection of specialized services contributing to health and well-being. There are advisors on sexual adjustment, on the emotional problems of young and old, on the prevention and treatment of illness and disability, and on many other complexities of man and his environment. Within this broad spectrum of specialization, the consumer must be prepared to choose rationally and intelligently. Each of the specialists has different professional qualifications. Many are entitled to use the title *doctor*. To many laymen, the term implies a medical education.

Historically, *doctor* meant teacher. In practice, however, the term is applied to persons in many different fields of activity, each of which require a prescribed course of study. Which of the doctors in Table 2.1, for example, are prepared and licensed to give medical treatment?

Obviously, all doctors are not qualified to administer to the health problems of the individual. Wide differences in both theory and practice exist even among the various specialties of the healing profession. Not all physicians possess the educational background and practical qualifications to prevent and treat all kinds of diseases. Most states require that a licensed physician have a minimum of three years of college, four years of medical school, and one year of internship and pass a state examination. Specialists need an additional two to six years' training beyond this minimum. A list of some of the common medical specialties is provided below. Although the general practitioner has not been considered a specialist in the traditional sense, more and more such physicians have postgraduate preparation of a specific nature.

Table 2.1   Not All Doctors Can Give Medical Treatment

Initials	Type of Doctor
*M.D.	Doctor of Medicine
N.D.	Naturopathic Doctor
D.C.	Doctor of Chiropractic
*D.O.	Doctor of Osteopathy
*M.O.	Medical Officer
D.M.D.	Doctor of Dental Medicine
L.L.D.	Doctor of Laws
Litt.D.	Doctor of Letters
D.D.S.	Doctor of Dental Surgery
D.V.M.	Doctor of Veterinary Medicine
D.P.H.	Doctor of Public Health
Ph.D.	Doctor of Philosophy
D.Sc.	Doctor of Science
Ed.D.	Doctor of Education
O.D.	Optometric Doctor

*Star Indicates licensed physicians.

Common Medical Specialties

Allergist. Diagnoses and treats body reactions resulting from unusual sensitivity to certain foods, pollens, dusts, or other substances.

Anesthesiologist. Specializes in the administration of anesthetics.

Cardiologist. Diagnoses and treats cardiovascular diseases.

Dermatologist. Diagnoses and treats diseases of the skin, as well as certain skin manifestations of constitutional diseases.

Endocrinologist. Treats diseases arising from disturbances of the secretion of the endocrine, or ductless, glands.

Epidemiologist. Specializes in the relationships of the various factors that determine the frequencies and distributions of an infectious process, a disease, or a physiological state in the human community.

Family practitioner. Specializes in general medicine; provides primary care.

Accurate medical advice? How do you know?*

The last time that I was really sick I thought that I was going to die. I had never experienced the symptoms before, but the pain was unbearable. It started with a dull pain in my lower back area, which became increasingly sharper as the day wore on. Finally, after two days of guessing, various diagnoses, and just plain fear, I went to the emergency room of Union Memorial Hospital. The intern did a blood test and urinalysis and asked the regular emergency room questions. Finally, after three hours of agonizing pain and waiting, I was told by the intern that he "thought" that I had gonorrhea. I was shocked; after all, it never happens to you.

To add to my physical pain, I had a mental one to deal with. The feelings of shame, guilt, and fear are seemingly natural ones in such a situation. I immediately proceeded to contact the people that I had had sex with within that past month. No one had contracted it.

Mad at being embarassed because I had to ask "have I burned you," I contacted the hospital and demanded to know the results of my urine and blood tests. They were evasive and took me through a great deal of bureaucratic crap before they gave my private doctor the results. They turned out to be negative, which meant that the initial diagnosis was wrong. The point is that this happened on two occasions within one month. I have never found out what the cause of my discomfort and pain was.

*The boxes throughout this book contain college students' anecdotal descriptions of health problems encountered by themselves or their friends.

FOUNDATIONS OF HEALTH SCIENCE

Gastroenterologist. Diagnoses and treats diseases of the digestive system.

Geriatrician. Specializes in preventing disease, prolonging life, and promoting health for persons past middle age.

Gynecologist. Specializes in medical and surgical treatment of diseases peculiar to women, primarily those of the genital tract, as well as female endocrinology and reproductive physiology.

Internist. Specializes in diagnosing and in internal medicine as distinguished from a surgeon or obstetrician.

Neurologist. Diagnoses and treats diseases of the nervous system.

Obstetrician. Specializes in care of women during pregnancy and childbirth and the period immediately following delivery. Gynecology-obstetrics is commonly a joint specialization.

Ophthalmologist (Oculist). Diagnoses and treats diseases and disorders of the eye and vision and prescribes glasses.

Orthopedist. Diagnoses and treats diseases, fractures, and deformities of the bones and joints by physical, medical, and surgical methods.

Otologist. Treats disorders and diseases of the ear.

Pathologist. Studies and interprets changes in organs, tissues, cells, and body chemistry.

Pediatrician. Specializes in the prevention, diagnosis, and treatment of diseases of children, usually up to the age of sixteen.

Physiatrist. Specializes in use of physical agents (heat, cold, water, electricity, manipulation, etc.).

Proctologist. Diagnoses and treats disorders and diseases of the colon, rectum, and anal canal.

Psychiatrist. Diagnoses and treats mental and emotional disorders.

Radiologist (Roentgenologist). Uses X ray, radium, and radioactive isotopes to diagnose and treat diseases.

Surgeon. Specializes in the treatment of disease by manual and operative procedures.

Urologist. Diagnoses and treats abnormalities and diseases of the genitourinary tract.

Criteria for Selecting Advisors

The choice of a competent medical or dental advisor should be considered in light of certain fundamental criteria. It should not be left to chance or delayed until an emergency situation necessitates a hurried selection. A family practitioner or internist ordinarily serves best as a family physician. The following suggestions might be of value in choosing a qualified dentist or physician. He or she should:

1. Be a graduate of an accredited medical or dental school. (Some schools do not meet standards established by the profession.)
2. Display a license to practice medicine or dentistry in the state in which he or she resides. (This demands the meeting of minimum qualifications and the passing of basic examinations.)
3. Maintain membership on the staff of a reliable and accredited hospital or clinic. (Most practitioners devote some time to community service or serve as regular staff members.)
4. Be an active member in good standing of learned professional societies. (Most competent practitioners participate actively in professional activities. They may be excluded from membership for malpractice or nonmedical reasons.)
5. Be involved continually in self-education activities: postgraduate studies, conferences, meetings, and other professional work. (Such self-improvement practices contribute to professional growth and increased skill, and a number of states require such studies for relicensure.)
6. Possess a good reputation in the community and among professional colleagues. (Ethical behavior, dependability, and professional integrity are important considerations.)
7. Have a background of supervised internship, clinical service, and experiences to provide necessary knowledge and skill, realizing his or her limitations for specialized care.
8. Maintain a hygienic, neat office with adequate modern facilities and equipment. (Flashiness and expensive furnishings, however, should not be overrated.)
9. Have a pleasing manner, a wholesome personality, and good habits of personal cleanliness and appearance. (A favorable impression and good interpersonal relationships should be considered.)

MEDICAL CARE COSTS

The annual expense for medical care in the United States has increased tremendously since 1950. The 1975 expenditures were 13.9% greater than those for 1974. It has been estimated that approximately 8 percent of total personal income goes to medical services.[9] This includes expenditures for physicians' services, hospital care, drugs and medications, dental care, nursing services, and other needs. In addition, about one-third of personal

Figure 2.6 The Medical-Care Dollar (Source: *Statistical Abstract of the United States, 1975.* Washington, D.C.: U.S. Government Printing Office, 1976, p. 71.)

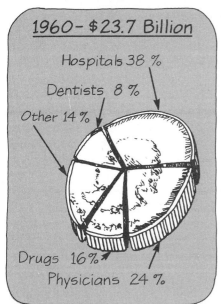

1960 – $23.7 Billion

Hospitals 38 %

Dentists 8 %

Other 14 %

Drugs 16%

Physicians 24 %

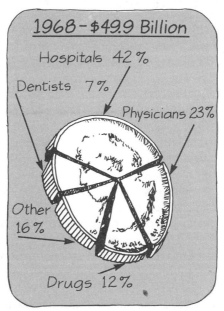

1968 – $49.9 Billion

Hospitals 42 %

Dentists 7 %

Physicians 23%

Other 16 %

Drugs 12%

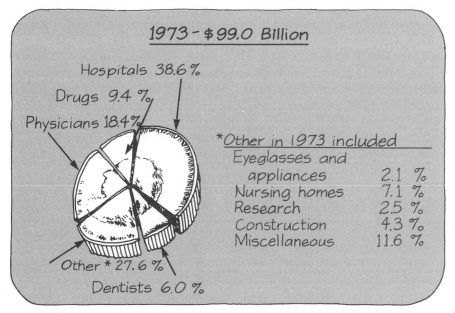

1973 – $99.0 Billion

Hospitals 38.6%

Drugs 9.4 %

Physicians 18.4%

Other * 27.6 %

Dentists 6.0 %

*Other in 1973 included

Eyeglasses and appliances	2.1 %
Nursing homes	7.1 %
Research	2.5 %
Construction	4.3 %
Miscellaneous	11.6 %

health care is reimbursed from government funds including Medicare and Medicaid.[10]

Various proposals have been made for alleviating the high cost of medical care. Current issues revolve around compulsory versus voluntary health insurance and the extent of federal subvention and intervention. These issues are discussed in Chapter 3.

The labor organizations contend that health insurance should be compulsory. Under such a plan, each person would contribute a small percentage of his or her income for comprehensive medical care. Health services would be coordinated in such a manner as to ensure adequate protection for all individuals. Opposing viewpoints hold that governmental control would surely ensue and that the quality of services and professional standards would suffer.

Programs in other countries illustrate different ways of meeting the complex problems of medical care. *State medicine,* as evidenced in the Soviet Union and Cuba, provides free or low-cost service for everyone. Physician and specialist education is provided free by the government, as are the facilities and equipment used in medical practice. The program is completely state or government-administered and controlled. Socialized medicine is comparable to a state system of medical care in many respects, except in the extent of governmental control. Socialized forms of medical practice, as found in Sweden, England, and parts of Canada, generally place the administration of the program with a professional group, but the cost is underwritten by the taxpayer. In addition to their participation in the socialized program, physicians are usually allowed to maintain private practices. There are distinct and rather obvious benefits and disadvantages to both state and socialized medical-care programs. Certain problems are frequently cited, notably the tremendous cost of providing adequate services to all. This has been due in part to the misuse and abuse of the system by hypochondriacs and health cranks. Some criticism has also been directed at the apparent decline in the quality of medical care.

CONSUMER HEALTH PROTECTION

The selection of health products, information, and services is, in the final analysis, a matter of individual responsibility. However, certain regulatory procedures afford the consumer protection. These consist of the local, state, and federal laws that control fraudulent health practices and the agencies and organizations that have been created to assure compliance with this legislation.

Government Protection

Legislation. Since ancient times, consumer health protection has been afforded by legal statutes. Early Mosaic and Egyptian laws governed the proper handling of meat and other foodstuffs. The Greeks and Romans sought to prevent the watering of wine. During the Middle Ages, the English Grocer's Company developed a system of public food inspectors, and in 1202 King John proclaimed one of the earliest food laws.

Efforts toward consumer health legislation were apparent early in the United States. A Massachusetts act of 1784 was the first general food law in this country; other colonies enacted similar provisions at a later date. National legislation first took place in 1848 with the passage of a law designed to control the importation of adulterated drugs. California enacted a pure food and drink law two years later, apparently as an outgrowth of practices during the Gold Rush. An 1897 Federal Tea Act authorized the establishment of standards regulating the purity and quality of all imported teas.

Food and Drug Administration. In 1906 the Federal Food and Drug Act was passed by Congress. This law provided for control over interstate commerce of drugs and made the adulteration of consumer products illegal. It also was an early attempt to prevent false labeling, the inclusion of inferior or harmful substances in foods and drugs, and the distribution of products under misleading brands or assumed names.

The Federal Food and Drug Administration, established in 1927 as a separate unit of the Department of Agriculture, was given responsibility for the enforcement of the Pure Food and Drug Law that was in existence at that time. Thirteen years later, the administration became a part of the Federal Security Agency. In 1953, it was transferred to the newly created Department of Health, Education and Welfare, becoming one of its major branches. The work of the Food and Drug Administration is tremendously broad and inclusive. Its principal task today is to enforce the Food, Drug, and Cosmetic Act and to assure protection against unfair competition by inferior or dishonestly labeled goods.

Laws are continuously being enacted to improve the safety of products. Some of the major provisions since 1960 are establishment of tolerance levels for the safe use of all pesticides, food additives, and colors used in foods, drugs, and cosmetics; requirement that warnings and antidotes appear on household products that are toxic, corrosive, irritating, flammable, strongly sensitizing, or radioactive or that generate injurious pressures, such as pressurized cans; immediate removal of a drug from the market when there is evidence of public hazard; and requirement that a new drug be *proved effective as well as safe* before being offered for sale. This last provision is economically significant in that an estimated 2,000 new drugs are tested each year for possible human use, and the manufacturers must do the testing!

The labeling of products has been greatly improved. Today labels must not be false or misleading and must stipulate such information as the name and address of the manufacturer, packer, or distributor; an accurate statement of quantity; adequate directions for use; and the common name and amount of active ingredients. The side effects must be listed by pharmaceutical companies in all advertising.

Effective enforcement of consumer legislation ensures public confidence in the quality and safety of purchases. In carrying out specific responsibilities related to policing the purity, quality, and labeling of foods, drugs, and cosmetics, the FDA:

1. Makes periodic inspections of food, drug, device, and cosmetic establishments and examines samples from interstate shipments of these products.
2. Assists industry in voluntary compliance with the law and in setting up controls to prevent violations.
3. Requires manufacturers to prove the safety and effectiveness of "new" drugs before they are put on sale to the public.
4. Tests safety and effectiveness of samples of insulin and of antibiotic drugs before they are sold. The manufacturers pay for these tests.
5. Enforces the law against illegal sale of prescription drugs.
6. Investigates therapeutic devices for safety and truthfulness of labeling claims.
7. Sets up standards of identity, quality, and fill of container for food products in line with the congressional mandate "to promote honesty and fair dealing in the interest of consumers."
8. Passes on the safety of food additives and checks to see that safety rules are followed.
9. Sets safe limits on the amount of pesticide residues that may remain on food crops and checks shipments to see that these limits are observed.
10. Passes on the safety of colors for use in foods, drugs, or cosmetics and, where necessary, tests and certifies each batch manufactured.
11. Checks imports of foods, drugs, devices, and cosmetics to make sure they comply with United States law.
12. Cooperates with state and local officials in the inspection of foods and drugs contaminated by floods, hurricanes, explosions, and fires and assists in removing damaged items from the market.[11]

To accomplish these broad functions, the Administration uses up-to-

FOUNDATIONS OF HEALTH SCIENCE

date scientific methods of analysis and inspection. It employs specialists in the fields of chemistry, microanalysis, human and veterinary medicine, pharmacology, bacteriology, entomology, and other sciences. It tests and evaluates the potency and efficacy of vitamins and drugs, investigates the toxicity of certain ingredients, studies the causes and prevention of food poisoning, and maintains controls over the processing, preserving, packaging, labeling, and storing of products. The FDA's budgeting staff includes inspectors who visit processing plants and factories that might be violating federal legislation. The inspectors, assisted by other employees, are required to sample some 100,000 factories and public warehouses and some 700,000 drugstores, public eating places, and other establishments that are subject to law. Only a fraction of the purchasable foods, drugs, and cosmetics, though, are checked in any given year. Domestic drug establishments are inspected once every two years, and food inspections are made about once every three or four years. A final important function of the administration is the preparation of evidence for cases of violation of law.

Since only a fraction of the purchasable foods, drugs, and cosmetics can be checked in any given year, fraudulent claims and questionable products may not be immediately discovered by the FDA. This is a reason for consumer health education. There may also be controversy about what constitutes sufficient scientific evidence to label a product safe or unsafe. Figure 2.7 suggests how consumers can help the FDA.

National Business Council for Consumer Affairs. The NBCCA was established in August 1971 by presidential order. It is composed of 116 top executives from all fields of business and has as its purpose "to advise government and their fellow businessmen on how business can voluntarily take a more active role in meeting the concerns of the consumer."

The Council is composed of seven subcouncils designed to help prepare guidelines for the business community and the public on major consumer problems. Some of these include advertising and promotion, packaging and labeling, warranties and guarantees, credit and other terms of sale, performance and service, product safety, complaints, and remedies. The guidelines are expected to serve as recommendations for action.

Occupational Safety and Health Act. In 1970 the Occupational Safety and Health Act was passed by Congress and with it was created the agency now frequently referred to as OSHA. This organization works actively to uphold the standards set forth in the legislation, which was designed to protect the health and safety of the American worker.

A number of other protective organizations have also evolved in recent years. Among these are the Consumer Protection Agency and the Office of Consumer Affairs. Industry and business has responded with such

Figure 2.7 When and How to Report to FDA

Consumers who report problems in sanitation, labeling, and safety of products regulated by FDA help the Agency to protect all consumers.

Such problems, reported by phone or letter, often lead to discovery and correction of violations, in some cases requiring recalls or criminal prosecution.

To insure prompt and thorough action on his report, the consumer must first determine if, in fact, it was the *product* that was at fault. Was it used as directed? Was it stored properly? If he finds the product was at fault, he should report the problem clearly and accurately to the FDA office nearest him, listed in this Consumer Guide, or to the Food and Drug Administration, 5600 Fishers Lane, Rockville, Maryland 20852.

The following should be included:

- Your name, address, telephone number.
- Clear statement of the apparent problem.
- As much detail as possible about the product label, including code marks.
- Name and address of store where purchased. Date of purchase.

Save whatever remains of the product or container for your doctor's guidance or possible FDA inspection. You should also report the problem to addresses on the label and to the store.

FDA has limited jurisdiction over certain consumer products. If you have complaints about any of the following, these are the Federal agencies to inform:

- Suspected false advertising—*Federal Trade Commission.*
- Meat and poultry products—*U.S. Department of Agriculture.*
- Sanitation of restaurants—*local health authorities.*
- Products made and sold exclusively within a State—*local or State health department or similar law enforcement agency.*
- Suspected illegal sale of narcotics or dangerous drugs (such as stimulants, depressants, and hallucinogens)—*Drug Enforcement Administration, U.S. Department of Justice.*
- Unsolicited products by mail—*U.S. Postal Service.*
- Accidental poisonings—*Poison Control Centers.*
- Dispensing practices of pharmacists and drug prices—*State Board of Pharmacy.*
- Pesticides, air, and water pollution—*Environmental Protection Agency.*
- Toys and other consumer products—*Consumer Product Safety Commission.*

FDA Consumer, 8:20, October 1974.

groups as the Major Appliance Consumer Panel and the National Advertising Review Board.

Federal Trade Commission. The Federal Trade Commission is primarily responsible for the regulation of unfair competitive methods and false or misleading advertising. With respect to consumer health, it assumes jurisdiction over foods, drugs, cosmetics, and therapeutic devices that are deceptively advertised, unfairly sold, or improperly distributed. Much like the FDA, the commission may rely upon court action in the prosecution of violators of the Federal Trade Commission Act and its amendments. In recent years, a number of cease-and-desist orders issued by the FTC have resulted in the elimination of false claims for certain products. In some

FOUNDATIONS OF HEALTH SCIENCE

cases, complaints have been initiated by individuals or by competitors producing a similar product.

The commission constantly studies advertising media—radio, television, magazines, newspapers, books, leaflets, billboards, and other mass appeals. However, because of the vastness of modern avenues of communication, the FTC has been unable to prevent all fraudulent advertising and deceptive practices.

U.S. Postal Service. The United States Postal Service is responsible for preventing the use of the mails for transmission of fraudulent health materials and devices. The selling of nostrums and the dissemination of false or misleading advertising through the postal system have met with severe penalties. By vigilance on the part of the postal inspectors, increased public action, and stronger legislation against violators, the Department discourages use of the mails by quacks and other questionable persons.

Department of Agriculture. The United States Department of Agriculture was at one time the principal governmental agency dealing with consumer health problems. Upon the establishment of the FDA, however, much of this responsibility was transferred. The two groups still cooperate closely. Today, the Department of Agriculture performs the formidable task of inspecting interstate and imported shipments of meat. It also controls agricultural procedures used in the planting, growing, and processing of foodstuffs. In recent years, it has questioned the improper use of insect poisons and other toxic substances and has been extremely active in analyzing the effects of radioactivity on farm products. DDT is now banned for some uses in agriculture.

State and local legislation. All states and many local communities have enacted legislation concerning consumer health practices. Many of these laws are patterned after federal acts and tend to complement and extend the benefits of national provisions. At the state level, the protection of health is often enforced by departments that provide for the health and safety of the population. Many states have established bureaus of food, drug, and cosmetic control as divisions of the state departments of public health.

A model law for state control of quackery in California deters the cancer quack by prohibiting fraudulent practice and by prescribing penalties for offenders. In general, it permits state officials to inspect facilities for cancer diagnosis and treatment, requires appropriate testing of new procedures, and demands accurate records.[12] Many other states have adopted similar legislation.

County and local ordinances reflecting concern for consumer health are found throughout the United States. By virtue of being able to exert greater direct control, agencies responsible for the enforcement of local legislation have been particularly effective in dealing with fraudulent health activities. For optimum results, however, a close operational relationship between local, state, and federal groups is essential.

Private Protection of Consumer Health

Numerous nongovernmental organizations and agencies have developed over the years to provide protection for the American consumer. Although hampered by a lack of personnel, insufficient operating funds, and legal restrictions, these groups serve as a strong force in the policing and enforcement of provisions relating to the health and safety of the public.

Professional associations. Public attention to problems of fraudulent health practice has been fostered to a great extent by the work of professional organizations. Although mainly interested in the improvement of standards pertaining to their particular professions, these groups collectively have contributed to the overall exposure of quacks, faddists, and cultists.

The American Medical Association has long been a leader among the professional societies. Its various committees—Councils on Medicine, Pharmacy and Chemistry, Drugs, Legislative Activities, and Foods and Nutrition—and the Bureau of Investigation of the association perform explicit consumer services. Members of each committee and the Bureau perform clinical investigations and testing and report upon various drug products, foods, and therapeutic devices. The American Dental Association, through several of its committees, is ever watchful for quackery within the dental profession. The American Dietetic Association helps combat nutrition misinformation and food fads, as does the American Home Economics Association.

The American Public Health Association has hit out against pseudo-scientific literature in the health sciences. The American College of Surgeons, along with the American Hospital Association, has been influential in the development of appropriate standards for hospitals and for proper surgical products. The American Pharmaceutical Association has adopted similar standards for drug dispensing.

Private agencies. Voluntary health agencies, such as the Arthritis Foundation and the American Cancer Society, work to eliminate fraudulent practice within their specialized areas. Since 1928, Consumers' Research, Inc., has provided unbiased scientific information on consumer products. Through open market purchase, testing, and evaluation of cost and quality, this organization rates products and reports the results in the *Consumers' Research Magazine*. The Consumers' Union, Inc., founded as a nonprofit organization about a decade later, performs a comparable testing and rating function to subscribers. It uses scientifically developed data on brand name comparisons and issues the monthly *Consumer Reports* and an *Annual Buying Guide*.

One of the most important consumer organizations in the United States is the National Better Business Bureau. This agency, working through more than 100 nonprofit local branches, affords protection services to communities throughout the nation. The various bureaus are supported by annual subscriptions from business and industry. The Bureau actively engages in combating fraud, false and misleading advertising, unfair competitive methods, and other forms of malpractice. It publishes educational materials, handles inquiries and complaints, and investigates activities reported to be fraudulent. In instances of violation of acceptable standards, the Bureau usually suggests correction to the offender before presenting the case to official law-enforcement authorities.

A number of business organizations concern themselves with consumer problems, many related to the health and safety of the public. Among these are the National Association of Consumers, the American Retail Federation, the National Consumer-Retailer Council, the Association of Food Chains, and the National Retail Dry Goods Association.

IN CONCLUSION

There are laws, regulations, and agencies that function to protect the consumer against quackery and fraud. However, consumers must assume the responsibility for selecting health products and services wisely and be discriminating in their acceptance of health information and commercial products. The old saying "you can't buy health or happiness" is no longer true. Everyone purchases health products and services that may promote or destroy their health and happiness. The *informed* consumer will be able to make wise purchases from today's vast marketplace.

Notes

1. Charles S. Cameron, *The Cancer Quacks*, U.S. Department of Health, Education and Welfare. Public Health Service, National Cancer Institute, PHS Publication No. 559 (Washington, D.C.: Government Printing Office, September, 1963), p. 2.

2. James Cook, *Remedies and Rackets: The Truth about Patent Medicine Today* (New York: W. W. Norton and Co., 1958), p. 25.

3. *The Arthritis Hoax*, Public Affairs Pamphlet No. 297 (New York: Public Affairs Committee, Inc., 1960), p. 1.

4. Cameron, p. 4.

5. Ibid., p. 6.

6. John P. McNeel, "Quack Medical Machines," *Popular Mechanics,* 120:220, October, 1963.

7. Better Business Bureau, *Facts You Should Know About Health Quackery* (Boston: Educational Division, Better Business Bureau, 1959), p. 2.

8. Richard K. Means, "Interpreting Statistics: An Art," *Nursing Outlook,* 13:35, May, 1965.

9. "Vital Signs," *Health/PAC Bulletin,* No. 67, November/December, 1975, p. 22.

10. "Hospitals and Clinics: Synergy," *UCSF News,* 1:13, February, 1974.

11. Food and Drug Administration, *FDA—What It Is and Does,* U.S. Department of Health, Education and Welfare, FDA Publication No. 1 (Washington, D.C.: Government Printing Office, February, 1965), p. 3.

12. Henry L. Garland and Henry LaCossitt, "California Outlaws the Cancer Quack," *Today's Health,* 37:30–31, 70–72, August, 1959.

FOUNDATIONS OF HEALTH SCIENCE

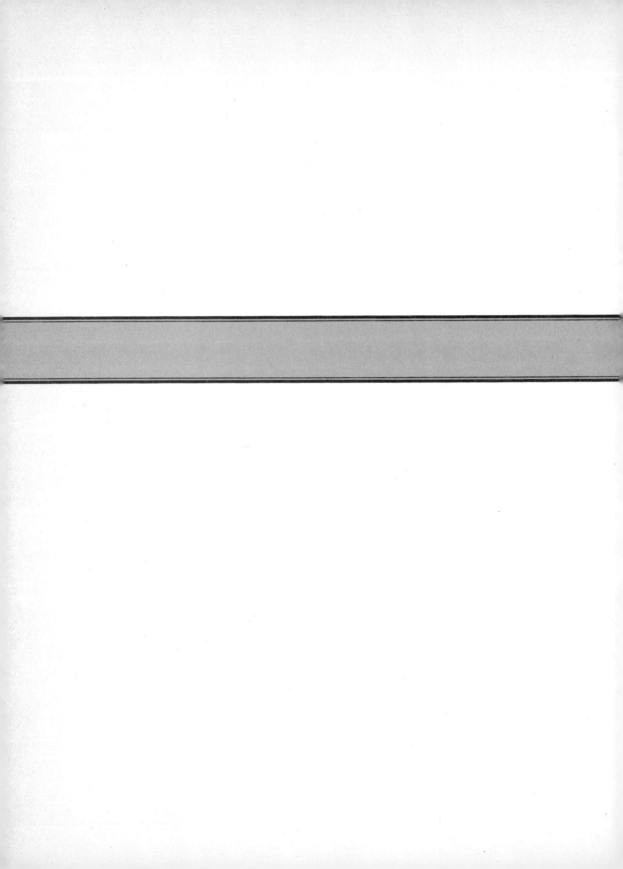

HEALTH MAINTENANCE

Health maintenance implies the incorporation of measures designed to prevent ill health and to promote optimal well-being. The responsibilities for the prevention of disease and debilitating conditions are both individual and professional. Assuredly, physicians and scientists must fulfill their roles, but equally vital to health maintenance are the actions that each person takes to obtain early medical care. These actions, or preventive measures, include having periodic medical examinations; obtaining necessary immunizations; protecting vision, hearing, and the teeth; keeping personal medical records, getting temporary care for acute conditions, and selecting health care services.

PERIODIC MEDICAL EXAMINATIONS

Periodic medical examinations are presumed to be one of the more important means of reducing illness and premature death or disability. Most persons between the ages of two and forty years should be examined every two to three years. Between forty and sixty years of age, an annual examination is preferable, and from sixty on, a semiannual examination is recommended. In a thousand examinations of supposedly healthy persons between the ages of forty and fifty-five, one physician found serious conditions in one-half of the examinees, including heart disease, diabetes, high blood pressure, ulcers, and tumors. The specific nature of the more common disorders is described in detail in later chapters.

There are two major types of physical examination. The first is a screening, in which select procedures are used to detect a specific disorder or to find those conditions commonly occurring in a specific age group. Examples of group screenings include glaucoma detection drives, communitywide checks for high blood pressure among blacks, and neighborhood checks for chronic respiratory disease (carried out through mobile units in shopping centers). Another kind of screening is the health appraisal conducted in schools and in industry. Its major objective is to determine the examinee's health status relative to school performance or job placement.

The second type of physical examination is the so-called complete physical conducted for prevention purposes. This is what most of us have in mind when we speak of periodic medical examinations. However, all practitioners do not give the same kind of complete physical, and many lay people do not know the difference between a screening, a partial examination, and a preventive examination. In addition, the procedures included in the so-called ideal preventive physical will vary with the age of the person

Useless Worry! Have Check-ups

My mother had a heart attack and died in my arms. I had always been healthy, except for hay fever, so when I began to repeatedly have a terrible pain in my chest I secretly feared I might have a weak heart. At my age, sixty-two, you really begin to worry about these things. I didn't want to go to a doctor and be put in the hospital for tests, but I knew sooner or later I would have to have a checkup.

One Saturday night the attack came on me, and I couldn't sleep. I still had horrible pains and was throwing up the next morning. Finally, my daughter took me to the emergency room. They did an EKG and told my daughter my heart was OK and I could go home, but that I should see my doctor for a good check-up. I did, and he told me I just have a hiatal hernia, and it was nothing serious although I shouldn't eat spicy foods or work too hard.

I only wish I had gone for the checkup earlier. There was no reason for me to suffer those painful attacks or to think I had heart trouble. For my peace of mind I'm now going to try to have a checkup every six months or whenever the doctor says.

being examined, his or her past medical history, and his or her present complaints. There are hundreds of tests the physician might do, some of which are possible only in a hospital setting. The routine procedures described here are the ones most commonly used in examining the average person. These are considered minimal by most prevention-oriented medical practitioners. There is a growing trend towards having either a physician's assistant or a nurse-practitioner conduct portions of the appraisals. The cost of the examination will average between $100 and $150. A specialist, such as an internist, may charge slightly higher than the general practitioner. If the physician does some of the laboratory work in his office, the price may be less. Averaged out over a two-year period, the cost is between $4 and $8 per month. Many health insurance policies still do not cover the cost of preventive medical care.

Health History

The most important part of the clinical examination is the medical history. It is what you tell that counts! First, the patient fills out a fairly standard form about past illnesses and present complaints, if any. Then the examiner interviews the patient, asking questions about his ability to get along with others, his family relationships (including sexual adjustment), and his job satisfaction. During the interview, the examiner goes over the questionnaire, since some answers can only be given in detail verbally. If the patient is a child, the examiner will ask questions about prenatal and birth conditions (rubella, toxemia of pregnancy, genetic disorders, prolonged or precipitate delivery, blood incompatibilities), growth and development, speech and communication skills, and school progress.

Clinical Examination

Following the health history, the patient disrobes and puts on a smock for the physical appraisal. Medicine is an art as well as a science, and experience and intuition give the physician the insight required for diagnosing levels of wellness. The examiner observes, sometimes using instruments to see inside body orifices; smells; palpates; and listens by tapping, using a stethoscope, or using a tuning fork. Some of these things may be done simultaneously, so the patient may not be aware of all aspects of the appraisal. The examiner weighs and measures the patient, takes his temperature, administers a tuberculin skin test, and makes the following checks of the body.

Skeleton. Posture, body alignment, shape and size of extremities, and gait are checked.

Skin and mucous membranes. Color, texture, presence of blemishes or lesions of the skin and mucous membranes of the eyes, mouth, and vaginal tract are checked. At this time the examiner will observe adequacy of subcutaneous tissue and muscle tone are checked. Examination may disclose clues indicating nutritional disorders, metabolic disease, infections, and pathology of the renal and cardiovascular systems.

Eyes. Ophthalmoscopic examination of the retina can reveal arterial changes that indicate diabetes, high blood pressure, hardening of the arteries, or syphilis.

Ears. Otoscopic examination can reveal a damaged ear drum, infection in the auditory canal, or the accumulation of wax that interferes with hearing.

Abdomen. Through palpation, the examiner evaluates size and shape of organs and notes presence of pain or discomfort. By tapping and by listening with a stethoscope the examiner can identify abnormal amounts of fluid, air, or solid tissue that could indicate cardiovasculorenal disease, neoplastic growths, or infection.

Mouth, nose, and throat. Observations may reveal signs of infections, allergic manifestations, precancerous lesions, and dental diseases. The color of mucous membranes may indicate good or poor nutritional status.

Heart and lungs. The examiner checks pulse and respiration and blood pressure. Examination techniques include tapping, stethoscopic examination (heart, breath sounds, and carotid artery), and pulmonary function tests.

Breasts. Both females and males are examined. The examiner should be sure women know how to do a monthly self-examination of their breasts.

Genitals. Pelvic examination in women includes a manual examination to determine the condition of the uterus and ovaries as well as the use of the speculum to see the vaginal tract and cervix. Examination of males includes palpation of testes for abnormalities. Both males and females should have a rectal check. In females, the examiner digitally palpates the uterus through the rectal wall. In males, the examiner palpates the prostate. A proctoscopic examination is done every several years to pick up precancerous conditions of the colon.

Nervous system. Reflexes are evaluated by tapping the elbow, ankle, and knee areas with a mallet and by brushing the abdomen and the soles of the feet with a sharp instrument. Ophthalmological examination of the eye can reveal abnormal pressures in the brain.

FOUNDATIONS OF HEALTH SCIENCE

Some laboratory tests are made at each visit, others are done every few visits, and a few are made if a specific disorder is present or if the physician wants to check clues further. Routine laboratory tests done at each examination include a chest X ray (primarily for neoplastic growths); a urinalysis for kidney dysfunction; smear tests to determine cervical, endometrial, and estrogen status in women; and a blood serology for syphilis, red and white cell counts, and hemoglobin. (Computers are being increasingly used for serological tests.) Periodic laboratory tests should include an electrocardiogram, pulmonary function tests, and tests for blood lipids and blood sugar.

Table 3.1 is a summary of routine procedures that should be included in a periodic physical examination.

Understanding Medical Findings

The concept of *normal* is not exact; it is one of degree or range. Findings falling outside of the normal range are considered evidence of possible

Table 3.1   Routine Procedures in a Periodic Physical Examination

Procedure	Type of Observation
Health and medical history	Familial diseases and disorders Past illnesses Present symptoms or status
Clinical examinations	Blood pressure, temperature, pulse, height, weight Palpation of subcutaneous tissue and abdomen Ausculation, or listening to sounds in chest, neck, and abdomen Eyes with ophthalmoscope and ears with otoscope Nose, mouth, throat Reflexes Posture Rectal, using palpation and proctoscope Pelvic and breast in women Tuberculin skin test Testes in men
Routine laboratory tests (at each examination)	Chest X ray Blood serology: syphilis, red and white cell count, hemoglobin Urinalysis Smear tests of cervix and endometrium
Periodic laboratory tests (every several examinations)	Electrocardiogram Pulmonary function tests Blood lipids Blood sugar

illness. For example, body temperature between 97 and 99 degrees Fahrenheit or 36 and 39 degrees centigrade is considered well within normal range, as is a pulse rate of between 60 and 90 pulsations per minute. To label any finding as abnormal, the physician compares it with the patient's reaction when he was presumedly well, besides comparing it with the so-called average range of the general population. This is one reason why data about health status accumulated during the presumedly normal young adult years are invaluable in assessing changes later in life.

Laboratory tests are never 100 percent accurate. A result can be a *false positive* (an indication that a disease exists when it doesn't) or a *false negative* (an indication that there is no disease when there is). When using tests that are not highly accurate, the physician may request that they be repeated. No diagnosis should be based on one test that does not agree with other findings of the examination.

The significance of blood pressure readings is not always understood. These readings are an indirect measurement of the elasticity of artery walls. The resistance between the vessel wall and the blood flowing through while the heart is resting is *diastolic tension,* and the resistance between the wall and the sudden surge of blood sent through the vessel when the heart contracts is *systolic tension*. Vessels with a consistently high diastolic tension or high diastolic and systolic tension interfere with circulation and ultimately cause heart, brain, and kidney damage.

An easy, well-known technique for measuring blood pressure involves use of the stethoscope and sphygmomanometer, although other devices are more elaborate and accurate. Arterial pressure is measured in millimeters of mercury (120 mm Hg means that the force exerted by the artery wall raised a column of mercury to the 120 mm level) The arm is constricted by a blood pressure cuff, and the cuff is inflated. When the pressure in the cuff is equal to the pressure in the artery wall, blood flows through the artery. This flow can be heard as a pulsating sound through the stethoscope. The level of mercury at this point of equalization and audible sound indicates the *systolic pressure.* When the level of pressure in the cuff is less than that exerted by the arterial wall during the resting phase of the cardiac cycle, the pulsating sound drops off markedly. This point of drop-off indicates the *diastolic pressure.* Blood pressure measurement is recorded as systolic/diastolic.

Changes in the systolic pressure result from exercise and emotional stress. If this reading is high, the examiner may recheck ten or fifteen minutes later. The diastolic level is the least affected by emotions and activity, so it is a more reliable index of normality or abnormality. The blood pressure range considered within normal limits is 110–150/60–90.

The mean arterial pressure is also used as a diagnostic aid. It is derived by dividing the sum of the systolic and diastolic pressures by two. A desirable mean is 100; when the mean is over 200, the heart is unable to circulate the blood satisfactorily. Few young adults have high blood pressure, so their blood pressure readings probably reflect their "normal." Such figures should be part of personal files for future reference.

Immunizations

It is a sad commentary on our health behavior that many of us do not have ourselves or our children immunized against communicable diseases, even though immunization is available, frequently without cost to nearly everyone in this country. Although immunization levels in 1974 were up slightly from those of 1973, almost one-third of the children entering school were inadequately protected. *Medical World News* reports that in 1974 the following percentages of children were adequately immunized: measles, 64.5%; rubella, 59.8%; mumps, 39.4%; polio, 63.1%; and diphtheria-pertussis-tetanus, 73.9%. Approximately 5.3 million of the nearly 13.2 million children aged one to four years were not protected.[1]

Vaccinations are one of the wonders of medicine, and diseases dreaded in the past are now almost completely eradicated. Existing vaccines and biologics are used to prevent some eighteen diseases. Immunizations should be started during the first year of life and updated during periodic medical examinations. Here are a few points to keep in mind regarding immunizations:[2]

Diphtheria, pertussis, and tetanus. Sporadic diphtheria cases in under-immunized populations confirm that infection is still occurring. An immunized person, even though protected, can still be a carrier and transmit the disease.

Poliomyelitis. A single booster dose of polio vaccine is recommended for adults if they plan to travel to areas where polio is endemic or if they live in a community that experiences an outbreak.

Measles. Properly used, vaccine is 95 percent effective, and there is no evidence of loss of protection with time. Because the number of unvaccinated children has increased, the incidence of measles has risen from a low of 23,000 cases in the 60s to 74,000 in the 70s.

Rubella. (German measles). Fifteen to twenty percent of women are still susceptible to rubella when they reach their childbearing years. If a woman is infected during pregnancy, the infection can cause the congenital rubella syndrome, which may result in severe abnormalities or death in the fetus or infant.

Mumps. Mumps vaccine provides durable immunity and can be given in combination with the vaccines for measles and rubella.

Exposure to Radiation

We are exposed to radiation from a variety of sources. Some are natural: cosmic rays; radioactive materials in the ground, air, and buildings; and radionuclides that normally occur in the body. Other sources are man-made—medical procedures, weapons fallout, nuclear energy industry, procedures in other industries, and color TV. More than 90 percent of man-made exposure to ionizing radiation, including 94 percent of gonad exposure, comes from medical and dental diagnostic sources.

Without the use of ionizing radiation in diagnosis and therapy, doctors could not provide the type of medical care we expect today.[3] But radiation produces biological changes that are usually undesirable and sometimes harmful. The harmful effect is related to the amount of exposure. We know that even the smallest amount can cause genetic change. As yet, we do not know the precise effect of specific doses. Any exposure to the gonads is undesirable, since alteration in the genetic structure of the ova and sperm can be transmitted to the next generation. Like other modalities of treatment (surgery and chemotherapy) radiation has good points and bad points. The bad points must be continually weighed against the good that radiation provides in preventing disease, disability, and death. Scientists are continuing to search for less dangerous means of diagnosis and treatment. Meanwhile, we can reduce the dangers of radiation ourselves by reminding physicians and dentists that we are concerned about unnecessary exposure and by not demanding an X ray when medical advice says it is not needed. We should also keep records of when and where we received either diagnostic or therapeutic doses of radiation.

Personal Medical Records

A complete medical record should be part of everyone's personal files. Few people will go to the same physician throughout their lifetimes, and it is not always possible to have records sent from one doctor to another, although most physicians will send them upon request.

The personal record should include the dates and findings of all laboratory examinations. (More and more doctors are taking the time to explain their findings. If your health adviser doesn't, *ask* him to do so!) It should also include dates of illnesses and accidents; dates and types of immunizations and medications prescribed; any reactions to a specific medicine or treatment; and dates of radiation therapy and the names and addresses of the person who administered it. A good plan is to update these records each year at income tax time or on one's birthday. Figure 3.1 is an example of one medical record form.

66

Symptoms of illness can develop at any time. When do they indicate a nonserious, transitory illness and when do they demand medical attention? This is not always easy to decide.

The configuration of various symptoms provides diagnosticians with clues. Physicians are helped immeasurably when patients describe their symptoms accurately, but examination can be upsetting, and frequently people forget everything they wanted to tell and ask the doctor. A carefully prepared record of symptoms should be made before seeing the physician.

Pain. Obviously, one does not go to a doctor with every minor ache and discomfort, but pain is a warning signal that can portend serious illness. Medical attention should be obtained when pain develops suddenly; persists for a day or more; is acute, sharp, stabbing, or piercing; and is unexplainable (muscular aches after unusual physical activity or an occasional headache after a tension-filled day is explainable). The physician will also want to know if the pain is continuous or intermittent and if an intermittent pain is correlated with any body process or activity such as eating, urinating, defecating, coughing, walking, or lying down.

Fever. Elevation of body temperature, fever, is an objective indication of illness, usually infection. Any rise in temperature of two degrees over one's

A needless scare—Don't wait

About three weeks ago, I became extremely sick. I haven't even had a sore throat in the last six years, so this really worried and upset me. I woke up on a Monday morning and when I went to the bathroom, I found blood in my urine and felt some slight pain. I didn't really start to worry until Tuesday night. By then, I was urinating every hour. I didn't want to tell anyone, because I thought that it would go away. By Thursday, I could hardly walk, and I was going to the bathroom every ten minutes. After dropping my mother off at work, I decided that I had better stay home from my classes. All day, I read medical books and other information and was thoroughly convinced that I had cancer. I picked up my mother from work and told her on the way home. She tried to keep me calm. I went to a gynecologist right away and found out that I just had a urinary tract infection.

Figure 3.1 Medical Record

Data	Year ( )	Year ( )	Year ( )	Year ( )
Physical Findings:				
Blood Pressure				
Electrocardiogram				
Chest X ray				
Pulmonary Function Test				
Blood Count				
Urinalysis				
Syphilis				
Blood Lipids				
Blood Sugar				
Other				
Illnesses and Accidents				
Medications and Reactions				
Radiation Therapy and Name of Radiologist				

Immunizations

Immunity for	Had Disease	Initial Series	Year Obtained	Boosters	
Recommended					
Diphtheria					
Whooping Cough					
Tetanus					
Measles					
Polio					
Influenza					
Rubella					
Mumps					
Special Needs					
Typhoid					
Paratyphoid					
Rabies					
Cholera					
Plague					
Encephalitis					
Yellow Fever					

Figure 3.1 Medical Record *(Continued)*

Typhus	——	——	——	——	——	——
Tuberculosis	——	——	——	——	——	——
Meningitis	——	——	——	——	——	——
Smallpox	——	——	——	——	——	——
Hepatitis A	——	——	——	——	——	——
Hepatitis B	——	——	——	——	——	——
Others	——	——	——	——	——	——
By Infection	——	——	——	——	——	——
(no vaccines)	——	——	——	——	——	——
Chicken Pox	——	——	——	——	——	——
Others	——	——	——	——	——	——

normal temperature is considered a fever. Rectal temperatures are one degree higher than mouth temperatures and are considered more accurate.

Bleeding. Bleeding from any body orifice—ears, nose, mouth, rectum, vagina (between menstrual periods), urethra, and nipples—is abnormal. Any wart or mole that bleeds may be a sign of cancer.

Sores. Sores that do not heal or keep coming back, rashes, boils, ulcers, or color changes are symptomatic of several chronic disorders including arterial disease, diabetes, and cancer.

Fatigue. Fatigue accompanies many systemic conditions as well as emotional disturbances. The development of that "tired feeling" may be so insidious that the victim is not aware of it until it becomes pronounced. Evidences of fatigue are inability to continue the daily routine without "forcing"; lack of energy that makes any unexpected task seem overwhelming; change in disposition; tiredness before even starting a job; and difficulty in concentrating on, or completing, anything.

Insomnia. Contradictory as it may seem, the person who is fatigued frequently suffers from insomnia. The healthy person will routinely go to sleep less than thirty minutes after retiring.

Weight change. Sudden gains in weight, such as five pounds overnight, are abnormal. Even if there is little weight gain, swollen hands and face first thing in the morning, as well as swollen ankles and feet at the end of the day, may be dangerously significant. Slow loss of weight without an accompanying reduction in caloric intake or increase in activity is also a sign of disorder.

Digestive changes. Serious digestive changes that might occur are sudden or gradual loss of appetite; difficulty in swallowing; persistent indigestion and/or heartburn; regurgitation; nausea; vomiting; increase in belching and flatulence unrelated to the ingestion of specific foods; alteration in bowel habits, such as constipation or diarrhea; and excessive thirst.

Respiratory changes. One of the most frequent maladies is the common cold. Symptoms of acute respiratory infections should disappear within a week or so, not linger for a month or more. Persistent sore throat, breathlessness, pain in the chest after exertion or when taking a deep breath, cough, continuous need to expectorate, and occasional difficulty in getting one's breath are significant symptoms, even though they may be transitory, that require medical attention.

Vision changes. Difficulties with vision result from problems with other organs and systems as well as the eyes. Vision problems include discoloration of the eye itself, double vision, inability to focus, seeing of spots, blurring, seeing of brightly colored lights, and pain in the eyeball. Reddened lids, crusting, and styes are other manifestations of disorder.

Neurological signs. Any sudden neurological symptom, such as mental confusion, convulsion, amnesia, numbness or paralysis, faintness or dizziness, and loss of consciousness, can indicate a number of serious conditions.

How to Get the Most Out of Your Doctor, or Rules to Make You a Better Patient

Except in emergencies, we should always make an appointment. In addition, Dr. William Nolen gives five do's and five don'ts of productive patienting.[4]

1. Do, when you call for an appointment, let the secretary or nurse know what the problem is. A complete physical examination takes much longer than a check on a sore throat.

2. Do organize your thoughts. An accurate history of your symptoms enables the physician to make a diagnosis more quickly. Write things down instead of trusting to memory.

3. Do cooperate with the type of examination the doctor suggests. Putting off a chest X ray or laboratory work or a pelvic to another time only means that you are not getting adequate care and may suffer in the long run.

4. Do ask questions. Some physicians may not give full explanations, and sometimes they may think you understand when you do not, so ask!

5. Do follow instructions. You have paid for them.

These are the five don'ts.

1. Don't take more time than was scheduled. For example, if you go in for treatment of a minor symptom, do not suddenly request a physical examination that may not be needed for that complaint.

2. Don't lie to the doctor or yourself. When symptoms suggest cancer, some people procrastinate about obtaining care and then are embarrassed to tell the physician how long they have had the symptoms. People also tend to be untruthful about such habits as smoking and drinking.

3. Don't ask for unnecessary pills.

4. Don't ask to be hospitalized unnecessarily.

5. Don't leave the office dissatisfied. Give the doctor a chance to explain the reasons for whatever it was that displeased you. As Doctor Nolen says,

> It takes two people, a doctor and a patient working together, to cure illness. This doctor-patient relationship must be warm and trusting if it is going to be productive. Nowhere is this relationship more subject to strain than in the hectic atmosphere of the office visit. The patient who works to make the office visit a success can help both herself and her doctor immeasurably.

And, believe me, doctors need that help.[5]

A Bill of Rights for the Hospitalized Patient

There is increasing concern that patients in hospitals be informed about their rights. More and more hospitals are posting "A Bill of Rights for Patients" in each room or are handing the newly admitted patient a copy of these rights. The Bill of Rights reprinted as Figure 3.2 is used by the University of California Hospital in San Francisco.

TEMPORARY CARE FOR ACUTE SYMPTOMS

When symptoms are acute, it may be necessary to do something to relieve pain and discomfort while waiting for the physician. A national health survey taken several years ago revealed that the general population was woefully ignorant about what to do when illness strikes. Some procedures are safe and effective; others may delay the physician in making a diagnosis and prescribing treatment; and a few are actually hazardous.

There are two cardinal rules. The first is *never take or give a medicine!*

Figure 3.2 A Bill of Rights for Patients

For a century the physicians of our faculty and our entire staff at U.C. have devoted their energies to the achievement of excellence in the care of patients. The following statement is a reaffirmation of our views toward your rights and responsibilities as patients. We wish to care for you in an atmosphere in which you are alert to our goals; and indeed, one in which you, as a patient, can help us in special ways to help you.

1 *You have a right to considerate and respectful care without regard to your sex or your cultural, economic, educational or religious background.*

2 *You have the right to know the name of the physician who has primary responsibility for coordinating your care and the names of other doctors who will see you, and their professional relationship.*

3 *You have the right to receive information from your physician about your illness, your course of treatment, and your prospects for recovery in terms that you can understand.*

4 *You have the right to receive as much information about any proposed treatment or procedure as you may need, to give your consent or to refuse this course of treatment. Except in emergencies, this information should include a description of the procedure or treatment, the medically significant risks involved in this treatment, alternate courses of treatment or nontreatment and the risks involved in each. You also have the right to know the name of the person who will carry out the procedure or treatment.*

5 *You have the right to participate actively in decisions regarding your medical care. This includes the right to refuse treatment, and to be informed of the medical consequences of failure to undergo the treatment. Your refusal must be in writing over your signature.*

6 *You have the right to privacy in your medical care and treatment program. Case discussion, consultation, examination and treatment are confidential and should be conducted discreetly. You have the right to be advised as to the reason for the presence of any individuals not directly involved with your care. (If you are not sure why someone is present, ask your doctor or nurse.)*

7 *You have the right to confidential treatment of all communications and records pertaining to your care and your stay in the hospital. You must provide your written permission before your medical records can be made available to anyone not directly concerned with your care.*

8 *You have the right to expect that the Hospitals and Clinics will make reasonable responses to any reasonable requests you may make for service.*

9 *You have the right to leave the hospital even against the advice of your doctors. If you do so, you will be asked to sign a 'Discharge Against Medical Advice' form which relieves the Hospitals and Clinics of responsibility under this circumstance.*

10 *You have the right to obtain information about the relationship of the University of California Hospitals and Clinics to other health care and educational institutions insofar as your care and treatment are concerned.*

11 *You have the right to refuse and are under no obligation to participate in any research project affecting your care and treatment.*

12 *You have the right to expect that you (or your family) will be informed by your physician or a delegate of your physician of your continuing health care requirements following your discharge from the hospital.*

13 *You have the right to examine your bill and receive an explanation of the charges, whether they will be paid by you, your insurance company, or others.*

14 *Where a person other than the patient is legally responsible for making medical decisions on behalf of the patient, all of the above rights to information and participation in decision making apply.**

*This list is an adaptation of "A Patient's Bill of Rights," developed by the American Hospital Association in 1973.

FOUNDATIONS OF HEALTH SCIENCE

Figure 3.2 A Bill of Rights for Patients *(Continued)*

No catalogue of rights can assure 100 percent the kind of treatment our patients will receive. A hospital has many functions to perform, including the prevention and treatment of disease, the education of both health professionals and patients, and the conduct of clinical research. All these activities are conducted with an overriding concern for our patients, and above all, the recognition of their dignity as human beings.

Success in achieving this assures success in the defense of your rights as a patient.

PATIENTS ALSO HAVE RESPONSIBILITIES

1 *Please keep your appointments with us. Let us know when you cannot, so that we can schedule another patient for that time. Be open and honest with us about instructions you receive concerning your health; that is, let us know immediately if you do not understand them or if you feel that the instructions are such that you cannot follow them.*

2 *It is your responsibility to tell your doctor about any changes in your health.*

3 *You have the responsibility to be considerate of other patients, and to see that your visitors are considerate as well, particularly with reference to noise and smoking, which can be very annoying to nearby patients.*

4 *You also have the responsibility to provide information necessary for insurance processing of your Hospitals and Clinics bills, and to plan for payment of your health care bills as soon as possible. In cases of financial hardship you should discuss with the Financial Counseling Office the possibility of financial aid to help in the payment of your Hospitals/Clinics bills.*

The University of California Hospitals and Clinics are interested in keeping you in the best health possible. If you feel you are not being treated fairly or properly, you have the right to discuss this with your doctor, nurse, unit manager, social worker or other health worker. You may also write to the Director, University of California Hospitals and Clinics, San Francisco, California 94143. All correspondence will receive prompt and personal attention.

This message reflects the interest and philosophy of the entire staff of the University of California Hospitals and Clinics.

"Bill of Rights for Patients," *UCSF News,* 1:15, February, 1974.

Medications can be harmful and can disguise symptoms. Aspirin, which allays pain and reduces fever, can significantly distort symptoms. It also can precipitate intestinal hemorrhage. Laxatives and enemas can cause intestinal ruptures, particularly in cases of appendicitis.

The second rule is to *keep the ill person in bed.* For a number of diseases bedrest is the major therapy. While in bed, the patient uses his energy to combat the illness. Activity raises metabolism, which may increase the disease process. Confining a patient to bed also serves to isolate him more or less from others.

Alleviation of pain and discomfort is of paramount importance to the victim, although not necessarily to the course of his illness. The emotional impact of just "doing something" helps appreciably. Going to bed, changing to sleeping apparel, and having someone take care of you is "doing something." In the case of acute pain, a safe analgesic is an ice bag applied to the affected area. Never use heat, since it may spread infection. If ice is not available, a wet cloth changed frequently is a fair substitute. As long as there is no vomiting or abdominal pain, soft, bland foods may be taken, either hot or cold as desired. Coffee, strong tea, and alcoholic beverages of any kind should be avoided.

A nonsweet carbonated beverage, such as ginger ale or plain soda water with a few drops of lemon juice, may reduce nausea. If there is vomiting, nothing should be given by mouth. The following measures will help reduce thirst and the bad taste after vomiting: rinsing out the mouth with water containing a dash of lemon juice; using any of the standard proprietary mouth washes; sucking small chips of ice, a few at a time, which melt in the mouth and keep it moist; or sucking on a small wedge of orange. If diarrhea is a symptom and there is no vomiting, plenty of bland liquids (milk, eggnog, jello, weak tea, or cream soups) should be consumed to replace the fluid lost in the stool. Fruit and vegetable juices may increase intestinal irritation and should be avoided.

An elevation in temperature, fever, is a sign that the body is fighting the disease. However, high fevers are not only uncomfortable but dangerous. The patient should be in a draft-free room with as few covers and clothes on as possible, since covering the body increases body temperature. Sponging with cool water and putting an ice bag on the head will reduce the temperature. Conversely, if there are chills, wrapping in warm blankets helps to bring the temperature up. Heating pads and hot water bags are dangerous when used with small children, the aged, and the unconscious.

If the patient has symptoms of an upper respiratory disease and is having trouble breathing, the room should be warm and the air moist. In case of severe problems with breathing, such as croup, relief can be obtained by going into a bathroom filled wth steam from running faucets. Patients with respiratory distress are usually more comfortable in a sitting

Each treatment involves some risk

The only time I was seriously ill was about four years ago. I was hospitalized for about a month and a half to have two operations performed on my back. At the time I was fairly young and didn't worry about anything because of the idea I had about doctors and surgeons being so great. However, when I think back on this experience and remember some of the things that went on, I realize how serious any operation is to most people. I could see this in the actions of my parents and other people close to me. I guess everybody expects the worst when it happens in your own family.

position. It is a fallacy that wide open windows and cold air increase the amount of oxygen available. Cold air can aggravate respiratory distress and make a heart attack worse.

At least one member of every family should be familiar with simple home nursing techniques and first aid procedures. Classes to develop these skills are available in many adult education programs sponsored by local high schools and by the American National Red Cross. Several good references on home care of the sick are available to the homemaker. Check with your family physician or with the local health department about classes and texts.

Table 3.2 is a summary of how to care, temporarily, for acute symptoms.

Table 3.2 Temporary Care for Acute Symptoms

Pain and Discomfort	Just doing something (e.g., going to bed, having someone take care of you) can make you feel better. Ice applied to the affected area is a safe analgesic. Never use heat! It may spread infection. As long as there is no vomiting or abdominal pain, soft bland foods may be taken. Coffee, strong tea, and alcoholic beverages should be avoided. *No* medicines such as aspirin!
Nausea	Nonsweet carbonated beverages or plain soda water with a few drops of lemon juice may reduce this unpleasant feeling.
Vomiting	Take nothing by mouth. Thirst and a bad taste in the mouth may be relieved by sucking ice chips or rinsing the mouth out with water mixed with lemon juice or a commercially prepared mouthwash.
Diarrhea	It is important to consume liquids if diarrhea is a symptom with no vomiting. Bland liquids, such as milk, eggnog, jello, weak tea, or cream soups, should be taken. Fruit and vegetable juices should be avoided.
Fever	High fevers can be dangerous. Stay in a draft-free room with as few covers and clothes as possible. Covering the body increases body temperature. Sponge the body with cool water and put an ice bag on the head to bring down the fever.
Chills	Wrap in warm blankets to raise body temperature. Don't use hot water bags or heating pads on the aged, on small children, or on the unconscious, since the heat may cause skin burns.
Upper respiratory disease	The room should be warm and the air moist. An upright position is the most comfortable. Cold air can aggravate respiratory distress and make a heart attack worse. Cases of croup or severe breathing problems can be relieved by sitting in a bathroom filled with steam from running faucets.

MAINTENANCE OF VISUAL HEALTH

Seeing is a highly complex process. Eyes are receptors and transmitters of stimuli. Interpretation of these stimuli is a cortical activity that is *learned*. Through visual, auditory, olfactory, and tactile experiences, meaning is attached to stimuli. This mental process is called *perception*. The nature of an object is recognized through the association of a memory of its qualities with the stimuli. If an individual does not perceive correctly, that is, his perceptions do not coincide with the true nature of the object, he suffers a problem even though the mechanical attributes of his body are physically normal. To perceive accurately, one needs a number of interrelated visual skills. Some of these are functional and others experiential.

Functional visual skills require that both eyes work in a coordinated fashion. They must move in the same direction simultaneously, and the lens and variable aperture systems must admit similar stimuli. Light rays reflected from an object go through the cornea, pupil, aqueous humor, lens, and vitreous humor to the retina. The amount of light admitted is regulated by the iris, the colored part of the eye. The muscle fibers in the ciliary body regulate the shape of the lens, which alters the angle of light rays so that they can finally focus upon the retina. This process of changing the angle of light is called *accommodation*. In the retina the nerve endings, cones, and rods are stimulated by the light to produce electrical impulses, which are transmitted to the brain via the optic nerve. (Rods and cones are highly specialized cells containing chemicals that form the light sensitive elements of the retina.) Any interference in these steps will cause distorted signals to the brain. If the eyes send dissimilar signals, the cortex will have difficulty in sorting and integrating them into an accurate representation of the object perceived. Skills of accommodation, focusing, and fixation can be improved with practice.

Experiential skills are gained through practice. A wide range of vision is necessary, for example, in order to read rapidly and to drive safely. With practice, one can increase awareness by attending to those stimuli entering from the periphery of the visual field. Determination of distance, speed, size, shape, and texture also comes through experience.

Care of Eyes

Eye examinations. The basis of all visual care, of course, is periodic evaluation by a specialist. Routine medical examinations do not include a complete vision check. Children should receive their first such check no later than when starting school. From then on it is desirable to have a reexamination at least every two years. Appearance of any of these symptoms indicates the need for immediate attention: persistent blinking, aversion to light, blurring of vision, spots before the eyes, inflammation of the eyes or eyelids, styes (inflammation of one of the sebaceous glands of the lid), sores on the eyeball or eyelids, pain in the eye, tearing (lacrimation), and a sandy or grainy feeling. Nonacute symptoms that appear over a period of time should also be checked: aversion to reading, running together of letters and lines, difficulty in seeing at a distance or up close, distortion of the face to see more clearly, persistent squinting, fatigue after continued eye work, continuous frowning, frequent errors in writing or in doing figures, constant headaches, holding of the head to one side, and inability to concentrate when doing close work.

Two kinds of vision specialists evaluate the condition of the eyes. *Ophthalmologists,* sometimes called oculists, are licensed physicians who specialize in the care of the eye and all its related structures. They diagnose all disorders of the eye, either of a functional and mechanical nature or of an organic and diseased nature. They may prescribe any appropriate medicine and use any modality of treatment from surgery to contact lenses. They are concerned, as members of the medical team, with diseases of other systems of the body that manifest themselves in the eyes—diabetes, toxemia of pregnancy, cancer, multiple sclerosis, hypertension, and syphilis are but a few.

An *optometrist,* the other type of vision specialist, has a minimum of six years' academic preparation in schools of optometry associated with accredited colleges and universities. Optometrists are skilled in the treatment of mechanical disorders of the eyes. They may use such modalities as lenses and visual training. They are also trained to recognize diseases of an organic or infectious nature and to refer a patient in such a case to the appropriate specialist.

An *ophthalmic optician* is qualified to make lenses and fabricate glasses upon the prescription given him by the ophthalmologist and the optometrist.

Visual fatigue. The human eye is mechanically structured to see objects clearly a number of feet away. The normally healthy eye can perform this task with little difficulty. Modern society requires that we use our eyes for near-point tasks such as reading, watching television, working with tools, and operating machinery. Even those with healthy eyes, after a period of doing near-point tasks, may complain of a burning, bleariness, and general feeling of tiredness.

Persons who are visually uncomfortable will eventually change their visual tasks. Students who lack visual skills have difficulty in school. They may be unable to concentrate on their studies; it may take them much longer to accomplish any near-point task, and they will be less efficient. Research has proved time and time again that improved visual skills increase reading comprehension and retention.

For comfortable use of the eyes in artificial light, the source of light should be steady (no flicker), uniform, nonglaring, and of adequate intensity. The major source of light on the printed page or other close work should come from behind. Direct glare of light into the eyes should always be avoided. Lamps should be well shaded, and bulbs should be frosted. It is better to work in a room that is reasonably well lighted throughout than to depend on "pinpoint" lighting on the work itself. In this respect, indirect lighting is better than direct lighting. *There is no conclusive evidence that work performed under conditions of poor lighting or improper posture, or for prolonged periods day after day, can cause structural changes.*

Plenty of sleep provides the best kind of rest. Alternating periods of study with activities that do not call for close work also helps. Even while working or studying, one can rest one's eyes by closing them from time to time or by looking away occasionally and focusing on some distant object.

Effects of the sun and sunglasses. A squinting reaction of the eyes under such conditions as bright sunlight is a good indication that the eyes need protection. Sunglasses will protect the eyes from the infrared and ultraviolet rays of the sun and act as a barrier against wind and glare. Cheap sunglasses made of plastic or brown glass cut down on the glare but absorb very little of the ultraviolet and infrared rays. They also distort light rays, making vision more difficult. On the other hand, the prescription-ground lens filters out from 20 to 80 percent of the invisible rays. Neutral colors— gray, green, and tan, in that order—are preferable.

One should never look directly at the sun. When the sun's infrared rays are focused on the retina, permanent burn damage and loss of vision may result. The effect is much the same as when a magnifying glass is used to burn a hole in paper with the sun's rays. Ordinarily, people don't look directly into the sun because it's too uncomfortable. But in the apparent twilight of an eclipse, there is great temptation to watch the darkening of the sun. The injurious rays from the portion still visible may inflict permanent damage, because the retina has no pain fibers to indicate that the eye has been overexposed. These rays will penetrate any kind of glass. Therefore, ordinary sunglasses are definitely risky, and even welder's goggles are not completely safe. Smoked glass and photographic or X ray film cannot be recommended either because "eclipse blindness" has occurred in persons using them as filters.

Emergency care. Cleanliness is of the greatest importance in the care of eye injuries. A slight scratch on the surface of the eye may become so seriously infected that the eyesight is lost. Because the tissues of the eye are extremely delicate, expert medical attention should be secured whenever there is an injury.

Dust, cinders, and other small particles of foreign material frequently lodge on the surface of the eyeball. The irritation thus produced results in a

FOUNDATIONS OF HEALTH SCIENCE

flood of tears that usually washes away the offending particle. Occasionally such particles get under the lid and cannot be dislodged by tears. In such cases, gently drawing the upper lid down over the lower one often dislodges the particle, and the accumulated tears wash it out. Rubbing the eyes only irritates the tissues and embeds the particle. Using dirty fingers or a soiled handkerchief may result in infection.

If tears do not wash out foreign matter, or if caustic liquids splash into the eyes, they should be immediately rinsed with a gentle stream of running water. *Never use boric acid or any kind of drops in an injured eye.* If any object has penetrated the eyeball, cover the injured eye (both eyes if possible), and obtain medical attention.

Eye exercises. If perceiving visually is a matter of skill development, will exercises help those with poor skills? The answer is yes and no! From time to time there is a wave of misleading advertising about eye exercises, alleging that they can cure every sort of eye defect. No exercise can alter certain structural defects, repair a damaged optic nerve, or correct eye disease such as glaucoma or cataract. The science of orthoptics, or vision training, is a highly technical field that involves a great deal more than what is commonly thought of as "exercise." Certain types of strabismus can be aided by exercise prescribed by an eye practitioner. Specific exercises can improve powers of perception. Courses in rapid reading are one example of this, as are the visual recognition training programs of the armed forces.

Visual Abnormalities

Abnormalities of vision and perception are classified in this book as defects and disorders. Defects pertain to irregularities in the anatomical structure of the eye that distort the reception of visual stimuli. Disorders are actual diseases of one kind or another. Eye problems of either type lead to physical, emotional, and social difficulties. At least 25 percent of the children starting school have a visual problem; by adolescence, 85 percent have some inadequacy in perception and/or visual skills.

Defects. Simply stated, *amblyopia* is seeing sharply with one eye and poorly with the other, although that eye is free from disease. The condition is commonly associated with the lack of balance and cooperation between the two eyes that result when, for example, one eye is turned inward or outward. Since the eyes are looking in two different directions, the child escapes the annoyance of seeing double by mentally shutting out the stimuli received by one eye. Unless treatment is started at once, the blocked-out eye will eventually lose its ability to function.

There are children whose eyes work in a synchronized manner but who have an optical imperfection of one eye. Since the distorted stimuli received by this eye cannot be reconciled with the clear stimuli received by the normal eye, the tendency is again to ignore reception by the defective eye. Since the good eye covers up for the faulty one, and some vision is present in the poor eye, the child may not be aware of any serious problem until the vision is tested.

In most cases, appropriate treatment, if started before the child is six or seven years of age, insures normal development of both eyes. Treatment for amblyopia includes glasses and pleoptics, which involves forced use of the defective eye. Techniques in pleoptics include using a special light to stimulate the child's poor eye, as well as ingeniously designed, toylike devices to perform various tasks that reinforce visual performance.

Myopia, or nearsightedness, is a very common development in school-age children. The point of focus is in front of, rather than on, the retina. It has not been proved that myopia increases because of poor lighting or posture. The near-point tasks required of life today probably aggravate an already-present problem that might otherwise have gone unnoticed. High degrees of myopia are a disadvantage. The condition seems to increase during adolescence, possibly as the result of increased demands on vision, growth, and pubertal changes. Myopia tends to stabilize eventually.

Hyperopia is farsightedness. The precise definition is ability to see clearly at a distance through a convex lens. Theoretically, the visual stimuli for near-point work focuses behind, rather than on, the retina. A moderate degree of hyperopia puts the individual at a disadvantage. He or she may suffer the symptoms of fatigue previously described. A person with a high degree of hyperopia may experience a great deal of discomfort and may be unable to perform either near or moderately distanced work with any degree of efficiency. The treatment for moderate and high degrees of hyperopia usually requires lenses.

Astigmatism is a distortion of the direction of the light rays so that they are not focused at a single point on the retina. The distortion results from unequal curvatures along the different meridians in one or more of the refractive surfaces in the cornea, or anterior or posterior surface of the lens. Small degrees of astigmatism may require no treatment; high degrees produce blurred vision. The effects can be compensated for by the application of lenses.

Strabismus is the medical term for crossed eyes. During their first year of life, infants may have difficulty in coordinating their eyes. If the children are treated early, exercise may be sufficient to assist them in using their eyes efficiently (proper binocular coordination). If the convergence or divergence continues past infancy, structural changes may occur in the extra-ocular muscles that move the eyeball. Once structural change results, surgery is required to equalize the muscle tension by either lengthening or shortening the muscles.

Strabismus interferes with focusing and produces a blurred or double set of images. The constant contracting of one or more muscles to produce proper binocular coordination causes stress and eye fatigue. Lenses may be prescribed in addition to exercise and/or surgery. The cause may be hereditary or congenital. Strabismus may also result from an accident or illness.

Color deficiency is a more accurate term than color blindness. The most common type is red-green deficiency, whereby the individual has difficulty in distinguishing red from green. Other types prevent differentiation of pairs of colors. Total color blindness is rare, and an individual afflicted with it can distinguish only shadings of gray and black. Tests for color vision include spot charts such as the Ishihara and Stilling color charts and isochromatic-type plates.

The inheritance of red-green color deficiency usually follows a sex-linked recessive pattern. The disability appears more frequently in men than in women; although only one girl in 100 will have color deficiencies, the disability is present in one out of every 10 or 12 boys. The disorder will not appear in a color-deficient man's son unless the boy's mother is color deficient or is a carrier of the gene for color deficiency. Consequently, the disorder is transmitted only rarely from father to son. More commonly, color deficiency is transmitted from an affected man, through his daughters (in whom the condition usually is not expressed), to about one-half of his grandsons.

The types other than red-green may be either inherited or acquired. In some instances, at least, total color blindness and pastel-shade deficiencies are thought to be inherited. The mode of inheritance is not known. Other causes are disease or injury of the retina or the optic nerve. Some people, notably men, may not have learned to differentiate between shades of color.

Disorders. Disorders of the eyes vary in symptoms and in cause. The major eye conditions causing blindness are retinal disease, cataract, and glaucoma in that order. Together, they account for half of all blindness. At age sixty-five and over, retinal disease is responsible for more than one-fourth of all blindness, and glaucoma and cataract each account for about one-sixth of the total.[6]

Retinal disease most often is the result of interference to circulation in the eye produced by arteriosclerosis, cardiac disease, and hypertension. In arteriosclerotic retinopathy the walls of the retinal arterioles become thickened. Hemorrhage may occur, and there may be white plaques in the retina due to insufficient blood supply. Treatment consists primarily of caring for the underlying cause.

Cataract is an opacity of the lens of any size or shape. Although a cataract is generally regarded as a disease of old age, it may occur at birth, in infancy, or in early childhood. In these cases surgical treatment may permit restoration of useful vision without complete removal of the lens. Medical scientists have spent much time and research investigating the mechanism of cataract formation, but it is still an unsolved problem. Causes of cataract include congenital rubella, injury to the lens, radiation, metabolic disease such as diabetes, chemicals, and senility. Although there is a hereditary tendency for the development of cataracts, not all victims have a family history of this disorder. Cataracts are not necessarily progressive, and all do not lead to blindness. Treatment, consisting of surgical removal of the lens, is at least 94 percent effective. After the eye has healed, a contact lens may be prescribed for the operated eye to produce improved binocular equalization. Figures 3.3 and 3.4 illustrate how a cataract interferes with vision.

Glaucoma is an increase in intraocular fluid pressure within the eye

Figure 3.3 Cataract: Imperfect Vision. The cataract victim sees much like this. Ninety per cent of those past seventy years of age have some degree of cataract. Simple, painless operations can reduce this type of visual problem in nearly all cases.

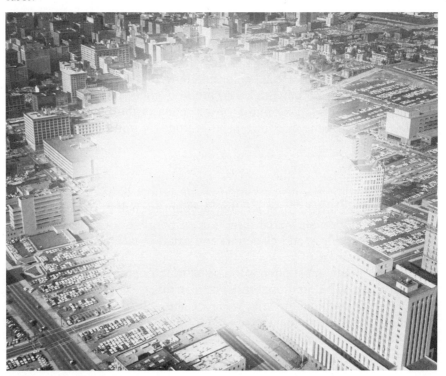

Figure 3.4 How a Cataract Interferes with Vision (from *Cataract: Fact and Fancy.* National Society for the Prevention of Blindness, Inc., 1963, p. 2). Courtesy of the National Society for the Prevention of Blindness, Inc.

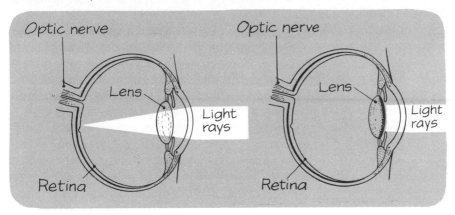

ball because of blockage or constriction of the outflow duct. Continued pressure may damage the optic nerve. The condition has many causes, some of which are unknown. Heredity seems to play a role in some cases of primary glaucoma. It usually occurs after age thirty-five and is more frequent in women than in men. Early symptoms include headache, blurred vision, rainbow-like lights, eye pain, and loss of peripheral vision.

Treatment depends upon the particular cause and stage of condition. Most cases are amenable to medication, but how the drugs work is not clearly understood. It may be necessary to cut a small hole in the iris (iridectomy) to relieve the increased pressure. Early detection is vital. A quick, painless test is available at many city and county health departments without charge.

Corneal Transplantation

In recent years, techniques have been devised by which a portion of defective cornea may be removed and a corneal disc from another individual substituted. Perfection of the methods of corneal transplantation has brought new hope to victims of corneal diseases. Patients have an excellent chance of regaining their vision through this procedure. One of the goals for transplant surgery is the restoration of transparency to a cornea that has been scarred by injury or burn.

Contact Lenses

The modern plastic corneal lens is smaller than a dime and is virtually undetectable. Since it floats on a layer of natural tears and is held in place by capillary action, it does not really touch the cornea. It moves with the eye, providing a greater field of vision than ordinary eyeglasses. The edge of the lens is smooth and polished; a slight bevel is on the inside to facilitate motility of the lens.

The success a person has with corneal lenses is commensurate with his need for them and his desire or motivation to wear them. Need may be visual, occupational, or cosmetic. Indications of visual need may be any high degree of refractive error. Contact lenses are used to great advantage by those who have had cataract operations and those with keratonconus (the cornea forms an irregular cone). However, some persons are unable to wear them because of irritation, insufficient tears, or irregularities of the cornea or eyelids. The lens is, after all, a foreign body. Psychological factors present a problem in some cases. The lenses are not usually prescribed for children. In children the cornea is more easily damaged. Also, the eyes may change so frequently that changing the lenses becomes costly.

MAINTENANCE OF HEARING

Early Detection of Hearing Loss

Early detection of hearing loss is the first requisite for hearing conservation. The majority of defects develop before a child starts school and during the elementary years. Parents should have their children tested before school enrollment so that any defects may be corrected or treated before too great a learning handicap develops. About 5 percent of the child population have hearing problems. Most states require routine testing of pupils in schools. In addition to formal examination, observation by parents and teachers is essential. Those most qualified to appraise hearing are the *otologist,* who has an M.D. degree and is a specialist in diagnosis and treatment of the ear; the *otolaryngologist,* who is also an M.D. but specializes in care of the nose and throat as well as the ear; and the *audiologist,* who may have an M.A. or Ph.D. degree and is a specialist in the nonmedical evaluation and rehabilitation of persons with hearing disorders.

The growing numbers of centers or clinics devoted to hearing disorders are enabling many more Americans to find help for their hearing loss problems.

Prevention of Hearing Loss

In planning an adequate program of prevention, one should stress the essential activities, since specific measures to prevent hearing loss are principally an individual matter.

1. Obtain medical attention for acute or chronic general infections and for local disorders of the ear, nose, and throat that might lead to middle ear disease.
2. Avoid forcing mucus from a head cold or sinus infection into the auditory tubes. Blow the nose gently, with both nostrils open.
3. Avoid intense sound or noise.
4. Destroy insects that get into the ear canal by instilling drops of oil.
5. Have hardened accumulated wax or foreign bodies in the external auditory canal removed only under the supervision of a physician.
6. Use measures to protect the head from severe blows that are a potential hazard in some sports and occupations.
7. Practice safe swimming habits.

Hearing Abnormalities

The organ of hearing is an intricate mechanism, and the hearing process itself is inadequately understood. The accepted explanation is that atmospheric sound waves collected by the *auricle* enter the *external canal* and cause the *tympanic membrane* to vibrate. This vibration, in turn, sets the *ossicles* of the middle ear (*malleus, incus,* and *stapes*) into vibration. These bones are in sequence and interdependent. Their action is like that of a fulcrum in that they increase the force of sound waves by about 60 percent. The third small bone, the stapes, rests against the membrane separating the middle and inner ears and transfers the vibrations through this membrane to the *endolymph,* the liquid in the inner ear. The inner ear contains cells known as the *organ of corti,* which convert the mechanical waves in the endolymph into electrical stimuli. These stimuli are sent by the acoustic nerve to each side of the brain, where the sound is finally interpreted. (See Figure 3.5.)

Any defect in conduction of sound along the way can cause reduced hearing, deafness, or a change in the pattern of sounds that are heard. Disturbance between the auricle and the acoustic nerve is labeled *conduction deafness.* Defects in the cochlea, the acoustic nerve, or the auditory reception center in the brain may result in *nerve deafness.* Conduction deafness may involve either one or both ears and produce impairment of hearing to varying degrees, but never total loss. Nerve deafness usually affects hearing on both sides and may be partial or complete. Mixed, or combined, deafness involves both types. Conduction deafness is often characterized by hearing loss in the low frequencies; nerve deafness results more often in perception loss of high or middle frequencies. In conduction deafness there is loss of volume, and loud speaking helps understand-

Figure 3.5 The Ear. Sectional diagram of the human ear. (Courtesy of Sonotone Corporation. Copyright 1953.)

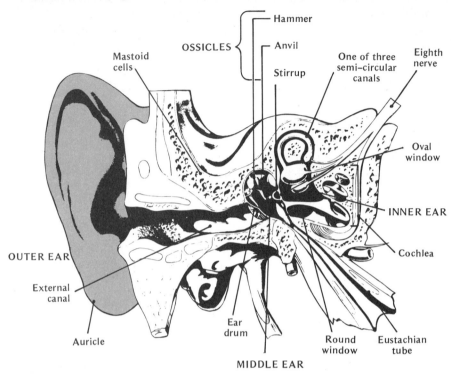

ing; in nerve deafness certain frequencies are not heard, so sound is distorted and loud speaking causes greater distortion. Persons suffering from nerve deafness may respond to loud speech by covering their ears. They may grimace with pain and complain of discomfort.

A diagnosis of type, cause, and extent of impairment is necessary because they influence the method of minimizing hearing loss. About 80 percent of all cases of impaired hearing are caused by interference in the conduction of sounds. This can be ameliorated by hearing aids and, sometimes, by surgery. In nerve deafness, the use of a hearing aid is limited, and surgery is rarely helpful. Regardless of the type or amount of loss, the emphasis should be on amount of hearing present. There are techniques that can develop remaining potential, improving the degree of perception.

Conduction deafness is the end result of infections, inflammations, otosclerosis, or obstruction of the ear canal. Common kinds of infections are measles, mumps, and whooping cough in children and colds and influenza at any age. Nerve deafness can actually be caused by longstanding conduction deafness, which makes the auditory nerve atrophy from disuse.

FOUNDATIONS OF HEALTH SCIENCE

More often, it results from aging, virus infections, concussion injuries, prolonged exposure to loud noises, and impaired circulation as in arteriosclerosis. Babies may be born with a hearing loss due to the Rh factor or to German measles contracted by a woman during the first week of pregnancy. Other factors responsible for hearing losses include blows to the ear, some medicines (including aspirin and quinine in individuals sensitive to them, and a few antibiotics), and radiation, Appraisals for hearing loss should include a complete physical examination.

Otosclerosis. Otosclerosis is a condition that immobilizes the stapes in the middle ear. The stapes is the smallest bone in the body (smaller than a grain of rice), but it is the key to normal hearing. A cementlike calcium deposit forms around the base of the stapes, acting as a plug and fusing the other two ossicles so that they cannot vibrate. Very little is known about the causes of otosclerosis. About 70 percent of the cases seem to be hereditary. It has been observed in young children, but its advance is usually slow, and people are rarely aware of it until they are in their twenties. Most reach middle years before they are noticeably affected.

Otitis Media. Otitis media (middle ear infection) is practically always caused by infections in the nose and throat. It is the most common disturbance of the ear in childhood and, consequently, the most common cause of earaches. Recent upper respiratory infection, hearing loss, a sensation of pressure or "water in the ear," and roaring tinnitus (buzzing) are common indicative complaints. Except in a few instances, a "running ear" means otitis media with a perforated ear drum. Such symptoms demand immediate medical care.

Swimming can constitute a hazard to hearing. Caps or ear plugs only partly protect the ears. Harmful organisms in contaminated water still can enter the auditory tubes through the nose and mouth. In addition, diving forces water into the tubes. This water may spread any pathogens present in the nose or mouth to the middle ear. Forcefully blowing the nose or attempting to "blow" water out of the ears *may cause damage.* Tipping the head to the affected side is usually sufficient to let any water drain out. If discomfort persists, getting medical attention is the safest thing to do.

Presbycusis. A majority of the twenty-two million Americans over sixty-five years of age in 1974 had some hearing difficulty. The increasing number of senior citizens in our society demands that we understand the physiological and psychological problems of the person with *presbycusis* (lessening of acuteness of hearing characterized by old age). Old-age deafness does not involve a volume loss. The persons hear, but they cannot distinguish what is being said; they have problems in discriminating between sounds.

Presbycusis has an emotional impact on the afflicted and their households. Classically, the hard-of-hearing practice "self-isolation," and because of their seeming inattention, they are frequently ridiculed by those around them. Counseling the elderly patient's family on the causes and effects of presbycusis will eliminate a great deal of turmoil and stress in the home, as well as contribute to the overall well-being of all members in the family.

MAINTENANCE OF DENTAL HEALTH

The science of dentistry has made remarkable progress in recent years. There are new and improved methods of diagnosis by means of X rays, high-speed drills, ultrasonic equipment, stronger materials for filling caries, and better techniques of oral surgery. Perhaps even more important has been dentistry's emphasis on preventive care—the use of fluorides to inhibit decay; pedodontics, or specialty care of children; orthodontics to remedy incorrect *bite,* or malocclusion; and oral hygiene to keep the mouth and teeth healthy.

Even so, oral disease affects 98 out of every 100 persons in the country. This rate has remained static for many years. At present, many of the adult population do not seek needed dental care, and more than one-half of school-age children are known to need treatment.

Regular Dental Supervision

Regular visits to the dentist are important. They include dental prophylaxis, X rays, and examinations using an explorer, or dental probe.

Dental prophylaxis. Dental prophylaxis is cleaning of the teeth by a dentist or a dental hygienist. It is part of regular dental care for both children and adults. Deposits of calculus (tartar), food, and other matter are removed from the crowns and necks of the teeth. These irritants are one of the causes of gum disease.

X ray examinations. Both children and adults should have regular dental X-ray examinations. This procedure enables the dentist to discover any abnormality that might affect the future health of the teeth and mouth. X rays help the dentist to detect such conditions as small cavities, decay developing beneath fillings, impacted (unerupted) teeth, and abnormalities of tooth roots.

Explorer examinations. The explorer or dental probe examination discloses cavities when they are just beginning. If cavities are properly filled when small, the progress of decay is arrested and the structure of the tooth is saved.

To postpone or neglect minor dental work is no economy. Major reconstructive work is expensive, and even the most skillful is not nearly as satisfactory as sound, natural teeth.

Dental Caries

The most widespread dental disease, especially in children, is dental caries, or tooth decay. It is as prevalent as the common cold. At least 95 percent of Americans suffer from tooth decay at some time during their lives. Dental caries may occur on various surfaces of the teeth, depending on the arrangement of the teeth and their structure. The crevices (fissures) and surfaces that are in contact with other teeth are the most vulnerable parts because they are the most difficult to keep clean.

Once a cavity has formed, the tooth can be restored only by removing the decayed material and replacing it with a filling. A decayed tooth cannot repair itself. Unless treatment is provided, decay proceeds from the enamel into the dentin and then into the pulp and nerve. When the pulp is exposed, infection occurs, and an abscess may form at the tip of the root. As the infection develops, the pressure may cause severe pulsating pain. Infection is often accompanied by fever, headache, and a general feeling of illness. Sometimes an abscess may form at the tip of the root without causing pain or giving the patient any sign that infection has been developing. Such cases are often discovered only by X ray, which will show the extent of the disease and aid the dentist in determining whether the tooth can be saved or must be extracted. (See Figure 3.6.)

Periodontal Disease

Periodontal diseases affect the soft tissues (gums), the periodontal fibers that hold the teeth in place, and the bone surrounding the teeth. The most common types of periodontal disease are gingivitis and periodontitis. Periodontitis that is accompanied by pus may be called pyorrhea.

In gingivitis (inflammation of the gums) the tissues become red and swollen, may pull away from the teeth, and bleed easily. Frequently gingivitis is neglected or undetected until it has reached an advanced stage, when treatment is more difficult. Some of the conditions that lead to gingivitis are accumulation of calculus; packing of food between the teeth; mouth breathing; and mechanical injuries resulting from improper brushing, use of toothpicks, or incorrect application of dental floss.

Figure 3.6 Anatomy of a Tooth

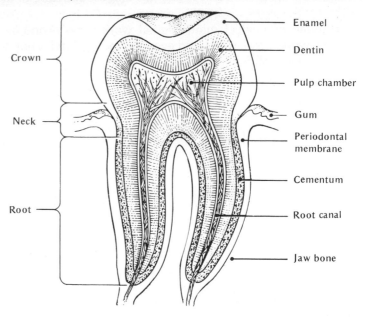

Periodontitis usually results from unchecked gingivitis. Inflammation spreads and the gums withdraw from the teeth, forming pockets that become filled with bacteria, food residues, and eventually pus. If the process is allowed to continue, the bony support of the teeth is destroyed, though bone destruction may occur very early in the course of the disease without many visible warning signs. (Adolescents may suffer periodontitis caused in part by an endocrine imbalance.) Eventually some or even all of the teeth may be lost. Regular visits to the dentist and good dental hygiene are the best measures for preventing periodontal disease. (See Figure 3.7.)

Oral Cancer

Mouth cancers account for about 5 percent of all cancers. As in other cancers, early detection reduces disability and death. Early cancers can mimic many innocuous conditions, such as cankers, burns, cuts, or infections. Investigators agree that smoking or chewing tobacco increases the risk of cancer. Nine out of ten oral cancer patients smoke, says Silverman. Excessive use of alcohol (more than five ounces daily) is also being indicted as contributing to this type of malignancy. Silverman stresses that any person having a sore in the mouth that does not heal in a reasonably

Figure 3.7 Periodontal Disease. Periodontal disease may affect supporting tissues of teeth if not treated early. (1) Calculus deposits at gum line cause irritation (gingivitis). (2) Gums become swollen and tender. (3) Inflammation spreads; pockets develop; and bacteria and pus form in pockets (periodontitis). (4) Gradually, gum and bone are destroyed, and the teeth become loose. (From *Today's Health*, 47:29, August, 1969.)

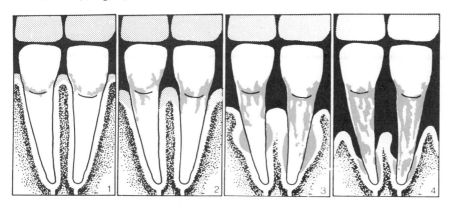

short time should seek an examination from a dentist or physician. He also states that "Dentists have a unique opportunity through routine mouth examinations to detect malignant growths while they may still be asymptomatic, innocuous and unsuspected."[7]

With surgery and radiation the five-year survival rates approximate 40 percent. However, a mouth cancer that is two centimeters at the time of diagnosis has twice the chance of cure as one that is larger.

Tooth Injuries

Injuries to teeth, especially the front permanent teeth, are common. They must be treated promptly if the teeth are to be protected and saved. If there is a blow to a tooth, whether or not there is an apparent break or fracture, X rays should be taken to make sure that no damage has been done to the jawbone or to the root of the tooth. Often, though no immediate injury is noted, the pulp of an injured tooth eventually dies. The pulp is most likely devitalized in a tooth that turns dark gray following injury.

If a tooth is fractured at the gum line or through the pulp chamber, it can be saved only by removing the pulp completely and doing pulp canal therapy. If a root of a tooth is fractured, the tooth and the root may have to be extracted. Sometimes if the root is fractured near the tip, a dentist may be able to surgically extract the tip and perform pulp canal therapy, thus saving the tooth itself.

If a tooth is knocked completely out of the mouth by an injury, it still may be possible to save it by a technique called reimplantation. Such a tooth should be wrapped gently in sterile cotton or gauze, soaked in alcohol, and rushed—with the victim—to a dentist. The dentist will do pulp canal therapy on the tooth to clean out its vital core, replace the tooth in its socket, and affix it with wires to its neighboring teeth. Usually antibiotics are given. If the time between the accident and the operation is short (ideally, within an hour) and proper sterile precautions are taken, there is every chance that the implant will succeed.

Malocclusion

Orthodontics is one of the most important developments in the field of preventive dentistry. By the use of braces, wires, springs, bands, and oral surgery, the orthodontist (a dentist who has taken special training) straightens teeth and supervises the correct growth and development of the jaws. Statistics show that about one child in three needs some orthodontic care. The purpose of orthodontics is to ensure healthy, attractive teeth that function effectively. It achieves this end primarily by correcting the bite (the way the teeth are placed in the mouth in relation to one another). How upper and lower teeth meet determines how a person speaks, bites, chews, and swallows food. The side-by-side relation of the teeth determines the amount of space between them, where decay can begin.

A poor bite—technically known as malocclusion—can be caused by a wide variety of factors. Some of them are:

1. Failure to insert a space maintainer when deciduous or permanent teeth are lost. The other teeth will "drift."
2. Too-late shedding of deciduous teeth. This causes permanent teeth to erupt in an irregular pattern, and upper and lower teeth do not mesh properly.
3. Irregular spacing of the front teeth. The teeth may be too small for the amount of jawbone they must occupy; an extra tooth may be present between the teeth, keeping them apart; a habit such as tongue-thrusting or prolonged thumb-sucking may force the teeth apart and keep them that way; or a large and heavy tissue band (the *frenum*) may interpose itself between the upper front teeth and prevent them from touching each other.
4. Irregular tooth positions caused by dental decay.
5. An impacted, or nonerupted, tooth. Any tooth that does not come through the gum causes the remaining teeth to shift and disrupts the

FOUNDATIONS OF HEALTH SCIENCE

way they intermesh. A partially erupted tooth that never rises to the proper biting level is likely to disturb the chewing pattern because the opposing tooth will grow down to meet it. The elongated tooth prevents proper grinding and meshing of the other teeth during chewing.

Malocclusions also may result from inherited tendencies to irregular or missing teeth; nutritional deficiencies, such as a lack of calcium or Vitamin D, resulting in poorly formed teeth or underdeveloped jawbones; glandular disturbances, which can affect the metabolism of calcium or the size of the jaws; or a severe attack of such childhood diseases as scarlet fever, chicken pox, or measles, which can interfere with bone development and affect the proper growth of the jaw.

Dental Prosthetics

Professionally defined, *dental prosthesia* is the science and art of providing suitable substitutes for the coronal (crown) portions of teeth, or for one or more lost natural teeth and their associate parts, in order that function, esthetic appearance, comfort, and health of the patient may be restored. The American Dental Association estimates that by the age of thirty-five, two out of three adults need replacements for one or more of their natural teeth.

Although preventive dentistry has advanced considerably in recent years, the premature loss of teeth is still a major problem. Methods of tooth replacement include the fixed bridge, the removable partial denture, the full crown to restore the crown portion of the natural tooth, and the full denture to replace all the natural teeth in the arch.

People with dental prosthesis, including upper and lower dentures, require yearly checks by their dentists. Tissues change over periods of time, and dentures gradually fit improperly. Dentures that irritate the gums, tongue, and soft palate are uncomfortable and could cause the chronic irritation that precipitates oral cancer. Yearly examinations of dentures can also prolong the life of these prostheses, reducing costly replacement.

COSMETIC SURGERY

Cosmetic surgery is by no means confined to the face, as some suppose. Often referred to as plastic surgery, it is actually reparative or constructive. Grafts and sections of tissues (such as skin, cartilage, and bone) are used to reshape, to form bridges, and to rebuild, as well as to cover blemishes. In the past, most cosmetic surgery consisted of repairing facial defects, as in rhinoplasty (plastic surgery of the nose); correcting harelips or cleft palates; and skin grafting. Now, plastic surgery is frequently used to modify a number of other undesirable physical characteristics, such as abnormalities of the ears, chin, bust, arms, and legs. Cosmetic surgery is expensive and must be performed by specialists, but it may be vital to happy, productive living, for defects that distort appearance are threats to the self-concept.

MEDICAL CARE DELIVERY

Ensuring effective medical care offers numerous problems, which are receiving top-level congressional consideration. These include insufficient numbers of physicians and qualified specialists in specific geographical areas (rural areas and ghettos), the high cost of a medical education, and the problems of establishing a practice. Many more preventive, curative, rehabilitative, and convalescent services are needed in most areas of the country.

In the past the main source of health services was in the office of the private physician. Today, there is increasing use of clinics. These are organized in several ways.

Group Practice

In this method of providing medical care, several physicians work together under a partnership type of agreement. They usually share office space; records and files; laboratory, radiology, other diagnostic and therapeutic equipment; and office personnel. Frequently such groups include a general practitioner and/or internist, a surgeon, a obstetrician-gynecologist, and a pediatrician.

Hospital Clinics

A second source of patient care is the outpatient department of a local hospital. The physicians providing service in this setting are either on the staff (approved by the hospital board of directors to treat patients in that hospital), or employed on a salaried basis. Emphasis is primarily on treatment of acute conditions that do not require hospitalization. The diagnostic and therapeutic services of the hospital are generally available. Presumedly this arrangement provides higher quality care more conveniently and at a lower cost than that available in non-hospital-associated laboratories. In 1970, 21 percent of all visits to physicians were in hospital clinics. People in large cities used such clinics more than people in rural areas.[8]

Health Maintenance Organizations

Another system of health care is the Health Maintenance Organization, HMO, which provides comprehensive services to a voluntarily enrolled population for a per capita prepaid fee. The HMO may be publicly or privately managed. Comprehensive services include primary care, emergency care, inpatient hospital care for acute conditions, inpatient and outpatient care for health maintenance, and rehabilitation for chronic and disabling conditions. The major difference between the HMO and hospital clinics or group practice is the HMO's major emphasis on maintenance of health and prevention of illness. Primary care, one of the essential elements in attaining these goals, includes health counseling and teaching. During the primary-care phase, when the patient is first seen, plans are made for total, coordinated care.

The federal government has promoted HMOs through funding and by making it mandatory that employers of twenty-five or more persons include in any employee health benefit plan the option of membership in a qualified HMO when one exists in the area. Basic health services mandated under federal regulations include physician consultant and referral services; inpatient and outpatient hospital services; medically necessary emergency care; short-term (not to exceed twenty visits) outpatient evaluative and crisis intervention mental health services; medical treatment and referral services for the abuse of, or addiction to, alcohol and drugs; diagnostic laboratory services and diagnostic and therapeutic radiologic services; home health services; and preventive health services, including voluntary family planning, infertility studies, preventive dental care for children, and children's eye examinations.

Special Clinics

Numerous special clinics concentrate on a specific health problem. Some clinics require full payment for services rendered, some charge on a sliding fee scale, a number are partially supported by the charity dollar, and increasing numbers are being financed by taxes. The last are usually under the auspices of the local health department. Cancer detection centers, family planning agencies, maternal and child health services, immunization clinics, and vision and hearing testing services are examples. One of the disadvantages of health care obtained in this manner is fragmentation. No one person is responsible for an overall view of the patient.

Despite the proliferation of clinic-type health care delivery systems, Bullough reports that "while it is important to improve clinic services, it is well to keep in mind that given a choice, many people apparently prefer a private physician."[9] Most care, either maintenance or therapeutic, is still obtained in the private doctor's office.

PROFESSIONAL STANDARDS REVIEW ORGANIZATIONS

To control the costs of medical care and to assure that the consumer is getting appropriate care, Congress in 1973 created a national system of Professional Standards Review Organizations—PSROs. These are regional groups comprising physicians, other members of the health professions, and sometimes lay representatives, who have the charge of assuring that federally funded institutional care is subject to effective peer review. The goal of such review is to "provide an efficient, humane experience for the patient; eliminate unnecessary procedures and duplication of effort; and get the patient diagnosed, effectively treated, and out of the hospital as soon as possible."[10] Two aspects of this process are utilization review and medical audit. The former covers the appropriateness of patient admissions, use of facilities, level of care, length of stay, and discharge practices. It involves examination of whether the care provided is medically necessary and assurance that the patient is receiving neither more nor less than is needed and that the care provided is of the highest quality. Medical audit is professional evaluation of the care given by specific institutions, comparing the actual care given a select group of patients with a set of predetermined standards of high quality care for that group.[11]

One of the outcomes of such reviews is that patients are being discharged from hospitals earlier. Sometimes they are transferred to less expensive facilities such as nursing homes or convalescent hospitals. It is possible for them to return directly to their homes if they can get special assistance from a visiting nurse, a home health aide, or a homemaker.

HEALTH INSURANCE

The costs of individual and family medical care are extremely uneven. High medical bills occur infrequently, but often all at once. One effective measure to eliminate uneven costs is the prepayment plan of health insurance. Under this system, unpredictable expenses of illness, accident, and medical care can be prorated over a period of time.

Voluntary Health Insurance

Voluntary health insurance plans, despite the diversity of individual policies, are generally of five basic types.

1. **Regular medical expense protection.** This type of protection usually pays for office visits or physicians' calls in the home or hospital. Most benefits do not begin until after the first several calls, and a maximum payment limit is ordinarily set for each illness.

2. **Hospital expense protection.** Hospital coverage is generally provided for a maximum period of perhaps a month or more. Services usually include hospital charges for room, board, laboratory tests, X ray, drugs, nursing care, anesthetics, operating room, and other miscellaneous or special service.

3. **Surgical expense protection.** This plan ordinarily provides surgical benefits before, during, and after an operation. Payments are usually made according to a predetermined fee schedule, with maximum limits set for each operation.

4. **Major medical expense protection.** This type of policy, available with different levels of coverage, is obtainable in several forms. It is frequently called *catastrophic* protection. The policies are often deductible. The patient pays the first $200 to $500, then possibly 20 percent of the remaining costs up to $10,000.

5. **Loss-of-income protection.** Such a plan guarantees cash benefits for a portion of normal salary during recuperation from illness or accident. It affords protection against loss of earning capacity and is sometimes called disability or indemnity insurance. Payments begin after a specified period of disability and continue up to a maximum time.

The benefits of the different types of protection can be combined into any desirable policy to meet particular needs. There are individual and group types of policies. Group policies often provide greater benefits at a lower cost, but they may also bind the policyholder to a particular form of protection.

Health insurance is available through a variety of sources, although insurance companies lead in the number of total enrollees. Nationwide, Blue Cross and Blue Shield are the most popular. The former has provided for hospital services since its inception in Texas in 1930. Blue Shield has supplemented this hospitalization with surgical benefits. It provides for claim payments depending upon individual income levels. Other national and local plans include the following: Ross-Loos in Los Angeles, the Health Institute of St. Louis, the Kaiser Foundation Plan, and the New York City Health Insurance Plan. Many colleges and universities provide low-cost group plans for students.

Misunderstood Facts about Health Insurance

The purchase of health insurance represents a significant portion of a person's financial outlay. Too frequently people do not understand what they are buying. Following are some of the common misunderstood facts about health insurance.[12]

All health insurance policies are not the same. Health insurance is a very general term. Policies usually pay for the cost of a wide variety of services and goods, and policies differ (sometimes greatly) in what they include. The most important buying factor in any health insurance plan is whether one purchases the coverage individually or as a member of a group. The most inexpensive is a group membership, which has fewer restrictions, more complete coverage, and lower rates. The savings may amount to as much as 20 percent.

You can obtain insurance even with a history of illness. Group policies do not rule out a person with a history of poor health. The insurance companies average costs in group coverage over the entire group, including those in good and poor health. Individual policies will cost more and may contain restrictive clauses for specific illnesses.

Payments are made primarily for sickness or injuries. Unfortunately this is usually true. Preventive care is not often covered, and the only diagnostic procedures usually covered pertain to present symptoms. However, some prepaid group practice plans (for example, Kaiser-Permanente, Health Insurance Plan of New York (HIP), and Health Maintenance Organizations) do include preventive care and diagnosis.

Frequent sickness and injuries will result in cancellation of a policy. Under group coverage your policy cannot be canceled without canceling the whole group. If you are individually insured, however, the company can do one of the following: insert a clause in the policy restricting payment for the illness causing the claims; raise your rates; or refuse to renew the policy at date of expiration. For an extra charge, it is possible to purchase policies that are guaranteed renewable.

Major medical policies providing for catastrophic illness should be a supplemental coverage purchased by all. Major medical insurance does not cover all illness, nor does it pay all the cost of such illnesses. Such policies usually have a top limit between $10,000 and $20,000, and you have to pay 20 to 25 percent of the initial cost of the care before the policy takes over. Policies are built around a system of deductibles.

In deciding whether or not to purchase major medical insurance there are other considerations. Major illness requiring long-term care can quickly wipe out years of savings. But how many Americans incur catastrophic health expenses each year? Meyers' study of 25,926 patients in 132 hospitals in 25 states found that:

1. Less than 9% of all patients surveyed had hospital expenses exceeding $2,000.
2. About 1.4% had hospital expenses exceeding $5,000. This translates to some 456,000 patients with catastrophic expenses, based on 1972 total admission figures of over 33 million.
3. About 0.3% of the patients surveyed had hospital expenses exceeding $10,000.
4. Only 0.8% of the U.S. population—or 1.6 million—have over $5,000 in total medical expenses each year.
5. The vast majority in this category are psychiatric or Medicare patients.
6. Less than two tenths of 1% (0.16%) of all Americans will incur catastrophic illnesses costing over $5,000.[13]

Disability insurance is the same as health insurance. This is not true. Health insurance reimburses you, or pays for, specific costs related to illness or injury. Disability insurance is protection against loss of personal income. Some employers provide for this, and some people are eligible for disability payment from Social Security. Be careful about how the insurance company defines disability—does it mean inability to return to your old job or another for which you are prepared, or does it mean inability to take any kind of job?

A good policy provides maximum coverage of services and time in the hospital. A good hospitalization policy provides at least sixty to ninety days of room and board at a rate equivalent to local hospital charges for a semiprivate room. But such charges account for only about 50 percent of the total bill; the remaining costs are for services not related to board or room. These include special diets; X rays; laboratory tests; operating and recovery room care; anesthesiology; medicines; special nursing; intensive care; and special treatments such as transfusions, enemas, surgical dressings, and intravenous infusions. Within a three-day stay in a hospital, these charges may boost your bill $500 to $1,000. For example, heart catheterization can easily cost $1,000.

The following question should be carefully answered before a health insurance plan is selected. Exactly what does a policy cover, and what are its "small print" exclusions? Some policies automatically expire when the policy holder reaches a certain age; others can be cancelled by the issuing company on any anniversary date. Many group policies terminate upon the policy holder's retirement or transfer to a new position. Most people consider a plan desirable if it provides for free choice of physician, specialist, and hospital; helps pay medical bills anywhere in the world, and covers major health needs. (See Figure 3.8, pp. 102–3.)

Government Health Insurance Programs

The two major government health insurance programs are Medicare and Medicaid. In 1975, Medicare and Medicaid helped meet the health care needs of 48 million Americans (almost one-fourth the total population), at a cost of $26.5 billion. Yet it is the consensus of many in the health care professions that while Medicare has insulated the aged from ruinous medical expenses, Medicaid has not provided good health care for the poor and near poor.[14]

Medicare. The initiation of Medicare represented one of the most sweeping changes in the Social Security system since it was created by the Wagner Act in the 1930s. Medicare actually consists of two health insurance programs for Americans sixty-five years of age or over who receive Social Security. Part A, the basic plan, is compulsory; part B, the supplemental plan, is voluntary, requiring a small monthly contribution by individuals who qualify. Extensive benefits are provided under each of the two plans.

The basic program includes hospital care, nursing home care following hospitalization, home health care after discharge from a hospital or nursing home, and outpatient diagnostic tests at the hospital. The supplemental plan provides for the payment of physicians, for home visitations, as well as payment for diagnostic tests and X rays, radioactive and X ray therapy, ambulance services, surgical dressings and splints, rental of medical equipment, braces, and artificial limbs. Both plans commenced operation in July, 1966, except for nursing home care, which began in January, 1967.

FOUNDATIONS OF HEALTH SCIENCE

Part A is automatic and free for almost everyone over sixty-five (even if he is not eligible for Social Security payments). Part B covers only those who sign up and pay monthly premiums. Part A is financed out of Social Security monies derived from payroll taxes, but part B is intended to support itself with matching federal grants. (The monthly fee has failed to keep pace with the cost of the program; it began at $3, was raised to $4, and is continuing to be raised.) Medicare incorporates devices borrowed from private carriers for sharing costs between the carrier and the insured party: coinsurance (the patient must pay a certain percentage of all bills) and deductibles (a specified initial amount is paid entirely by the patient).

The hospitalization deductible was originally $40, but in ten years it rose to $84, while the per diem hospital coinsurance for the sixtieth to ninetieth days rose from $10 to $21. The 98 percent who have part B must also pay the first $60 in doctor bills (up from the original $50) and 20 percent of all charges thereafter. There are numerous gaps in coverage. In 1970 Medicare paid for 64 percent of the doctor bills for the elderly, but by 1973 it paid for only 53 percent. (Doctor bills represent only a portion of medical care costs.) Figure 3.9 illustrates the rise in medical care costs for the aged and that proportion of costs covered by Medicare.[15]

Medicaid. Medicaid is a more comprehensive program of medical care assistance. Sponsored by the federal government, it is available primarily to women and children. The program is designed to provide services to the indigent and those lacking sufficient financial resources. Medicaid differs from Medicare in three major ways, all of which have been worked to Medicaid's disadvantage. First, Medicaid is administered by the states separately. The federal government pays 50 to 83 percent of the costs of the program but has little control beyond setting guidelines. (Medicare is nationwide, with uniform standards.) Second, because it is an assistance program rather than an insurance program, Medicaid in most cases pays the provider of services directly, thus increasing paper work for doctors, whereas Medicare reimburses the patient (unless both doctor and patient prefer direct payment from the government to the doctor). Third, Medicaid requires a test of each patient's eligibility—a proof of need. Each state sets its own eligibility requirements, within federal guidelines and is responsible for reexamining recipients' eligibility at least once every twelve months.

There is little doubt that within the next several years some form of comprehensive health care legislation will be negotiated at the national level, extending coverage to all Americans. Some view this as a definite move to socialized medicine, while others hesitate to make such an assumption. Current issues center around compulsory versus voluntary health insurance and the extent of federal subvention and intervention.

Figure 3.8 Does Coverage Meet Your Needs? (Source: *Today's Health,* 47:55, December, 1969. Published by the American Medical Association.)

Before purchasing or renewing your voluntary health insurance, examine the contract. To see if it meets your needs and your ability to pay, determine the answers to the following questions:

What inpatient hospitalization benefits are covered? Is deductible payment required? How much? Are benefits provided for intensive care?

What outpatient hospital services are covered?

How many days of hospital care are covered for each illness? Are the covered days limited to one period of hospitalization? Are there limitations on readmission to a hospital for the same illness?

Are there any limits on choice of hospital or other place of care?

Does coverage provide for payment based on surgeons' and physicians' usual and customary fees?

Are surgical procedures covered wherever performed? If payment is subject to a schedule of benefits, what provisions are there for operations not specifically listed? Are fractures and dislocations covered? Oral surgical procedures?

How much of a surgeon's bill is paid by the insuring organization? Are there provisions for the services of consultants?

Are there any limits on choice of physician?

What benefits are provided for daily hospital visits by the attending physician?

Are there provisions for office or house visits? Is deductible payment required for these visits?

Are there provisions for concurrent services of more than one physician?

What provisions are made for radiation therapy, diagnostic x-rays, laboratory tests, anesthesia services?

How soon after family membership begins are maternity benefits effective? What are the benefits for normal delivery? For abnormal or complicated delivery? For out-of-hospital birth? [For abortion?]

In a major medical contract, does the deductible amount apply per illness, or is it based on the calendar year? Is co-insurance payment required? How much?

What is the maximum amount payable for each illness? Can maximum benefits be restored after recovery from an illness?

Is coverage provided for services of a registered nurse? Of a licensed practical nurse? Are nursing benefits limited to periods of hospital confinement?

What benefits are provided for services in an extended care facility? What is the maximum number of days? Must this follow hospitalization within a specified period of time?

Are hospital benefits provided for nervous and mental disorders? Are there deductible or co-insurance amounts? Are there benefits for psychiatric treatment in a doctor's office? In a hospital outpatient facility?

In a prepaid group practice plan, what benefits are provided? What provisions are made for out-of-area emergency care?

What family members are covered under a family plan? Are newborn babies covered from birth? To what age are dependent children covered? Are there provisions for older dependent children? For full-time students? Is a child covered if married?

Can an individual apply for separate coverage after becoming ineligible for dependent coverage? Is there a time limit on this application? What provisions are made for continued coverage of dependents if the primary insured is over age 65? If the primary insured dies?

(Continued on next page)

Figure 3.8 *(Continued)*

Is there a waiting period before accident benefits begin? Before coverage of certain illnesses or operations? Are these periods acceptable in light of the family's medical history?

Is there a waiting period following discharge from a hospital before eligibility for readmission is restored?

Is coverage provided for injuries or illnesses which occurred or began prior to the contract's effective date?

Are there provisions for chronic diseases?

In a group contract, can the insured convert to another form of coverage on termination of employment?

Are there any restrictions on conversion for any circumstances? Is there a time limit?

Can the contract be cancelled? By whom? Under what conditions?

Are there any exclusions other than the common ones?

If covered under more than one contract, are benefit payments restricted?

Is the insuring organization authorized to do business in your state?

Does coverage apply equally to health care services anywhere in the United States? What benefits are available for health care received outside the United States?

According to proposed bills, the federal government would pay the hospital or the physician directly. Many of the proposals have built-in controls on quality of care, such as requirements for a professional standard review council, establishment of minimum standards for health personnel and organization, compilation of a generic list of drugs, and provision of a utilization review program. When a bill proposes utilization of private carriers, the carrier may be required to provide certain types of coverage at reasonable premiums. Some bills include incentives to encourage preventive health care and the formation of HMOs and provide funds to develop health manpower.

Figure 3.10 is a summary of current proposals.

The labor organizations contend that health insurance should be compulsory. Under such a plan, each person would contribute a small percentage of his income for comprehensive medical care. Health services would be coordinated to insure adequate protection for all individuals. Opposing viewpoints hold that governmental control would surely ensue and that the quality of service and professional standards would suffer.

Programs in other countries illustrate different ways of meeting the complex problems of medical care. *State medicine,* as evidenced in the Soviet Union and Cuba, provides free or low-cost service for everyone. Physician and specialist education is provided free by the government, as are the facilities and equipment used in medical practice. The program is completely state or government administered and controlled. *Socialized medicine* is comparable to a state system of medical care in many respects, except in the extent of governmental control. Socialized forms of medical

Figure 3.9 Averaged Medical Care Costs among Aged—Percentage Reimbursed by Medicare

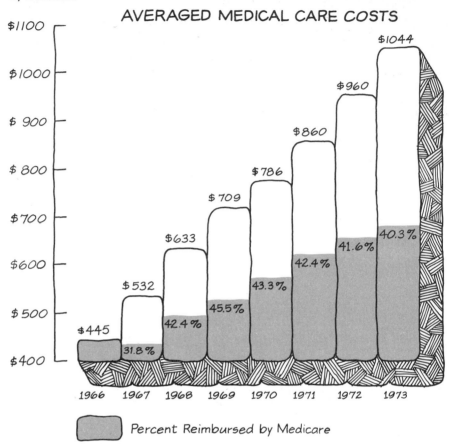

AVERAGED MEDICAL CARE COSTS

("Ten years of Medicare and Medicaid," *Medical World News,* 16:64, March 10, 1975.)

practice, as found in Sweden, England, and parts of Canada, generally place the administration of the program with a professional group, but the cost is underwritten by the taxpayer. In addition to their participation in the socialized program, physicians are usually allowed to maintain private practices. There are distinct and rather obvious benefits and disadvantages to both state and socialized medical care programs. Certain problems are frequently cited, notably the tremendous costs involved in providing adequate services to all. This has been due in part to the misuse and abuse of the system by hypochondriacs and health cranks. Some criticism has also been directed at the apparent decline in the quality of medical care.

Present National Health Insurance includes an Employer Plan paid for

FOUNDATIONS OF HEALTH SCIENCE

Figure 3.10   National Health Insurance Proposals

Health Security Act   S3(HR 22)   Kennedy/Griffiths

CONCEPT	National Health Insurance administered by federal government deletes Medicare but not Medicaid. Covers all U.S. citizens and aliens.
COVERAGE	Physician, in- and outpatient hospital care, home health, optometry, podiatry (dental to be gradually phased in), devices and appliances, drugs with limitations, outpatient psychiatric care with limitations.
FINANCED	No deductibles or coinsurance or waiting periods. 3.5% of employer's payrolls, 1.0% of employees' wages, 2.5% from self-employed, balance (50% of costs) from general revenues.

Health Care Insurance Act   S444(HR 222)   Hansen and Hartke/Fulton and Broyhill

CONCEPT	Voluntary—called medicredit. All under 65 eligible. Those with no federal income tax would not have to pay. Continue Medicare.
COVERAGE	To qualify, a health care policy must provide (1) limited period of hospitalization and nursing, drugs, blood, appliances, maternity care, psychiatric care, physical therapy with $50 deductible; (2) home health services, outpatient hospital care including X rays and laboratory services, subject to 20% coinsurance on first $500 of expense; (3) medical care by physicians in hospital and office—20% coinsurance; (4) limited dental care; and (5) catastrophic coverage.
FINANCED	Federal government would pay health insurance premiums for poor and allow income tax credits for all others toward purchase of private insurance plans.

National Health Insurance and Health Improvements Act   S915   Javits

CONCEPT	National health insurance by gradually expanding Medicare (eliminate Medicare B), Medicaid to continue. Eventually to cover everyone.
COVERAGE	Hospital and posthospital. Physician and related services including outpatient diagnostic services, home health services, and physical therapy. Maintenance drugs for chronic conditions, annual physical examinations, and dental care for children.
FINANCED	Taxes on employer and employees, general revenue. Federal administration using private carriers. Use of deductibles and coinsurance.

National Health Care Act   S1100(HR 5200)   McIntyre and Burleson

CONCEPT	Give financial aid to state health care insurance plans for the poor and uninsurable. Increase income tax deductions for costs of private health coverage (private policies must meet specified standards).
COVERAGE	Private policies must provide limited hospitalization, home health services, diagnostic tests, outpatient surgery and radiation, well-baby care, unlimited physician services, catastrophic coverage. State plans for the poor and uninsurable would include dental care for children, prescription drugs, maternity, family planning, physical therapy on coinsurance basis.
FINANCED	Employer and employees through premium payments to private insurance companies. State pool plans through partial payments for near poor, federal matching funds from general revenues.

National Health Insurance Proposals, Brief Outline of Pending Bills, Committee on Finance, United States Senate, May 2, 1974. Washington, D.C.: U.S. Government Printing Office.

(Continued on next page)

Figure 3.10 *(Continued)*

Health Rights Act   S2756   Scott and Percy

CONCEPT	Two separate insurance programs: (1) a federally administered inpatient plan to cover costs of catastrophic illness and (2) an optional health maintenance plan administered by private insurers under contract to the government. Would pay for inpatient benefits above a "health cost" ceiling and for outpatient above a specified deductible. Replaces Medicare.
COVERAGE	Inpatient care, psychiatric hospital services (limited time), secondary care services, post inpatient home health services. Outpatient plan would include physician services, diagnostic exams, limited physical exams, prenatal care, well-child care up to four years of age, physical therapy, home health services, some psychiatric visits, dental care up to age eleven years, long term maintenance drugs.
FINANCED	Social Security payroll taxes, general revenue, individual premium payments.

Comprehensive Health Insurance Act   S2970(HR 12684)   Packwood, Mills, Schneebeli

CONCEPT	Health insurance available to all through three separate plans: (1) mandated Employee Health Insurance Plan (EHIP), (2) Assisted Health Insurance Plan (AHIP) for low income and others not eligible for EHIP, and (3) Modified Medicare.
COVERAGE	Hospital services; physician services; outpatient prescription drugs; mental health including limited in- and outpatient care; preventive services for children including vision, hearing, and dental care; prenatal and maternity services; home health services; extended care; blood and blood products; prosthetic devices; dialysis; X rays, laboratory tests, etc.
FINANCED	Deductibles and coinsurance, employers and employees paying for premiums; Federal subsidies, payroll tax, general funds. Use of private carriers.

Comprehensive National Health Insurance Act of 1974   S3286(HR 13870) Kennedy and Mills

CONCEPT	Covers everyone except those on Medicare. Medicaid extended to include long-term care and outpatient drugs.
COVERAGE	Inpatient services, physician care, home health services, extended care, mental health (both in- and outpatient), outpatient prescription drugs for specified chronic conditions, dental care for children, well-child care to age six, prenatal care and family planning.
FINANCED	Payroll taxes and general funds. Administered by Social Security. Utilizes private carriers, deductibles, and coinsurance.

National Health Standards Act of 1974   S3353   Fannin

CONCEPT	A two part national health insurance program that would require employer-purchased health insurance and would replace Medicaid with federally purchased health insurance for low-income persons. Continue Medicare. All employers must provide an approved health insurance plan (cost to employer to be 50% of premium). Employers of more than twenty-five employees must provide option to join an HMO.
COVERAGE	Inpatient, physicians' services, outpatient X ray and laboratory services, prescription drugs, physical therapy, outpatient psychiatric care, extended care, medical devices and appliances, ambulance.
FINANCED	Employer and employee contributions, use of private carriers, state set up insurance pools to provide coverage for low income and self-employed.

Figure 3.10 *(Continued)*

Low-income costs to come from federal revenue. Utilizes deductibles and coinsurance.

National Health Care Services Reorganization and Financing Act   HR 1   Ullman

---

CONCEPT	Continue Medicare but expand to catastrophic coverage. Low income and medically indigent covered by Medicare. Employers must provide employees with private health insurance covering at least Medicare level. Health Care Corporations (HCC) to be established in every geographic area with a State Health Commission responsible for setting up the HCC and for enforcing regulations pertaining to providers, HCCs, insurance carriers, etc.
COVERAGE	Gradual expansion of benefits to ultimately provide these comprehensive health care benefits: screening tests and exams, immunizations, well-baby care to age five, dental care to age seven, visual care to age twelve, physicians' services, outpatient diagnostic services, hospital care, supplies and drugs on outpatient basis, ambulance, mental illness, alcoholism, drug abuse, prostheses, home health services, extended care and nursing home care.
FINANCED	Payroll taxes and general revenues, coinsurance, employer pays 75% of premium and employees 25%.

National Comprehensive Health Benefits Act   HR 11345   Staggers

---

CONCEPT	Comprehensive health care benefits for everyone; continue Medicare and Medicaid.
COVERAGE	Physician care, hospital care, laboratory and radiological services, limited mental health services, home health care, preventive health services. Ultimately would cover screening tests and exams, immunizations, well-child care to age five, dental to age twelve, vision to age fifteen, family planning, drugs, ambulance, alcoholism and drug abuse, prostheses, home health services, extended care and nursing home care, and ambulatory diagnostic procedures.
FINANCED	Employer 75%, employee 25%; general revenues. Administered by a newly created State Health Commission. Some coinsurance. Utilize private carriers but federal government would control directly with HMO.

---

by employers and employees. Employers must offer their full-time employees a plan for which the employer contributes the major share of the cost. Employers with more than twenty-five workers are also required to offer their workers the option of joining a Health Maintenance Organization in areas where approved HMOs exist.[16]

IN CONCLUSION

It is our personal responsibility to maintain the health levels of ourselves and our dependents. Such responsibility involves having periodic medical examinations, obtaining recommended immunizations, knowing when to obtain professional advice, getting treatment for emergency conditions, and selecting appropriate health care delivery systems. Within the next several years, this nation will have some type of national health insurance program; however, it is doubtful that any such program will meet all medical and health care needs.

We need help in assuming our responsibilities. Many physicians are still not informing patients in detail of their health status, yet Boyd says, "it is the patient who must assume ultimate responsibility for his health behavior."

> It is the moral responsibility of the health professional to return to the citizen both his right and his responsibility for health. One doctor has attempted this by making out two copies of his medical report on a patient. He writes both in plain language, deleting all mystifying code words. When he hands the report to his patient, he says, "This report is about you and your health condition. It is your life. I cannot make you healthy; I can only assist. You must take charge of your own health." What a change this would be if adopted widely! The health professional becomes an aide, a resource person, in the health process. The citizen becomes the final bearer of his health responsibility.[17]

Notes

1. "Immunization Levels Inch Up, but 'Conquered Diseases' Remain a Threat," *Medical World News,* 16:86, September 22, 1975.

2. Byron John Francis, "Current Concepts in Immunization," *American Journal of Nursing,* 73:646–649, 1973.

3. Charles F. Eason and Barbara G. Brooks, "Should Medical Radiation Exposure Be Recorded?" *American Journal of Public Health,* 62:1189–1193, 1972.

4. Abstracted from William Nolen, "Rules to Make You a Better Patient," *Today's Health,* published by the American Medical Association, 51:41, 42, 66, 67, April, 1973. Reprinted by permission of the author's agent, Lurton Blassingame. Copyright © 1973, American Medical Association.

5. Ibid., p. 67.

6. "Profile of Blind Persons," *Statistical Bulletin,* 54:11, July, 1973.

7. Sol Silverman, "Oral Cancer Expert's Advice," *UCSF News,* 3:2, September, 1975.

8. "Science and the Citizen," *Scientific American,* 226:40, February, 1972.

9. Bonnie Bullough, "The Source of Ambulatory Health Services as It Relates to Preventive Care," *American Journal of Public Health,* 64:588, June, 1974.

10. "Hospitals and Clinics: Synergy," *UCSF News,* 1:13, February, 1974.

11. Ibid.

12. Based on Gerald M. Knox, "Ten Misunderstood Facts about Health Insurance," *Better Homes and Gardens,* 46:39, 40, April, 1968.

13. " 'Catastrophic' Illness: How Common?" *Medical World News,* 16:127, 128, February 24, 1975.

14. "Ten Years of Medicare and Medicaid," *Medical World News,* 16:64, March 10, 1975.

15. Ibid.

16. "Health Insurance Plan Resurfaces," *Medical World News,* 14:97, September 21, 1973.

17. Tom W. Boyd, "What's Wrong with Public Health?" *Environmental News Digest,* 41:9, January-February, 1975.

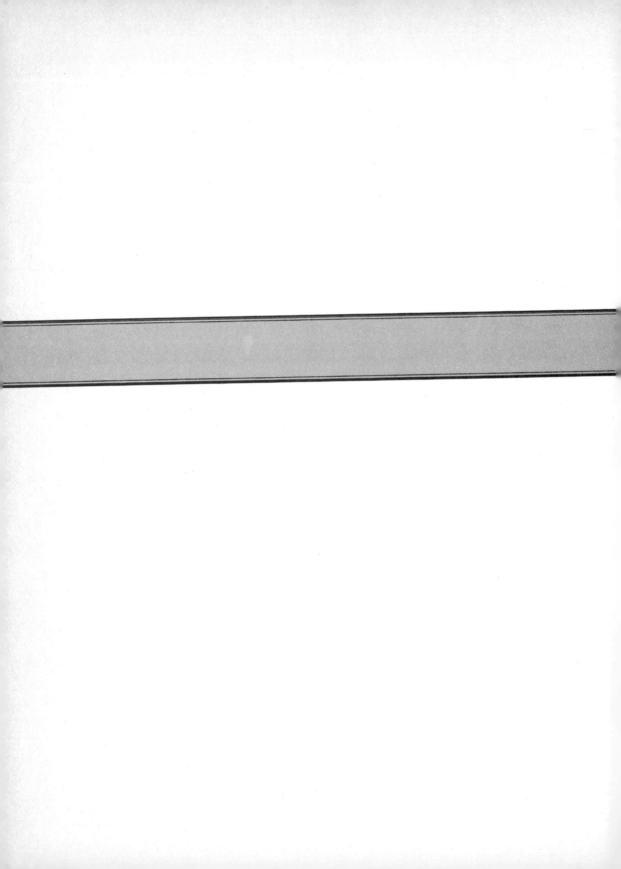

PHYSICAL FITNESS

chapter four

Physical fitness implies a condition of readiness. Readiness enables the individual to meet the demands of life more effectively. Since each person has innate differences in his or her physical and emotional capacities, and since each requires his or her physical and emotional self to perform different tasks, no single standard can be used to judge the physical fitness of all. The professional athlete, the bus driver, the secretary, the salesman, the engineer, the teacher, the housewife, and the relatively sedentary college student all require different degrees of physical fitness to fulfill their responsibilities and to function effectively. Whatever one's present pursuits or future aspirations, physical fitness is an important ingredient for success. It can never be completely separated from other elements of total well-being.

Total fitness in modern society is not dependent upon physical capacity alone. It intimately involves the cultivation of a number of basic and interrelated qualities and potentialities. The fit individual possesses:

Optimum organic health consistent with heredity and the application of present health knowledge

Sufficient coordination, strength, and vitality to meet emergencies, as well as the requirements of daily living

Emotional stability to meet the stresses and strains of modern life

Social consciousness and adaptability with respect to the requirements of all of life

Sufficient knowledge and insight to make suitable decisions and arrive at feasible solutions to problems

Attitudes, values, and skills that stimulate satisfactory participation in a full range of daily activities

Spiritual and moral qualities that contribute the fullest measure of living in a democratic society.[1]

Total fitness, then, is a combination of the basic components that are implied by the term *health*. It means a state of optimal well-being. Physical fitness is but one important facet of total fitness, or health.

CONCEPTS OF PHYSICAL FITNESS

Authorities who have attempted to conceptualize and appraise physical fitness have identified three common elements—physical growth and development, organic soundness, and motor condition. These elements incorporate such positive characteristics as strength, agility, cardiovascular and respiratory efficiency, endurance, emotional stability, skill, sensory alertness, and coordination. Accordingly, a healthy person with optimal physical fitness:

> . . . can carry out his usual everyday tasks without undue fatigue and have enough reserve energy left over to enjoy his leisure; to meet emergencies such as an accident, illness, an operation, or a disaster; and to engage in activities requiring reasonably prolonged, vigorous physical effort when necessary or desired.[2]

A biologist at Springfield College in Massachusetts defined physical fitness as "work capacity." He asserted that:

> Physical fitness is the capacity to do work. It is determined by strength, endurance, and coordination. Each of these components in turn is founded upon the underlying biologic bases of age, sex, health status, and anatomic and biochemical condition. Furthermore, it is characterized by a high degree of specificity which changes with growth and development. Both the measurement and practical application of fitness are strongly affected by motivation.[3]

There are basic hereditary differences in capacity for physical fitness, involving such matters as neuromuscular coordination, reaction time, emotional balance, somatotype, and the like. However, no matter what one's hereditary endowment, everyone has the capability of improving his or her skill, stamina, and strength, unless prevented by serious disease.[4]

An understanding of physical fitness is dependent in part upon some knowledge of the structure of the human body. For those that need a brief review, an explanation is in the appendix.

EXERCISE AND HEALTH

Why should we be concerned about the role of exercise in promoting and maintaining health? Patterns of living in the United States have altered in recent years. No facet of American life has remained static amidst the scientific, technological, social, economic, and cultural innovations of the century.

The development of automation and the availability of labor-saving devices have meant that many muscle-building tasks are now unnecessary.

Each in his own way

I tried to gain weight and strength by lifting weights. I tried and did gain weight (twenty pounds) by weight lifting. I lift three times a week, Monday, Wednesday, and Friday. For a period of a year I have done very well in putting weight on the upper part of my body. I did this to have more physical size when playing contact sports.

I tried to keep my lungs and legs in shape by running one to one and one-half miles every night. This was after the soccer season, so I was able to start running the distance without becoming too exhausted. After a week, I ended each run with a 200-yard sprint. At the end of these runs I was exhausted but was able to regain regular breathing within fifteen minutes. This exercise lasted only one month as I was un-able to motivate myself as I had for the soccer season.

I tried to build up my legs and endurance by riding a bicycle. I started out riding the length of my road and back—four miles—and then adding a little more. I got to about eight miles easily even with hills. It didn't work too well because if I visited somebody and stayed until it was dark, I didn't like to ride in the dark. So I went back to using the car.

In high school I competed in all three running sports over a span of three years. I was skinny and gained twenty pounds during my first year. I also greatly increased my strength and endurance. My main objective was to have fun; improved fitness came along with it.

Population changes and urbanization are producing overcrowded cities, schools, playgrounds, and recreation centers. There is less room for strenuous, lively, and varied physical activities. Since it is possible to function at many jobs and occupations without good levels of fitness, people are not motivated to maintain the degree of vigor that produces a feeling of well-being and prevents future degenerative disease. See Table 4.1 to determine your level of fitness.

Effects of Exercise

Physical activity produces organic vigor. Muscles, nerves, and organs perform more efficiently when they are stimulated to function at maximal levels. When the organs and systems of the body are not exercised, they lose their ability to work and may atrophy. It has been said that "the body is the only machine that breaks down through disuse." Extended periods of inactivity cause lessened body tonus and result in weakness, flabbiness, and lethargy.

Table 4.1 What Is Your Level of Fitness?

The following exercises can be performed by either a man or a woman. They are designed to partially evaluate minimal levels of strength, endurance, and flexibility. The performance scale is calculated for an average college-age student.

Exercise	Description	Average Score	Your Score
Toe Touch	Legs straight and together. Touch toes and hold as long as possible.	Hold for 10 seconds	
Step Test	Use stable chair. Step up on chair, then down, at rate of 24 steps per minute for three minutes. Rest one minute and check pulse for 30 seconds.	Average pulse: 55–56	
Prone Arch	Lie face down on floor, extend arms to side. Arch back, arms, and legs, keeping chest off floor. Hold position for count of three. Repeat as many times as possible.	12 times	
Jump and Reach	Mark highest point you can reach on wall. Standing sideways next to wall and bending knees, jump as high as possible. Measure distance beyond mark.	15 inches	
Push-ups	Lying face down on floor, push up by straightening arms. Keep back straight. Lower body until only the chest touches the floor. Men rest weight on hands and toes; women on hands and knees. Do as often as possible.	Men: 15 times; Women: 12 times	
Knee-Bent Sit-up	Hook toes under couch or low object while lying on floor. Bend knees and clasp hands behind head. Keeping back straight, come to sitting position as often as possible in one minute for women and 1$\frac{1}{2}$ minutes for men.	Men: 45 times; Women: 25 times	

Body functions. Exercise has a favorable influence on metabolic processes. It requires increased fuel and oxygen and a more rapid disposal of waste products; the heart, lungs, kidneys, skin, intestines, liver, and other organs work harder. This work, exercise if you will, of the circulatory, digestive, respiratory, excretory, and nervous systems improves performance. Muscular activity, therefore, contributes to the improved functioning and vitality of the body system.

Some people believe that exercise is a good way to lose weight. Certainly it is an important part of any weight-control program. However, a person of medium weight who desires to shed a pound of fat through exercise alone must expend 3,500 calories—for example, by running for more than an hour.

Studies have revealed that additional values related to well-being are derived from exercise. Regular physical activity not only produces desirable organic alterations in the lungs and circulatory system, but also promotes an increase of strength, bone density, and muscle size. There is good evidence to suggest that well-planned exercise can significantly delay the aging process.

Some of the relationships between health and exercise are presented in *Exercise and Fitness,* a booklet published by the American Medical Association:

> There is no longer any doubt that the level of physical activity does play a major role in weight control. Maintaining a good caloric balance between dietary intake and energy output requires a sound approach to both food consumption and exercise. There is some evidence to suggest that exercise has a beneficial effect on metabolic functions that combat obesity, in addition to burning calories. The high mortality rate associated with being overweight suggests that obesity contributes to organic degeneration.
>
> The relation of physical activity to mental health should not be overlooked; from this standpoint, the ability to be engrossed in play is basic. Pleasurable exercise relieves tension and encourages habits of continued activity. In fact, muscular effort is probably one of the best antidotes for emotional stress. Fortunately, such a variety of activities is available that everyone should be able to find some from which he gains pleasure as well as exercise.[5]

Exercise and cardiovascular disease. A good deal has been written concerning the effects of exercise on the heart and circulatory system. A lack of proper physical activity is frequently cited as a related cause of cardiovascular disease—by far the number one killer in the United States. A multitude of research studies support this belief. Investigators report a definite correlation between inactivity and a high incidence of cardiovascular ailments. Microscopic examinations of arteries of inactive people and those who had regularly participated in vigorous activity revealed less hardening and fewer atherosclerotic plaques in artery walls of the active people, as well as an increase in the size of the lumen in both arteries and veins. (The lumen is the space in the interior of a tube such as an artery or vein. Atherosclerotic plaques are deposits of fat-containing materials.)

Proper exercise helps to keep healthy hearts healthy and prevent the onset of disorders. Also, physical activity may lessen the severity of a heart attack, make recovery more likely, and hasten rehabilitation. There is no evidence to suggest that reasonable amounts of exercise will damage the healthy heart.

The Method of Exercising

In order for any regimen of exercise to be effective, it must accomplish two objectives. First, to maintain a specific level of efficiency, the tissue, organ, or system must be required to perform at its present capacity daily. Second, to increase development, the muscle system and vascular system must be taxed beyond their normal performance. This means placing additional stress on the body daily to improve its level of efficiency. Physical educators say that to be of general benefit any activity should be sufficiently strenuous to increase respiration and pulse and produce sweating. The minimum period of exercise time is about fifteen minutes. Sporadic strenuous activity is probably more harmful to the body than insufficient exercise.

The concept of endurance fitness was perhaps most strongly stimulated by the book *Aerobics,* by Kenneth H. Cooper, which was published in 1968. It received wide circulation when it was excerpted in several popular periodicals, including *This Week Magazine* and *Reader's Digest.* In his book Cooper differentiated between different perspectives of fitness. He believes that without activity the body will deteriorate and is more vulnerable to certain chronic disorders. Cooper also claims that muscle fitness is too limited and one should strive for endurance fitness. Desirable activities are those which will improve the work capacity of the lungs, heart, and blood vessels. Endurance is related to the amount of oxygen consumed. Those activities requiring more total body effort use more oxygen.[6]

Cooper, then, emphasizes increased use of oxygen as a way to fitness. He has analyzed the oxygen requirements for various types of activity, assigning a "point value" to them. Those activities yielding two points in his system are presented in Table 4.2.

Other publications on fitness stress the significance of jogging or running as one good way to improve and maintain well-being. One such book, *Jogging, Aerobics and Diet,*[7] obviously incorporated several modern ideas.

FOUNDATIONS OF HEALTH SCIENCE

Many jogging celebrities—such as Billy Graham, John V. Lindsey, William Proxmire, and George Romney—have been featured in national magazines. Although this form of exercise rates high on the list of desirable activities, some people prefer more competitive types of exercise that offer equal health benefits.

Whatever form exercise might take, it should be part of any health regimen. This is particularly important during the college years when students spend large amounts of time sitting in classes. The selection of, and participation in, physical activity is largely a matter of personal desire. The factors that influence a person's choice of exercise are age, type of occupation, sex, physical condition, and individual reactions to activity. Exercise should be adapted to accommodate these variances. Ideally it should provide for the vigorous use of the large muscles of the trunk, arms, and legs, especially for those who do not do enough of this type of movement as a part of their daily routine.

Table 4.2 Aerobics Point System Equivalents

| Alphabetical Listing of Activities Yielding Two Points | | |
Activity		Duration and/or Distance
Basketball	14	minutes
Cycling	2	miles in 6–8 minutes
Fencing	20	minutes
Football	20	minutes
Golf	12	holes (no motorized carts)
Handball	14	minutes
Hockey	14	minutes
Lacrosse	20	minutes
Rope Skipping	8	minutes (continuous)
Rowing (2 oars)	12	minutes (20 strokes per minute)
Running-Walking	1	mile in 12–14$\frac{1}{2}$ minutes
Skating (roller or ice)	30	minutes
Skiing	20	minutes
Soccer	20	minutes
Squash	14	minutes
Stationary Running	7$\frac{1}{2}$	minutes at 450–525 steps per min.
Swimming	250	yards in 4–6 minutes
Tennis (singles)	1$\frac{1}{2}$	sets
Volleyball	30	minutes
Walking	2	miles in 29–40 minutes
Wrestling	5	minutes

From *Aerobics* by Kenneth H. Cooper. Copyright © 1968 by Kenneth H. Cooper and Kevin Brown. Reprinted by permission of the publisher, M. Evans & Co., Inc., New York, New York 10017. Note differences in types of activity and extent of participation. The physically fit young adult should expend 30 points per week.

Not everyone can excel in athletics, but most people can obtain satisfaction and value from some form of physical activity. Badminton, skating, dancing, bowling, tumbling, tennis, volleyball, and basketball are strenuous; sports that require less action include golf, table tennis, archery, fishing, and hunting. Numerous recreational pursuits can provide enjoyment and pleasure, in addition to the benefits of vigorous participation. Examples of such activities are swimming and diving, tennis, hiking and mountain-climbing, skiing, handball, and bicycling. The person who has never learned to play and to perform at least moderately well in some motor capacity has missed a vital experience of living.

Conditioning exercises—calisthenics, gymnastics, setting-up exercises, and isometrics—can contribute too. Isometric exercises in particular have become quite popular and widely accepted. An isometric contraction takes place when you exert a force against resistance that does not move. It is like unsuccessfully pushing a stalled automobile. An isotonic contraction takes place when you exert muscular force against resistance that does move; you succeed in getting the automobile to move.

Isometrics, then, are performed on an immovable object and are based on muscle contraction. They may be done as self-resistive exercises, such as placing the palms of the hands together and pushing them in opposition to one another. *Isometrics do not contribute to the development of stamina and endurance,* which are important accruements of isotonic, or traditional, activities. However, they can develop specific groups of muscles. They do not require special equipment and can be performed in limited space.

Running, walking, and cycling clubs are becoming popular for all ages. Running increases cardiac output and is a particularly good form of exercise for people in high coronary risk groups. Two additional benefits obtained from running are a redistribution of weight and a loss of inches around the waist. If there is no increase in calorie intake, a person who runs regularly will lose weight.

Fatigue: A Body Warning

Fatigue is an intricate body condition that affects the total organism. It may have multiple causes and affects the body in different ways. Generally it is the body's manner of forcing a slowdown following continued stimulation, exertion, or sustained physical or mental effort. It is the body's warning that prevents us from expending all our resources and gives us a chance to recoup. It may be used, though, as an escape mechanism to avoid work or stressful situations.

There are many different types of fatigue. Auditory fatigue may develop following overexposure to noise, especially high frequency sounds. Visual fatigue is frequently due to overstimulation of the retinal receptors of the eye. Muscular fatigue, indicated by a lessened ability for muscular contraction, results from previous use. Continuous stimulation of nerve cells, causing a depletion of their energies and the accumulation of waste products, may bring about nerve fatigue. Mental fatigue appears to be psychological rather than physiological, however, and is related to boredom, failure, discouragement, or lack of interest.

Fatigue can be viewed in another way. General fatigue is a gradual decrease in performance as a result of previous effort. It is marked by a deterioration of efficiency, timing, and effectiveness.

The treatment of general physical fatigue is relatively simple. It can be alleviated by rest, relaxation, and sleep. Sometimes a warm bath or massage will help to effect recuperation.

Chronic fatigue has more profound effects on the body, including irritability, exhaustion, shortness of breath, difficulty in sleeping, restlessness, constipation, and a loss of weight. Chronic fatigue may be caused by extended periods of work, insufficient rest and sleep, poor nutrition, excessive worry, or other poor health practices.

Immaturity, emotional instability, and many organic disease states predispose the body to overwhelming fatigue after disproportionately slight exertion or exposure to relatively minor stress. Boredom, loneliness, financial and domestic worry, mental conflicts, frustration, bright light, loud noise, pain, and bad weather are also predisposing and complicating factors. So too are malnutrition, hypoglycemia, hyperthyroidism, and alkalosis. (The last two are associated with increased muscular excitability.)

Chronic fatigue is an accumulatory process over a long period of time, and usually demands time and a new schedule for complete recovery. (Chronic fatigue produced by severe underlying anxiety or emotional conflict is complex and difficult to relieve. The fatigue state is overcome only when the anxiety is dissipated.)

The use of stimulant drugs to mask tiredness, or sleep-producing substances to promote rest, can be dangerous. This is discussed in a later chapter.

SLEEP, REST, AND RELAXATION

Fatigue in its various forms indicates the need for periodic cessation of activity. Intervals of sleep, rest, and relaxation are essential if the body is to operate with optimal effectiveness.

Sleep

Poets, philosophers, and men of science have long extolled the benefits of, and need for, sleep. It has been called the "restorer of life," the "preserver of sanity," and the "refresher of the soul." Yet, despite the tremendous progress made in understanding the nature of man and his being, there is no single accepted scientific explanation of sleep—what it is, why it is necessary, and how it is caused.

Sleep is a normal state that involves the diminution of sensation and thought and periodically interrupts our waking activities. Natural sleep is the best way to recuperate from fatigue and restore energy. Although adults vary somewhat in the amount of sleep they require, most need an average of seven to nine hours. Awakening refreshed in the morning is usually a sign of a sufficient amount of sleep.

A number of physiological changes normally occur during sleep. In general, all metabolic processes decrease. The heart slows down to fifteen to twenty beats each minute, breathing rate is deceased approximately four to six respirations per minute, the blood pressure drops and perspiration increases, the liver stores up glycogen for later conversion to blood sugar, and activity or body movement decreases markedly, although not entirely. It is estimated that a person makes between twenty and sixty major body movements during a normal night's sleep.

Problems Related to Sleep Loss

Since the body normally possesses its greatest resilience and adaptability in youth, college students feel that they can safely disregard the need for adequate sleep. To do so occasionally may involve no great danger. Over a long period of time, an accumulated loss of sleep may have serious results. Tension, irritability, and depression are among the emotional consequences of prolonged sleep-cheating, and physical results include a loss of coordination, poor timing, muscular fatigue, and visual problems.

Some people build up a sleep debt because they are unable to fall asleep when they go to bed. Such unfortunates may lie awake hours, night after night, unable to fall asleep. The reasons for insomnia are many, but the most common are irregularity of sleeping hours, neuromuscular tension, overeating, worry, frustration, indiscriminate use of stimulants (such as coffee or tea), and overexertion immediately before retiring. In some instances, as in the case of deep-seated emotional problems, counseling might be necessary to discover and remove the cause of sleeplessness.

Because the inability to sleep is such a common problem, a variety

Figure 4.1 Sleeping Aids. An increasing number and variety of gimmicks and devices are available to facilitate sleep and lull the insomniac to slumber.

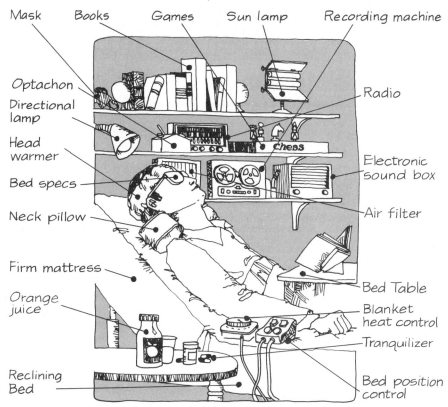

Mask   Books   Games   Sun lamp   Recording machine

Optachon
Directional lamp
Head warmer
Bed specs
Neck pillow
Firm mattress
Orange juice
Reclining Bed

Radio
Electronic sound box
Air filter
Bed Table
Blanket heat control
Tranquilizer
Bed position control

and quantity of slumber aids and relaxation devices have appeared on the market. One machine emits the soothing qualities of waves breaking on the seashore. Another scientifically blends all sounds into what is advertised as "white sound." Other machines hum, like air conditioners. In addition, there are ear plugs, "his and her" reading lights, and hospital-type beds.

The sleeping pill business has become a lucrative industry in the United States. Although many of these preparations are subject to rigid prescription regulations, illegal and indiscriminate use still result in numerous health problems and many accidental or suicidal deaths each year. Sleeping pills should be used as a last resort and only under medical supervision.

People vary in the length of time it takes them to fall asleep. This may be anywhere from a few seconds to thirty minutes. For those who take even longer, the procedures listed below may be beneficial.

1. Routine preparation for sleep, done methodically and habitually, is conducive to falling asleep.
2. Activities prior to routine preparation should be soothing and of a repetitive nature. Tepid baths or showers (neither extremely hot nor extremely cold), a warm drink, and a few stretching exercises are physically relaxing.
3. Loose fitting night clothes, light coverings, a cool but not cold room, and an adequate-sized bed in a quiet, dimly lit room help sleep.
4. Soothing music, a nonstimulating book, and gimmicks such as counting backwards also promote sleep by preventing "thinking too much."

Rest

The reduction of motor activity and the cutting down of sensory stimulation is an accepted definition of rest. It is characterized by a period of inactivity, quiet, and meditation. Its chief purpose is recovery from fatigue and reduction of tension. Rest differs from sleep in that the conscious mind is still functioning during rest.

Different people require different amounts of rest, depending on their activity and fatigue. A balanced program of living demands rest at certain intervals if the body is to be capable of efficient performance.

Relaxation

Not all people find the same activities relaxing, and an activity that is relaxing on one occasion is sometimes not on another. Generally, however, relaxation provides a change of pace that helps to reduce everyday tension and the stresses of living. Activity is required, but in a reduced amount.

A number of colleges and universities offer courses on relaxation, and many articles and books have been written on the subject—rightfully implying that relaxation is partially a matter of training. The ability to relax can be cultivated, and it usually results in improved efficiency and increased enjoyment of life.

Undoubtedly the best procedure is to attempt to prevent excessive fatigue by the maintenance of a high level of fitness and mental health, sufficient rest and sleep, and adequate nutrition. Helpful too is a well-planned rhythm of daily routine, including provision for change-of-pace activities. Despite the pressures and problems of modern college life, it is possible and important for students to develop a personal schedule designed to cope with fatigue hazards. Constructing a time budget is a technique that many who "never get done" find of value. See Figure 4.2.

FOUNDATIONS OF HEALTH SCIENCE

Figure 4.2 Action Analysis

Activity[a]	Time Alotted (hours)						
	Mon	Tue	Wed	Thu	Fri	Sat	Sun
Chores							
Eating							
Studying							
Church							
Socializing							
Relaxation							
Employment							
Classes							
Exercise							
Recreation							
Sleep							
Grooming							
Hobbies							
Transportation time							

24 hours per day

[a]Some activities (such as recreation, exercise, and hobbies) might be combined in the same time period.

POSTURE AND BODY MECHANICS

The manner in which we stand, sit, and walk helps to determine the impressions that others form about us. This position, or bearing, of the body is known as posture and influences total well-being. It includes activities such as reclining, sitting, standing, bending, squatting—in fact, all bodily positions or movements.

Good Posture

Good posture is usually the result of proper habits in early life. It depends in large measure upon the development of the vertebral column and the harmonious functioning of the large muscles of the body. Good posture helps to reduce or prevent strain and fatigue, reflects attitude and personality, affects appearance, aids in the mechanical use of the body, and is presumed to promote organ efficiency.

For some of the more fortunate, good posture comes naturally and without special attention. Others, however, achieve such a state only through concentrated effort. These people, some of them handicapped through illness or physical defects, have attained functional posture by persistently following carefully regulated programs of exercise and relaxation designed to promote general health and correct particular problems. Although the early years are most important for the correction of postural defects and the promotion of good posture, persons of college age can still improve their carriage and bearing.

Sedentary activities, in which the large muscles of the body are not used, may allow decreased tonus and precipitate postural difficulties. Fatigue may also affect mechanical effectiveness. Poor vision or hearing sometimes results in compensations such as tilting the head to one side or thrusting it forward.

Structural Defects

Although at birth a baby's spine is straight, normal anterior-posterior curvatures develop as the child grows. In other words, a side view of the skeleton of a normal adult will show a very limited S-shaped vertebral column. When the spine is viewed from the back, it is straight.

Continuous use of the body in an abnormal position can result in permanent structural change. An exaggerated outward curvature of the upper back region, commonly called "humpback" and technically known as *kyphosis,* is an anterior-posterior defect that can result from poor sitting habits. Another is *lordosis,* or hollow-back, which is an exaggerated forward curvature of the lumbar region. Some authorities state that the wearing of high-heeled shoes tilts the pelvis forward, causing lordosis. *Scoliosis* is a lateral curvature defect that may be either single or compound, occurring in the upper or lower back region or both. It is presumed to be caused, frequently, by standing on one leg or using only one side of the body to carry heavy materials. Persistent habits of this nature cause the shoulder on the side used to drop and the hip to raise. Other defects are bowlegs, stoop shoulders, knock-knees, paunchy abdomen, stiff neck, and pigeon toes.

The correction and care of serious postural defects should be conducted under the supervision of an orthopedist. Postural defects cause discomforts such as back and neck pain, muscular strain, and fatigue. The defects may place undue stress on particular joints. It is hypothesized that this is a factor in the development of arthritis.

Foot Problems

The feet bear and help balance the entire weight of the body in standing and locomotion. Foot troubles of various kinds produce poor posture. The direct effects of aching, tired, or malformed feet are well known.

Each foot consists of twenty-six bones arranged in the same basic pattern as the bones of the hand and wrist. These bones are connected by ligaments to form two arches. The longitudinal arch runs lengthwise of the foot. The transverse arch extends across the foot just behind the toes. These arches provide strength and flexibility to the feet and help to cushion the impact of body weight when one is walking, running, or jumping. In some cases of flat feet, where the longitudinal arch is lacking or has broken down, walking and other movements involving body weight on the feet are painful.

Proper foot care is prerequisite to efficient functioning, since poor foot hygiene may give rise to a number of complicating problems. The foot and ankle are susceptible to strains and sprains; the foot is also susceptible to corns and bunions. Improperly fitting and inappropriate shoes can cause these. High-heeled shoes for women and pointed-toe shoes for both men and women have apparently aggravated such conditions. Spiked heels offer little supporting surface, and all heels that are too high tend to throw the body weight entirely onto the transverse arch. Platform soles and "earth shoes" can also promote foot and postural difficulties. Platform shoes impede flexibility of the foot so that jarring of the body is increased. Because of reduced flexibility, there is also greater danger of falling. Earth shoes cause the heels to bear most of the impact of body weight when walking, which may produce pain in the heel.

LEISURE TIME AND RECREATION

The worthy use of leisure time is a goal proposed by ancient philosophers and recognized through the years as basic to the very existence of civilizations. A study of history reveals that the progress of nations declines as the amount of available leisure increases. A number of contemporary philosophers suggest that if humanity does not destroy itself through destructive technological advances, it may well succumb to the dangerous misuse of free time. The close relationship between work and play in the maintenance and promotion of well-being may well be the key to survival in the space age.

The changing scene in modern America has provided time for leisure to an unprecedented extent. Dulles describes the nature of these changes in the first half of the twentieth century.

The people of no other country and no other age had ever had anything like the leisure, the discretionary income, or the recreational choices of the American people in mid-twentieth century. It was overwhelming. Science and the machine had reshaped traditional patterns into hundreds of new forms. Something had undoubtedly been lost, but also a great deal had been gained. Working men and working women—factory operatives, plumbers, waitresses, bank clerks, farm-hands, stenographers, storekeepers, subway guards, mill-hands, garment workers, office boys, truck drivers— found countless pleasures and amusements readily available that had once been restricted to the privileged few. The democracy had come into its recreational heritage. It had achieved both leisure and the means to enjoy it.[8]

There are innumerable varieties of recreational pursuits. Some require active participation and others are passive, or of a spectator nature. Choice is motivated by personal likes, enjoyment, and satisfaction. Raking leaves or mowing the lawn, for example, can be a form of recreation to some people, while to others it is drudgery. The effect is largely dependent upon personal needs, desires, and motivations. It is also related to such factors as occupation. A postman would probably not want to go hiking or mountain climbing on his day off. For the normally sedentary college student and adult, recreation should involve vigorous activities.

IN CONCLUSION

Bauer has expressed the philosophy underlying the cultivation of physical fitness for living.

Fitness is like a jewel. In the rough, it is undistinguished in appearance and without obvious value. It may even fail of recognition. Most of us, like jewels in the rough, possess the basic attributes of fitness undeveloped and unused. They need to be uncovered, just as a fine jewel needs to be split, cut, and polished, before its color and sparkle are discernible through its many facets. Then, if each facet is perfect, the inner fire is revealed in all its priceless beauty. But let one facet be at fault, and the gem is flawed; its beauty marred; its value reduced.

You are the craftsmen, the jewelers, as it were. It is for you to take the rough stone, cut and shape and polish it, and make of it a precious gem.[9]

Notes

1. "Fitness for Youth: Statement Prepared and Approved by the 100 Delegates to the AAHPER Fitness Conference," *Journal of Health—Physical Education—Recreation,* 27:8–9, December, 1956.
2. Howard S. Hoyman, "Our Modern Concept of Health," *Journal of School Health,* 32:256, September, 1962.
3. Clifford E. Keeney, "Work Capacity," *Journal of Health—Physical Education—Recreation,* 31:30, September, 1960.

4. James L. Whittenberger, "Physiologic Aspects of Physical Fitness," *American Journal of Public Health,* 53:793, May, 1963.

5. Joint Committee of the AMA and AAHPER, *Exercise and Fitness* (Chicago: American Medical Association, 1964), p. 6.

6. Kenneth H. Cooper, *Aerobics* (New York: Bantam Books by arrangement with M. Evans and Company, 1968), pp. 9–14.

7. Roy Ald, *Jogging, Aerobics, and Diet* (New York: Signet Book, New American Library, 1968), p. 191.

8. Foster Rhea Dulles, *A History of Recreation* (New York: Meredith Publishing Co., 1965), p. 397.

9. W. W. Bauer, "Facets of Fitness," *Journal of Health—Physical Education—Recreation,* 31:25, September, 1960.

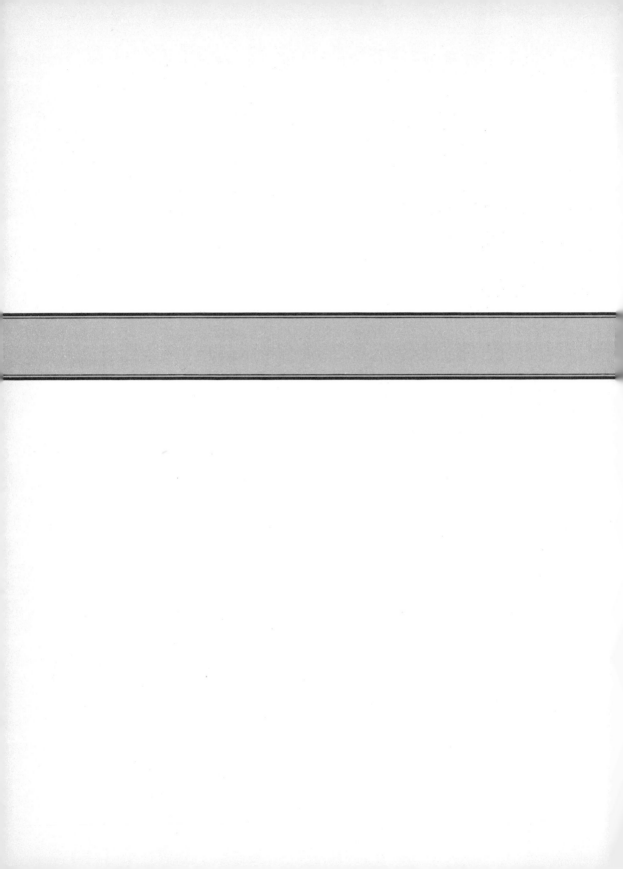

THE SCIENCE OF NUTRITION

chapter five

What does eating mean to you? Is it a way to stay alive, a chance for fellowship and sociability, a way to celebrate an event, a means of soothing hurt feelings and relieving depression, a display of affluence and importance, an indication of love and security, a means of showing your independence, an occasion of self-denial, something to fear because you might become ill, that which is your right, or something to enjoy? Chances are *eating* means a number of things to you. The values we have about food and our eating patterns are largely determined by our family, friends, and cultural group. These patterns are difficult to modify.

A newspaper columnist recently said that in the United States there is more food than in any other country in the world and more diets to keep us from eating it. People spend millions of dollars each year on pills, capsules, tonics, appetite stimulants and depressants, and special foods to do special things. People are food conscious but not nutrition wise. They often lack an appreciation of the relationship between nutrients and physical and emotional health, and they are misled by custom, incorrect information, and beliefs in fallacies and superstitions.

Eating is a pleasurable experience. Meals and refreshment periods are a means to sociality and conviviality. Of secondary importance to most people is eating to provide the necessary nutrients and energy for growth, maintenance and repair of tissues, and activity. Patterns of eating are influenced by culture, family background, knowledge of the science of nutrition, and philosophy about nutrition behavior.

According to the U.S. Food and Drug Administration Office of Nutrition and Consumer Sciences, the population as a whole has a good state of nutrition, except for the widespread occurrence of obesity. Segments of the population with problems are primarily those with inadequate income.[1] But, independent surveys do not corroborate these findings. A recent ten-state nutrition survey revealed that an unexpectedly large number of children were malnourished and a surprisingly large number from poor families showed retarded growth. Other findings included the following: there was little variation in nutritional quality relative to family income or race; iron deficiency was prevalent in boys and girls from infancy through adolescence (but there was little relationship between deficiency and family income); children from economically advantaged families

There are diets, and diets, and diets

Last year, I decided that I was too fat, so I proceeded to go on a seven-day diet with my older sister. We figured that if we both went on the diet, we could stick to it. We would both eat at the same time, when we weren't working, to help our morale on sticking with the diet. The diet was the type in which the amount of food is reduced so that on the fourth day nothing is consumed but liquids and then it builds back up so that the seventh day is like the first day. I made it through the third day and then decided I was starving; so I quit. My sister went on until about the fifth day, when she almost fainted. That was the first and last "official diet" for me.

———

I have for the past eight years attempted without success to formulate a vigorous dietary program. Unfortunately, I have not researched the field of nutrition, and, therefore, I have not been able to maintain a "good" diet.

Usually I would make myself a promise to have breakfast every morning. I always broke that promise. Also, I made the pledge to have a "balanced" lunch. That promise, too, was broken. Dinner—that's right, you guessed it—was often missed and if not missed was often unbalanced!

I'm going to give up and just eat. If I get fat, then I'll go to a doctor to get some pills to diet.

———

I've been trying to improve my diet. I've gone for several-month intervals as a vegetarian. I totally abstained from any meat, poultry, or fish. I became very conscious of trying to balance my diet with proteins and vitamins other than those supplied by meat. Because of this diet, I watch everything I eat.

FOUNDATIONS OF HEALTH SCIENCE

tended toward obesity; median thickness of subcutaneous fat increased directly with family income; children from wealthier families were taller and heavier than those from poor families; and black boys and girls tended to mature earlier and showed skeletal and dental advancement sooner than white or Spanish-American youths (a finding that suggests the need for different standards in assessing nutritional status among racial groups).[2]

In a nation with a food supply as abundant as ours, these findings seem unbelievable. In part they show lack of knowledge about what constitutes "good nutrition."

Most people ascribe to a common sense approach in food selection and eat to live rather than live to eat. Some individuals are very conservative in their nutrition behavior and spend much time, energy, and money in selecting foods that *always* provide maximal value. They minimize social and sensual pleasure. Unfortunately, there is a sizeable group of people who are nutrition faddists. Their behavior is not always based on scientific evidence, and they become emotional about their way of life. These people tend to impute almost magical properties to special foods and believe diet is a panacea for disease. Quacks prey upon the faddists and extort millions of dollars each year from the gullible for worthless nostrums and special concoctions.

The best insurance one has against the pervasive influence of the quacks is to understand the scientific principles underlying good nutrition and to apply these to daily living. A scientific background can help us become more critical of nutrition information we hear and read. How many of the misconceptions in the list below do you believe to be true?

1. Oleomargarine is less fattening than butter.
2. Large doses of Vitamin C prevent colds.
3. Eggs, oysters, and olives promote fertility.
4. A meat diet will cause weight loss.
5. The "drinking man's diet" works.
6. Vitamin B cures hangovers.
7. All food additives poison foods.
8. Hot cereals are more nutritious than cold cereals.
9. Salt and water are fattening.
10. Exercise causes weight gain.
11. Honey, a natural sugar, is more nutritious than table sugar.
12. We should not eat alkaline and acid foods at the same time.
13. Toast is less fattening than bread.
14. Dark bread is more nutritious than white bread.
15. Organically fertilized foods are more nutritious than chemically fertilized foods.

16. Fresh foods are more nutritious than frozen or canned foods.
17. Foods stored in open cans can cause ptomaine poisoning.
18. Eating before bedtime causes overweight.
19. Placing hot foods (roasts) in the refrigerator can cause harmful toxins to develop.
20. Fried foods are indigestible.
21. Everybody needs milk.

All of these are myths, but more than one-third of the average college students believe one or more of them.

The science of nutrition has its basis in chemistry, biochemistry, and physiology. In *Stedman's Medical Dictionary*, nutrition is defined as a process ". . . consisting in the taking in and assimilation through chemical changes (metabolism) of material whereby tissue is built up and energy liberated; its successive stages are known as digestion, absorption, assimilation, and excretion. . . ." There are levels of nutrition just as there are levels of wellness. Optimal nutrition exists when foods containing the nutrients necessary for body maintenance, repair, and growth are ingested and the nutrients are efficiently utilized physiologically. A general understanding of what nutrients do and the kind of foodstuffs that supply generous amounts of specific nutrients enables normally healthy persons to select diets that meet the needs of themselves and their families.

CALORIC NEEDS

Foods provide fuel, or energy, required by the body for overt muscular activity referred to as work or exercise, for internal operation of the organs and processes, and for maintenance of body temperature. Energy requirements of an individual are based not only on activity levels but on sex, age, size, type of body tissue, endocrine activity, environment, state of health, and specific dynamic action of the food ingested.

The energy needs of an individual and the energy supplied by foods are measured in *calories*, which are defined as the amount of heat required to raise the temperature of one kilogram of water (2.2 pounds) one degree centigrade. Through laboratory experiments, the caloric values in commonly used foods have been computed, as have the number of calories necessary to accomplish involuntary and voluntary activity.

Overt muscular activity accounts for one-fourth to one-third of the energy needed. Persons who do hard manual labor may exceed this proportion, but the sedentary types of occupations such as office work, studying, or teaching do not require a great deal of energy. The number of calories needed per hour to do some common activities are given in Table 5.1.

Basal Metabolic Rate

The minimal amount of energy or number of calories needed to carry on the physiological process of the body is known as the *basal metabolic rate*. Several laboratory tests can determine this accurately, and an approximate rate can be computed easily. The basal metabolic rate in adults is about one calorie for every 2.2 pounds of body weight per hour. This averages out to about 1,400 calories for a woman and 1,700 calories for a man, and accounts for the major number of calories required per day.

Size, shape, and age also influence that basal metabolic rate. Physiological functioning requires a more or less stable internal body temperature. Since heat is constantly being lost from the body surface, it must

Table 5.1 Caloric (Energy) Expenditure in Relation to Activity

Activity	100 Lbs.	120 Lbs.	140 Lbs.	160 Lbs.	180 Lbs.	200 Lbs.
Sleeping	40	50	55	65	70	80
Sitting still	60	75	85	95	110	120
Standing relaxed	70	85	95	110	125	140
Dressing or undressing	80	95	110	125	145	160
Talking or singing	80	95	110	125	145	160
Eating	80	95	110	125	145	160
Typewriting rapidly	90	110	125	145	160	180
Driving a car	95	115	135	150	170	190
Dishwashing or ironing	95	115	135	150	170	190
Studying or writing	100	120	140	160	180	200
Light exercise	110	130	155	175	200	220
Working in yard	150	180	210	245	270	300
Moderate exercise	185	220	260	295	335	375
Walking fast	200	240	280	320	360	400
Vigorous exercise	290	350	405	465	520	580
Swimming	320	385	450	510	575	640
Running fast	370	445	520	590	665	740
Very severe exercise	400	480	560	640	720	800

Figures given refer to the number of calories expended for each hour of activity in relation to different body weights. Approximate caloric expenditure for activities not specifically listed can be estimated by using the table as a guide. Other variables, such as age and sex, are not taken into consideration.

constantly be replaced; the larger the body surface, the greater the amount of heat lost. People who are short and stocky have less body surface than those who are tall and lanky; therefore, they need fewer calories. More calories are required to maintain muscle than to maintain adipose tissue. Consequently, a muscular person may have a rate as much as 5 percent greater than someone the same weight, size, and shape who is "soft and flabby."

Caloric needs decrease with age. For example, people thirty-five years of age require about 250 calories per day fewer than they needed when they were twenty. Moderate climates, in contrast to very cold climates, reduce needs by as much as several hundred calories per day, since much less heat is lost.

A number of people believe that by eating lots of meat they will burn up calories and lose weight. However, a high protein diet such as the average person might follow will not in itself cause weight loss. To be digested, absorbed, and utilized by the body, different kinds of foods require different amounts of calories, or energy. This requirement is called *specific dynamic action*. Protein by itself has a much higher specific dynamic action than do fats and carbohydrates. But meat, fish, fowl, eggs, and cheese, which make up the so-called high protein diet, are composed of varying amounts of protein, fats, carbohydrates, minerals, vitamins, and nondigestible substances. They are not just protein. For most diets, including the so-called high protein ones, the specific dynamic action requirement is about 6 percent of the daily caloric needs.

Computing Daily Needs

If a person's weight remains relatively stable, and if he or she weighs within five pounds of the norms indicated in Table 5.2, daily caloric intake is most likely adequate. If the person's weight is not within this recommended range, then caloric consumption should be adjusted to caloric needs.

To determine frame size, measure the circumference of either wrist. In each category, the wrist size, of both men and women increases with height. (See Table 5.3.)

NUTRIENTS

The elements in foods that are required for the maintenance and growth of the body are called nutrients. These are the carbohydrates, comprising starches and sugars; the proteins, made up of amino acids; fats, consisting of fatty acids; vitamins; and minerals. Although not called nutrients as such, water and cellulose are also necessary to life. Most foods contain more than one nutrient, but vegetables, fruits, and cereals are primarily sources of carbohydrates, and meats, fish, and fowl are mostly

Table 5.2 Desirable Weights

	Weight in Pounds According to Frame (In Indoor Clothing)			
	HEIGHT (with shoes on) 1-inch heels Feet Inches	**SMALL FRAME**	**MEDIUM FRAME**	**LARGE FRAME**
Men of Ages 25 and Over	5 2	112–120	118–129	126–141
	5 3	115–123	121–133	129–144
	5 4	118–126	124–136	132–148
	5 5	121–129	127–139	135–152
	5 6	124–133	130–143	138–156
	5 7	128–137	134–147	142–161
	5 8	132–141	138–152	147–166
	5 9	136–145	142–156	151–170
	5 10	140–150	146–160	155–174
	5 11	144–154	150–165	159–179
	6 0	148–158	154–170	164–184
	6 1	152–162	158–175	168–189
	6 2	156–167	162–180	173–194
	6 3	160–171	167–185	178–199
	6 4	164–175	172–190	182–204
	HEIGHT (with shoes on) 2-inch heels Feet Inches	**SMALL FRAME**	**MEDIUM FRAME**	**LARGE FRAME**
Women of Ages 25 and Over	4 10	92– 98	96–107	104–119
	4 11	94–101	98–110	106–122
	5 0	96–104	101–113	109–125
	5 1	99–107	104–116	112–128
	5 2	102–110	107–119	115–131
	5 3	105–113	110–122	118–134
	5 4	108–116	113–126	121–138
	5 5	111–119	116–130	125–142
	5 6	114–123	120–135	129–146
	5 7	118–127	124–139	133–150
	5 8	122–131	128–143	137–154
	5 9	126–135	132–147	141–158
	5 10	130–140	136–151	145–163
	5 11	134–144	140–155	149–168
	6 0	138–148	144–159	153–173

For girls between 18 and 25, subtract 1 pound for each year under 25.

Metropolitan Life's Four Steps to Weight Control, courtesy of Metropolitan Life Insurance Company, 1969.

Table 5.3 Frame Size

Frame Size	Wrist Size	Height
Small	5$\frac{1}{2}$" or less	5'2" or under
	6" or less	5'3" to 5'4"
	6$\frac{1}{4}$" or less	5'5" to 5'11"
Medium	5$\frac{1}{2}$" to 5$\frac{3}{4}$"	5'2" or under
	6" to 6$\frac{1}{4}$"	5'3" to 5'4"
	6$\frac{1}{4}$" to 6$\frac{1}{2}$"	5'5" to 5'11"
Large	5$\frac{3}{4}$" or more	5'2" or under
	6$\frac{1}{4}$" or more	5'3" to 5'4"
	6$\frac{1}{2}$" or more	5'5" to 5'11"

protein. Milk, milk products, eggs, nuts, and legumes are rich in carbohydrates, proteins, and fats. Most foods contain vitamins and minerals, but some have more of certain vitamins and minerals than others.

Carbohydrates (CHO)

Foods rich in carbohydrates are the main source of inexpensive energy, and they often supply many vitamins and minerals. Among the diet-conscious population in the United States, some of the carbohydrated foods have a poor reputation because of their high caloric value per serving. Examples are breads and other cereal products, potatoes, legumes, and nuts. Nevertheless, these foods are valuable adjuncts to a meal, since they are inexpensive sources of valuable minerals and vitamins. Legumes and nuts are also good sources of some of the amino acids.

Carbohydrates are made up of carbon, hydrogen, and oxygen. They are classified as sugars and starches. Some of the simple sugars need no digestion and can be absorbed directly into the blood stream. This is why honey, grape juice, and very ripe fruits are often called "quick energy foods." Starches and complex sugars must be broken down into simple sugars before absorption. These simple sugars are either circulated in the blood stream in the form of glucose for immediate use by the tissues; stored as glycogen, an animal form of starch; or converted into adipose tissue. A ready supply of glucose must be constantly available for the brain and nerve cells, which cannot use any other form of carbohydrate. A very small amount of the absorbed sugars are converted into glycogen. The liver can store as much as 100 grams of glycogen and the muscles 200 grams. The glycogen is released as glucose if the glucose level in the blood falls. Sugars not sent into the blood or stored are converted into adipose tissue.

FOUNDATIONS OF HEALTH SCIENCE

One of the more complex sugars, sucrose, is known to us as table sugar (refined, raw, and brown sugars are more or less the same). Sucrose is not necessary in the diet, and there is growing evidence that it may be harmful.

Some commercials say we need sugar for quick energy. But "quick" energy obtained from such a source can have "rebound". The sugar (sucrose) readily breaks down into glucose, a form of sugar used by the body. There is always glucose—usually called "blood sugar"—in the blood stream. In healthy people, a complicated interaction of hormones keeps the level of the blood sugar fairly constant. When you eat something like table sugar or starch, glucose is released during digestion. This is then absorbed from the alimentary canal into the blood and the level of blood glucose rises. Immediately, however, there is an outflow of hormones, especially insulin from the pancreas. The effect of this is to lower the level of glucose toward its normal level—sometimes even below normal, so that less glucose is available to meet physiological needs—by converting it into glycogen.

Glucose and sucrose are by no means identical. They have different chemical structures, and affect the body differently. When the word *sugar* is used for both the sucrose in food and the glucose in blood, the crucial differences between sucrose and glucose are hidden.

Concentrated forms of sugar, if used excessively, can cause irritation of the intestinal tract and can be a factor in the incidence of dental caries. They may also dull the appetite or promote satiety (feeling of fullness) to the point that foods with other nutrients are omitted from the diet. Table sugar (whether refined or raw), honey, syrups, and molasses contribute *only* energy. Despite what some people believe, they contain little or no vitamins and minerals, as any food composition table in a standard nutrition text will show. The traces of minerals in molasses and honey are negligible. These sweeteners can be used in place of other concentrated forms of carbohydrate to please the palate and provide variety.

According to Yudkin, sucrose (table sugar) may be a precipitating factor in several chronic diseases, particularly coronary heart disease, diabetes, and ulcers. In fact, Yudkin believes that it is sucrose, not saturated fats, that is involved in the development of atherosclerosis. His hypothesis is that some people have a special sensitivity to sugar. When such persons consume sucrose, these changes take place: insulin levels rise, platelets in the blood become sticky and clump together, and cholesterol and triglyceride levels increase.[3]

In an article written for *Family Health*, Mayer of Harvard University states definitely that we should "scale down our sugar intake." These points are emphasized:

1. Table sugar is not a traditional food historically; it has only recently been introduced into the diet, particularly among westerners.
2. The findings of Yudkin are controversial, though they probably apply to a select group of people who are particularly sensitive to carbohydrates.
3. Though it may be difficult to eliminate table sugar (sucrose) completely from most diets, people can select foods low in sucrose, such as non-sugared cereals, fresh fruits, and fruits canned in their own juices.
4. *The body does not need sucrose!*[4]

Insufficient carbohydrate intake results in the use of proteins or fats to supply energy requirements, and since energy needs take precedence over all other needs, valuable and expensive proteins may be used for this purpose rather than for growth and repair. Carbohydrates, then, "spare proteins" to do the things that only proteins can do. If neither carbohydrates nor proteins are available for energy, body fat is used. The use of adipose, or fat, tissue to supply *all* energy (this happens in fasting) results in the accumulation in the blood of incompletely oxidized products that upset the electrolytic balance in the body, causing illness.

It is necessary for people to consume carbohydrate foods daily. Diets consisting entirely of high protein foods and/or fats can result in malfunctions. The exact daily requirement for carbohydrates, including cellulose, has not been established. Studies show that man can function when extremely wide variations are consumed.

Protein

Protein is necessary to build and repair tissue. It is the solid matter of muscles, organs, and body fluids. Every cell and nearly all body fluids contain protein. Proteins are composed of amino acids, which are made up of a carboxyl, or acid, group (COOH) and an amino, or basic, group (NH_2). Nitrogen, the key element in proteins, differentiates them from other substances. Twenty amino acids are commonly found in proteins. These can be combined in many ways and with other substances into almost infinite numbers or kinds of proteins. Different species synthesize different amino acids, which they then use to build proteins. There are eight out of the twenty that humans *cannot* synthesize but must ingest as such; they are referred to as "essential amino acids." (Children have an "essential" requirement of nine or ten amino acids.)

Foods, consequently, are classified according to the degree to which they provide all eight, or are *complete*. The *complete protein* foods, having highest biological value, are able to maintain life and promote growth. This group includes eggs, milk, meat, poultry, and fish. *Partially complete protein foods* will maintain life but will not promote growth. Plant sources of these include the seed foods, such as nuts, many cereals, and legumes. Totally *incomplete proteins,* such as those found in corn and gelatin, are incapable of supporting life.

For the body to obtain maximum biological value from proteins, all twenty of the amino acids must be available at the same time. Most people in the United States use plant proteins to supplement the more expensive dairy products and meats. *Plant proteins are utilized maximally only if some complete protein is eaten at every meal.* Casseroles made with milk and cheese, cereals served with milk, and bread made with milk or eggs supply complete proteins. Meals consisting of fruits and vegetables alone are usually of poor biological value. Vegetarians eat meals of good biological value only by planning carefully to include specific combinations of foods. Those who exclude meat from their diets frequently use a lot of milk, cheese, and eggs to obtain complete proteins.

At present, it is not possible to enrich foods with synthetic amino acids to supply those that are missing. The ratio of one amine to another seems to be a factor in whether or not the body can use each efficiently. Researchers are continuing to study such supplementation, so it is quite probable that enrichment will be possible in the future. Since the majority of the world's population subsists on vegetable sources of amino acids, protein deficiency is widespread, particularly among children, who need it for growth and repair. Extreme deficiencies result in a syndrome known as *kwashiorkor,* found in such underdeveloped countries as Africa. This occurs most commonly in infants after weaning. It is characterized by retarded growth and development, spindly legs and arms, protruding abdomen, or "pot belly," mental apathy, edema, diarrhea, skin lesions, change in color of hair, and symptoms of the vitamin-deficiency disorders.

In the United States, protein deficiencies are not usually so severe; they are most apt to be manifested by nutritional edema, an accumulation of fluid in the legs at the end of the day. This symptom can be observed in people who are ignorant of the science of nutrition, cannot afford to purchase protein foods, are in poor health, or have no incentive to eat. Pregnant women and elderly people are the ones most apt to suffer this type of deficiency. The recommended dietary allowance in the United States is approximately 65 grams of protein a day for men and 55 for women. Since the consumption of meat in this country has increased, there is concern about excessive protein intake. In metabolizing protein the body produces urea and other nitrogen-containing compounds that must be eliminated. Excessive protein intake could put a strain on the kidneys. A number of animal studies indicate that this could be harmful.

Fats

Fats are almost as widely available as carbohydrates. They are organic compounds made up of carbon, hydrogen, and oxygen, plus a few molecules of other elements. They differ from carbohydrates in the proportion of oxygen (much less) to hydrogen and carbon. Some of the fatty acids are labeled essential—*linoleic, linolenic,* and *arachidonic.* Lack of these fatty acids will cause failure in growth and reproduction, dermatitis, and poor utilization of fats. Linoleic acid must be consumed as such, since the body cannot synthesize it. It is plentiful in seed oils, such as cottenseed, corn, soybean, and, to a lesser extent, peanut oil. These oils are widely used in making oleomargarine and salad dressings.

The terms *saturated* and *unsaturated* are used to describe fatty acids. Saturated fatty acids have no double bonds between the carbon atoms; that is, they contain as much hydrogen as the carbon atoms are capable of holding. Unsaturated fatty acids have double bonds that are capable of holding more hydrogen atoms.

Why are unsaturated fatty acids considered more desirable than saturated acids? First, the three essential acids, linoleic, linolenic, and arachidonic, are unsaturated. Since linoleic cannot be synthesized by the body, foods containing it must be included in the diet. Second, there is evidence that some people who eat diets high in saturated fatty acids have increased levels of serum cholesterol. If their diets are changed to include a high proportion of unsaturated fats, the cholesterol level decreases. (The evidence does not indicate that healthy people consuming moderate amounts of fat will effect a lowering of serum cholesterol by using only unsaturated fats. Nor is there any proof that eating eggs from chickens fed special foods will lower cholesterol levels.)

Liquid fats such as the vegetable fats, especially safflower oil, are primarily unsaturated, while the solid fats found in meat, lard, and butter are saturated. Hydrogenation of oils to make the numerous shortenings used in cooking increases the amount of saturated acids.

The coffee-cream substitutes, or whiteners, may contain even more saturated fatty acids than milk, and their mineral and vitamin content is considerably less than that of milk and cream. These substitutes are not recommended for use by children as replacements for milk.

One of the pathological conditions related to cardiovascular disease is *atherosclerosis.* In atherosclerosis, plaques of a calcified nature develop in arterial walls, causing rigidity and inelasticity that interfere with circulation and cause the heart to work harder. Cholesterol is found in these plaques, and affected persons have higher levels of serum cholesterol than do the non-affected. The mechanism that causes the deposits is unknown, and biochemists are not sure that cholesterol is the major villain, since other compounds are involved too. The body synthesizes cholesterol whether or not it is ingested. However, for individuals who have a serum cholesterol level that is in the upper normal range or is abnormally high, physicians recommend a diet that limits, or even completely omits, saturated fats, eggs, milk products, and organ meats.

Fats, which have twice the energy (nine calories per gram) of proteins and carbohydrates, are often the main constituent of foods that an overweight population eats too much of. (The so-called rich gravies and sauces, spreads, and desserts are usually high in fat and, consequently, high in calories.) Therefore, fats have been labeled "bad." However, they are vital to life.

Fats provide a padding for such organs as the heart, kidneys, liver, and spleen. This padding helps to keep organs in proper anatomical position so that they can function correctly. It also protects them against injury. (In the obese person, however, the fatty tissue around an organ may be so thick that it constricts the organ and interferes with its function.) Fat is a necessary component of the sheath surrounding and protecting nerves, and it insulates the body, preventing rapid changes in body temperature due to excessive heat loss. Fat people, being well insulated, suffer more readily from heat than do thin people, and thin people are more uncomfortable when it is cold.

If lipids are not available in conjunction with carbohydrates to provide energy, precious proteins will be used for energy rather than for growth and repair—so fats, like carbohydrates, are protein sparers. They are also carriers of the fat-soluble vitamins, A, D, E, and K.

Digestive functions are facilitated by fats. They lubricate the digestive tract and depress the secretions of the stomach, which delays its emptying and retards feelings of hunger. This delaying action enables food to pass gradually from the stomach to the small intestine; consequently, the end products of digestion are absorbed more slowly. This helps to maintain blood sugar at an even level.

As a rule, fats are completely digested if they are properly used. Burned fats interfere with digestion, since cooking at too high a temperature results in the decomposition of glycerol, which can irritate the digestive tract mucosa. Soft fats, such as butter, burn at very low temperatures. Hard fats, such as lard and the hydrogenated vegetable fats, require high temperatures before this decomposition occurs. Foods are digested more slowly when they are covered with fat; but if the frying temperature is low, the foods may absorb so much fat the digestion is too retarded. The consequences may be digestive upsets.

In planning for daily dietary needs, there can be a wide range in the percentage of calories provided by fats. Some common sense rules about fats are listed below.

1. The essential fatty acids are available in unsaturated fats only, so the diet should include some of these daily.
2. People with high cholesterol levels should keep the intake of saturated fats to a minimum, possibly 4 percent or less of their caloric needs.
3. Until more is known about the relationships between saturated and unsaturated fats, cholesterol, and atherosclerosis, those with a family history of high cholesterol level, high blood pressure, or coronrary heart disease should reduce their intake of saturated fats and high cholesterol foods.
4. Since fats are high in caloric value, reduction in daily intake can prevent overweight and obesity.

Vitamins

Vitamins, their discovery, and the application of knowledge about them have been both a boon and a bane to man. In the United States, the deficiency diseases, such as scurvy, beriberi, and pellagra, are seldom seen anymore. But the quacks and faddists have a field day with "subclinical deficiencies," "depleted soils," and "subminimal nutrition." Just how these conditions can be detected, proved, or corrected no one is quite sure, but "they" say "vitamin and mineral supplements plus organically grown foods will correct the problem." Evidence from research sponsored by different governmental agencies and by large universities indicates that these statements are not valid.

Vitamins are organic compounds that are found in very small quantities in foods. They are essential for maintenance and growth of the body. No one vitamin is more or less valuable than another. They function as catalysts, or enzymes, in the metabolism of carbohydrates, proteins, and fats. The body cannot synthesize most of the vitamins, so they must be obtained from food. Each has different functions, and for the body to work effectively all must be available.

Normally healthy persons will have no difficulty in obtaining the necessary amounts of vitamins if they eat a wide variety of cooked and raw foods. Ordinarily, it is not necessary to use vitamin supplements. The water-soluble vitamins used in excess of body needs are excreted in the urine. The fat-soluble vitamins may be stored in the body, and if consumed in excessive amounts they can produce toxic effects. In time of physical or emotional stress or disease, a person's physiological needs may be increased. Vitamin supplements might then be prescribed by a physician. The one desirable routine supplementation is the daily use of vitamin D by infants, growing children, and pregnant and lactating women.

FOUNDATIONS OF HEALTH SCIENCE

The fat-soluble vitamins are A, D, E, and K. The body can store a large amount of vitamin A. These vitamins are able to withstand the usual cooking temperatures, so only slight losses occur in food preparation. Long periods of cooking reduce the amounts more than rapid cooking. The water-soluble vitamins are C and those compounds known as B-complex. These are affected by heat and cooking because they are easily oxidized. Fifty to 75 percent of the vitamin B-complex content can also be lost when cooking water or drippings are discarded. There are fifteen or more different factors in the B-complex; however, if the daily diet includes recommended amounts of riboflavin, thiamine, and niacin, there is little danger of deficiency in the others. Studies indicate that smokers have appreciably lower blood levels of vitamin C. A summary of the vitamins, important sources of each, their functions, and the effects of deficiencies is in the Appendix.

Minerals

Minerals are constituents of all tissues, bones, nerves, muscles, and blood. They function in regulating such body processes as muscular contractions, nerve irritability, water balance and acid-base equilibrium, and metabolism. A deficiency of one of the minerals can alter how others are used.

If diets include foods that provide the requirements for calcium, iron, and iodine, the other mineral needs probably will be met. Although people seem to be most concerned about "iron deficiency anemia" and "tired blood," calcium is the mineral most frequently deficient in the diets of Americans. It is difficult to provide this mineral in sufficient amounts unless milk or its products are consumed daily (butter does not contain calcium). Iron deficiency is more common among women than among men, since slight amounts of this mineral are lost during menstruation.

Among children iron deficiency anemia is a common type of nutritional anemia. Yet this condition is needless, for the cause is known, testing is easily done, and prevention is possible. Years of experience have proved that the school-aged child who is malnourished learns less and is less responsive to stimuli.

Normally, a fruit or vegetable that contains appreciable amounts of a particular vitamin or mineral will always contain about the same amount. If the soil is deficient or the seed of poor quality, the crop yield or size of the fruit or vegetable itself is smaller. There is no scientific evidence that foods grown on soils fertilized by chemical fertilizers have less vitamins or minerals than crops fertilized by manure or the so-called organically grown foods.

"Choice" appearing fruits and vegetables look and taste the same regardless of the technique used to produce them. The less expensive, inferior-appearing grades available in many markets are also nutritious. Crops that are picked when they are at the peak of ripeness and are used as quickly as possible after picking have the highest levels of nutrients. Produce that is frozen or commercially canned at its peak is equal to fresh and may have even greater value than fresh produce that is not used for several weeks after harvesting or is improperly cooked.

Iodine is found in seafoods and in plants that have been grown in iodine-rich soil. In areas where the soil lacks this mineral and seafoods are not available, there is a danger of goiter, cretinism, thyroidtoxicosis, and thyroid cancer. This problem is easily prevented by using iodized salt. A summary of minerals, their functions, and food sources is in the Appendix.

Dietary Allowances

By what criteria are diets judged to be adequate? In 1943, the Food and Nutrition Board of the National Academy of Sciences, a private non-profit organization of scientists concerned with the general welfare, published the first Recommended Dietary Allowances. This is periodically revised when research indicates that changes must be made.

A copy of the most recent revision is in the Appendix. This standard, accepted by both government and nongovernment groups, is used to plan and evaluate diets. It can be used by individuals as a basis for self-evaluation, although good nutrition can be achieved very simply by making sure that foods from the basic groups listed in Figure 5.1 are included in the daily diet. Nutrition textbooks contain lists of the amounts of nutrients in various foodstuffs, so it is relatively easy to compute whether or not the foods consumed during a week's time approximate the amount of nutrients recommended.

In planning for nutritional needs, it is not necessary to eat an adequate diet every day or at every meal; one day of poor selection will not lead to a deficiency disease the next day. Recommended amounts of nutrients are merely guides; individual needs vary.

Milk is often touted as the "perfect food." As you will note in Figure 5.1, nutritionists recommend that people of all ages consume milk daily. It is an inexpensive source of protein of high biological quality and is one of the best sources of calcium. However, it is high in cholesterol and saturated fatty acids, so those with blood lipid problems and potential cardiovascular disease should limit the amount they drink to no more than two glasses per day, and they should drink nonfat milk.

For most children, milk in moderate amounts has no untoward effect

Figure 5.1 A guide to good eating. This is the foundation of a good diet. Use more of these and other foods as needed for growth, for activity, and for desirable weight. (Adapted from "A Guide to Good Eating," courtesy of National Dairy Council.)

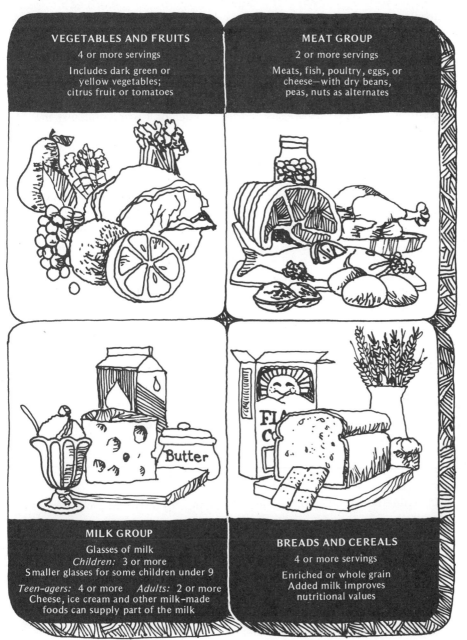

VEGETABLES AND FRUITS

4 or more servings

Includes dark green or yellow vegetables; citrus fruit or tomatoes

MEAT GROUP

2 or more servings

Meats, fish, poultry, eggs, or cheese—with dry beans, peas, nuts as alternates

MILK GROUP

Glasses of milk
Children: 3 or more
Smaller glasses for some children under 9

Teen-agers: 4 or more   *Adults:* 2 or more
Cheese, ice cream and other milk-made foods can supply part of the milk

BREADS AND CEREALS

4 or more servings

Enriched or whole grain
Added milk improves nutritional values

and is beneficial. According to the Committee on Nutrition of the American Academy of Pediatrics, milk should be restricted for (1) the child with nutritional iron deficiency, (2) the child who won't eat, and (3) the child who tends to be constipated. Those children drink milk *instead* of eating a balanced diet. Milk is low in iron and vitamins such as C, and it lacks the fiber content (or roughage) necessary for normal intestinal action.

Elimination of milk is recommended only for the child with congenital lactase deficiency, galactosemia, or allergy to milk protein. There is no evidence that the prevalence of coronary heart disease in later years is decreased by limiting cholesterol early in life or that milk intake per se is a contributing factor in obesity. Some physicians do recommend that the child whose parents have a history of high blood lipids and cardiovascular disease be tested for abnormal blood lipids; if the child has evidence of abnormality, dietary management may be instituted as a preventive measure.

Lactose intolerance and milk allergy are the major medical considerations against universal milk drinking. Lactose intolerance due to abnormally low levels of the enzyme lactase is reported to affect 70 percent of the blacks and about 25 percent of the overall population in the United States. Among most people the intestinal production of lactase drops rapidly after the age of two. Those with limited lactase activity have difficulty in digesting milk, and seven in ten of these have some discomfort—cramps, bloating, fullness, and occasionally, diarrhea—when taking as little as eight ounces of milk.[5]

Eating Patterns

An examination of American eating patterns reveals that more and more meals (40 percent reported in 1970) are eaten away from home, fewer meals are eaten by all members of the family together, there is greater and greater reliance on convenience foods for meals, and increasing amounts of snack foods are being eaten between meals. The Department of Foods and Nutrition of the American Medical Association has presented this description of the eating habits of the middle-class American family:

> Breakfast, once a family meal, is thrown together hastily and individually by each family member old enough to do so.
> Dad skips lunch if he is too busy or may have a business luncheon with martinis. If Mom feels guilty about the sweet roll at mid-morning she skips lunch, or dines on a package of Daughter's liquid breakfast drink; Junior and Daughter eat a hot lunch at school, but on weekends may continue the snacking begun after breakfast.

FOUNDATIONS OF HEALTH SCIENCE

Mom slips in another cup of coffee and a dessert at mid-afternoon when a friend drops by, while the kids come home from school and reach for the potato chips.

Mom valorously but vainly tries to maintain a "no-snack period" of at least an hour before dinner. In actuality, snacking goes on until dinner arrives on the table.

Mom whips dinner together in about 20 minutes from a variety of convenience foods. Unlike Americans of 25 years ago, the family spends not more than 30 minutes eating dinner before disappearing into individual activities. Alternatively, the main course may be purchased from a franchise food "carry-out" outlet, with various snack foods providing the balance of the meal.

Snacking begins soon after dinner ends, and continues to bedtime.[6]

One government survey disclosed that the use of convenience foods was increasing most rapidly in low-income households. Some nutritionists believe that convenience foods and snack foods contribute to malnutrition among the poor, since some of these foods are not adequately nutritious. When a combination of meat, cereal products, and vegetables is bought as one dish, it is difficult even for the informed homemaker to determine its nutritional adequacy. While the consumption of potatoes is increasing, Americans are not using fresh potatoes but frozen French fries and processed potatoes, which contain fewer nutrients than fresh. More and more people are selecting an inadequate diet, eating snacks that provide little but pleasant taste and calories and avoiding the foods high in vitamins, minerals, and amino acids.

Overall, however, food quality is better than it was twenty-five years ago. There is little danger from bacterial contamination, since we have better facilities for storing foods commercially and in the home. The use of vegetables has increased slightly. The biggest change in the American diet is the marked increase in the use of meat—beef especially, but also chicken and pork. There is a reduction in the use of cereal products. People are serving macaroni, rice, and beans, which are good sources of protein. In the future, we can expect to see more soybean products replacing meat.

Food Labeling

State and federal laws require specific information on the labels of packaged foods to enable the purchaser to evaluate and compare products. The Food and Drug Administration acts require that label information be conspicuously displayed and that it be written in terms the ordinary consumer is likely to understand. The size of type, location, and format are specifically prescribed. The following information must appear:

1. Name and address of manufacturer, packer, or distributor
2. Net weight or volume
3. Form of product (whole, chopped, etc.) and a listing of the ingredients unless it is a standardized food)
4. Presence of artificial flavoring, coloring, or chemical preservatives
5. Notification that the product is an imitation
6. Notification that food is enriched or fortified

Under FDA regulations, the nutritional information panel must appear on foods that are enriched and fortified and foods for which a nutritional claim is made. The panel must follow a standard format and appear to the right of the principal display panel. Nutritional information must include the size of a serving and the total number of servings in the container; the number of calories per serving; the weight in grams of protein, carbohydrate, and fat per serving (fat content by degree of saturation and amount of cholesterol and sodium is optional); and the percentage of the U.S. Recommended Daily Allowance (U.S. RDA) of protein, five vitamins, and two minerals provided by one serving. Percentages of the U.S. RDA for an additional twelve vitamins and minerals may also be listed. Figure 5.2 is an example of two nutrition panels, one for rice and one for dried cereal.

OBESITY

It is estimated that from 25 to 45 percent of us are officially obese (more than 20 percent overweight). Obesity is one of the most difficult nutritional problems with which we must cope. The causes are complex and not well understood. There is much theory and too few facts! Although the consumption of more calories than are required to provide for the output of energy results in the accumulation of fatty tissue, the satisfactory loss of weight usually requires more than just reducing caloric intake. Less than 10 percent of the people who lose weight are able to maintain the loss.

What is the nature of obesity? Is there a difference between one who is overweight and one who is obese? People who weigh at least 10 percent more than the recommended level for their specific height, age, and sex are considered overweight. Since bone size and muscle mass account for individual variations, the person who is large-boned and muscular should be heavier than the person who is small-boned with little muscular tissue. Obesity refers to the amount of fat tissue in the body. Unless an

Figure 5.2 Nutrition Panels

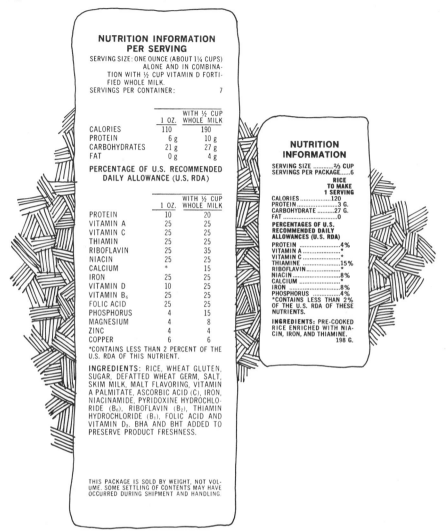

**NUTRITION INFORMATION
PER SERVING**
SERVING SIZE: ONE OUNCE (ABOUT 1¼ CUPS)
ALONE AND IN COMBINA-
TION WITH ½ CUP VITAMIN D FORTI-
FIED WHOLE MILK.
SERVINGS PER CONTAINER: 7

	1 OZ.	WITH ½ CUP WHOLE MILK
CALORIES	110	190
PROTEIN	6 g	10 g
CARBOHYDRATES	21 g	27 g
FAT	0 g	4 g

**PERCENTAGE OF U.S. RECOMMENDED
DAILY ALLOWANCE (U.S. RDA)**

	1 OZ.	WITH ½ CUP WHOLE MILK
PROTEIN	10	20
VITAMIN A	25	25
VITAMIN C	25	25
THIAMIN	25	25
RIBOFLAVIN	25	35
NIACIN	25	25
CALCIUM	*	15
IRON	25	25
VITAMIN D	10	25
VITAMIN B₆	25	25
FOLIC ACID	25	25
PHOSPHORUS	4	15
MAGNESIUM	4	8
ZINC	4	4
COPPER	6	6

*CONTAINS LESS THAN 2 PERCENT OF THE
U.S. RDA OF THIS NUTRIENT.

INGREDIENTS: RICE, WHEAT GLUTEN,
SUGAR, DEFATTED WHEAT GERM, SALT,
SKIM MILK, MALT FLAVORING, VITAMIN
A PALMITATE, ASCORBIC ACID (C), IRON,
NIACINAMIDE, PYRIDOXINE HYDROCHLO-
RIDE (B₆), RIBOFLAVIN (B₂), THIAMIN
HYDROCHLORIDE (B₁), FOLIC ACID AND
VITAMIN D₂. BHA AND BHT ADDED TO
PRESERVE PRODUCT FRESHNESS.

THIS PACKAGE IS SOLD BY WEIGHT, NOT VOL-
UME. SOME SETTLING OF CONTENTS MAY HAVE
OCCURRED DURING SHIPMENT AND HANDLING.

**NUTRITION
INFORMATION**
SERVING SIZE ....⅔ CUP
SERVINGS PER PACKAGE......6

	RICE TO MAKE 1 SERVING
CALORIES	120
PROTEIN	3 G.
CARBOHYDRATE	27 G.
FAT	0

**PERCENTAGES OF U.S.
RECOMMENDED DAILY
ALLOWANCES (U.S. RDA)**

PROTEIN	4%
VITAMIN A	*
VITAMIN C	*
THIAMINE	15%
RIBOFLAVIN..................	*
NIACIN	8%
CALCIUM	*
IRON	8%
PHOSPHORUS	4%

*CONTAINS LESS THAN 2%
OF THE U.S. RDA OF THESE
NUTRIENTS.

INGREDIENTS: PRE-COOKED
RICE ENRICHED WITH NIA-
CIN, IRON, AND THIAMINE.
198 G.

individual is grossly overweight—30 percent above the recommended
level—it may not be possible to detect obesity by weight alone. Since
about 50 percent of fatty tissue is subcutaneous, it is possible to measure
skin fold to detect obesity. The physician may use either thumb and fore-
finger or calipers to measure a fold of skin picked up over the lower rib
cage. If the width is more than one inch, there is an excess of adipose
tissue. Another rather simple technique is to subtract girth, or waist measurement, in inches from height in inches. If the difference is less than

thirty-six inches, there is excess adipose tissue. There are precise clinical measurements; however, observation, palpation, and scales give quite accurate diagnoses.

Characteristics of Overweight and Obese People

Numerous studies of overweight and obese people reveal that they have common characteristics: a history of obesity in the family; an obese parent; a history of childhood obesity (children who are fat at four to five years and adolescents who gain weight at fourteen to fifteen years of age tend to stay overweight or obese); a history of low expenditures of energy, less activity than people of average weight, and more standing still and sitting; and a tendency to do most eating in the late afternoon and evening. Women are overweight more often than men. Overweight people are likely to be passive and dependent and poorly equipped to handle stress, have little ability to withstand extensive self-deprivation, are not well accepted by their peers, and are frequently underachievers. They tend to skip breakfast and eat more fat than other people. Fats should provide about 30 to 35 percent of the daily caloric needs, but among the obese, fats may provide 40 to 50 percent of the needs.

Etiological Factors

The direct cause of overweight and obesity is, of course, eating more calories per day than are expended in work or energy. Excess calories may be derived from any type of foodstuff—carbohydrates, proteins, or fats. Serving for serving, though, fats produce about twice as many calories as do either carbohydrates or proteins. Overweight can be controlled by reducing caloric intake and increasing activity. The consistent consumption of 100 calories more per day than are needed will result in a gain of 10 pounds per year. Consuming approximately 100 calories less per day than are needed will result in a loss of 10 pounds per year. There are few exceptions to this mathematical fact. The problem is not how to lose weight but how to get a person to eat less and exercise more.

Lack of exercise. There is an energy output difference between those who are overweight and those who are average or thin. Studies measuring the amount of overt movement reveal that people who are obese expend much less energy in everything they do. They tend to move more slowly, use the minimal number of motions required to do a task, and stand still and sit more. These activity patterns do not change when such people

FOUNDATIONS OF HEALTH SCIENCE

lose weight. Consequently they use less calories than do their counter-parts who maintain average weights.

Jules Hirsch and Jerome Knittle, obesity experts at Rockefeller University, found that "obesity in young rats was a result of too many fat cells, while adult-onset obesity was due to an increase in the size of preexisting fat cells."[7] The rate of fat cell development is greatest from birth to two years and from eight to twelve years. By age sixteen, the number of cells is fixed.[8] More than 80 percent of all obese children become obese adults. How this knowledge can be utilized is not clear. One question being researched is, Do particular foods affect fat cell development?

Endocrine disorders. Endocrinological disorders such as thyroid deficiency can be controlled only under medical supervision. They contribute to less than 5 percent of the cases of obesity. There is evidence that some persons may have a hereditary defect in metabolism by which acetates are used to synthesize fats, which are then stored as adipose tissue, rather than used to produce energy. However, in the majority who are overweight and obese, the cause is not metabolic or genetic in origin; it is overeating.

Habit. Habit is a frequent cause of overeating. This is particularly true of those who gain weight with age. As people get older, their metabolic rate decreases, as does their energy output. They need to eat less, but since the amount of food consumed is determined more by habit than by body requirements, they may continue to eat the same as they did in their twenties.

Food may be used to control childrens' behavior. They may be disciplined by being deprived of food or desserts. This equates foods, particularly those of high caloric content, with reward. And then we continue to reward ourselves as adults by overeating or eating too many desserts and other sweets.

Nutritionists, in an extensive study of 3,444 preschoolers, at all socio-economic levels, in twelve states, discovered that some mothers implant bad eating habits, causing their children to overeat. Such children frequently become obese adults. Twenty-three percent of the parents in this study used food as a reward for good behavior; 10 percent held back food as punishment; and 29 percent used food as a pacifier. Mothers who overestimated food needs tried to force children to eat too much. Another frequent practice when a small child dawdled at meal times was forcing the child to clean up his or her plate before doing anything else.[9]

Sherrel Hammar, a professor of pediatrics, believes the trend toward early introduction of solids is leading to overweight in infants. Infants are doubling their birth weight at a much earlier age than infants did several decades ago. The most popular baby foods have too many calories and possibly too much salt. They are prepared to please the palate of the mother rather than the needs of the infant.[10]

Effects of Obesity

Overweight and obesity contribute to physical illness as well as emotional illness. It is unfortunate that adults, for the most part, are not motivated to lose weight by the fear of the relationship of overweight to the increased incidence of heart disease, arteriosclerosis and atherosclerosis, diabetes, gout, and gallbladder disease. Impaired circulation can be the result of excess weight that must be moved. Fat deposits in the lungs and in and around the heart can also interfere with respiratory and cardiac efficiency. The body suffers not only from lack of oxygen, but also from accumulation of waste products. In an attempt to compensate for these, the body may build extra red blood cells (polycythemia), which make the blood so thick that circulation is further impeded.

Reducing Regimens

People who are not more than 10 percent above the normal weight for their size and age can safely reduce their caloric intake to modify weight. Increasing activity will improve their success in losing. If they do not change their pattern of eating and exercise, they will regain and have to do it all over again. People who are more than 10 percent overweight should have a medical examination to determine possible causes of overweight. It is improbable that they can lose weight successfully without medical and/or supportive treatment. Drastic and rapid loss of weight can be harmful, resulting in disorders ranging from mild irritability to severe neurosis, avitaminosis, protein deficiency symptoms, and ulcerative colitis.

Most people do not want to reduce the amount of food they eat or give up eating certain kinds of foods. Neither do they want to increase the amount of physical activity they do per day. They continually search for an easy way to lose weight. Some of the "diet crutches" they use can help, some do not help, and some are harmful. Crutches do not lead to reeducation; when the crutch is cast aside, weight is usually put back on.

Formula diets. A popular aid to reducing is the formula diet. Formulas come in bottles and cans in a variety of flavors. Such a diet provides approximately 1,000 calories per day and meets the body's needs for nutrients and some energy. Additional requirements for energy are obtained from the breakdown of adipose tissue. The so-called advantages of a formula

FOUNDATIONS OF HEALTH SCIENCE

are that it provides the essential nutrients, that it is convenient, and that there is little temptation to eat one more bite. The disadvantages are that it does not provide emotional satisfactions, it is quickly digested and does not produce satiety, and it does not contain the roughage necessary for proper functioning of the intestinal tract. Because of some of these factors, the manufacturers now make the formula in solid forms, such as cookies, and they advertise their use for one or two meals per day rather than in place of all other foods.

Noncaloric sweeteners. Another crutch is the noncaloric sweeteners, like saccharine, which enable the eating of foods in much larger amounts than if they were sweetened with sugar, honey, or syrups. There is a psychological value in low-calorie products that allow the reducer to eat foods similar to those others eat: he or she does not have to be obviously different. Many low-calorie products are available in restaurants and are prepared in a variety of ways. Some people object to their flavor. Even unsweetened food contains calories, of course, and if consumed in large amounts can add considerably to the day's total.

Pills and nostrums. No nostrums available over the counter have lasting value in producing weight loss. They contain either a sugar-like substance that allays feelings of hunger or a bulk-like product that creates a feeling of satiety. The instructions that accompany such reducing aids nearly always prescribe dietary changes in addition to the nostrum. These crutches are rarely harmful.

Some medications reduce the feeling of hunger and step up metabolic processes. These are supposedly available only by prescription. They should be used only under the *continuous* supervision of a physician. Such compounds produce nervousness, depression, high blood pressure, insomnia, and other undesirable effects if their use is not carefully controlled. A physician, after careful examination, may prescribe hormones if they are indicated; if there is evidence of an abnormal accumulation of fluids in the body, the doctor may prescribe diuretics to be taken either by mouth or by injection.

Special diets. Potentially harmful techniques include some of the fad diets that have short periods of popularity: the drinking man's diet of steak and alcohol; milk and bananas; cottage cheese and oranges; hard-boiled eggs and tomatoes; and a home-concocted formula of salad oil, sugar, and egg. Any of these, if used for longer than several weeks, produce nutritional deficiencies.

Although not a diet, the practice of drinking no water and using no salt is equally dangerous. Mild limitations of salt and water can account for temporary weight changes of several pounds. This is not an alteration of fat tissue. The change is due to water loss. Drastic limitations that result in continued loss of fluids can have serious consequences to all body cells.

Publicity has been given to prolonged periods of fasting. This, too, is dangerous. It may result in permanent physical damage even when it is done under careful medical supervision.

It is a misbelief that foods eaten before work are used for energy and foods eaten before sleeping turn to fat tissue. Weight control is a matter of calories, not spacing meals. People who eat all of their meals late in the day and gain weight gain primarily because they consume more calories.

Of recent popularity are the low-carbohydrate diets, or the high fat–high-protein diets. High-fat diets are not very palatable, and they trigger an abnormal body response called ketosis. Ketosis occurs when a quantity of fats are digested without a concomitant digestion of carbohydrates. There is a buildup of acetone. Acetone is one of the chemical compounds grouped as ketones. When ketones flood the system in excessive quantity, they suppress the appetite, so less calories are consumed. Ketogenic diets result in acidosis. It is a fallacy that we can eat all the protein we want and lose weight. Proteins and fats not used to build and repair body tissues are converted to sugars; if the sugars are not required to meet energy needs, they, in turn, are converted to fats. Some of the effects of a low-carbohydrate diet are fatigue, apathy, dehydration, calcium depletion, kidney disorders, elevated blood lipids, and postural hypotension with ensuing dizziness and fainting. If followed for any length of time, the low-carbohydrate diet may result in permanent damage to the cardiovasculorenal system.

Eating Patterns of Overweight Versus Normal Persons

Other differences between eating patterns of obese and normal persons have been found. Obese people literally do not know when they are physiologically hungry. Rosenstock reports on the following findings from studies done by Stanley Schacter, a psychologist. Using gastric motility as the criterion of hunger, normal subjects reported hunger that coincided with motility 71 percent of the time, but obese people reported it only 48 percent of the time. Twenty-nine percent of the normals did not know whether or not they were physiologically hungry, while 52 percent of the obese did not know.[11] A second finding was that if a normal person was induced to believe he was hungry even though his stomach was full, he did not eat as much as did the obese under the same circumstances. "The obese recognize neither physiological signs of hunger nor

FOUNDATIONS OF HEALTH SCIENCE

physiological signs of satiation." A third finding was that "the obese person eats little when the food and circumstances of eating are uninteresting or dull. The eating behavior of the overweight person is triggered more by external stimuli than internal stimuli.[12]

Rosenstock concludes that if these findings are true, then teaching over-weight individuals "self-control about eating" may have some degree of success. Two techniques are involved. The first is to introduce barriers to eating. One barrier might be to keep only foods in the house that require preparation and then only prepare one portion at a time. Another barrier might be to take only a small amount of food at a time and put down eating utensils until the food is chewed and swallowed. The whole process of eating becomes less automatic.

The second technique is to assure the "experience of immediate and continued success in exhibiting self-control."[13] Detailed records should be kept concerning the quantities and circumstances of all food intake and weight fluctuations and progress. Success in losing is proof of self-control that reinforces continued control.

In addition to the development of self-control, the following principles of nutrition can aid in planning effective reducing regimens:

1. A moderate increase in exercise not only burns up a small number of calories but also creates a feeling of well-being through improved circulation and muscle tone. It also takes the mind off eating. It does not physiologically increase appetite.
2. The first two or three days of decreased food consumption are the most uncomfortable as far as physical feelings of hunger and emptiness are concerned.
3. Fats and proteins should be included with each meal, not only for better nutrition, but also for their satiety value. Eating low-calorie vegetables and fruits that are high in water and cellulose content contributes bulk and a temporary feeling of fullness.
4. The desirable meal pattern varies with each individual. Some people have less of a tendency to snack if they eat five or six small meals than if they eat two or three large meals.
5. After several weeks of dieting, the body adjusts to a different level of intake and weight loss may cease. It may be necessary to reduce caloric intake further. The cessation of weight loss may also be the result of an unusual retention of fluids in the tissue. This condition requires medical assistance. Most people who persist in following their prescribed diet will start to lose again.

The person trying to lose weight might borrow a bit of philosophy from Alcoholics Anonymous. Live one day at a time; just diet today. Each day that less food is eaten than is required for energy needs is an accomplishment. As in the case of the alcoholic, we look at the obese and say, "If you had willpower you could lose weight." But it usually takes more than willpower to lose weight. Like that of alcoholism, the etiology of obesity is obscure and complex. Many answers are still being sought. Mayer states:

> In the long run, what we can hope for from research is a better definition of the various syndromes leading to or associated with obesity. We also hope for a systematic investigation of their etiology and pathogenesis and specific treatments. Meanwhile palliative treatment—a good diet and exercise—is all we can hope to do.[14]

This chronic condition is frustrating, and the prognosis is only fair. If the attitudes toward those afflicted were ones of compassion and encouragement rather than condemnation and derogation, the outlook might be better.

UNDERWEIGHT

Problems of those who are underweight are also difficult to correct. Such persons should base their efforts to gain weight on the same nutrition principles as do the obese. They need to eat frequent meals when they are not fatigued and select foods that are high in calories but low in satiety value. The physiological consequences of underweight are not as serious

Fat is beautiful for some

I am perfectly happy being fat. I have lots of friends—no dates, but lots of friends. I am a good cook, and I'm happy most of the time. But sometimes I find myself overreacting to things. It is important to me that other people view me as intelligent, and I'm not afraid to voice my opinions. So I do express myself —wrong or right, I make my voice come through loud and clear.

I love my family, but all their attempts of offering me money to help correct my weight problem rub me the wrong way. Fat is beautiful. I resent all attempts to change me. I like me the way I am. Who says thin has to be "in" and fat has to be "out"?

Leave me alone. I am happy, really I am. If by bugging me you try to show your love, then I don't want your kind of love. Real love would be accepting me as I am, whether you agree with me or not.

FOUNDATIONS OF HEALTH SCIENCE

as those of overweight, and some degree of underweight is desirable. But the person who is 20 to 30 percent below the average of his or her size and age should be examined medically and should plan a dietary regimen based on professional advice.

DISORDERS OF THE DIGESTIVE TRACT

Disorders of the digestive tract are common. Some are serious and some are minor even though distressing. The number of advertisements for antacids and laxatives makes one wonder if anyone is free from indigestion, heartburn, or constipation. What are the causes of such conditions, and how can they be remedied?

Indigestion and Heartburn

Indigestion and heartburn are characterized by regurgitation accompanied by a burning sensation in the throat, belching, a feeling of fullness and distension, nausea, and abdominal pain. These symptoms can be mild or sufficiently severe to keep the sufferer awake at night. The causes may be dietary indiscretions or such conditions as gastritis, ulcers, cancer, cirrhosis, nephritis, and gallbladder or heart disease.

Dietary indiscretions. The most common cause of discomfort is dietary indiscretion. Overeating too much fatty or "rich food" at one time, and using foods fried in fats at too low a temperature or at a temperature so high that cooking fats or oils burn—all can contribute to indigestion. From experience, people know which kinds of foods seem to upset them, and it is certainly common sense to avoid these. When one is tired, emotionally upset, or under constant tension, the digestive process may be interrupted, and discomfort can result. An occasional use of antacids such as bicarbonate of soda or one of the commercial products will not be harmful. Persistent discomfort should be checked medically. If untreated, symptoms or a disease causing them may become intractable.

Gastritis. Some of the serious disorders affecting the upper portion of the intestinal tract include gastritis, ulcers, and cancer. All three may have the same symptoms. Acute gastritis may result from the ingestion of poisons, drugs, alcohol, or too much food. It should have medical treatment, for it may become chronic. Too much or too little gastric acid may be a factor in gastritis. In most instances, there is *hypoacidity*, which cannot be corrected by self-treatment with antacids or by using foods high in fat.

Constipation

An appreciable number of people worry about the functions of the colon. It is a fallacy encouraged by the advertisers that a "daily bowel movement and regularity" is the normal pattern for all people at all times. Much better criteria of normality are freedom from distension, comfort in defecating, and a soft, formed stool. Abnormal stools can be watery and streaked with mucus or dry and hard. Any sign of blood is a danger signal, as is a persistent change in bowel habits. Functional constipation is most commonly the result of poor habits. It is best to prevent or correct this problem by:

1. Eating a diet containing some roughage such as is found in most fruits and vegetables.
2. Drinking eight to ten glasses of liquid daily.
3. Responding to the urge for defecation and maintaining regular habits of evacuation.
4. Participating in some vigorous activity or exercise each day, which helps maintain muscle tone of the intestinal tract.

During illness and emotional tension, the normal bowel action is apt to be disturbed. Occasionally use of a laxative can relieve a distended, or full, feeling. However, laxatives or enemas should never be used when there is abdominal pain.

Food Poisoning

Another type of intestinal disorder is caused by the contamination of food by parasites, such as bacteria, amoebas, and worms. In the United States, it is rare to find typhoid, dysentery, tuberculosis, diphtheria, botulism, or hemolytic streptococcus being spread by food. However, improper storage of foods in restaurants and homes is still a cause of food poisoning, and while people seldom die from it, many become acutely ill. The exact number of food poisoning cases in this country each year is not known, but estimates range from three to ten million cases. Most of these cases can be prevented by:

Keeping food clean
Keeping food hot
Keeping food cold
Not keeping food very long if it can't be kept hot or cold[15]

Keep food clean. Food must be prepared in clean areas, in a clean manner, and with clean equipment—cutting boards, grinders, can opener, mixer, and utensils. Food should be stored in areas free of vermin and rodents, off the floor, and covered to prevent contamination. Wash your hands before preparing food, cover and wear rubber or plastic gloves if you have a skin infection.

Keep food hot. Hot foods must be kept at a temperature of 140 degrees Fahrenheit or higher. All pork, poultry, and eggs that are dried or frozen must be thoroughly cooked. When using prepared products like cake mixes that contain dried eggs, do not lick the spoon.

Keep food cold. Cold foods should be kept at a temperature of 45 degrees Fahrenheit or less. Prepared foods should be chilled as rapidly as possible. Don't let foods come to room temperature before refrigerating.

Don't keep food too long. Don't keep food for more than four hours if it can't be kept hot or cold. Dishes made with eggs, milk, and salad dressings are particularly dangerous. Custard pies, cream pies, macaroni, and potato salad must be kept refrigerated. *Infectious bacteria in food can double every fifteen to thirty minutes when food is not kept sufficiently hot or cold.*

Sources of food poisoning. Staphylococcus and nonhemolytic streptococcus are the two kinds of bacteria that cause the most trouble. These organisms are prevalent in the air and on the skin. Staph is a common cause of skin infections such as boils, and strep may be carried in the throat. When foods are in the temperature range of 40° to 140°F the pathogens multiply and excrete toxins. Symptoms of illness from staphylococci will develop in five to six hours. The toxins cause diarrhea, nausea, vomiting, and severe

All is not food poisoning

The last time I can remember any semi-serious sickness to anyone close to me was when four or five members of my household were stricken with a stomach virus at the same time. I felt very bad at the time because it was my night to cook, and my dinner was blamed. Although I found out later we didn't have food poisoning, it ruined everyone's ability to eat sweet and sour pork. It was a very unpleasant sickness for all of us, but it felt good to be sick with plenty of company.

cramping. If symptoms are allowed to persist, the victim can become severely dehydrated. Once the toxins develop in a food, it takes high temperatures to destroy them.

Some plants, such as toadstools and hemlock, contain chemical poisons. Shellfish may be a source of poison during specific seasons of the year. Frozen food that has thawed will deteriorate in flavor and consistency, so it is best not to refreeze it. Even if the frozen food has not been opened, there is no assurance that some pathogenic bacteria are not present. Any frozen foods that have been allowed to reach room temperature should be treated in the same manner as fresh foods—stored under refrigeration and eaten within a few days.

Molds formed on foods in the home are usually not harmful. Food that has started to decompose is rarely dangerous if it is still palatable. Ptomaines are nitrogenous products resulting from decomposition. There is no evidence that their ingestion has ever caused human illness. Such decayed foods are unappetizing, but not intrinsically harmful.

Trichinosis. Trichinella infection is more common in the United States than in most other parts of the world. In a 1970 study W. J. Zimmerman and I. G. Kagan found that 2.2 percent of Americans, or some 4.4 million, were infected.[16] The trichina worm most often infests hogs, and the cycle is perpetuated by the feeding of raw garbage to swine. The worms enter the human digestive tract as larvae coiled inside cysts in improperly cooked pork. The larvae mature and copulate, and the embryos migrate to muscle cells, where they grow and become encysted. A severe infection causes fever, muscular pain, blood disorders, and sometimes death by interfering with breathing. The danger to people is primarily from sausages that are eaten uncooked. Cooking all garbage fed to hogs or, better still, preventing the use of garbage as a food, plus microscopic examination of the pork when the pig is slaughtered, would do much to eliminate trichinosis.

Diet and Disease

A number of diseases other than avitaminosis are related to diet. The most common are dental caries, certain gastrointestinal disorders, and the previously mentioned cardiovascular diseases.

Caries. One thing that has been scientifically established is that sugar can promote tooth decay, or caries, and gum disease. Sugar by itself does not cause the problem. Tooth decay and gum disease are related to dental plaque, a sticky, colorless film of harmful oral bacteria that form on the teeth. The combination of sugar and the bacteria in the plaque produces

FOUNDATIONS OF HEALTH SCIENCE

acids that attack the tooth enamel. Sugar in foods that are retained in the mouth because of their consistency are more dangerous than sugars in sweetened beverages. Dentists say that the amount of sugar consumed is not as important as the form (sticky foods that adhere to the teeth are worse than nonretentive foods) and the frequency of between-meal usage.[17]

Gastrointestinal disorders. There is little evidence that the common gastrointestinal disorders are better controlled or cured with special diets than with normal diets. Ulcers have been traditionally treated with a bland diet, but there is no reason to believe that a bland consistency, color, taste, or odor of a food as it enters the mouth is related to its action on the GI tract. People with peptic ulcers should avoid caffeine and alcohol, but otherwise they can eat anything that does not seem to cause distress. Neither is there much evidence that special diets are helpful for gallbladder disorders, regional enteritis, ulcerative colitis, diverticulitis, or other colonic conditions.[18] Patients with diverticulitis benefit more from a normal diet plus extra roughage than from the traditional low-residue, or low-fiber, diet.[19]

> This is not to say that there may not be temporary, acute flare-ups that call for special attention to diet until the episode diminishes. A physician should certainly be consulted during such periods.[20]

Cardiovascular disease. The relationship between cholesterol and cardiovascular disease has been mentioned a number of times. A controversial hypothesis is that lack of dietary fibers, roughage, may be a factor in producing or contributing to ischemic heart disease, occlusive vascular diseases, varicose veins, hemorrhoids, and deep-vein thrombosis. There is experimental evidence that dietary fiber plays a significant role in the prevention of cholesterol gallstones, and the control of obesity, and that it lowers serum cholesterol.[21] In addition, according to Kenneth Heaton, a British physician, as the fiber content of diets goes down, sugar content goes up. Heaton also believes that sugar is a factor in cardiovascular disorders.[22]

Vitamin C is being promoted in England as being antiatherosclerotic. Constance Spittle postulates that vitamin C mobilizes cholesterol from the arteries and enhances its transport to the liver, where it is converted to bile acids. According to Spittle, very large doses of this vitamin will remove cholesterol deposits in arterial walls. Vitamin C exerts another antiatherosclerotic effect by repairing weakened areas in the arterial walls that could act as a focus for cholesterol deposits.[23] The role of vitamin C in tissue repair is well accepted; its relationship to cholesterol has not been widely studied.

One goal of the American Heart Association is to change American patterns of eating by lowering cholesterol and raising polyunsaturates in food choices. The Prudent Diet calls for "reduced calories," from an average of 3,200 to 2,400; "reduced total fat," from 40 percent to 35 percent or less; "increased polyunsaturates, twice as much polyunsaturated fats as saturated fats;" "reduced dietary cholesterol," 300 milligrams or less daily; "adjusted carbohydrate," about 50 percent of total calories from this source derived from complex carbohydrates such as grains, fruits, and vegetables; "reduced salt intake," from today's average of 14.5 grams a day to 5 grams a day; and "stabilized protein intake," 12 to 15 percent of each day's calories.[24]

Corey, a nutritionist at Harvard, recommends the following to reduce dietary cholesterol:

1. Limit drastically the use of pork or pork products that contain high amounts of invisible animal fats.
2. Cut down on the number of times you serve beef, and cut down the size of the portions; trim off all visible fat, and use lean ground beef.
3. Rely primarily on chicken, fish, and veal for animal sources of protein.
4. Increase amounts of unsaturated fats by using vegetable oils and margarine; avoid butter and hydrogenated oils.
5. Use more fortified nonfat milk and fortified buttermilk instead of whole milk; eat cottage cheese in preference to other kinds of cheeses.
6. Limit eggs to three a week including those used in the preparation of baked products (one egg yolk equals 250 mg of cholesterol).[25]

NUTRITION QUACKERY

Despite the abundance and the excellent quality of food available in the United States, there is a constant campaign to discredit the nutritional value of products found in the average market. Because they lack information, too many people are susceptible to the pitch of the faddist and some overzealous promoters of vitamin and mineral supplements. Some faddists are also quacks.

Faddists may go to any length to follow their dietary choices. They are unduly concerned with eating foods that contain the greatest possible amount of nutrients. They emphasize maximal nutritional values and may not consider likes, availability, or cost to be important. They discount the fact that use of a wide variety of foods can provide for the needs of the average person more easily and pleasantly than simple foods.

Faddists are usually emotional about their beliefs, and "proper diet" becomes a cult. The beliefs of these cultists often may not be based on tenable hypotheses. For example, some insist on eating meats at one meal, fruits and vegetables at a second, and cereals at a third. In reality, this schedule reduces the availability of nutrients, since optimal usage is possible only when the essential amino acids, fatty acids, vitamins, minerals, and carbohydrates are digested at the same time. The faddist frequently attributes great values to specific foods. These are panaceas such as virgin honey, brewer's yeast, yogurt, raw sugar, molasses, and wheat germ.

Health educators and scientists of the Food and Drug Administration state that the most common myths propounded by quacks and faddists fall into six groups.

1. That all diseases are due to faulty diets
2. That food supplements and special foods are needed for good nutrition
3. That processed food is not nutritious
4. That depleted soils produce depleted food
5. That "natural" is good and "synthetic" bad
6. That manufacturers and food processors are poisoning foods with additives

Vitamin and Mineral Supplements

Frequently, dietary supplements are advocated as a cure-all for disease. Supplements have their place in medical treatment, and under conditions of stress, malabsorption, and severe deficiencies the physician will prescribe them. At present there is no scientific evidence that they improve the nutritional level of the average healthy individual who eats a variety of the basic foods. Neither can these supplements substitute for a varied diet. There are many trace elements in foods that are necessary for health that are not contained in these pharmaceutical preparations. Since these elements are present in such abundant amounts in food, there is no need to "bottle" them. The role of many trace elements in promoting biological existence is not clearly established.

Trace elements are inorganic elements such as copper, manganese, zinc, cobalt, aluminum, and chromium. They act as catalysts in body processes and are needed for regeneration of red blood cells in certain forms of anemia. Philip White says, "The probability of encountering a deficiency of the trace nutrients in the United States seems very, very remote, as our infants and children are fed a variety of foods and protected from severe infections of long duration."[26] In several studies, those found to have a deficiency have been infants and children who had subsisted on severely restricted diets in countries such as Lebanon and Egypt. These children suffered "near starvation made worse by infection and diarrhea, which causes such a tissue depletion of minerals and other nutrients that the physiological significance of the trace minerals (those needed by the body in quite small amounts) and the less well-known vitamins become manifest."[27]

We do know that vitamins will not cure diabetes, high blood pressure, baldness, arthritis, or flat feet.

Under new Food and Drug Administration regulations, only nineteen essential vitamins and minerals can be included in products marketed as dietary supplements. These nutrients must be in quantities that range from 50 to 150 percent of the U.S. Recommended Daily Allowances, no more or less. These percentages are sufficiently potent to be nutritionally effective without exceeding reasonable limits. Ingredients with no recognized nutritional value, such as bioflavonoids, rutin, and inositol, must be excluded from such supplements. Any food, vitamin, or food supplement containing nutrients in excess of 150 percent RDA is classified as a drug and must be dispensed on a prescription-only basis. Overdoses of vitamins can cause disorders.

It is possible to achieve a nutritious diet from foods available in the marketplace. The majority of us probably do not require supplements, but there is nothing hazardous in taking supplements as defined and controlled by the new regulations. There are a number of fallacies propounded by the faddists about certain of the vitamins.[28]

Vitamin C. Vitamin C has long been recommended as effective in preventing colds. Acceptable scientific evidence disputes this. Controlled studies do show that vitamin C may modify the symptoms of a cold. Excessive amounts can produce gastrointestinal disturbances.

Vitamin D. Vitamin D can accumulate in the tissues, and excesses may lead to deposition of calcium in the soft tissue, as well as bone changes. There is some evidence that too much vitamin D can be a factor in the development of heart disease. More than 400 units per day, the amount in one quart of fortified milk, is not considered safe. More than this amount should be taken under medical supervision only.

Although no special claims are made that more than 400 units per day are desirable, there has been a trend in recent years for food manufacturers to add Vitamin D to various foods. This may be done "purely to promote a product's superiority over other similar products, or in the belief that if a little is good, more is better."[29] The Council on Foods and Nutrition sees no justification for adding Vitamin D to any foods other than milk and margarine.[30]

Vitamin E. Probably no other vitamin has been credited with doing so much. There is no scientific evidence that it will do any of the dramatic

FOUNDATIONS OF HEALTH SCIENCE

things being claimed or that large supplements are needed for the treatment of disease. It does not grow hair, prevent graying, cure skin problems, prevent ulcers, or increase sexual potency.

The amount of vitamin E needed by most people appears to be satisfied by the average, well-balanced diet. This vitamin is plentiful in food—particularly leafy vegetables, whole-grain cereals, and vegetable oils. Some of it is lost in food preparation because of prolonged exposure to heat. So far it has not been possible to specify exactly how much vitamin E humans need, because deficiencies do not produce any recognizable clinical symptoms. The RDA is a hypothetical requirement based on the usual daily intake, rather than a clinically established requirement.

Deprivation of vitamin E has never produced identifiable symptoms of disorder in adult humans. (This statement is based on an extensive examination of the current medical literature and an evaluation of human studies including those that show the normal intake of the vitamin to be adequate). Some premature infants suffer from a deficiency that produces anemia and skin irritation. There is evidence that when oxygen must be administered to premature babies, Vitamin E supplementation will reduce the chance of vision impairment from retrolental fibroplasia. Breast milk, in comparison to cow's milk, is high in vitamin E.

Repeated studies in England and the United States reveal that vitamin E produces no benefits for angina patients. There is also no evidence from controlled studies that it will heal skin blemishes, soften dry skin, erase wrinkles, or act as a deodorant.[31]

Natural, or Organic, Foods

A natural, or organic, food means a product produced without pesticides and herbicides, with natural composts as fertilizer, and without additives. Of the few studies made, evidence suggests there is no difference between organic, or natural, foods and other kinds. The organic people say that processed food is of no value. But unless we eat food raw (and some things are inedible or indigestible raw), all foods are processed in some way. Even the organic food may be processed by extracting, purifying, heating, fermenting, concentrating, dehydrating, cooling, or freezing.

Food faddists recommend the use of natural foods rather than synthetic. They distrust all chemicals. But acetic acid is the same thing as vinegar, and ascorbic acid is the same thing as the vitamin C in an orange. The value of a nutrient remains constant, whatever its form, according to reputable scientists.[32]

The same reasoning is applicable to the use of fertilizers—manure versus chemicals. Fertilization primarily affects yield. The mineral content of food depends on what is in the soil, whether it be essential minerals or toxic metals. The nutrients in the plant depend on its access to organic matter and to sunlight. There is no significant difference between organic matter in a commercial fertilizer, such as phosphate deposits, and organic matter in the form of ground-up rocks and limestone.[33]

However, we do not know the long-term effects of additives and pesticides. Ecologists recommend that it would be wiser to reduce the use of these substances whenever practical.

THE NEW VEGETARIANS

Among the young generation, many are turning to vegetarianism. Vegetarians range from disciples of exotic spiritual or religious sects to people who are very conservative in their religious beliefs. They may live like most of the rest of the population or they may be members of a commune. Many believe that "they can purify their bodies and souls through a new religion and a life style whose essential element is vegetarianism."[34] These new vegetarians are

> usually well educated, self-reliant, socially mobile, and reflect a middle- and upper-class background that is not strongly influenced by ethnic origins. Their diet justification resolves around spiritual purification, mind expansion, health "maximization," ecologic law, gluttony avoidance, and opposition to killing and aggressive behavior.[35]

Unfortunately, despite their intellectual and critical approaches to diets, they sometimes misinterpret facts. Their interpretations of the findings of scientific research in nutrition, which is often taken out of context, leads to severe nutritional deficiencies. They rear their children in their beliefs, since "in their view, it is diet manipulation that gives man ultimate control over his life in terms of creating mental, physical, and spiritual changes that guarantee health, happiness, and well-being."[36]

The new vegetarians endow some foods with curative powers and fear practically every item condemned by folklore. They believe that pork is unclean; red meat leads to aggression (it contains blood); fertile eggs (from hens that have access to a rooster) are better than nonfertile eggs, since they are "natural"; fortified, pasteurized, or homogenized milk is unnatural; and processed, refined, hydrogenated, or fortified foods are poisonous, as is anything containing additives.

Malnutrition among vegetarians does not result from lack of availability of proper food, but from the elimination of certain foods for philosophical reasons. Those who exclude all animal products including dairy products and eggs risk vitamin B deficiency and iron deficiency anemia, lack of protein and the essential amino acids, and insufficient calcium. Children reared on such diets display the typical symptoms of retarded growth and development, including delayed walking, mental apathy, marked abdominal distension, decreased muscle mass, hypotonicity, anemia, and rickets, among other abnormalities.

The cult most apt to produce malnutrition is the Zen macrobiotic group. Members who are fanatical in their dietary practices suffer from scurvy, hypoproteinemia, anemia, hypocalcemia, emaciation, and loss of kidney function. The last condition is the result of the belief that one should not ingest too much fluid and thus overwork the kidneys. The diet is high in sodium, which increases the need for fluids. This compounds the problem.

"Believers in the Zen macrobiotics doctrine hold that there is no incurable disease, that man has unlimited potential for mental, spiritual and physical development. Thus, one who eats wisely and lives morally and in harmony with nature will enjoy mental tranquillity and health and find eternal happiness."[37] The diet is composed of 60 to 90 percent cereal grains, mainly brown rice. According to proponents of the movement, "if one's thoughts are right, one's body can literally change vegetable to animal matter, carbohydrate to sugar, sugar to protein, foods to blood, sodium to potassium, potassium to calcium, sodium to magnesium, magnesium to iron, and so on."[38] A diet of vegetables, grains, beans, and seaweed, for example, supposedly strengthens a person's ability to transmute. Meat, milk, fruits, and drugs destroy transmutation ability.

EATING WISELY AND WELL

Applying the principles of the science of nutrition to living is not complicated. One does not have to spend time each day calculating whether or not one has consumed the necessary nutrients. If weight does not vary more than several pounds from normal from one month to the next, the necessary number of calories are being consumed.

In general, the correct proportions of carbohydrates, proteins, fats, vitamins, and minerals can be obtained by eating a wide variety of foods (including raw and cooked fruits and vegetables) daily and cooking foods in a way that preserves their nutritional value. Storing cooked food in tightly covered containers under refrigeration will assure their safety. As Darla Erhard, a dietician, says

> The human body is obviously a marvelous organism. Despite all our standards of nutrition, it can apparently adapt and survive in a manner

that no one can prophesy on a variety of diets containing different levels of nutrients.[39]

Notes

1. "The State of Nutrition Today," *FDA Consumer*, 7:13, November, 1973.
2. "Academy of Pediatrics Release Comments on National Nutrition Survey," *Nutrition Today*, 8:33, January/February, 1973.
3. John Yudkin, *Sweet and Dangerous* (New York: Peter H. Wyden, Inc., 1972), pp. 172 and 173.
4. Jean Mayer, "Scale Down Your Sugar," *Family Health*, 6:24, 74, 75, April, 1974.
5. "There's a Fly in the Milk Bottle," *Medical World News*, 15:30, May 17, 1974.
6. James L. Breeling, "Are We Snacking Our Way to Malnutrition?" *Today's Health*, 48:50, January, 1970.
7. "When to Start Dieting? At Birth," *Medical World News*, 14:31, September 7, 1973.
8. Ibid.
9. Clifford B. Hicks, "Eat! Says Fat Little Johnny's Mother," *Today's Health*, 48:48–50, February, 1970.
10. "When to Start Dieting? At Birth," pp. 32–33.
11. Irwin M. Rosenstock, "Psychological Forces, Motivation, and Nutrition Education," *American Journal of Public Health*, 59:1993, 1969.
12. Ibid.
13. Ibid., p. 1994.
14. Jean Mayer, "Obesity Control," *American Journal of Nursing*, 65:113, June, 1965.
15. "Food Borne Diseases," *UCSF News*, 1:1, February, 1974.
16. "The Garbage Sickness," *Scientific American*, 229:56, December, 1973.
17. Lou Joseph, "Foods and Drinks that Will Cause You the Fewest Cavities," *Today's Health*, 51:41, October, 1973.
18. Philip L. White, "Smart Eating," *Today's Health*, 52:8, July, 1974.
19. "Roughage in the Diet," *Medical World News*, 15:35, September 6, 1974.
20. White, "Smart Eating."
21. "Roughage in the Diet," p. 36.
22. Ibid., p. 38.
23. "A Vitamin Answer to Atherosclerosis?" *Medical World News*, 15:64h, September 13, 1974.
24. "The Prudent Diet: Vintage 1973," *Medical World News*, 14:35, August 10, 1973.
25. Joyce E. Corey, "Dietary Factors and Atherosclerosis: Prevention Should Begin Early," *Journal of School Health*, 44:511–514, November, 1974.
26. Philip L. White, *Let's Talk about Food* (Chicago: American Medical Association, 1970), p. 68.
27. Ibid., pp. 67–68.
28. "The Food Fad Boom," *FDA Consumer*, 8:5–12, December, 1973–January, 1974.
29. White, "Smart Eating," p. 62.
30. Ibid.
31. "Vitamin E—Miracle or Myth?" *FDA Consumer*, 8:24, July–August, 1973.
32. "The Food Fad Boom," p. 7.
33. Ibid., p. 8.

34. Darla Erhard, "The New Vegetarians, Part I," *Nutrition Today*, 8:4, November/December, 1973.

35. Ibid., pp. 5–6.

36. Ibid., p. 6.

37. Darla Erhard, "The New Vegetarians, Part II," *Nutrition Today*, 9:20, January/February, 1974.

38. Ibid., p. 23.

39. Erhard, "The New Vegetarians, Part I," p. 12.

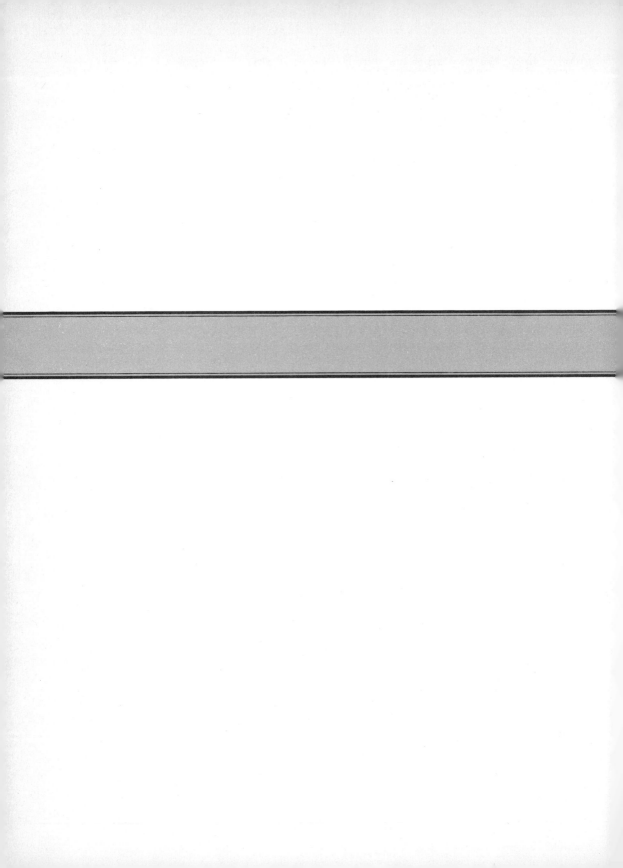

EMOTIONAL HEALTH

chapter six

The emotionally or psychologically healthy individual is one who has learned to cope effectively with himself and his environment. Since the environment is in a constant state of flux and the individual is continuously developing and changing, psychological effectiveness or good mental health is an ongoing process and not a static achievement. The term "mental health" is really a description of behavior. If a person's social and personal behavior appears to be reasonably well integrated, he appears to be reasonably happy, and society generally approves of his behavior, his means of coping with himself and his environment are looked upon as effective and he is said to be psychologically healthy or well adjusted.

Psychological health, then, is a complex process involving ways of thinking, feeling, and behaving. It has a personal as well as a social dimension. The attitudes, ideals, values, and self-concept of the individual are involved along with the values, ideals, and customs of society. The congruence or reconciliation of personal attributes with cultural values involves learning. Learning to cope with oneself, relate effectively to others, and deal effectively with one's environment are lifelong processes.

ADJUSTMENT

There are so many dimensions and criteria of adjustment that we question the usefulness of this concept as an overall characterization of a person. Instead of trying to decide what good adjustment really means, it is better to accept the fact that there are many facets and dimensions of the adjustment process. Following is a series of questions concerning each dimension:

1. How much is the person distracted or bothered by constant environmental factors to which the average or the "ideal" person normally becomes accustomed?
2. To what degree is the person fighting irremediable social circumstances in his life?
3. Does this person's trouble stem from social nonconformity or from rigid overconformity?
4. To what extent are these activities satisfying experiences?
5. How well are individual needs and desires being satisfied?
6. To what extent is the person realizing his potentialities?

We must also consider adjustment to what, adjustment in what way, adjustment in what dimension, and adjustment according to what standards? Within this context it is meaningless to try to indicate a level of adjustment as a single value. For purposes of discussion, seven dimensions of adjustment are now described.[1, 2]

The Selective Awareness Dimension

It is not the quantity or intensity of sensory input that determines the effectiveness of adjustment. Adequate adjustment requires appropriate

This person could use some help

In the past five years I've tried to improve the fact that I worry too much. I worry about what I've done, what I am doing, and what I will do. I see my father, who is a worrier, and hope I don't have his physical problems later in life. He has high blood pressure and has had two heart attacks. I've tried to remove worry from my mind knowing that it does me no good and will change nothing, but my luck hasn't been good—I still seem to worry a lot.

FOUNDATIONS OF HEALTH SCIENCE

selectivity. We are bombarded by more sensory impressions than we can possibly assimilate. In order to survive and be effective, we must perceive when danger is or is not present. We must distinguish between relevant and irrelevant, threatening and benign. We must tune out that which has no relevance and give priority to that which is maximally relevant.

Throughout life each of us is continually bombarded by an ever-changing flow of stimuli. Because of limitations imposed by our attention span as well as by our available time and energy, we are continually selecting those stimuli to which we will respond. If we respond to A, we cannot respond to B. If we attend to this, we cannot attend to that. If we indulge one interest, a competing interest must be deprived. If we are perpetually concerned with trivia, we will never meet up with the more socially important and personally satisfying aspects of life. There has never been a time in which so many components of the universe were capable of making such an impact on mankind. With space being compressed daily by airplanes, missiles, and satellites, with the barriers of distance eliminated by telephone, telegraph, radio, and television, each of us is potentially in touch with a rapidly expanding environment.

Because of the perpetual bombardment of our senses by competing stimuli, it is essential that the well-adjusted person be discriminating. Survival and effective living require that we be sensitive to our environment, but maximum sensitivity to the significant aspects of one's universe requires selective unresponsiveness as well. A high level of attentive concentration on significant problems also implies selective inattention. The selective responsive dimension can be extended to include what has been called the efficient perception of reality. This concept, according to Maslow, involves distinguishing spurious from real, fake from genuine, and dishonest from honest.[2]

This person helped himself

I try to be more concerned about myself and less concerned with other people's feelings. When I thought of others, I was used and manipulated by them instead of being myself and tending to my own needs and wants. I always wondered what other people were thinking of me and what I did. The people that I associated with were the cause of my problem. I don't see these people anymore. I have tried to seek out just a few good friends for healthier relationships. I have my own mind now and am not subject to others' beliefs. I find that my own reasoning and thoughts are perfectly good and I don't worry as much about what other people think as I once did.

Another characteristic of the psychologically healthy person is the quality of detachment. This characteristic includes concentration, productive absent-mindedness, and the ability to be solitary without discomfort. These characteristics imply the presence of habits of responding and not responding, attending and not attending, and the ability to discriminate between essential and nonessential elements of an environmental complex. Rogers calls this an "openness to experience,"[3] but for most effective living this openness must be selective.

Attitudes toward Self and Others

Some psychologists have labeled the way a person perceives himself (his self-concept) and others the central concept in adjustment. The general idea is that each person rather early in life develops a general idea of the kind of person he is and then tends to act in accordance with this self-image. People differ in the degree of permanence, stability, and consistency with which the self is organized. A well-integrated, fairly stable, and personally satisfying self-concept is conducive to optimum adjustment.

The self-concept also implies the complementary concept of *others*. This concept includes a series of expectancies—the social ought's and should's. When a person becomes so other-directed that his acts are continually monitored in terms of "what will other people think of me," he cannot be true to himself, he cannot feel free. He is a slave to the social oughts and cannot function optimally. On the other hand, when one has developed an overrigid set of values (conscience), is completely self satisfied and has a principal defense of self-righteousness buttressed by the conviction that in every way he is always right, he is similarly reduced

Perfection is not always the most satisfactory goal

Tests used to really make me sick. I try not to worry about them now. I go into class thinking that I know what I know and I just try to do my best. I don't try to get A's in everything anymore.

———

I used to plan ahead as to what my friends and I would do during the weekends. Whenever we would take a trip I would always make sure that every detail was planned. Now, I just take the weekends as they come. Everytime I planned something big, I would get too involved. If something didn't turn out just the way I planned it, I would get very upset and take my anger out on somebody. Now I make plans, but not down to every picky detail.

in his capacity for optimum functioning. Compulsive and rigid behavior can be either inner- or outer-directed and controlled.

Ideational flexibility, ability to deviate from conventional restraints and restrictions without being socially insensitive to others, a tolerance of ambiguities, an adequate self-concept with a certain degree of self-dissatisfaction, which characterize highly creative individuals, are also components of the attitudes toward self and others that are conducive to optimum adjustment.

Acceptance of one's self and others, as well as the rest of the individual's entire phenomenal world, are part of this component of adjustment. Cultures differ greatly in what they consider to be the optimal range along the acceptance–striving-for-change scale.

It is quite probable that the ideal American adjustment range will be close to the rejection-of-the-status-quo end of the theoretical acceptance–striving-for-change scale. Each individual functions at some point or range on such a hypothetical scale. Well-adjusted people have reasonably satisfactory self-concepts and accept themselves as they are without thinking very much about the matter. They recognize their own shortcomings without excessive concern. They strive for self-improvement. In doing so they remain problem centered and are not defensive in their motivation. They feel sufficiently guilty concerning their improvable defects to do something about them, but they do not spin their wheels in the quagmire of self-incrimination and anxiety. The discrepancy between their self-concept and their concept of the ideal can be admitted without its constituting an excessive threat. Their self-satisfaction is such that they do not need to pose or be on the defensive.[4]

The well-adjusted person accepts other people. He sees human nature as it is, not as he would prefer it to be. He has a set of values and a moral code, but he can still accept, associate with, and even like people who violate that code. He may not approve of what others do; he may try to change them in ways that he considers desirable, but his concern for them as individuals worthy of consideration and help is not contingent upon their being like him nor upon their conforming to his own conception of what is desirable. The well-adjusted person has an abiding faith in the improvability of people but he neither demands nor expects perfection. He can perceive the worst in human beings without feeling revolted or disgusted.

The well-adjusted person finds the world a pretty good place to live in, but considers that it is still subject to improvement. He neither accepts the world as the best of all possible places nor does he perceive it as hopeless. He does not close his eyes to the world's imperfections and take refuge in passive contemplation. His world is one more of promise than of threat.

A satisfactory position in this dimension requires a reasonably acceptable self-concept (self-acceptance), a high degree of acceptance of others, and a comfortable relation with reality. The ideal for this dimension seems to demand a warm and profound relating of oneself to others (empathy). This involves an ego-extension and an identification with other people. That goes considerably beyond acceptance and tolerance. The well-adjusted person lives comfortably with himself and with others.

A person's self-regarding attitude is a focal component of personality that functions as an important dimension of adjustment. What a person believes about himself—his self-concept—constitutes a kind of internalized road map for living. The self-concept serves as the central focus of his personal life-style and his pattern for social living. One's self-image is developed principally from the reflected appraisals of the significant others in his life. A well-defined, satisfactory, consistent, and stable self-concept is an important dimension of adjustment.

Autonomy

The autonomy dimension of adjustment is currently receiving a critical reevaluation. Many people believe that conformity has a repressive effect on self-realization and creativity. The reaction against those social forces contributing to conformity has sometimes taken the form of a compulsive non-conformity, that can become just as rigid and compulsive as conformity. Both extreme adjustment patterns are handicapping and maladaptive.

What works for some is not the best for all

I was at this college last semester. I transferred here from a community college and found that things at the university are quite different. It was very difficult to get to know people and I didn't seem to fit in anywhere. My classes weren't really what I wanted because I got closed out of the courses I really wanted, so I just took courses because they were required.

After a while I just said the heck with it and dropped out and found a job. I have friends outside of college now and am taking a couple courses and still working. For me this seems to work better. I just hate trying to fit in and play that college routine. At least this way I feel I'm running my own life, have my own place and a few real good friends. To me this is the real world, not the college world where you have to act like everyone else and have a big social life.

The overconforming person is excessively conservative. He has been punished for deviating from socially approved patterns of behavior so often that even the perception of something different, either in himself or in others, is threatening. His social anxiety keeps his behavior within such narrow limits that he is unable to be spontaneous and creative except in restricted socially approved ways.

The compulsive nonconformist is just as limited and socially determined as the extreme conformist. When the social norm dictates neatness, he is slovenly; when others are serious, he is frivolous; when fashion demands formality, he is casual. The nonconformist lacks freedom, flexibility, rationality, and adaptability although he sees himself as free, independent, original, and creative.

Sometimes what passes for nonconformity within the larger cultural context is really conformity to the values and expectancies of a subculture. The adolescent may defy the social dictates of the dominant adult culture in order to be accepted by a peer group whose approval is important to him. The hippie is a conformist within his own culture. His defiance of the broader social conventions is the price of admittance to the inner circle that demands rigid conformity to its own code. This means that social conformity and nonconformity have to be judged within their appropriate contexts.

The well-adjusted individual is both conforming and autonomous in selective ways. Individual and social efficiency, productivity, and creativity require a large amount of social conformity. Maximum concentration on significant problems requires habitual absent-mindedness and a disregard of irrelevant stimuli. Habituation of the tremendous number of daily activities relieves one of the necessity of making daily decisions concerning these acts. This leaves the person free to explore new approaches to significant problems in a special area of competence.

Nonconformity is most likely to be productive in areas where an individual is most knowledgeable. To go off the beaten path in all directions in the hope of becoming creatively productive is not a very fruitful procedure. The artist is most likely to produce promising innovations in the field of art; his attempt to produce advances in chemistry by randomly mixing solutions on the chance that something uniquely useful may be produced is not likely to be fruitful. Because a creative architect must deviate from conventional architectural forms to be productively creative, it does not follow that nonconformity in the way he dresses and talks, or in the kind of car he drives, is an equally promising form of deviation.

Studies of creative people show that such people, early in life, possess the skills and interests necessary to their later achievements. Architects are good at drawing even in childhood. Creative mathematicians have a talent for mathematics. These creative people also have a very high level of interest in their special area of competence. Nonconformity in a person's special area of competence is most likely to be creatively productive.

The emphasis placed by Allport, Maslow, and Rogers on individual autonomy and self-direction as desirable personality traits may or may not be a plea for social nonconformity. The overconscientious person has a high degree of individual autonomy and self-direction. He has internalized a moral code which functions in a very rigid, autonomous fashion. Such a person feels that he is entirely right in all that he does, but his autonomy is maintained at the expense of others' welfare and his own long range social effectiveness. Self-direction is not an unqualified good. Autonomy needs to be tempered with social sensitivity and social perceptiveness. The psychopath may be highly autonomous but he is not an effective social being. Healthy autonomy requires a selective detachment from one's culture.

Personal Integration

The ideal level of personality integration is that of an intermediate position between the extremes of diffusion and disintegration, and rigidity, closure, and self-containment. A lack of personal integration is characteristic of expedient, amoral, and disassociative neurotic people. The well-integrated personality functions as an articulated system with sufficient flexibility to interact with the ever changing requirements of reality. Fact and value are satisfactorily integrated. Life is lived as a whole, with an encompassing view of one's own life and culture. The capacity for change and flexibility of behavior are reconciled with the demands of stability and personal integrity. A unifying philosophy of life operates as a stabilizing influence and provides meaning to one's existence. An inner core of beliefs, socially relevant skills, and personally acceptable attitudes, provides a consistency between the self-concept and external behavior. However, these personality components are not fused in such a way as to preclude the development of new configurations as a result of new experiences.

Creative activity requires both stability and instability of personality organization. It involves the capacity to engage in loose, unregulated thinking (divergent thinking) and the ability to return to critical and regulated thought (convergent thinking). Fanciful, unregulated thinking can occur only when the individual is free of the anxiety and guilt that such thinking commonly arouses. Creativity requires a well-balanced and nicely modulated relating of reality tied and autistic processes, in the same way that adjustment in general requires the balancing of stable and integrated personality components with flexible ones.

FOUNDATIONS OF HEALTH SCIENCE

Self realization, as a distinctly human trait, has been a central concept for many of the humanistically oriented writers. This trait has been called self actualization,[5] self realization,[6] competence,[7] and existential orientation.[8] For Rogers, self actualization is the motivational construct. The organic drives such as food-seeking and sexual satisfaction, and the sensorimotor drives such as exploration, are all basically motivated by the actualizing tendency. For Maslow, the need for self actualization is the highest in his hierarchy of drives (physiological, safety, affection, esteem, and self-actualization).

A basic assumption of self actualization theorists is that human nature is inherently good. Rogers says, "The basic nature of the human being is constructive and trustworthy. When freed of defensiveness and open to experience, his reactions may be trusted to be positive, forward, and constructive." This is a restatement of the ancient doctrine of man's inherent goodness. According to such a conception, man is born without sin. He aspires to goodness and moves toward perfection. All human evil is of exogenous origin. It is the betrayal of man's inherent nature by unfortunate environmental circumstances. Man is misled by the false goals of society. If he can only be kept free from the fetters of society he can reach unlimited heights of satisfaction and achievement. If this sounds familiar, it is because it has been stated and restated by others throughout history, most notably by Rousseau when he said, "Let us lay it down as an incontrovertible rule that the first impulses of nature are always right. There is no original sin in the human heart. . . . Leave the germ of his [the child's] character free to show itself; do not constrain him in anything, so you can better see him as he actually is. . . . Man is by nature good, only our institutions have made him bad.[9] Rousseau eloquently poured out his invectives against artificiality, insincerity of fine manners, snobbishness of higher social classes, callous extravagances of the rich financed by exactions from the poor, and impoverishment of human life by the replacement of sentiment and intuition with science and logic. Man can only be saved by abandoning the blind alleys of philosophy and science and returning to the honesty, naturalness, and simplicity of nature. These sentiments have been echoed and reechoed throughout the ages.

It is obvious that the humanistic concept of self-actualization assumes the same things that Rousseau postulated in the eighteenth century. Growth is a self activated, self directed, and internally regulated process, which, if permitted, will unfold in accordance with a prearranged design. A maximally permissive environment facilitates this development by not interfering with the direction dictated by this spontaneous motivation.

Social learning theorists consider the principal components of self-actualization a socially learned process whereby the person reinforces his own achievement and progress toward highly valued goals. This process includes:

1. the development of internalized standards of excellence (levels of aspiration, ideals, value systems, concept of an ideal self);
2. self evaluation of one's present status and rate of progress with regard to these standards;
3. psychological tension because of any perceived discrepancy between present status and the ideal (cognitive dissonance); and
4. positive or negative effect (satisfaction or dissatisfaction) incident to progress toward, or behavior consistent with or inconsistent with, these standards of excellence.

According to such a conception, self realization consists of moving toward the realization of one's ideals and behaving in ways that are consistent with these standards. Behaving in these ways is being true to one's best self, moving in the direction of being the best that one is capable of being, being truly human, and being a good person, to use the terms of the humanists. Moving away from these standards is being false to one's self, being less than human, being bad or conscience stricken when the principles involved are moral ones.

High self-actualizers are individuals who receive positive self reinforcement because they tend to perform those classes of responses, entertain those thoughts, and experience those impulses and feelings that are consistent with achieving goals which they value most highly. Self administered reinforcements outweigh the influence of social and material rewards and punishments in governing behavior. Freedom consists of achieving and developing in ways we perceive as most worthwhile.

The social learning concept, like the humanistic one, grants that man is the only self-actualizing organism. As far as we can tell, man is the only animal who is critical of his own actions. He is acting uniquely when he looks at his proposed ways of behavior, his wishes, desires, feelings, and impulses, evaluates them, and labels them as good or bad. Such a conception of self-actualization does not deprive the idea of any of its essential characteristics. However, the concept does deny its innate origin, its universal nature, and the infalliability of its standards of excellence in terms of which self-actualization is viewed.

Environmental Mastery

Maslow refers to this dimension as problem-centering. He insists that persons displaying optimal adjustment focus strongly on problems outside themselves. Allport refers to this characteristic as the ability to lose oneself in work or play. People high in this dimension have missions in life, significant tasks to fulfill, movements or activities that enlist their time and energy. These individuals live and work within a large frame of reference. The problems and movements in which they became immersed tend to be social, moral, and philosophical ones rather than more immediate and specific day to day tasks. Being concerned with a wide frame of reference and a total commitment often imparts to them, a certain serenity and a lack of anxiety over immediate concerns. For this reason, it is possible for such people to maintain a certain quality of detachment and to remain relatively undisturbed by the minor irritations and shortcomings that produce turmoil in others. Since they are more problem- than ego-centered, they are more concerned with the problem itself than with their own wishes and hopes with reference to the situation. Vance has claimed priority for this characteristic as a criterion of good mental health.

Rogers has listed two general conditions that he considers to be favorable to creative activity: psychological safety and psychological freedom. Acceptance of the individual is one of the most important factors conducive to psychological safety. Creative children, as a group, are aware of those traits which their culture, teachers, and peers value highly, but they do not want these traits for themselves.

Highly creative people deviate from the cultural norm, and they recognize this fact. It follows from the very nature of creativity that creative activity must be different; it must be deviant behavior. When acceptance of the person is conditional upon conformity, creative people will be devalued as individuals, and their deviant ideas will be discouraged. Therefore, a society that provides a wide variety of socially approved roles for its citizens will be accepting of the deviant creative individual. In a culture that is highly tolerant of a minority of one, the deviant person can be what he is without posing or pretending. He does not feel less worthy because he is different. In a nonthreatening social environment, the creative individual will have a low level of anxiety. His principal sources of motivation will be the positive satisfactions of exploration and discovery rather than the reduction of anxiety. When this person feels psychologically safe, he is not afraid to develop and express his divergent ideas.

When the creatively deviant individual associates with people who are able to understand and appreciate his world, he can be comfortable and need not waste time and energy protecting himself. He can be divergent without being defensive. He can be a nonconformist without suffering social disapproval.

Psychological freedom, described by Rogers, is in many ways a consequence of psychological safety. Some of the characteristics of the person who is psychologically free are:

1. He is able to accept himself for what he is without fear of being laughed at or ridiculed
2. He can give at least symbolic expression to his impulses and thoughts without having to repress, distort, or hide them
3. He can handle percepts, concepts, and words playfully and in unusual ways without feeling guilty
4. He sees the unknown and the mysterious either as a serious challenge to be met or a game to be played

Many people believe that the prevailing cultural and educational climates in America today are not rewarding creative people commensurately with their potential value to society. They suggest that to promote creativity, we need to provide a more friendly and rewarding environment for the encouragement of creative activities. To accomplish this will require us to cease equating ideational divergence with mental illness. We will have to recognize the value of a wide diversity of talents, encourage children to perceive things in unconventional ways, increase our tolerance of people who perceive and think in ways that are different from our own, and develop specific methods for teaching and for encouraging creativity.

MOTIVATION AND ADJUSTMENT

The wants, wishes, desires, and purposes of the individual are motivational factors. Each person must develop, for himself, means for their satisfactory attainment or resolution. Behavior designed to cope with one's motives and the environmental influences that may assist or impede their satisfaction has been called *adjustive* behavior. The development of effective coping behavior has been called *adjustment*. Motivation and adjustment are closely related. Motives derive from social-cultural learning and are subject to modification with experience. Means of coping with motives and with the environment are also developed through experience. Thus, it can be seen that adjustment involves physical, motivational, and learning components.

Motives are connected with the wants, wishes, desires, and purposes of the individual and the manner of their attainment. They may be classified according to the goals or purposes that behavior is intended to achieve. The motives of man are many and varied. It has become conventional to group motives into categories for purposes of discussion. All such classifications are arbitrary and derive principally from the opinion of those doing the classifying.

A classification system that is usable within the context of psycholog-

FOUNDATIONS OF HEALTH SCIENCE

ical health divides the social motives into two large groups—the *affiliation-oriented* and the *prestige-oriented*.

Affiliation-oriented Motives

The affiliation-oriented motives constitute the most basic of the socially directed behavioral forces. They represent a series of continuums ranging from a desire to be with other people rather than to be alone (gregariousness), at one end, to a preference for the presence of people with whom we have a common language and interest (social interaction) as contrasted with "foreignness," to a preference for people with whom we have had previous pleasant experience (friends) as compared with strangers, as intermediate categories, to a desire to have continued intimate contact with our loved ones, at the other extreme. The series of social relationships encompassed by the affiliative motives range in their degree of affectional or emotional involvement from minimal (gregariousness) to the most intimate of emotional ties as found in the parent-child, husband-wife relationships (love).

Derivation of the affiliation motives. Although the evidence is not entirely consistent, affiliative motives are probably learned. They develop as the result of the child's inevitable contacts with people. In infancy, other people are the food givers, the warmth providers, and the irritant removers. People are the source of the child's principal satisfactions. Because of the association of people with the satisfactions of the child's organic sources of drive, the physical contact with the sight and sound of people become desirably pleasant in themselves.

As the result of this early and continuing conditioning, we come to desire the company of other people. We are especially motivated to perpetuate our contacts with those acquaintances, friends, and loved ones with whom our associations have been pleasant. We become gregarious. We feel lonely when deprived of human contacts and strive to reestablish them. The fact that solitary confinement is generally considered to be a severe form of punishment is evidence of the universality and strength of the affiliative motives. Harlow's studies showing that young monkeys develop affectional motives to mechanical surrogate mothers that serve as sources of food, warmth, and contact, support the contention that the affiliative motives are learned.[10]

As the child develops, he comes to attach differential meanings to various social cues. Because certain postures, gestures, facial expressions, and sounds regularly precede or accompany either positive or negative reinforcements (rewards or punishments), they come to have particular ideational meanings and emotional associations for the child. For example, a smile, a light tone of voice, and a rising inflection regularly accompany patting and playing with the child; a frown, a threatening tone of voice, and a falling inflection either precede or accompany the withdrawal of affection, spanking, and other forms of punishment. The facial expressions and vocal cues alone come to operate as substitute stimuli in place of the original stimuli with which they have become associated.

When facial expressions, gestures, and words have acquired either positive or negative emotional values, they operate as motivational factors in themselves. Thus, the child does those things that will obtain for him smiles, words, gestures, and other signs of commendation, and he tends to avoid those things that result in the withdrawal of commendation and the administration of reproof. The child tries to avoid words of criticism because these words have become emotionally loaded as a result of their associations with either punishment or the withdrawal of approval.

Significance of affiliative motives. The affiliative motives are seldom manipulated purposely. However, they are frequently involved without this fact being recognized. The affiliative motives constitute the differential that causes a student to work hard for the teacher he likes and to refuse to do so for the one he dislikes. If we are commended by parent, teacher, or friend our affectional relationship with that person is likely to continue or increase in intimacy. On the other hand, blame, reproof, and scolding may signify rejection, withdrawal of affection, and partial social isolation. In our culture we receive love and social acceptance as a result of engaging in culturally approved activities. As a result we develop a tendency to behave in conformity with the desires of those whose good opinion we value and whose association we seek.

Once affectional relationships have become established, they become powerful motivating devices in themselves. Behavior is modified to ensure continued affective relationships. The prospect of disruption of personal-social relationships acts as a deterrent to certain kinds of behavior just as the prospect of establishing or continuing a specific affiliation is an impetus to other kinds.

Prestige-oriented Motivation

People not only want to associate with other people, they also want the approval of others. We all like to receive the recognition, the applause, and the acclaim of our fellow man. This desire for status in the eyes of others represents the motive for prestige. Very early in life children learn that many of life's sweetest satisfactions derive from the elevation or maintenance of status with other people. When we learn to derive satisfaction from the maintenance of prestige for engaging in personally and socially acceptable behavior, prestige does not represent a serious problem. However, if we cannot develop behaviors that are worthy of prestige in the eyes of others, serious problems may arise. Ideally, prestige motivation should represent a desire to achieve in personally satisfying and culturally approved areas and to be recognized for the achievement.

People tend to be motivated to engage in activities that will produce achievement in areas that are revered by the culture. The motive to achieve in these areas has been termed the achievement motive and the strength of such a motive has been measured among various groups in the culture.[11]

Our culture is a tremendously competitive one, and people living in it develop an almost universal desire to outdo their fellow men. There is hardly an aspect of our culture that does not bear the imprint of competitive striving. Children become committed to the competitive race for superiority, and their competitive tendencies may become so strong that they never really escape from the commitment to rigorous striving as a way of life.

Social relationships are permeated with competition. It is interesting to reflect on the social conversations in which one has engaged in the past few days. How many of these started as idle, social chit-chat and degenerated into a duel for supremacy between the participants? One person relates an incident of interest, whereupon the next individual tells of some event more interesting, startling, or superior to the first. The person whose story is more interesting, more unusual or superior in any way to the other's adds an increment to his feelings of prestige. After all, the story was superior and he borrows some of the superiority of the story for himself. It is proverbial, in storytelling situations, that the first person doesn't have a chance. The temptation to compete in such situations is very great, as witness the fact that in a group situation one rarely hears related *only one* joke or funny story. Someone usually has another that must be told, and so on, until many have joined the competition.

When competitive striving in social situations becomes too exaggerated, there develops a tendency to derogate and belittle others. The tendency to retell and exaggerate malicious gossip, make petty remarks, and criticize others is probably motivated by a desire to make oneself appear better or more virtuous than others. If many of our acquaintances can be said to be dull or dishonest our own lack of virtue in these areas may not be so personally painful. When this tendency to derogate others is carried to the extreme, we look for the shortcomings of others, gloat over their mistakes, and revel in their misfortunes. Such behavior, of course, is representative of inadequate adjustment and may be considered to be psychologically unhealthful.

People's efforts to get others to notice them, to regard them as distinctive, to obtain excellent school grades and honors, to become skilled technically or artistically, to climb the social ladder, to get their names in print, and to cultivate the acquaintance of the great and the near great are all partially if not dominantly prestige-motivated. When obtaining the attention of others is a prerequisite to establishing status with them, attention-getting behavior becomes rather common. The obtaining of attention may become a substitute for the establishment of prestige because the two are invariably associated with each other. Attention-getting behavior can thus become well established and we deceive ourselves, but usually not others, by mistaking attention for status. Excessive personal idiosyncrasies in dress, speech, manner, and other nonconformities can thus become personally deceptive means of substituting attention for prestige.

Status and status symbols. Symbols of prestige vary from culture to culture and from generation to generation. When people expend reasonable effort in approved ways to attain status or superiority in those areas that the culture values highly, their behavior is recognized as healthful and is approved. Children growing up in the culture learn of those things that are worthy of prestige and also acquire the culturally approved means of their attainment.

In modern American culture competitive success is idealized to an extreme degree. People growing up in the culture become committed to striving strenuously and persistently. The following expressions and exhortations are illustrative of this commitment:

1. Whatever you do you must do with all your might
2. There is nothing that you can't do if you only want to badly enough and try hard and long enough
3. If at first you don't succeed, try, try, again
4. Hitch your wagon to a star
5. There is always room at the top
6. Never give up
7. Never be satisfied until you are at the top
8. Onward and upward

Although we recognize that all of these statements are not strictly true and may be amused by them, we may recognize also that they represent an

FOUNDATIONS OF HEALTH SCIENCE

American philosophy. As a result of this philosophy, the typical American develops an enormously competitive striving for superiority. This undoubtedly has its values in a vigorous and expanding economy and a progressive technology. Inevitably, it also leads to widespread discontent, dissatisfaction, frustration, and discouragement. For a person with limited capacities and resources, adopting a hitch your wagon to a star philosophy may set the stage for feelings of futility, disappointment, and guilt incidental to the ultimate realization that he is not going to fulfill his destiny.

Individual and cultural differences in prestige values. With very young children prestige may derive largely from appearance. The child is cute or attractive or the opposite, quite irrespective of sex. As boys mature, prestige becomes more a matter of physical power than appearance. The largest, the strongest, the fastest, and the best fighter becomes the one with the most prestige. Most girls soon renounce reliance on physical power in favor of appearance. To be beautiful, to be lovely, or to be adorable is to achieve prestige.

In adolescence, status becomes tied up with the attaining of independence and self-sufficiency. Independence from adult control becomes a mark of status and maturity. Many young people obtain this status because of their own self-sufficiency and apparent lack of need for adult approval. Frequently, adolescent leaders are those who are independent of adults and self-sufficient enough not to actively seek either adult or peer approval. Other adolescents emulate their adult-independent behavior and seek approval from their peers and adolescent leaders. Independence of adult authority is a symbol of maturity that has great prestige value. It marks the individual as being self-sufficient, competent, and independent. Much of the adolescent rejection of certain adult values and behavior stems from the prestige value of being independent. A difficult task for the adolescent is to discriminate between those adult values and behaviors that should be perpetuated and those that should be discarded. In the quest for independence, the temptation to reject the entire adult world rather than selective aspects of it that have become outmoded is sometimes very great. The healthy person learns to make these discriminations and becomes effective in producing cultural change.

People differ widely in the relative values they attach to intellectual, social, athletic, and other achievements. Typically, they place greater value on the types of proficiency that they themselves have or can develop. All-around or over-all superiority is not necessary for the development or maintenance of an acceptable self-concept or for the attainment of satisfactory status with others.

A principal source of disturbance in old age is the deflation of the self-concept incidental to the aging process. If the elderly person continues to receive social recognition and esteem, the loss of physical power and stamina does not entail loss of satisfaction with living. Life is still worthwhile. If our self-satisfaction has been exclusively tied in with physical prowess or attractiveness, the physical deteriorative effects of aging may be devastating to our self-concept. The development of interests and values that will permit prestige to derive from a variety of sources may be some insurance against loss of prestige and consequent deflation of the self-concept.

Cultural differences in those things that are prestige enhancing are bound to exist. For the most part whatever behaviors, attributes, or possessions are revered by the culture will come to be revered by the people in that culture. Thus, persons of one cultural background may get prestige from achievements, behaviors, attributes, and possessions that are quite different from those of another cultural background.

ADJUSTING

Whenever anything occurs to disrupt motivated behavior the individual is said to be *frustrated*. Frustration can be conceptualized as a response to the disruption of ongoing behavior. It is a response that has stimulating properties, causing the organism to make further responses. The responses elicited by the stimuli of frustration are called *adjustments*. Adjustment, as such, is not evaluative or conformative. Whatever response is made to the frustrating situation is termed *adjustive*. It may be socially or personally desirable or undersirable from an evaluative point of view and it may be socially conformative or nonconformative, or it may have combined elements of both. The adjustments (responses) that are made are dependent upon a great number of factors including previous experience, the source of the frustration, the strength of motivation, and the ability of the individual to cope with the situation. Adjustive or adaptive responding ranges from very simple and uncomplicated to extremely complex.

Frustration can be produced by a variety of situations. The basic situations can be classified as thwarting, delay, and conflict. See Figure 6.1, "Frustration by Thwarting."

Frustration by Thwarting

Interference with motivated behavior (or what one wants to do) in almost any fashion can be considered thwarting. Any prevention of a re-

Figure 6.1 Frustration by Thwarting. An organism (S) is motivated to approach (1) a goal. It encounters a barrier (2), is thwarted and tries various responses (3). One response successfully gets around the barrier (4).

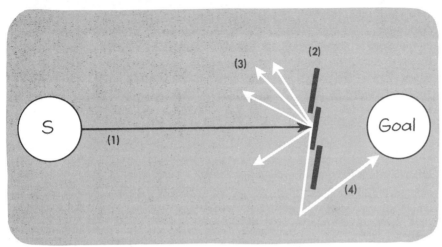

sponse or interference with the occurrence of motivated behavior results in frustration. In the learning situation presented to a hungry rat in a maze, there are barriers between the animal and food. Frustration of a minor sort occurs as the result of these obstructions. Minor frustrations are an inevitable and necessary part of learning. If thwarting in the learning situation is temporary and can be overcome by appropriate behavior, learning will take place. Thwarting that is prolonged and cannot be resolved readily or at all is intense, and can interfere with learning.

Society places many rules, regulations, and restrictions on behavior. The setting of unattainable standards by parents is frustrating to a child.[12] Some thwarting of infants and children is inevitable, but it can safely be said that much of adult thwarting of children is not necessary for the welfare and protection of the child. The unnecessary thwarting of children's activities stems from the thwarting experienced by the parents and their own consequent frustrations.

Personal sources of thwarting. Obstacles to performance that produce frustration may include our own physical characteristics. The physically clumsy or inept, for example, cannot do well in games calling for physical agility. The person who is physically ill cannot engage in physically strenuous activity. The physically handicapped can be severely frustrated by their disabilities. Some physical characteristics serve as thwarting agents, not because of actual restriction, but because of the personal or social value placed on the possession of the characteristic. Skin blemishes in either a man or a woman may act as thwarting agents and prevent the establishment or maintenance of satisfactory social relationships.

Although unattractive physical characteristics may be a deterrent to effective social interaction, it is probably true that the person's self-*characteristics,* operates as the more effective barrier to socialization. A concept, *his own evaluation of himself as a person possessing these* person with a poor self-concept can lack self-confidence, which in turn leads to anxiety over personal failure. This anxiety, then, can be a thwarting agent.

Social sources of thwarting. The source of much frustration is social in nature. A person may want to become a member of a particular group, club, or society and be prevented from doing so by religion, race, or economic status. Attending college may be interrupted or prevented by economic or social barriers. Legal restrictions, such as laws about driving or marriage, may operate as social barriers.

Thwarting frequently results from the behavior of other people. Others do not always behave in the way that is most conducive to the satisfaction of our motives. Their behavior is designed to satisfy their own motives rather than ours, and the resultant behavior may constitute a barrier to the satisfaction of our motives. The frustration of adolescents by the behavior of their parents has received a good deal of attention in our culture. Adolescents also frustrate their parents. Girl friends thwart their boy friends. Brothers and sisters can be sources of frustration to each other. Teachers frustrate students and students frustrate teachers. The listing of persons who act as thwarting agents for other persons could be extended almost indefinitely.

Frustration by one circumstance or another is a lifelong process. Some frustrations occur at all ages; others are peculiar to a specific age. The desire to be independent and free from the restraint of living with one's parents results in frustration when independence is unattainable because of lack of money, immaturity, or family responsibilities. Many people would like to travel and see the world but are thwarted by economic considerations, social circumstance, or emotional involvements. People are frustrated when they want to get a job and employment is unavailable, or they do not possess the necessary training or experience.

The desire to get a college education may be thwarted by a number of factors. Admission requirements are high and one cannot qualify, or economic or social circumstances make a college education unattainable. The wish to marry can be thwarted by a host of factors, including age, financial insecurity, emotional insecurity, inability to establish affectional relationships, and physical illness. As life moves along one may want to retire but not be able to because of personal responsibility and social obligation. Or a person may want to work beyond retirement age but finds that employment is impossible because of a legal restriction or physical infirmity.

Frustration by Delay

When a response has regularly been reinforced or successful and now the reinforcement is delayed or is not available, the consequences are frequently those of frustration. The period of delay may vary from being only momentary to an indefinite period of time. If the delay is momentary there is only a slight break in the ongoing behavior of the organism. This slight delay in receiving reinforcement precipitates frustration. The reaction is emotional and the ensuing behavior is affected.

The frustrations of waiting until you are old enough can probably be recalled by most people. It is easy to recall the frustration produced because we were not old enough to get a drivers license or not considered mature enough to have our own apartment.

Frustration resulting from delay in achieving sexual reinforcement is prominent among adolescents in our culture. Stimulation for sexual activity is strong and its expression must be delayed. Autosexual behavior is frowned upon in our society and other sexual contacts are forbidden. The adolescent is told he must wait until a certain age, when marriage is permissible, to engage in heterosexual activities. Other means of sexual expression are punished. Sexual frustrations as a source of personality problems have received a great deal of attention from clinical and personality theorists. Clinical evidence indicates that these frustrations have important dynamic influences on personality.

Frustration by Conflict

Conflict is a descriptive word used to identify those situations in which a person is motivated to behave in two incompatible ways. In thwarting, attainment of a motive is blocked by some barrier and the situation must be adjusted to by some means. In conflict, the individual is confronted by equally desirable or equally distasteful situations between which he must choose.

Most people find that their conflicting motives are not perfectly counterbalanced, fortunately, since exactly counterbalancing motives would result in their doing nothing at all to resolve the situation and tension would remain undiminished. Conflicts are most usually of such a nature that one motive is stronger than the other. Even so, most people occasionally find themselves suffering from the demands of conflicting motives, which can lead to difficulties in personal adjustment.

Lewin describes conflict as an interaction between an individual and his environment.[13] His system of concepts is useful in the understanding of conflicts. People respond to things in their psychological environment and learn to be either attracted or repelled by them. The tendency for an object or situation to either attract or repel the person serves as the basis for the person's responses. The degree to which an object elicits approaching or avoiding responses from the individual is its *valence*. Objects toward which an individual makes approaching responses are said to have *positive valence*, and objects that evoke avoiding responses have *negative valence*.

A person's response to each aspect of his environment is either to approach it or to retreat from it, unless a given object has zero valence for him. The strength of the response tendency is a function of the valence of the object and its psychological distance. A distant goal is usually approached less strongly than a similar one close at hand. A threat that is close at hand evokes stronger avoidance responses than one that is not immediate or imperative.

Four types of conflict situations may arise between the tendencies to approach and to avoid objects.[14] The *approach-approach conflict* occurs rather frequently and is usually rather readily resolved. When two alternative goals are equally or nearly equally attractive, conflict results. Slight fluctuation in motives or in the environment usually cause such situations to be resolved without too much difficulty. Approach-approach conflicts are apparent when we must decide which TV program to watch, which motion picture to attend, what to order from a menu in a cafe, and in other similar situations where the same motive would be satisfied by either decision. There are more complicated approach-approach situations, in which one motive must be satisfied at the expense of the other.

It may be impossible to be a member of one social group and do good work in school at the same time. Some social groups are so active that they interfere with study time; some groups are disdainful of academic endeavor and thus make it difficult, if not impossible, for a member to be socially acceptable and academically prepared at the same time.

Avoidance-avoidance conflicts are those produced when the individual must choose between two unpleasant alternatives. As he approaches one it becomes more unattractive and so he withdraws. As he approaches the other its negative qualities become more and more apparent and he tends to avoid it too. For example, failure versus tediousness of study. A student may vacillate for a short time, then resolve that study is absolutely necessary. He finds himself easily distracted and frequently tempted to do other things. He may spend much time daydreaming or

192   FOUNDATIONS OF HEALTH SCIENCE

avoid the unpleasant task by lengthy and elaborate preparations for study. These are devious ways to escape the situation.

The resolution of conflicting motives of the avoidance-avoidance type is difficult. In such a situation as the one described, in which the student wants to avoid study and to avoid failure at the same time, psychological distance becomes an important factor. Failure of a test or failure in a course is not as immediately imperative as the unpleasant prospect of study. The student neglects his study because it is the closest of the two unattractive alternatives. This does not satisfactorily resolve the conflict, because he will still suffer anxiety over the possibilities of failure. But his behavior is controlled by the strength of his motives at the moment. His motivation to avoid the whole unpleasant situation may be stronger than either the motive to avoid study or to avoid failure. When this is the case this avoidance motive will dominate, and the person will tend to escape the whole affair, at least for the moment. He cannot approach either undesirable activity so he removes himself from the situation.

When a single object or situation possesses characteristics that tend to attract and to repel the individual at the same time, it has both positive and negative valence—*approach-avoidance*. The tendency to approach and the tendency to avoid are in conflict. Such conflict situations are relatively common. Wanting to marry but not to assume responsibilities is such a situation.

Approach-avoidance conflicts are not resolved by escape. If the person withdraws, his fear and tension are temporarily reduced but he still wants to approach the favorable aspects of the situation. His motives to approach are active when he is farther from the conflict. As he approaches the situation his fears are reactivated. A vicious circle of conflict is thus established. The person is in almost a constant state of fear and tension. When motives to approach and to avoid are nearly evenly matched, the individual may vacillate between the two motives, and tension is maintained at a high level.

Double approach-avoidance conflict situations involve two complex stimuli. That is, each of the two stimuli elicit both approach responses and avoidance responses. If the choices are multiple rather than just two, the conflict would be more appropriately designated multiple approach-avoidance. However, it is conventional to refer to all of these complex situations as double approach-avoidance.

Conflict situations that develop in the course of living are frequently of a complex nature. The woman with two suitors between whom she must choose probably illustrates multiple approach-avoidance conflict. Both men may be attractive to her, but one is more talkative, one is more economically secure, one is taller, one has a better sense of humor, or one is more aggressive than the other.

SOURCES OF FRUSTRATION

There are a great number of potential sources of frustration in everyone's life. It would be impossible to discuss or even to list all of them. Two common sources of frustration are given brief consideration here.

The Family

The family exerts a powerful influence on its members. It is the source from which much emotional strength can come as well as a possible source of frustration and emotion-arousing experiences. Chronic disagreement and quarreling by parents can leave a child emotionally exhausted. The entire home atmosphere is one of anxiety and tension. It never lets up. It is always there. The child becomes insecure. The mother's good is the father's bad and vice versa. Home life is essentially unhappy and tension-producing.

Harsh or overly restrictive discipline causes emotional strain in children. The child who cannot engage in the usual activities of his age group because of parental restrictiveness will resent the parent and feel like an outsider in groups with which his friends can identify. When harsh discipline is common, genuine fear and deep resentment can ensue. This may result in constant anxiety and apprehension.

Children from broken homes have more problems of adjustment and have more serious problems in general than other children.[15] Studies have not indicated whether the broken home as such is anxiety-producing or whether the familial lack of harmony that led to and followed the divorce or separation was the main cause of the emotional stress. Whether a child comes from a broken home or not it has been found that family conflict has a pronounced effect on the offspring of various ages[16] and social class.[17]

In an increasing number of families both parents are employed outside the home. Research has not answered the question of whether or not the mother's place is in the home. A study by Clancy and Smitter indicated that elementary school children whose mothers were employed full time outside the home have more serious problems than others.[18] The reasons for the mother's employment outside the home may be significant factors. It is possible that many of the homes studied were broken homes and the mothers were the sole support of the family. In such cases there would be the combined effects of a broken home and a working mother. Another study dealing with adolescents indicates that the relationship between children and their parents was better when the mother worked part time than when the mother did not work outside the home at all or was em-

FOUNDATIONS OF HEALTH SCIENCE

ployed full time.[19] *The basic feelings of acceptance and understanding in the parent-and-child relationship are probably more important variables than the mother's employment as far as emotional climate is concerned.*

Studies of the effects of separation from parents[20] and of attachment behaviors in infancy[21] attest to the importance of consistency of infant-adult interactions in the life of the child.

Sex

The restrictive attitude of American culture toward sexual behavior among children and adolescents causes sex to be a potent source of emotional disturbance. Boys and girls in our culture frequently learn that sex is immoral, dirty, or shameful. Our society condones only a minimum of sexual stimulation and advocates abstinence until after marriage. In spite of the teachings of the culture, adolescents engage in a wide variety of sexual behavior. Kissing and petting are extremely common, as even the most naïve adult observer will report. According to Kinsey, 95 percent of boys have had their first orgasm by the age of fifteen, and by the age of twenty, 71 percent of males and 40 percent of females have engaged in intercourse.[22] Condoned or not, adolescents engage in homosexual behavior, masturbate, and have intercourse. Sexual activity is far more abundant in adolescent males than in females. Feelings of guilt and shame for engaging in sexual activities that are not condoned by society in general can have serious consequences. The person can and frequently does feel that he is immoral, weak, and sinful.

A counselor could help with this not unusual problem

A family problem is really messing me up now. I am twenty years old and the oldest of three children. My parents separated some years ago and I have increasingly become the go-between. Whenever my father has something to tell my mother he tells me to take the message to her. Whenever it is time for my father to give us the support money, my mother makes me go after it. Whenever my mother is upset with my father for any reason I have to relay that message. I feel like they are running me around like a messenger boy. My mother leans on me too much because I'm the oldest and the only boy. I would like to cut out and go live on my own, but my mother couldn't handle things. I feel trapped between my parents who are supposed to be grown ups.

Ignorance of sex and sexual functioning can cause great anxiety in the young female when she first menstruates or in the young male when he has a nocturnal emission. When these functions are not understood they can be frightening and cause prolonged anxiety.

Retardation of sexual development in young people can cause emotional strain. Immature boys and girls may be embarrassed and humiliated to have to dress and undress in the locker room in front of boys or girls the same age and in the same grade who are more fully developed. They may also worry about the possibility that they are not going to develop. Or they may have developed early and worry that there is something physiologically wrong.

Many children learn to fear sex and sexual responses from the earliest training they receive. The child whose experiences at home with the topic of sex have been to hear it whispered about, denounced as immoral, and cautioned against rather than referred to as good, normal, and healthy can hardly be expected to go through adolescence without considerable anxiety about it.

Lack of social skills—not knowing how to become acquainted with the opposite sex—can be a source of sexual conflict too.

HABIT PATTERNS

Man learns to respond to thwarting, to delay, and to conflict in various ways. These ways of responding become routinized through being reinforced and repeated. When they have become well-established habit patterns they are called *mechanisms*.

In learning to respond to situations that threaten our self-respect or prestige, the first response is typically to simply withdraw from the situation. This is usually not very satisfactory, and when the situation persists the response is varied in an attempt to find a more successful solution. The individual's behavior at this point is typically that of trial and error. Almost any response that will reduce the tension and anxiety will be tried. First one kind of behavior and then another is tried until something is found that is satisfactory. On one occasion the person may act shy and withdrawn; on another he may be bold and overaggressive; and on still another he may attempt to give excuses and explain away his faults. The behavior that is most successful in reducing his anxiety will be repeated, and each time it is repeated it is reinforced until it becomes a well-established pattern. In the future, when a comparable situation arises, the person will behave in the way in which he has learned to behave, without any particular attempt at direct problem solution.

FOUNDATIONS OF HEALTH SCIENCE

It should be pointed out that we do not deliberately set out to learn a particular way of satisfying our needs. By trial and error we discover some behavior that reduces our anxiety. This behavior is repeated because it is reinforced. The person is not aware that this is the way he has learned or that his behavior is an attempt to maintain self-respect or prestige. There are a number of ways in which people commonly behave to reduce anxiety arising out of frustration.

Aggression

Aggression is a typical reaction to frustration and is normal and usual. A typical reaction might be to attack the frustrating object directly. Small children typically attack the frustrating object in their environments directly and immediately. They hit what gets in their way. Children from lower socioeconomic groups are more likely to continue to express their aggressions directly than children from the middle and upper social classes.[23]

Much, if not most, aggression engaged in by people is indirect. Direct aggression is so frequently not rewarded, or actually punished, that indirect means for the expression of aggressive tendencies are substituted. In our culture, direct aggression toward parents, teachers, and other authority figures is discouraged. The child typically relieves his tensions caused by frustration on objects in the environment that are not in and of themselves threatening to him. He may bang a toy, kick a door, or throw a book.

Displaced aggression may result in scapegoating. A scapegoat is an innocent individual, or group, blamed for the frustrations of others. Minority groups are frequently used as scapegoats when other groups of people are frustrated.

Withdrawal

Some people learn to adjust to social situations through withdrawal. Such a habit of adjustment is probably learned in the same manner that other social responses are learned. The individual has found this kind of behavior to be rewarding. Withdrawing is a relatively easy response to make. It probably requires less effort than aggressive behavior and it is rather immediately rewarding. Withdrawal can act as a kind of insurance against social failure. If we do not try we cannot fail. As far as some people are concerned, it is better never to have tried at all than to have tried and failed.

A word of caution is in order here. Not all who enjoy solitary activities or who are less socially inclined than the average are to be considered maladjusted. Those who are precariously adjusted are those who exhibit withdrawing behavior that results from intense anxiety or fear.

Loneliness

A defense against conflict, tension, and anxiety is to build a shell of emotional passivity around oneself. When active emotional involvement in interpersonal relationships is found to be too threatening and anxiety-arousing, one may become cold, detached, and aloof as a protective device. Rebuffed by associates, betrayed by friends, jilted by a lover, one withdraws from all emotional involvements. Since giving affection carries the risks of further rejection and disappointment, a solution is neither to accept nor to give affection.

Such defenses may make it possible for the individual to meet others with a superficial correctness. The social amenities are observed. Many acquaintances are made and superficial friendships are formed, but whenever genuine affection begins to develop, the person feels threatened and retreats to less emotionally involved relationships. Such a person is often lonely and feels a need for love but is unable to give or accept it when the opportunity arises. Individuals so motivated may have a wealth of social contacts but still remain affectionally isolated and lonely.

When one feels lonely or lonesome as a result of unsatisfactory personal-social relationships, it is easy to begin to think of oneself as less than adequate and to feel depressed. The world becomes a pretty bleak place and even those personal-social contacts that are maintained tend to be devalued as superficial and meaningless. Such loneliness leading to depression may become severe enough so that personal devaluation and feelings of hopelessness develop to the point where self-destructive behavior may ensue. On a personal basis, active, open, realistic involvement with others in the affairs of the culture can do much to allay the feelings of isolation and depression that are so destructive of self-worthiness. Acceptance of one's self and others as well as the rest of the world is a goal toward which mentally healthful striving is directed.

Daydreaming

In daydreaming the individual engages in the imaginary satisfaction of his motives. When thwarting is persistent, severe daydreaming is likely to become a principal means of need satisfaction. Daydreaming requires little effort. The content of the fantasy is known only to the daydreamer;

therefore it cannot be criticized by others. Fantasy is a normal part of the lives of children.

People who are seclusive in nature have less of an opportunity for overt social expression and are thus likely to engage in fantasy more than the socially active individual. This may become the predominant mode of tension reduction for the shy and reserved individual. Fantasy can be very rewarding. It can be used as a direct satisfier of basic motives or as a compensation for the frustration of failure.

Regression

Regression is engaging in behavior that is characteristic of a much younger person. Such responses to frustration are immature and seldom constructive. The reoccurrence of thumb-sucking, the loss of previously acquired toilet-training habits, diminished verbal skill, and infant-like behavior frequently occur when children of preschool age are frustrated by the birth of a new member of the family or by other familial disruptions. Adults also respond to frustration by regressive behavior. The husband who grumbles and picks up the evening paper without comment because dinner is not ready precisely on time is pouting—a response that may be somewhat cute in four-year-olds but is hardly becoming to a forty-year-old. The wife who behaves in an emotionally immature fashion—is peevish or uses tears as a means of getting what she wants—is behaving in a childish way. These kinds of behavior can appropriately be called regression.

Rationalization

Rationalization is the giving of socially acceptable reasons for one's behavior. People frequently find that the responses that they make can be interpreted as appropriate for more than one motive. At times the real motive for performing a particular act is not socially acceptable. Rather than lose prestige and self-respect by having it believed that his behavior was instigated by an unacceptable motive, a person tends to deceive himself and attempts to deceive others by ascribing his behavior to some more culturally desirable motive. This allows him to maintain his self-respect because it cannot logically be proved, usually, that his motives were other than the most socially acceptable ones.

With the tremendous emphasis in our culture on competitive success, rationalization becomes necessary. We learn very early in life that we must get ahead in the world and at the same time that we must be careful to observe the social mores. These two motives are frequently in conflict.

When this happens we deceive ourselves and others by our rational explanations.

It is sometimes difficult to tell the difference between the deliberate attempt to deceive others and rationalization. In rationalization the person is convincing himself of the appropriateness of his behavior. *Blaming the incidental cause* is a common rationalization. The boy who fails to get a hit in the ball game complains that his favorite bat was not available. The student who is not prepared for today's lesson may blame his classmates because they were using the references when he wanted them. The student who fails a test may insist that the reason for this is that his parents entertained the night before and he did not have time to review. These and similar explanations contain an element of fact and are therefore defensible. The whole truth might indicate that the real reasons were much more personal and less defensible.

With practice, we can become quite adept in rationalizing behavior and in deceiving others. When an individual comes to believe his own rationalizations, he forgets what the real and original motives were and loses sight of the fact that his behavior is face-saving and ego-inflating. Rationalizations then become habitual, unconsciously motivated—a way of life. Verbal expressions of appropriate motives for socially inappropriate behavior are learned because they are rewarded.

There are a goodly number of behaviors whose development can be understood through essentially this same pattern of learning, reinforcement, social deception, and self-deception. The usual mechanisms, such as projection, identification, sublimation, withdrawal, aggression, daydreaming, regression, compensation, and repression, are to be viewed as usual habits of responding. But they are habits that can get out of hand and become dominant and consistent ways of behaving that are detrimental to society and to personal effectiveness.

Repression

Situations that arouse guilt, fear, anxiety, and shame are often forgotten very readily. This selective forgetting of unpleasant experiences is the phenomenon of repression. Experiments by Wallen[24] and Shaw[25] demonstrate that if an event is in disagreement with our social evaluation of ourselves or is derogatory in nature, it will arouse conflict and anxiety. One way of adjusting to such self-threatening situations is to forget them. If we inhibit the recall of an experience because to recall it would bring about anxiety, the experience can be said to be repressed. We can learn to avoid situations that would serve as cues to the recall of the anxiety-producing memory. Eventually, the person can become quite skillful at avoiding cues

FOUNDATIONS OF HEALTH SCIENCE

to anxiety-producing memories. Repression is successful and is reinforced by the reduction of anxiety.

Repression is not a very satisfactory form of adjustment because it does not solve a problem. It merely serves to keep anxiety within limits by inhibiting responses that are anxiety-producing. It does not provide a means of satisfying social motives. It may cause the person to avoid having experiences in the area of his anxiety that would tend to be motive-satisfying. When a person develops a generalized habit of using repression as adjustment, he is likely to become maladjusted. Repression is basic to the formation of phobias (irrational fears) and compulsions (irresistible urges to perform certain acts).

Identification

The process of enhancing our feelings of personal worth through identifying strongly with an illustrious person or institution is called identification. The individual, through identification, takes on some of the prestige and esteem of the person with whom he identifies. Identification does not come about as the result of deliberate effort. The person is usually not aware that he is identifying with anyone or anything, nor aware of the adjustive purposes that his identification serves.

Each generation of teenagers seems to have a hero with whom identification is strong. They identify with a movie star or television performer whose successes are theirs and whose setbacks are keenly felt by them. The achievement of individual aspirations is often accomplished by identification with a group that represents the achievement. Exclusive organizations such as fraternities and sororities are especially likely to satisfy needs for prestige and self-esteem through identification with collective status. People also identify themselves with their possessions. They take pride in the family car or the family home; their self-regard and prestige are ministered to by display or even by the mere act of possessing.

Projection

A person who perceives in others the motives that he himself is concerned about is using projection as an adjustive technique. When concerned about a particular trait or motive that is characteristic of himself he is likely to perceive this trait in others. Normal individuals use projection as a mechanism of behavior.

A student who is inclined to copy his neighbor's work may interpret the slightest glance of one classmate at another classmate as evidence that copying or cheating is occurring. A student who fails an examination projects the responsibility for failure on the test, which he says was unfair. Projecting blame or responsibility for failure to achieve is a way of sparing oneself the anxiety of personal failure and loss of prestige. Such minor projections are common to most people. They may, however, become very serious maladjustive forms of behavior. They can lead to delusions of persecution. A *delusion* is a belief that is grossly false. Delusions are characteristic of certain psychotic and neurotic individuals.

Compensation

Compensation is the overdevelopment of a behavior. When the individual is unable to succeed in a particular area, he overemphasizes achievement in another area. This is a form of substitution of one thing for another. This protects the person from self-criticism and resultant anxiety. It may serve as a kind of distractor since if one overachieves in an area, the overachievement is more noticeable than the fact that he is deficient in some area.

The scholastically inferior student may compensate for his academic weakness by developing himself physically, by behavior that attracts attention, or by becoming the leader of a gang. The physically inferior individual may substitute academic achievement for lack of athletic prowess. Though this may serve immediate purposes, compensating behavior can interfere with all-around development of the individual. The area most needing development in the person is likely to be neglected. Frequently areas of deficiency can be improved.

Compensation can occur for both real and imaginary deficiencies. Compensations for imaginary deficiencies are unfortunate because this behavior can rob the individual of opportunities for achievement in areas in which he really could achieve. In this sense they are more personally damaging than real deficiencies. The person with a real deficiency is actually prevented from achievement by this deficiency.

IN CONCLUSION

Although personal satisfaction and happiness are seldom listed as criteria or dimensions of adjustment, no conception of the good life entirely disregards them. We conceive of happiness as the accompaniment or consequence of life processes functioning at optimum points in terms of the other dimensions of adjustment. Pleasure seeking as a life goal is

FOUNDATIONS OF HEALTH SCIENCE

universally belittled, but personal satisfaction and happiness are considered to be the incidental outcome of activities directed at something quite different. The person who is appropriately selective in his responses to his environment, whose acceptance versus attempted modification efforts are realistic, and whose self-realization motives are adequately met will be a happy person.

The person who is open to experience and who perceives the world as dominantly friendly, who is not afraid of his own thoughts and feelings, and who is open to external reality will find life worth living.

Notes

1. J. M. Sawrey and C. W. Telford, *Adjustment and Personality* (Boston: Allyn and Bacon, 1975); E. T. Vance, "Social Disability," *American Psychologist,* 28:498–511, 1973.

2. A. H. Maslow, "Self-Actualizing People," in *The Self,* ed. C. E. Moustakas (New York: Harper and Brothers, 1956).

3. C. R. Rogers, *On Becoming a Person* (Boston: Houghton Mifflin, 1961).

4. G. Allport, *Pattern and Growth in Personality* (New York: Holt, Rinehart, and Winston, 1961).

5. A. H. Maslow, *Motivation and Personality,* 2nd ed. (New York: Harper and Row Publishers, 1970).

6. C. R. Rogers, "The Actualizing Tendency in Relation to Values and to Consciousness," in *Nebraska Symposium on Motivation,* ed. M. R. Jones (Lincoln: University of Nebraska Press, 1963).

7. R. White, "Motivation Reconsidered: The Concept of Competence," *Psychological Review,* 66:297–333, 1959; D. Zern, "Competence Reconsidered: The Concept of Secondary Process Development as an Explanation of 'Competence' Phenomena," *Journal of Genetic Psychology,* 722:135–162, 1973.

8. R. May, *Love and Will* (New York: Delta, 1973).

9. W. Durant and A. Durant, *Rousseau and Revolution* (New York: Simon and Schuster, 1967).

10. H. F. Harlow, "The Nature of Love," *American Psychologist,* 13:673–685, 1958; "The Heterosexual Affectional System in Monkeys," *American Psychologist,* 17:1–9, 1962.

11. J. W. Atkinson, J. R. Bastian, R. W. Earl, and G. H. Litwin, "The Achievement Motive, Goal Setting and Probability Preferences," *Journal of Abnormal and Social Psychology,* 60:27–36, 1960; D. C. McClelland, *The Achieving Society* (New York: D. Van Nostrand Company, 1961); J. Veroff, J. W. Atkinson, S. Field, and G. Gurin, "The Use of Thematic Apperception to Assess Motivation in a Nationwide Interview Study," *Psychological Monographs,* 74, no. 12, 1960. (Whole No. 499.)

12. A. Amsel, "The Role of Frustrative Nonreward in Noncontinuous Reward Situations," *Psychological Bulletin,* 55:102–119, 1958.

13. K. Lewin, "Behavior and Development as a Function of the Total Situation," in *Manual of Child Psychology,* 2nd ed., ed. L. Carmichael (New York: John Wiley & Sons, 1934), pp. 918–970; *A Dynamic Theory of Personality* (New York: McGraw-Hill Book Co., 1935).

14. C. I. Hovland and R. R. Sears, "Experiments on Motor Conflict: I. Types of Conflict and Their Modes of Resolution," *Journal of Experimental Psychology,* 23:477–493, 1938.

15. N. Clancy and F. Smitter, "A Study of Emotionally Disturbed Children in Santa Barbara County Schools," *California Journal of Educational Research,* 4:209–218, 222, 1953; H. Reyborn, "Guidance Needs of Students from Broken Homes," *California Journal of Education Research,* 2:22–25, 1951.

16. A. J. Ferrera and W. D. Winter, "Decision-Making in Normal and Abnormal Two-Child Families," *Family Process,* 7:17–36, 1968.

17. T. Jacob, "Patterns of Family Conflict and Dominance as a Function of Child Age and Social Class," *Developmental Psychology,* 10:1–12, 1974.

18. Clancy and Smitter, "A Study of Emotionally Disturbed Children."

19. F. I. Nye, "Marital Interaction," in *The Employed Mother in America,* ed. F. I. Nye and L. S. Hoffman (Chicago: Rand McNally, 1963).

20. B. M. Lester, M. Katelchuck, E. Spelke, M. J. Sellers, and R. E. Klein, "Separation Protest in Guatemalan Infants: Cross-Cultural and Cognitive Findings," *Developmental Psychology,* 10:79–85, 1974.

21. L. J. Cohen, "Father, Mother, and Stranger as Elicitors of Attachment Behaviors in Infancy," *Developmental Psychology,* 10:146–154, 1974.

22. A. C. Kinsey, W. B. Pomeroy, and C. E. Martin, *Sexual Behavior in the Human Male* (Philadelphia: W. B. Saunders, 1948); A. C. Kinsey, W. B. Pomeroy, C. E. Martin, and P. H. Gebhard, *Sexual Behavior in the Human Female* (Philadelphia: W. B. Saunders, 1953).

23. R. J. Havighurst and H. Taba, *Adolescent Character and Personality* (New York: John Wiley & Sons, 1949).

24. W. Wallen, "Ego Involvement as a Determinant of Selective Forgetting," *Journal of Abnormal and Social Psychology,* 37:20–39, 1942.

25. F. J. Shaw, "Two Determinants of Selective Forgetting," *Journal of Abnormal and Social Psychology,* 39:434–445, 1944.

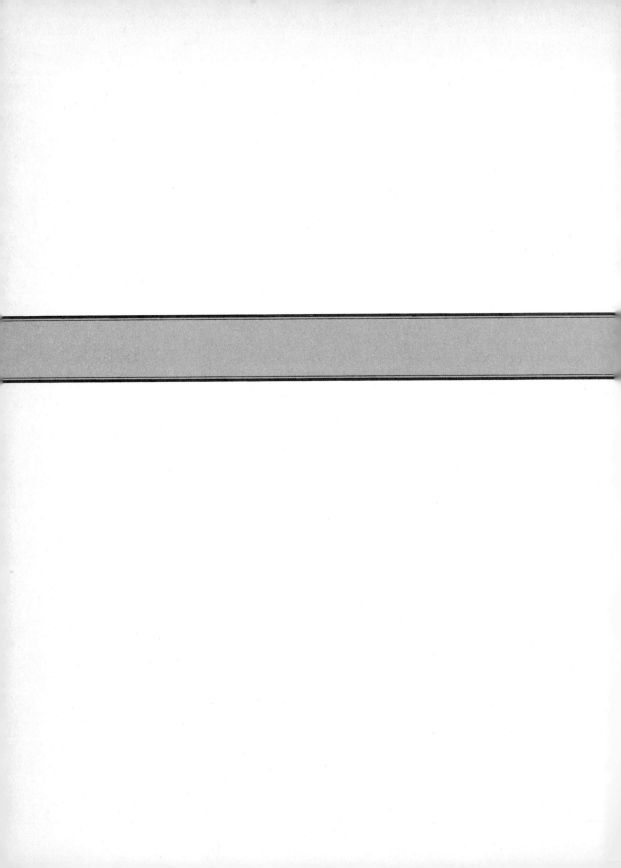

PEOPLE WITH PSYCHOLOGICAL PROBLEMS

chapter seven

Professional help is sought by many people. Those who seek help have a tremendous variety of problems ranging from difficulty in studying to severe neurotic or psychotic disturbances. It is a common misconception that only people who are seriously disturbed seek or need counseling. Many people need help to deal with problems that are completely rational in nature but for which they are unable to find solutions. Some people contact a counselor about a problem that is of minor importance to them but causes discomfort or inconvenience.

EMOTIONAL DISTURBANCES

Minor mental illnesses and emotional disturbances tend to be great in number. Roughly one-half of the general medical practitioner's patients suffer from some kind of emotional disturbance, and nearly one-third of hospitalized medical and surgical patients are either neurotic or psychosomatic cases.

In addition to the number of people who are severely disturbed to the extent that their illness can be recognized by laymen as well as professionals, there are many who suffer from less severe and less obviously incapacitating frustrations, conflicts, and anxieties. Some people who on the surface seem to be reasonably happy and well-integrated are really suffering psychologically and are in need of help in order to regain mental health. Under the surface many people carry burdens of personal feelings of inadequacy, fear, sorrow, and discontent that make their lives miserable and their social utility extremely limited. They may behave in only slightly eccentric ways and their basic unhappiness and unproductiveness goes unnoticed by friends and associates.

The hail-fellow-well-met and the shy may both be in need of professional help if they are eventually to live complete and full lives. The aggressively hostile, the seclusive and fearful, the depressed, the anxious, the woman hater, the man hater, the boisterous, the sensitive, the heavy drinker, the antisocial, the chronically fatigued, the self-disparaging, and others displaying behaviors that are symptomatic of distress are frequently not recognized as being in need of psychological help.

Emotional stress, of course, is a part of life. It is probable that most people learn to live with it quite adequately. When stress becomes excessive, or when the means of coping with it have not been acquired, serious problems may arise. Personal relationships may suffer, inefficient work habits may develop, personality traits that are socially handicapping may appear, and the emotional stress becomes greater and greater. In trying to resolve these problems, additional stress is generated. Very frequently people in such situations need the help of a psychologist or psychiatrist to establish effective means of dealing with their problems and to become reasonably happy and competent.

The number of psychiatrists and clinical psychologists in the United

Sometimes all we need is a friend to listen

After an abortion, a friend of mine became very depressed. It became so serious that she couldn't sleep and she cried about almost anything. One night at a party she drank too much and started talking about her deep feelings. Several times she mentioned dying as an escape from her guilt and her boyfriend's threats to leave her. After that night, she could talk openly about the abortion and her feelings about it to me. Together we started figuring out what she should do and how to get started again. She is now better adjusted. Sometimes she even makes jokes about the past, but when we talk seriously she still regrets having been put in a situation with a boyfriend who didn't really care.

FOUNDATIONS OF HEALTH SCIENCE

States is totally inadequate to meet the need for competent therapists. The cost of providing adequately trained persons and adequately equipped facilities is high, but the cost of not providing adequate psychological and psychiatric services may be even higher in economic and social loss as well as in terms of human suffering. So popular have the services of psychotherapists become in the past few years that it can certainly be said that psychotherapy is used not only to treat and restore but it has become a means, for many people, of working toward self-fulfillment. Psychotherapy, for some, has become part of a way of life.[1]

People with problems that center around feelings of inadequacy, inability to concentrate or study, irrational fears, social incompetence, marriage, relationships with their parents, relationships with their children, sex, money, feelings of depression, inability to make friends, compulsive behavior, nightmares, insomnia, psychosomatic reactions, tics, delusions, hallucinations, and a host of other personal and interpersonal factors comprise the clientele of any psychotherapeutic clinic. A few examples may serve to illustrate the variety of problems for which professional psychotherapy is sought.

Don F., a senior in high school, had no idea what he wanted to do after graduation. He felt certain that he did not want to enter his father's business, but beyond that he had no plans. His parents were very concerned about his apparent lack of purpose, and his father contacted a psychotherapist to seek help for Don.

A young lady, Mary M., went to see a clinical psychologist at her college counseling center. She had difficulty in talking about her problem, but finally indicated that she had a younger sister at home with whom she had never gotten on very well, As a matter of fact they appeared to dislike each other intensely. Mary felt guilty for not liking her sister and angry at the same time. The younger sister was going to be a freshman at the same college next semester, and their parents wanted the two girls to share a small apartment. This presented an almost intolerable situation for Mary. She wanted to talk about her relationship with her sister and with her parents.

A young man, Jerry T., sought help with a problem that was embarrassing and made him feel inadequate. He thought that he might be a homosexual even though he had had no homosexual experiences. He was unable to be comfortable with a girl on a date. He had stopped dating because he felt frightened and guilty whenever he found himself alone with a woman. His friends were constantly trying to line him up with a date. He felt he must have some help with his problem.

Betty L., a college sophomore, was a good student. She had studied diligently her first year at college and had earned good grades. She started her second year in the same fashion but became very interested in a young man whom she started dating. He was a senior and he wanted to marry her. Betty felt that she should finish college, but she had been getting poor grades since she started to go steady with this young man. She was afraid that she would be a bitter disappointment to her family if she did not finish college. She also felt that if she did not marry this young man she would be unhappy. She sought the help of a psychotherapist.

Kathleen A. sought help with the following problem. She was the daughter of an industrial executive. Most of her childhood had been spent in the care of a nurse or governess and, later, at boarding school and summer camp. Her younger brother, whom she barely knew, had been treated similarly. He was now in a military school for boys. Kathleen and her brother, who was now fifteen years old, had corresponded rather regularly for the past year and a half. They had both looked forward to spending the Christmas holidays at home, but the parents had decided that they would take a trip to Mexico for the holidays and had informed the children that they should not come home for Christmas. Kathleen had then asked that her brother come to visit her for Christmas. This was arranged. During the time they spent together it became obvious to both Kathleen and her younger brother that they did not know or like their parents very much. After her brother had returned to school, Kathleen thought about her brother and herself a great deal. She came to the conclusion that neither she nor her brother were loved by their parents. This, she decided, she could live with, without too much difficulty. Her concern was that she herself might become like her parents. She said she had never felt any great fondness for anyone and wondered if she were capable of ever loving anyone. She said she would not want to have children and treat them as shoddily as she felt she had been treated. Her father had been married previously and she was born to his first wife. She had never known her real mother; she also said that she was quite certain her mother was pregnant with her before she was married and that her father may or may not have been her real father. She was unhappy, confused, and angry that she and her younger brother were in their present situation.

If one reads between the lines in the cases that have just been presented, it becomes apparent that the problems brought to a psychotherapist are many times more complex than they appear to be initially.

Don's lack of purpose and desire to avoid involvement in his father's business was confirmed. He was very bitter toward his father and his own adjustments were very precarious. Mary's problems were no less serious than Don's. Jerry's problems reflected his own feelings of guilt for some earlier behavior with women and an unfortunate attitude toward sex. His case turned out to be quite an involved one. Betty and Kathleen both had problems involving parental relationships. They were different problems, but both were serious and complex.

FOUNDATIONS OF HEALTH SCIENCE

The examples presented do not represent bizarre or unusual cases. More serious cases of disorganized behavior, from sexually deviant involvements to referred cases of individuals who compulsively set fires, steal, or commit other crimes, come to the attention of psychotherapists. Fully developed neurotic and psychotic patients are, of course, a part of the clientele, but patients of this nature are frequently thought to comprise the majority of psychiatric patients. Cases like the ones that have been described are probably more representative of the patients seen in an outpatient clinic than are the more seriously disorganized. The very seriously disturbed frequently need the protection provided by a hospital and require constant supervision, care, and treatment.

Loneliness

To be *lonesome* is not an absolute consequence of being alone. A person can be lonely in a crowd if he feels he is surrounded by people with whom he has or feels little in common. He can also have this feeling if he thinks people are rejecting him. Loneliness can be a form of self-pity deriving from an elevated feeling of self-worth and therefore a devaluation of associates. It can also be a result of a devaluation of the self in comparison with others.

There can be little doubt that all of us experience the feelings of loneliness at one time or another. Perpetual feelings of loneliness and isolation accompanied by self-devaluation can lead to the sadness and seriousness of depression. Most periodic loneliness can be overcome by renewed efforts toward socialization and achievement. Feelings of loneliness and mild depression can be treated psychologically. Professional help from counselors and psychotherapists can redirect thinking and behavior to be less self damaging and more optimistic.

Learned Helplessness

Expectancies concerning the consequences of our acts, and beliefs concerning the causes of those consequences, have been established as important determiners of motivation, learning, and achievement.[2] There are two types of these expectancies. One is the expectancy of either negative or positive reinforcements following particular acts. The second refers to the extent that we perceive ourselves as the important causal agent in determining outcomes. If we believe we are responsible for the outcomes of our own acts, we are displaying internal reinforcement responsibility. If we attribute the outcomes to other forces (other people, the external environment, or chance) we are displaying external reinforcement responsibility.[3] Some of the more extreme outcomes of building up minimal expectancies of positive reinforcement and maintaining low levels of perception of personal control of behavioral outcomes, have been conceptualized as learned helplessness.[4]

The phenomenon of learned helplessness was first observed in experimental animals. It was noted that administering inescapable trauma to both animals and man often resulted in their subsequent failure to make any overt response even in situations where the punishment was avoidable.[5] In other situations, animals who were subjected to less traumatic punishment would not become immobilized, but would take the punishment while simply whining or howling. The animals seemed to give up; they had learned that they were helpless. Subsequent experiments produced learned helplessness in many subjects, ranging from cockroaches to college students.

Depression

Seligman proposed that passivity, the most prominent symptom of depression, can be the result of our prior life experiences in controlling our environment.[6] According to this interpretation, depressed people make fewer responses. They become apathetic. When they do respond, they do not expect to succeed. They misinterpret success as failure, and they perceive any success as pure chance. The depressed person perceives himself as a born loser.

Research studies obtained results consistent with this interpretation of depression. Subjects were given either soluble problems sufficiently easy to ensure success or insoluble problems, which are harder to solve, and then subsequently provided with either success-possible or success-impossible additional tasks. The response decrements and persistence in the face of repeated failure characteristic of these subjects, were then related to their scores on an Intellectual Achievement Responsibility Scale in one study[7] and to scores on the Beck Depression Inventory in the other.[8] The results of these studies showed that subjects who had the greatest work decrements and the least persistence following failure were those who took less personal responsibility for the outcome of their actions (externals). Those who accepted more responsibility for the behavioral outcome (internals) persisted longer and showed less work decrement following failure experiences. The depressed subjects perceived success and failure (reinforcement) as more independent of their personal efforts and acts than did the nondepressed subjects. Also, as predicted, the depressed subjects showed less change in expectancies of success following success experiences than did the nondepressed subjects. The more depressed the subject, the greater tendency to perceive success and failure as independent of action. Depression had a persistent and predictable perceptual-distortion affect on the consequences of the acts.

The results of these studies are consistent with the clinical observation that depressed people selectively forget or devalue success experiences and have a high expectation of failure.

Also in connection with these research findings, Seligman suggests that the life histories of people resistant to depression probably contain extensive success experiences; they have been able to control and manipulate many of the sources of satisfaction in their lives.[9] Such people are able to view the future optimistically.

An unpredictable world without mastery produces vulnerability to pessimism. Pessimism and depression can be the result of an affluent society where reinforcements (things and experiences) are received independently of the behavior of those who receive them—a kind of goodies from heaven attitude. Rewards and punishments that come independently of one's efforts, can induce an attitude of learned helplessness and depression.

Suicide

Suicide ranks among the eight leading causes of death in the United States. In 1973 about 25,000 people in this country took their own lives and the death rate was 12 per 100,000 people. The rate in 1960 was 10.6.[10] Self-inflicted deaths are more frequent among males than females, al-

Those with severe psychological problems do get well

My father walked out on us when I was in elementary school. At the time my Mom was in the hospital for another operation. My grandmother didn't tell my mother about my father's leaving until she came home from the hospital. It was awfully hard for my Mom to take. My sister and I were cared for by our grandmother for a long time; we moved in with her. I remember my Mother being sick for a long time and then later we moved back to our own apartment. During that time my Mother didn't do anything for us, my grandmother did everything. Now I know that my Mother was in a deep depression and was seeing a psychiatrist. Today she is a totally different person. She is well-adjusted and can accept any stress that faces her.

though the difference in rate has been narrowing in recent years. The suicide rate among males in the age range fifteen to twenty-four is five times that for females.[11] The ratio of male to female suicides increases as their age increases. This is also true for the suicide rate in general. More females than males attempt suicide but they are not as successful. Males usually attempt suicide by more violent means than females, which may account for their higher suicide rate.

Although suicide can be a result of severe mental illness, it is not true that "You have to be crazy to kill yourself." Unless, of course, by crazy we mean that one is only a bit emotionally disturbed or has personality problems. Most people who are psychotic do not kill themselves. It is not true either that all those who commit suicide are psychotic, although suicide rates are high among depressive psychotics, those with involutional melancholia, and some schizophrenics.[12] The causes of suicide among the psychotic are not grossly different from the causes of suicide among the nonpsychotic.[13] It is rather self-evident that the potentially suicidal person has severe problems for which, under stress, he does not possess adequate personal defenses. Studies of suicide attempters indicate that a feeling of rejection was of importance and that suicide attempts are frequently made after criticism by important persons in the individual's life.[14] Broken homes during childhood seem to be a predisposing factor to a later suicide attempt[15] and family disorganization[16] may be of major concern.

Although some suicidal attempts may be insincere, may constitute histrionic attempts at attention getting, may be an attempt to frighten someone with whom the person is in close contact, or may represent pleas for help, pity, and favors, not all suicide attempts fall in these categories.[17] Suicide is final; attempts at suicide cannot be ignored or belittled. Intervention by others is imperative for the prevention of suicide. A person beset by difficulties may see his life drifting from bad to worse, or from poor health to helplessness. He sees himself as a burden or potential burden to others. He concludes that the only responsible action that can be taken is that of self destruction. This person needs some kind of intervention in order to survive. Another person may simply abandon responsibility for his own existence and depend upon the intervention of others if he is to survive. If there is no intervention, life can be perceived as not worth living.

The potential suicide is often psychologically immature and lonesome, with a low self regard and inadequate personal defenses.[18] Intervention can impose temporary external controls, provide support for inadequate psychological defenses, show the person that he is not alone in the world and that someone *does* care, provide temporary human companionship, and an opportunity to talk about himself and thus release some tension and anxiety. He must learn to direct his anger to some other objects,

FOUNDATIONS OF HEALTH SCIENCE

events, or persons, and eventually to live happily and without the feelings of hostility, self-devaluation, and rejection that have proven so damaging. The potential suicide must be helped to feel wanted, needed, and deserving of affection and attention.

MENTAL ILLNESS

We all know that mental illness exists. We know that the problem of mental illness is extensive. But we do not always accept the fact that mental illness, like any other illness, could and does happen to us, our families and associates. Mental illness frequently produces frightening behavior, and our concept of the mentally ill person is distorted. As with a disease that is induced primarily by physical factors, early detection of severe emotional disorders can lead to more effective treatment and rapid rehabilitation.

The purpose of the following discussion of the extent and nature of mental illness is to make you more aware of the many types of mental illness and to help you understand what they are, recognize their symptoms, and realize that they can be treated.

PSYCHONEUROTIC DISORDERS

Psychoneurotic disorders range in severity from slightly impairing effective functioning to being almost completely incapacitating. The terms *psychoneurosis* and *neurosis* are interchangeable. There are four classical forms of psychoneurosis: neurasthenia, hysteria, anxiety neurosis, and

Depression has many causes and many faces

A friend of mine is burdened with depression although he won't admit to it. He has been receiving welfare and unemployment assistance for over a year. I think the problem lies in the fact that his job fluctuates with the economy. Ever since he began this particular job there have been stretches of unemployment for months at a time.

He must support a wife and a child with this uncertainty. Along with this primary problem I think there is a second one. They overuse alcohol and other drugs such as marijuana. I think this overuse of drugs stems from the environment in which they live—that of a city apartment dweller's crowded, lonely existence. Lately my friend has begun questioning his own existence and contemplating suicide.

phychasthenia. The symptoms of the mentally ill person often do not fit into any one category.

Neurasthenic Reactions
(asthenic reactions)

Neurasthenia and *hysteria* have much in common with some psychosomatic disorders. The lines between them are not sharply drawn. Neurasthenia is characterized by a rather indefinite and changeable set of symptoms, including vague aches and pains, a constant state of fatigue that is unrelieved by rest, hypersensitivity to minor irritants, and hypochondriasis. Fatigue is usually the dominant symptom and because of this fact the newer term "asthenic (weakness) reaction" is in some respects a more suitable designation. Neurasthenia literally means a "nervous weakness," which suggests, erroneously, that the condition is organic rather than functional in origin. The following case is fairly typical.

An unmarried male, age thirty-two, complains of the following symptoms. He suffers extreme fatigue and finds it impossible to work for more than twenty or thirty minutes at a time. The fatigue is present in the morning just as much as it is during the rest of the day. He has a poor appetite and suffers from indigestion, which he describes as sour stomach, gas, heartburn, and constipation. He has frequent headaches and blurred vision, which make it impossible for him to read for any length of time. Periodic back pains prevent him from sitting or standing in comfort. He has ringings and buzzings in his ears that are highly distracting. He is very irritated by ordinary noises. The ticking of the clock, the traffic noises, and the slamming of doors keep him hunting for quieter living quarters. He is sure that he has some obscure malignant illness. Repeated physical examinations have been negative, and various tonics and dietary supplements have been tried with only short-term improvements. This man has become a health food faddist and is sure that he would have died except for his special diet.

The neurasthenic symptoms are thought to originate from sustained emotional tensions, but the individual ascribes his discomfort to physical ailments. These symptoms of physical illness permit the person to escape from his problems, his responsibilities, and environmental stresses.

Hysteria

In many ways the hysterical symptoms are the most dramatic of the psychoneurotic behavior patterns. The more bizarre forms of hysteria seem to have gone out of style. Hysteria is much less common today than twenty-five or fifty years ago, whereas psychasthenias seem to be more common. Hysteric reactions may be motor, sensory, and epileptiform in nature.

The motor symptoms of hysteria include functional paralyses, which may involve one or more limbs or a whole side of the body. Other motor symptoms are total inability to speak (mutism), inability to speak above a whisper (aphonia), tremors, and tics (involuntary spasms of localized muscle groups). Occupationally related motor disorders, like writer's cramp, may also be symptoms of hysteria.

Sensory symptoms include several varieties of functional anesthesia. Blindness may involve one or both eyes, the right half or the left half of both eyes, or the visual field may be restricted (tunnel vision). Functional deafness can occur. Functional loss of skin sensitivity (cutaneous anesthesia) of various types has also been reported.

Hysterical seizures may also occur. These are usually epileptiform but not truly epileptic in nature. Occasionally hysterical twilight states are experienced. In these conditions the person is confused and slightly disoriented. His experiences seem to have an unreal and dreamlike quality.

A newer term for hysteria is conversion reactions. The name derives from the hypothesis that anxiety that cannot be manifested or resolved in overt behavior is converted into or manifests itself in the blocked or distorted function of some body organ. According to this hypothesis, conversion reactions are anxiety-linked and represent the somatic equivalent of the internal emotion. Anxiety typically precedes the appearance of the hysterical symptoms and diminishes on their occurrence. Consequently, hysterical symptoms are sometimes spoken of as anxiety equivalents. Hysterical syndromes can be considered to be defensive and anxiety-reducing.

Dissociative reactions. Dissociative reactions are a different form of neurotic manifestation. The common form of dissociative reactions are (1) amnesias, (2) fugues, (3) dual or multiple personalities, and (4) somnambulisms. In all of these cases, there is a blocking off of a part of one's memories, experiences, activities, or life from the main current of one's existence.

In hysterical *amnesia* there is a partial or complete inability to recall or recognize past experiences. Although amnesia is often referred to as a loss of memory, it is not a failure to retain but an inability to recall or recognize. The fact that amnesias are often only temporary and the forgotten experiences can usually be recalled under hypnosis or narcosis indicates that the failure is not one of retention but of recall.

The inability to recall in amnesia is selective and usually involves ego-related material, such as one's identity, one's relatives and friends, and the events or a segment of one's past. Motor skill and habits are usually retained. The amnesic individual can still talk, walk, write, and play a musical instrument. The individual may function quite normally except where the segments of past experiences for which he is amnesic are concerned.

When the amnesia also involves a fleeing or running away it is called a *fugue*. A person may wander away from his home or community, or he may travel by train, car, bus, or plane and then find himself in a strange place, not knowing who he is, where he is, or how he got there. Such cases are frequently reported in the daily newspapers.

A soldier may suddenly find himself several miles behind his line of duty, traveling away from his battle station, with no knowledge of who he is, how he happens to be where he is, or where he is going. An unhappily married girl leaves home to go shopping, boards a bus, and finds herself two days later, in a strange city, with no awareness of her own identity and no recollection of her past life. A boy whose fantasy life is filled with adventure may awaken to find himself a member of a crew, aboard ship, and headed for the South Pacific with no knowledge of how he got there or who he is.

In *somnambulism* (sleepwalking) the individual, in a dreamlike or trance state, does bizarre and inappropriate things in a purposeful fashion but, in his normal waking state, has no recollection of the events. Sometimes these somnambulisms are reenactments of past events in the person's life, or they may represent the actual or symbolic carrying out of an act that the individual would like to perform but is unable to do in his ordinary waking state. The somnambulism may represent an attempt to escape from either real or imagined danger.[19]

Dual or multiple personality represents the most dramatic form of dissociation. While Robert Louis Stevenson's Dr. Jekyll and Mr. Hyde are, of course, fictional, many less spectacular actual cases of dual or multiple personality have been studied and documented.

In the case described by Lipton, Maud was a happy, extroverted, noisy individual who wore gaudy, striped, high-heeled, open-toed sandals, used excessive makeup, painted her fingernails and toenails deep red, and wore girlish red ribbons in her hair.[20] She used poor English, had a limited vocabulary, and childish handwriting. She chain-smoked, had no sense of right and wrong, and felt no guilt over her promiscuous sexual behavior. In contrast with Maud, Sara, the alternate personality, was quiet, sedate, and depressed. She dressed demurely and used no makeup or nailpolish. Her favorite color was blue. Sara was a mature, intelligent woman who used good English. She did not smoke, was very awkward when she tried, and had marked guilt feelings concerning her previous sexual misdemeanors.

From the girl's previous history, it appears that the appearance of the

FOUNDATIONS OF HEALTH SCIENCE

dissociated personality, Maud, enabled Sara to gratify her sexual and other frivolous desires without Sara's conscious knowledge and without guilt feelings. The evidence suggests that Sara changed to Maud whenever her sexual desires and guilt feelings concerning her previous sexual behavior became too threatening. The alternate personality operated as a defense against excessive anxiety and served as a means of resolving a conflict.

Anxiety Neurosis (anxiety reactions)

Although the state of chronic anxiety characteristic of anxiety neurosis is not a defensive reaction, it is a form of neurosis and is discussed here along with the other neurotic reactions. Chronic anxiety may precede the development of other neurotic defensive reaction patterns or it may continue indefinitely due to the partial or complete failure of defenses to develop. A typical case points out some of the characteristics of the anxiety neuroses.

The subject complained of being afraid. He was afraid all or most of the time. He could not say what he was afraid of, but he had a rather constant feeling of impending disaster without knowing why. The fear, or more accurately anxiety, varied in intensity from situation to situation. He was most disturbed when he was alone or in crowds. He felt least anxious when he was with some member of his immediate family, preferably his wife. He wanted his wife to be with him all the time. If she was not with him he wanted to know she was either at home or immediately available. When he was at work and knew his wife was at home he could feel reasonably comfortable, but if he knew she was away and he did not know where, he would become quite disturbed. Having one of his little children with him was preferable to being alone.

The subject was afraid to go places by himself. As it neared time to go home from work, his anxiety would mount to such a pitch that when he started for home he would be in a panic, feeling sure that something terrible would happen to him on the way. He dreaded crossing street intersections because he was sure he would never get across alive. In crowds he would sigh repeatedly, become tense, and find some excuse to move on. He could no longer drive his car; his wife usually drove for him.

The subject recognized the irrationality of his feelings but could do nothing about it. He knew all about the statistics of personal accidents and realized the low probabilities of any of his fears being realized, but facts and information did not help. He would say, "I have a fine wife and two wonderful children. I have a good job, some money in the bank, and a nice home clear of mortgage. I should be a happy man, but actually I am miserable all the time."

Over a period of six years he apparently never had any other neurotic symptoms. His general health remained good. He had no other bodily complaints or symptoms. He had no specific phobias, compulsions, or obsessions. His persistent anxiety seems to fit the classical picture of anxiety neurosis or anxiety reaction.

The level of anxiety in such neuroses is pathological in the sense that it is out of all proportion to its cause. It is unrealistic and is often so recognized by the individual. It is often free-floating in the sense that the anxiety is rather constant, although varying in intensity, and is not stimulus- or situation-tied. The anxiety state is often described as a fear and is ascribed by the sufferer to a specific cause or situation. This assigning is an attempted rationalization and the causes ascribed to it and the objects to which the emotion is attached shift from time to time and are not the real causes of anxiety.

Psychasthenia (phobic and obsessive-compulsive reactions)

The classical symptoms or forms of psychasthenia are phobias (morbid or pathological *fears*), obsessions (unwanted, irrational, persistent *thoughts*), and compulsions (forced repetitive *actions* performed despite the person's recognition of their inappropriateness or irrationality). In phobias the emotion of fear is the dominant element; in obsessions the ideational component is foremost; in compulsions the act or the impulse to act is predominant. All three of these may be present in varying degrees and in all possible combinations.

The number of possible *phobias* is almost infinite. Medical dictionaries often list several hundred. The names of the phobias are derived by attaching the Greek name indicating the thing feared to "phobia"; thus we have *claustrophobia,* a fear of closed places, *acrophobia,* a fear of heights, and *agoraphobia,* a fear of open places.

Some examples of phobias follow. A soldier is so afraid of closed places that he will spend the night in an open truck under fire rather than remain in an enclosed safe dugout. A grown woman is extremely afraid of cats, dogs, and any other small household pets. A fifteen-year-old boy has an intense fear of open places. He becomes panic-stricken whenever he finds himself alone in any large open area. An adult male becomes very disturbed whenever he has to go alone more than a few blocks from his home. A young man has a strong fear of being attacked from behind.

While the forms of phobias are legion, they do have some common features. Most phobias originate from early, childhood experiences. The phobia-inducing experience has some element of shame or guilt connected with it. It is anxiety-laden. The original experiences that gave rise to the

FOUNDATIONS OF HEALTH SCIENCE

phobia have been forgotten. (They cannot be recalled.) The phobic object often symbolizes the real cause of fear; some phobias are generalized conditioned fear responses; and phobic reactions are perpetuated because they operate as defenses and are anxiety-reducing.

An *obsession* is a *thought* or *idea* that keeps recurring and cannot be shaken off. An obsessive idea is usually coercive, irrational and to some extent anxiety-laden. For example: a mother is continually bothered by the idea that she may harm or even kill her baby, whom she dearly loves. A widow is obsessed with the idea that if she had given her husband a certain medicine he would not have died. A commuter is obsessed with the notion that he will lose his commuter's ticket. He keeps thinking about losing it, looks into his pocket every few minutes to reassure himself, and heaves a great sigh of relief when the conductor has punched it. Obsessions typically occur in combination with compulsions, and so the two are usually combined into the obsessive-compulsive reactions.

Compulsions are coercive, recurrent *acts* or *impulses* to act in rather specific ways. Compulsive acts are automatisms over which we have little control. The person is quite aware of what he is doing or feels compelled to do, he recognizes it as irrational, silly, or even dangerous, but he is unable to either stop doing it or get rid of the impulse to perform the act. The impulse is sometimes situation-tied to the extent that it occurs whenever the situation is right. At other times the impulse or tendency to act seems to build up spontaneously until the act is performed. Performing the act affords the sufferer a measure of relief.

The catalog of compulsions or compulsive-obsessive reactions is as long as that of the phobias. They range all the way from having to count

Most can adjust to such an experience—it takes time

My cousin was raped at the age of thirteen by two men about twenty-one and twenty-two years old. The two men were tried in court and both received eight year sentences, serving only about two or three years at the most. This was a traumatic experience for her. Shortly after, she began to see a psychiatrist regularly. After about three months of psychiatric help, she noticed in the paper that the two rapists were out of prison for good. This brought about nightmares and other haunting fears. At the age of sixteen she dropped out of school and began using drugs of all kinds, marijuana, pills, LSD. She recently lost her job and still seems to be restless and messed up from the whole terrible happening years ago.

Figure 7.1 Effects of Changing Thresholds for Psychosomatic Reactions. Under normal conditions only individuals E and H will display psychosomatic symptoms, while under emotional stress individuals B, F, I and L will also respond. The rest of the individuals—A, C, D, G, J, and K—will not react psychosomatically. The height of each individual's column is his constitutional susceptibility or reactivity.

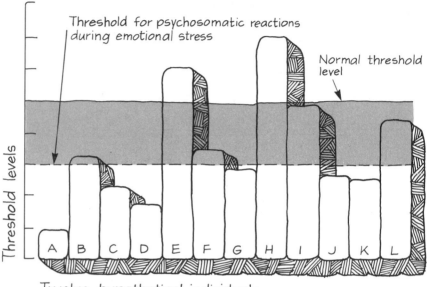

steps, posts, and cracks in the sidewalk to criminal acts such as kleptomania (compulsive stealing) and pyromania (compulsive fire-setting). All of the manias are technically compulsions.

As previously indicated, combinations of phobic and obsessive-compulsive reactions are more common than the pure forms. For example, a person may have a mysophobia (a morbid fear of dirt); he is obsessed with the idea that he is being contaminated with dangerous germs by everything he touches, and he has an accompanying hand washing compulsion. These elements are all consistent and mutually supportive.

Adjustment by Ailment

No one will admit that he wants to be ill. Illness is bad by definition. However, illness, or symptoms of illness, have advantages for the individual. Some personal and social advantages of illness are as follows:

1. Illness operates as a socially acceptable excuse for evading many of life's problems.

2. It serves as a means of avoiding responsibility and provides a plausible excuse for the absence of achievement.
3. Illness is a means of obtaining a relaxation of discipline and of avoiding blame and punishment.
4. Increased attention, sympathy, and care are normal consequences of being ill.
5. Bizarre, unusual, or baffling illness may provide a patient an increment of uniqueness or status.
6. Illness may be perceived as a punishment that relieves anxiety springing from a sense of guilt.

Illness, or the development of the symptoms of illness, may be either consciously or unconsciously motivated. *Malingering* is the conscious feigning of illness or physical disability. It always involves deliberate deception. In the conversion reactions (hysteria), neurasthenia, and less certainly in the psychosomatic disorders, the motivation for illness is largely unconscious. It is quite possible that habitual conscious malingering may gradually shift to the more unconsciously motivated hysterical, neurasthenic, and psychosomatic manifestation.

The child who pretends to have a headache in order to avoid school attendance when he is unprepared is malingering. The girl who feigns illness on the night of her dreaded recital is doing likewise. There are few people who have not sometime pretended that they were sick as a means either avoiding threatening and potentially unpleasant situations or of obtaining special considerations of some sort. In cases involving disability claims or lawsuits for compensation following accidents, the possibility of malingering is always present.

Malingering is a conscious maneuver designed to defend one's status and either prevent ego-deflation or contribute to one's status. It is a means of obtaining protection, exemptions, special privileges and rewards via deliberate deception.

PSYCHOSOMATIC DISORDERS

If the term is taken literally, the category of psychosomatic disorders is a very broad one. The term can be used to refer to any disturbance in which functional (usually emotional) maladjustment results in organic changes or dysfunction of some physiological system. This broad definition would include every disorder in which psychic (functional) and somatic (organic) factors both play a part. This is practically everything a person does. In practice, the term is not given such a broad meaning.

In common usage, the psychosomatic disorders are those organic dysfunctions having functional (usually emotional) causes. The term is further limited to the malfunctioning of those organs or parts of the organs controlled by the autonomic nervous system, the smooth muscles and glands of the body. Psychosomatic disorders involve the gastrointestinal tract, the circulatory, respiratory, and genitourinary systems, and other regulatory processes that are controlled directly or indirectly by the autonomic nervous system. The classical neurotic syndromes (hysteria, neurasthenia, and psychasthenia) are not considered psychosomatic illnesses, although the line between these two groups is often a tenuous one.

The conditions that are most commonly recognized as psychosomatic in nature are: the common allergies (eczema, hay fever, asthma), ulcers, colitis, and hypertension (high blood pressure).

Organic and Functional Aspects

There is still considerable difference of opinion as to the exact role played by the emotional as contrasted with the organic sensitivity factors in the precipitation of allergic reactions. These facts are evidence that emotions are precipitating factors in allergic reactions:

1. Allergic patients do not always react to the allergens to which they are sensitive.
2. Sensitive patients often develop typical allergic attacks when there is no evidence of the presence of the provoking allergen.
3. The allergic reactions of many patients vary directly with their emotional states.

In many cases, the relationship between emotional tension and allergic reactions is so marked as to indicate a causal relationship between the two. Suggestions and expectation can also induce typical allergic reactions in susceptible people. For example: hay fever in rose-pollen-sensitive people may be brought on by the sight of an artificial rose and asthma may be induced by the sight of a dust cloud on a movie screen. The evidence indicates that in psychosomatic allergies reactions both organic sensitivity and emotional factors are usually involved. The emotional conditions affect the general resistance of the person to disease and his reactiveness to allergic agents or inflammatory processes.

The other side of the picture can also be demonstrated, since there are nonpsychogenic allergies. The injection of an allergen into a sensitive subject can induce a reaction in a person who is ignorant of the nature of the injection and who will not react to similar injections of allergens to which he is not sensitive. The sensitivity of some people is so great that a minimal amount of the allergen itself, without any lowering of the threshold of reactivity by emotions, will cause reaction. Such individuals will react to the allergens whenever they are present, even in very small quantities. The emotional state of the person may influence the extent of the reaction but is not necessary for its induction. The allergic reactions in such people are not called psychogenic or psychosomatic.

Not all people react alike to stress, but in susceptible individuals experiencing psychosomatic disorders, the arterioles and other small blood vessels of the skin dilate, the mucous membranes swell, especially those of the nose, and the gastrointestinal tract dilates. The involved tissue becomes engorged with blood, swells, and becomes turgid. Such engorged and swollen tissues are particularly susceptible to the allergen.

Unrelieved feelings of hostility, resentment, and guilt have been shown to be associated with increased activity, increased blood supply, swelling, and, at times, small hemorrhagic lesions of both the stomach and the colon. Such lesions are considered to be the forerunner of peptic ulcers and ulcerative colitis. The involvement of the mucous membranes of the nose, sinuses, and bronchial tubes in emotional responses have been demonstrated in many cases of psychosomatic asthma and hay fever. Chronic hypertension (high blood pressure), acne vulgaris, and many chronic headaches (particularly some migraine headaches) are also often psychosomatic in origin.

Many of the bodily aspects of emotion are protective and defensive reactions to stress. However, some of these preparatory responses are not appropriate to the actual situation and become persistent chronic preparations for crises that never arise. Psychosomatic disorders are the results of persisting emotional disturbances and can be considered as natural concomitants or consequences of these disturbances.

The Problem of "Organ Selection"

There is only speculation and hypotheses as to why the psychosomatic disorders take the form of gastrointestinal disturbances in some people, eczema in others, and asthma, hay fever, or chronic hypertension in still others. One suggestion is that each individual has an inherent weakness, vulnerability, or sensitivity in a given organ or system of the body. The person with a weak digestive system develops ulcers or colitis, while the one with weak lungs develops asthma. This hypothesis assigns no specificity to the emotional components; the selection is entirely in terms of differential organ vulnerability.

On the other hand, there is the emotional specificity hypothesis. Each type of psychosomatic syndrome is thought to result from a specific emotion. According to the specificity hypothesis, there is high correlation between type of organic (somatic) disorder and type of emotional disturbance. Up to the present no such correlation has been demonstrated.

It is claimed that during psychotherapy the psychosomatic symptoms may shift from one system to another—from migraine headache to asthma to eczema. Cases have been reported in which similar symptoms have apparently shifted spontaneously. In times of war the case histories of servicemen suffering from psychosomatic disorders indicate that the psychosomatic syndromes seem to hold back or prevent the development of more severe neurotic or psychotic personality disorganizations. These latter observations suggest that the psychosomatic reactions constitute a form of defensive adaptation.

PSYCHOSES

Many psychotics display neurotic behavior prior to the onset of the more severe patterns of psychosis, and many neurotics evidence mild delusional behavior that properly would fall in the psychotic category. It appears profitable to think of neuroses and psychoses on a continuum of severity and of personal disorganization. Psychotic behavior is extremely variable, but there are some symptoms that seem to be common to psychotics. Many, but not all, psychotics have one or more of the following symptoms: hallucinations, delusions, and amnesias.

Hallucinations are disorders of perception. The individual involved may see things that others do not see, hear things that others do not hear, and feel things that others do not feel. Hallucinatory behavior may involve any of the sensory modalities and vary in the degree to which the behavior is incapacitating.

Delusions are beliefs that are grossly false. A person may feel that he is powerful and wealthy, or that he is some notable person (delusions of grandeur); or he may feel that he is being persecuted or punished by others (delusions of persecution). He may believe that some part of his body is malfunctional or missing (somatic delusions). Any belief that is grossly false according to the accepted standards for reality can be considered delusional.

Amnesias are disorders of memory. They have been discussed early in this chapter. Psychoses associated with aging and other deteriorative processes frequently have amnesias as a part of their symptoms. Amnesia can serve the psychological purposes of avoiding recall of painful or embarrassing experiences. It further provides an excuse for the avoidance of personal and social responsibilities.

FOUNDATIONS OF HEALTH SCIENCE

There are many subvarieties of schizophrenia that exhibit a tremendous diversity of symptoms. Some workers are so impressed by this that they doubt the usefulness of a single category for all forms of the disorder. However, the majority of workers feel that the different varieties of schizophrenia have enough in common to justify giving them a common name, and assume that the many forms have a common origin.

There are some lines of research that indicate that organic and biochemical factors are either contributory or basic causes of schizophrenia. However, this psychosis has traditionally been classed with the functional as opposed to the organic psychoses.

Schizophrenia is generally conceived of as a disturbance of one's relationships with people. As a result of these disturbances the individual withdraws from social participation, retires into himself, and lives largely in his own private world of thoughts and fantasies. This withdrawal is accompanied by a general, and often progressive, personality disorganization, and a breakdown of rational thinking and adaptive behavior. Whether the personality disorganization, bizarre ideation, and irrational behavior are the result of unsatisfactory relationships (defenses against threats) or the disturbed social relationships and withdrawal are caused by the personality, ideational, and behavioral disorganization is still in doubt. The consensus seems to favor the first of the alternatives—that disturbed social relationships are primary factors and that the social withdrawal and inappropriate affect, disturbed ideation, and bizarre behavior are their natural consequences.

Historically, four subgroups of schizophrenia have been recognized:

Simple schizophrenia is characterized by a gradual loss of interest that

All are not cured

A cousin of mine, a boy age fifteen, underwent severe withdrawal after the death of his father. His father's death was not the sole cause but triggered his reaction. He has been in and out of hospitals and various rehabilitation groups for the past four years. Recently a doctor related his condition to a physical hormone imbalance. As yet I don't know if his recent treatments have shown any change. Nothing else has worked and he has been going through hell for four years. He has tried drugs, religion, institutions and group therapy to no avail. He is constantly worried about something and has become rather difficult to live with because of his rash judgments and actions. Where does someone like this go from here?

progresses to the point of general *emotional apathy*. Affected individuals become increasingly ineffective in social relationships, until a complete social withdrawal occurs. The level of mental functioning declines until the person gives the superficial appearance of being mentally deficient.

The *paranoid form* of schizophrenia is characterized by delusions, usually delusions of persecution. Less often, delusions of grandeur may be present. The delusions typically have a recurring theme but are unsystematized and variable in their manifestations. They are frequently accompanied by various auditory and visual hallucinations. The patient's life becomes centered around these hallucinations, with resulting erratic, unpredictable, and occasionally dangerous behavior.

The *hebephrenic schizophrenic* shows severe disintegration of the personality, with repression to a childish level of behavior and withdrawal into a fantasy world. Facial grimacing and silly giggling or laughter are common. Inappropriate affect is a dominant feature of this form of schizophrenia.

When motor symptoms become dominant features of the disorder, it is called *catatonic schizophrenia*. The individual may remain motionless in stereotyped positions or postures. Sometimes he shows a waxy flexibility in which he will maintain any posture or position in which he is placed until fatigue forces him to modify it. Some catatonic individuals are very negativistic and resist any instructions or suggestions given them.

Characteristics of schizophrenia. Individuals diagnosed as schizophrenic tend to have certain common characteristics. The schizophrenic breakdown usually comes as the culmination of a history of unsuccessful social and personal adjustments. The typical childhood home atmosphere is described as oppressive, hostile, inconsistent, and either subtly or directly dominating or indifferent. Such a background is conducive to withdrawal as a defense.

Disturbed family relations and unhealthy family patterns are common with schizophrenics. Their mothers frequently have been found to be perfectionistic, moralistic, rejecting, dominating, overanxious, and over-possessive.[21] The fathers of schizophrenics are described as inadequate and either indifferent or passive.[22]

A relative lack of social give-and-take necessary for normal reality testing is found in the social history of many. The lack of normal family relationships results in a failure to develop the necessary social skills and emotional attitudes for healthy social participation. The preschizophrenic often acquires unrealistic conceptions of his own social roles and develops a self-concept considerably at variance with others' conceptions of him. Because of a lack of constant checks on his own frame of reference there develops an ever widening gap between him and other people. His

228   FOUNDATIONS OF HEALTH SCIENCE

thought and language patterns become progressively more individual and he becomes an emotional stranger in a strange land.[23] The schizophrenic's thinking regresses from an abstract, conceptual level to a primitive concrete form.[24]

Manic-depressive Psychosis

Schizophrenia accounts for around one-half of the total of psychotic persons. The remainder is composed of a great variety of disorders. The principal functional disorder other than schizophrenia is *manic-depressive psychosis.*

Manic-depressive psychosis is characterized by disordering of affect. This individual may be emotionally involved in a state of depression. The world is a sad and lonely place for him, and he becomes lethargic, inactive, and ideationally impoverished. Another possibility is that he will become overexcited, hyperactive, and even violent. Sometimes he may fluctuate between periods of depression and mania. During his manic periods he may be elated, hyperactive, do foolish things, make big plans, make bad investments, and suffer from delusions of grandeur. When the condition is one of depression the individual may sit for long periods of time, suffer from delusions of persecution, or become suicidal. The most common form that manic-depressive psychosis takes is depression.

Involutional Melancholia

A condition of *agitated depression,* or *involutional melancholia,* may occur as a concomitant to menopause. The symptoms are typically those of the depressive form of manic-depressive psychosis. With increasing knowledge of endocrine functioning this condition can now be much more adequately treated than in the past. A combination of hormonal and psychological treatment is effective in most cases. It is difficult to classify involutional melancholia as either functional or organic. There are predisposing elements of both involved.

Organic Psychoses

Organic psychoses are psychoses where the cause appears to be a basic underlying organic pathology. The symptoms of such disorders vary with the nature and extent of the physiological and neurological involvement. Such psychoses may result from addiction to the use of alcohol and some drugs. *General paresis* is a form of psychosis resulting from long-standing untreated syphilitic infection. Psychoses produced by such infections may take a variety of forms. The patient may become expansive and manic, or depressed and agitated, or may deteriorate to the point of decreased intellectual functioning characteristic of mental deficiency. *Encephalitis* and *meningitis* may both produce psychosis and/or intellectual deterioration. *Brain tumors* and *brain damage* can produce psychotic reactions that vary with the nature and extent of the damage produced.

Toxic deliria is a psychosis that may accompany infectious diseases such as diphtheria, pneumonia, and typhoid fever. It may also result from uremia, pernicious anemia, or the absorption of some drugs, metals, and gases. Such conditions, though severely disturbing at the time, are usually temporary and clear up when the toxin or the disorder is corrected. Certain nutritional deficiencies and endocrine disturbances can produce psychotic reactions, as can a number of traumatic events.

By far the most numerous of the organic psychoses are those associated with aging. The *psychoses of old age* may be of the nature of simple deterioration or they may include paranoid reactions, delirium and confusion, depression and agitation, as well as a mild form of mania. Amnesias are particularly common among the aged. Their recall of recent events becomes rather seriously impaired and they come to dote on the past.

ANTISOCIAL OR PSYCHOPATHIC BEHAVIOR

Antisocial personalities are not really classifiable as neurotic, psychotic, or mentally retarded. They are characterized by a marked deficiency in ethical and moral development and an inability to follow accepted and approved modes of behavior. These individuals frequently get into trouble, are most insistent on their own rights and privileges and are negligent of others', profit little from experience, and maintain no real loyalties or affections for others. This omnibus category of individuals includes people from all walks of life and educational levels. The range of severity of the disorder runs from an insensitivity to the welfare of others to overt crimes of violence, rape, prostitution, delinquency, and other crimes. Few such persons find their way into mental hospitals; some are in penal institutions; the majority, although they may be constantly in conflict with authority and frequently in social and personal difficulty, are outside of institutions.

The symptoms of antisocial personalities are complex and variable. Typically the individuals appear to be spontaneous and likeable on the surface. They may be seductively friendly if it serves their purposes. They seem to live for the present with little regard for the past or future and with an utter disregard for the happiness or welfare of others. They are emotionally immature, irresponsible, and impulsive.

The dynamics of antisocial behavior are not at all well understood. Some investigators emphasize the role of inheritance, injury, and other constitutional factors in the development of the behavior. Others attribute the causes primarily to inappropriate social learning deriving from family and community patterns of living. There is some evidence in support of each position. No doubt some juvenile delinquency derives from psychopathic disorder. However, much of delinquency would appear to derive from social and cultural factors, in that most juvenile delinquents abandon their delinquent behaviors when they reach adulthood and become reasonably productive citizens.

Treatable constitutional factors have really not been isolated; therefore current therapy is principally of a psychological or sociological nature. The patterns of behavior, once acquired, are highly resistant to change, and current treatment programs are not very effective. Research emphasis on preventive procedures might yield information on the origins of these difficulties. In view of the rather bleak picture of current treatment, this may be the more profitable area of investigation.

TREATMENT

The various theories of personality have been generated in large part from the experiences of psychotherapists in dealing with clients and their problems. In that the clinical practice and observations of the psychotherapists evolve into viewpoints relative to personality, it can readily be understood that personality theories and psychotherapeutic procedures are closely allied. A general orientation of some procedures is presented in the discussion that follows.

Psychoanalytic Approaches

In psychoanalytic approaches to psychotherapy, concepts of levels of awareness are significant for therapy. The conscious level consists of those thoughts and ideas which the person is aware of at the moment. The preconscious is composed of those ideas which the person is not aware of at the moment but that can be voluntarily recalled. The unconscious consists of memories and ideas that the person has forgotten and cannot recall. The unconscious was perceived by Freud as comprising the bulk of the personality. Much of the forgotten material had a strong motivational influence on the person's behavior.[25] Psychoanalysis emphasizes the importance of the previous experiences of the person, with particular regard to psychosexual development. Instincts or genetically determined impulses to actions are directing agents for the libido, or life energy. Much of our early experience is unconscious but still remains motivational in character.

Great emphasis is placed on the motivational aspect of the unconscious, which contains much forgotten and repressed material. Techniques for uncovering the repressed material and bringing it into consciousness have been developed. Much time is devoted to these processes in psychoanalysis. The recall of much unconscious material may be psychologically painful for the patient, and he may resist attempts to bring some of it into consciousness. Resistance designates both an inability and a reluctance to recall repressed desires and ideas. Freud developed psychoanalysis to overcome resistance and bring the patient's conflicts and anxieties into consciousness. Freud viewed the overcoming of resistance as the key factor in bringing about permanent change in the psychic life of the patient.

Prominent among the techniques for uncovering repressed material is free association and dream analysis. Psychoanalysis is usually a lengthy process. Because it does take a great deal of time and involves an analyst and a patient in a one-to-one situation, psychoanalysis can be quite expensive.

Client-Centered Therapy

Client-centered therapy has also been termed *phenomenological, self theorizing,* and *nondirective.*[26] The system is based on a phenomenological point of view and on confidence that the individual has the capacity for growth or self-actualization. The work of therapy is designed to release the patient from threat and conflict and to permit growth to occur. Emphasis is placed on the differences between the client's perceived self and his behavior. When the person begins to perceive himself as behaving in a manner consistent with his self-concept, he begins to feel more secure and adequate. If the discrepancy between the perceived self and actual behavior becomes too great, it creates threat. The person may protect himself against this threat through the use of defense mechanisms.

The client in client-centered therapy is presumed to have the capacity for growth toward self-actualization. The client is the center of the process. The attitude of the therapist is permissive and accepting in order to reduce threat to a minimum. The therapist is neither coercive nor authoritarian. Rogers emphasizes the importance of the attitude of the therapist and indicates that this is more important than technique.[27] In the absence of threat, the client is able to accept parts of himself that he previously could not accept or of which he was unaware. In accepting himself realistically, he is capable of accepting others and becoming a more self-actualizing person.

Emphasis in therapy is upon freedom for the client to discuss those facets of his problem or personality that he wishes to discuss. The therapist assists in this matter by trying to reflect the feelings of the client. The therapist attempts to understand and view the world as the client does. The climate of the therapeutic situation is of vital importance and is characterized by the therapist's warmth, sincerity, sensitive understanding acceptance of the client, and regard for him as a human being. The therapeutic relationship is of greater importance than the direction of the discussion that takes place.

Various self theorists have been active in the development of therapeutic procedures. There are differences among them, but the basic principle of self-actualization is typically central to their procedures.

Behavior Modification

Modification of behavior through conditioning procedures has received a great deal of investigation in recent years. Wolpe modeled a system of psychotherapy upon the results of laboratory research with cats.[28] Cats were given electric shocks in their feeding cages. It was observed that following this treatment they would refuse to eat anywhere near their cages. This behavior was interpreted as comparable to the generalization of anxiety in human patients. Anxiety, conditioned to the feeding cages, was generalized to the whole room which interfered with the eating response outside the cages. The cats were then treated by feeding them in a room a considerable distance from the place in which they had been shocked. They displayed no anxiety. The feeding of the animals was brought closer and closer to the original place where they had been shocked. The gradual nature of the approach to the original feeding area was maintained in order not to upset the eating responses. Eventually the animals were capable of eating within the room where they had previously been shocked and finally within the original feeding cages. The cats were cured of their neuroses in this manner. By strengthening the eating response, the response of anxiety was inhibited. Wolpe described this process as one of reciprocal inhibition.

Therapy sessions have been organized for human patients according to the same principle used with the cats. Through interviews, a hierarchy of situations that produce anxiety in the patient is established. Starting with those situations that produce little anxiety, the situation is arranged so that some positive response takes place; anxiety is replaced by this positive response. The patient works up through the hierarchy by making some positive response to the situations until eventually he is able to replace his irrational neurotic responses with appropriate ones. The use of the conditioning procedure in psychiatry has been proven successful.

Another group of investigators has followed procedures and principles developed by Skinner. He attacked the assumption that behavior disorders were a reflection of some internal conflict or sickness.[29]

So-called neurotic behavior is conceived of as maladaptive behavior that is acquired through a process of conditioning and is capable of being modified by a number of laboratory techniques. There is no complex and no illness. Treatment is directed entirely toward the behavior of the individual. This is in sharp contrast with dynamic psychotherapy, with its emphasis on hypothetical underlying complexes, disease processes, and illness. Behavior therapy constitutes a rejection of traditional psychodynamic personality theories. Conceptions such as insight, lifting of repression, and unconscious processes and urges, are rejected as unnecessary to the modification of behavior. The treatment problem becomes one of altering the reinforcing environment so that adequate behaviors are maintained, effective new behaviors learned, and inadequate behaviors extinguished. Behavior therapy consists of the application of principles of learning to the treatment of disordered behavior. This has been accomplished in a wide variety of areas using a variety of techniques.

Counterconditioning, response inhibition, operant conditioning with positive reinforcement, social reinforcement, avoidance conditioning, and extinction procedures have all been employed as procedures for the modification of maladaptive behavior. It has been traditionally believed that when attention was given solely to modification of disordered behavior, the behavior could be modified, but other inappropriate behaviors would appear. This is known as symptom substitution. Contrary to the traditional belief, there is little evidence that symptom substitution actually happens.[30]

The number of psychologists contributing to this expanding area of treatment is imposing. The behavior therapies are being expanded continuously, and their success has created challenging new possibilities for the effective treatment of behavior disorders using scientific procedures. The science of psychology and the practice of clinical psychology are becoming more mutually supportive and interdependent.

Further Procedures

Means have been devised to assist mentally ill and emotionally disturbed people to regain adequate mental health. Some of these procedures are used by psychotherapists as a routine matter; others are designed for

FOUNDATIONS OF HEALTH SCIENCE

special purposes and special problems. Occupational therapy and physiotherapy are valuable adjunctive services in psychotherapy.

The problem of a shortage of adequately trained psychotherapists has led to a number of innovations in therapy. One such innovation has been that of limiting the time that the patient may see his therapist. Patient improvement in time limited therapy has been reported to be favorable.[31] However, most attempts to find an answer to the perennial problem of clinic waiting lists and therapist shortages have depended upon the treatment of patients in groups.

Group Therapy

The procedure known as group therapy has developed out of scarcity of trained psychotherapists, the great number of individuals seeking assistance, and the belief on the part of some psychotherapists that working through one's problems within a group, rather than in an individual therapy situation, provides a more real, life-like atmosphere in which the patient can interact with others.

In group therapy a psychotherapist can see more than one patient at a time. Thus the patient-hours of contact with a professional therapist are vastly expanded. Interaction with other people in a situation designed to be therapeutic can serve a real function. The security provided by a group of people can be enough so that certain patients, who normally would have extreme difficulty in relating to a professional psychotherapist in a one-to-one relationship, may be able to function in a group. They can derive psychological benefits that would take a great deal more time and effort in individual therapy. In some circumstances a patient may be seen on an individual basis until he is emotionally strong enough to function in a group.

The Group

During the late 1960s group interaction situations were devised in great number. To be in a group became the popular thing to do. Groups were formulated in schools, industries, churches, and clinics. They were formed for the training of managers, for personnel workers, for various psychiatric reasons, and for social reasons. The names given the group processes were extremely variable. Names such as sensitivity group, encounter group, basic encounter group, and T group, became familiar to a great many people.

By the time the 1970s arrived, there had been little actual research on how a group should or could function best and on what the actual outcome of these group interactions was. Some people reacted with great enthusiasm and almost fanatic acceptance of the group processes as being the most vital of the social interactive exercises that resulted in self-enlightenment, increased self-understanding, greater love for others, and increased personal happiness. Others contended that most groups provided an essentially emotional experience that had the scientific status of a Midwestern, Protestant revival meeting of the 1920s. The group was an emotion laden experience, with short-lived results.

According to Rogers, none of the research on group experience is very precise.[32] Most early investigations report that changes in attitude, behavior, and self-concept occur. A reasonable number of those changes persist over time. Extensive investigations of various kinds of groups do not report such favorable findings. It is reported that nineteen percent of the individuals involved in various groups changed in a negative way or become casualties during the group session.[33] This negative impact of the process is nearly twice as great as that reported for other psychotherapies (Bergin and Garfield, 1971). Moreover the results of what favorable changes do occur appear to be relatively short-lived. Growth groups of various kinds have become so numerous and so many people have become involved that the American Psychological Association has developed a set of guidelines for psychologists conducting growth groups. *Those anticipating entering a group of some kind should find out in advance who is leading it, what his qualifications are, what is expected to transpire in the group, and various other items of information important to the individual. Moreover, participation in any group should not be the result of coercion or persuasion. Participation should be voluntary and as much information as possible about the group and its functioning should be obtained before making a commitment to participate.*

The group experience has developed as a result of the feelings of loneliness, isolation, and alienation that arise in contemporary life. Rogers points out that "the person who is involved in a basic encounter with another is no longer an isolated individual."[34] The group may serve other purposes such as handling tensions arising from familial and cultural conflict. Social and personal feelings of fulfillment may be provided by group interaction. Obviously, the group is used for reasons other than those of restoring or training people to live in the society effectively enough to keep from being labeled as disturbed.

Family Therapy

The treatment of people with problems is often difficult. The family situation within which the patient must live or to which he must return is often quite unsatisfactory. When this is the case, the progress of therapy can be slow and tenuous. In recognition of the familial-social nature of

FOUNDATIONS OF HEALTH SCIENCE

many problems of behavior, some therapists have turned to working with the whole family rather than only the psychologically disturbed member.

When behavior is viewed as a result of interactional experience, the necessity for understanding familial interaction processes becomes rather self-evident. There are a variety of approaches to family therapy. They may range from working exclusively with the family as a unit, working with the patient alone plus working with the family, to working with a number of families at the same time. The journal *Family Process* is devoted to the understanding and treatment of families of psychiatric patients. This Journal provides a source of current information on developments in this area.

Medical Treatment

Recently, advances in the field of medical treatment of emotional disturbances have been particularly noticeable. Biochemical and pharmacological treatment has received more attention than any other medical approach. Some drugs have been developed that have been particularly effective with tense and anxious patients. The variety of drugs now available has reduced the frequency with which surgery for the relief of symptoms in psychiatric patients is performed. Shock therapy in the form of electric, insulin, or Metrazol shock has been used less frequently since the advent of tranquilizing drugs.

The drugs most frequently used in the treatment of behavior disorders are tranquilizing drugs; these are used extensively in the control and treatment of patients in mental hospitals. Their use for out-patients in both medical and psychiatric institutions also has become a rather common practice. It is probable that in and of themselves they have no real influence on the causative factors in emotional disturbance, but they are very effective in the relief of symptoms. Certain patients who would not otherwise be amenable to psychotherapy can be treated with such medication.

Drugs that have exciting or arousing effects are used with some psychiatric patients. Drugs are used in analysis in order to permit the patient to express feelings that he ordinarily would be afraid to express, such as deeply repressed experiences and feelings. Hypnosis is used for the same purpose by some psychotherapists.

IN CONCLUSION

Neuroses can be treated in a variety of ways. Medical, psychological, and sociological treatment procedures may be employed. Treatment is an individual matter and must be fitted to the needs of the patient. The use of drugs of various kinds have been employed as effective adjuncts to various psychological and sociological treatments. The number of effective psychotherapeutic procedures that may be utilized is rather large, and research continues in the development and evaluation of various psychotherapeutic techniques.

Most colleges and universities have counseling centers or psychological clinics that are available for students with emotional problems, vocational problems, and problems of adjustment. Metropolitan communities have services available through family service agencies, community psychiatric clinics, and private agencies and practitioners.

The general prognosis for psychoneurotic disorders appears to be good, although there are no definitive studies that clarify what the psychiatric status of the young adult neurotic can be expected to be ten to twenty years later. It is estimated that some 40 to 60 percent of people with neurotic problems resolve their problems and develop greater maturity of behavior with or without therapy. Although methods of evaluating the outcome of therapy are not uniform or very good, it is probably a safe estimate that about 90 percent of neurotics show apparent recovery or marked improvement as a result of treatment.

With increasing information, improving techniques, and changing attitudes toward mental illnesses, care and treatment become more successful in assisting the mentally ill to live more effectively. Prognosis for schizophrenia and other psychotic disorders is becoming increasingly favorable. Most schizophrenics now can be treated and recover sufficiently to live reasonably happy and productive lives. This represents a great deal of progress over the past fifty years.

Notes

1. P. London, "The Psychotherapy Boom. From the Long Couch for the Sick to the Push Button for the Bored," *Psychology Today*, 8:62–69, 1974.

2. C. S. Dweck and C. Reppucci, "Learned Helplessness and Reinforcement Responsibility in Children," *Journal of Personality and Social Psychology*, 25:106–116, 1973.

3. J. Ducette and S. Walk, "Cognitive and Motivational Correlates of Generalized Expectancies for Control," *Journal of Personality and Social Psychology*, 26:420–426, 1973; S. J. Nowicki and B. R. Strickland, "A Locus of Control Scale for Children," *Journal of Consulting and Clinical Psychology*, 40:148–154, 1974.

4. M. E. P. Seligman, "Fall into Helplessness," *Psychology Today*, 7:43–49, 1973; W. R. Miller and M. E. P. Seligman, "Depression and Perception of Reinforcement," *Journal of Abnormal Psychology*, 82:62–73, 1973.

5. Miller and Seligman, "Depression and the Perception of Reinforcement."

6. Seligman, "Fall into Helplessness"; M. E. P. Seligman, "Submissive Death: Giving Up On Life," *Psychology Today*, 7:80–85, 1974; M. E. P. Seligman, *Helplessness* (New York: W. H. Freeman, 1974).

7. Dweck and Reppucci, "Learned Helplessness and Reinforcement Responsibility in Children."

8. Miller and Seligman, "Depression and the Perception of Reinforcement."

9. Seligman, "Fall into Helplessness."

10. *Statistical Abstracts of the United States, 1975* (Washington, D.C.: U.S. Government Printing Office, 1976), p. 64.

11. Ibid., p. 61.

12. L. L. Dublin, *Suicide: A Sociological and Statistical Study* (New York: Ronald Press, 1963).

13. R. Kastenbaum and R. Aisenberg, *The Psychology of Death* (New York: Springer Publishing Company, 1972).

14. N. Tabachnick, "Observations on Attempted Suicide," in *Clues to Suicide,* ed. E. S. Shneidman and N. L. Farberow (New York: McGraw-Hill Book Co., 1957).

15. I. R. C. Batchelor, "Suicide in Old Age," in *Clues to Suicide,* ed. Shneidman and Farberow (New York: McGraw-Hill Book Co., 1957).

16. J. Tuckman, W. F. Youngman, and B. Feifer, "Suicide and Family Disorganization," *International Journal of Social Psychiatry*, 12:291–295, 1966.

17. L. R. Wolberg, *The Technique of Psychotherapy* (New York: Grune and Stratton, 1964).

18. Kastenbaum and Aisenberg, *Psychology of Death.*

19. J. C. Coleman, *Abnormal Psychology and Modern Life,* 3rd ed. (Glenview, Ill.: Scott, Foresman & Company, 1964), pp. 217–218.

20. S. Lipton, "Dissociated Personality: A Case Report," *Psychiatric Quarterly*, 17:35–56, 1943.

21. E. R. Clandy, "A Study of the Development and Cause of Schizophrenia in Children," *Psychiatric Quarterly*, 25:81–90, 1951; R. V. Freeman and H. M. Grayson, "Maternal Attitudes in Schizophrenia," *Journal of Abnormal and Social Psychology*, 50:45–52, 1955.

22. J. L. Despert, "Schizophrenia in Children," *Psychiatric Quarterly*, 12:366–371, 1938; G. L. Hajdw, "Contributions to the Etiology of Schizophrenia," *Psychoanalytic Review*, 27:421–438, 1940.

23. R. B. Ellsworth, "The Regression of Schizophrenic Language," *Journal of Consulting Psychology*, 15:387–391, 1951; M. Whiteman, "The Performance of Schizophrenics on Social Concepts," *Journal of Abnormal and Social Psychology*, 49:266–271, 1954.

24. J. S. Kasanin, "Developmental Roots of Schizophrenia," *American Journal of Psychiatry*, 101:770–776, 1945.

25. S. Freud, *A General Introduction to Psychoanalysis* (New York: Liveright, 1920).

26. C. R. Rogers, *Client Centered Therapy* (Boston: Houghton Mifflin, 1951).

27. C. R. Rogers, *On Becoming a Person: A Therapist's View of Psychotherapy* (Boston: Houghton Mifflin, 1961).

28. J. Wolpe, *Psychotherapy by Reciprocal Inhibition* (Stanford, Calif.: Stanford University Press, 1958).

29. B. F. Skinner, *Science and Human Behavior* (New York: Macmillan, 1953).

30. J. M. Grossberg, "Behavior Therapy: A Review," *Psychological Bulletin*, 62:73–88, 1964.

31. G. A. Muench, "An Investigation of the Efficacy of Time-Limited Psychotherapy," *Journal of Counseling Psychology*, 12:294–299, 1965.

32. C. R. Rogers, "The T-group Comes of Age," *Psychology Today*, 3:27–31, 58–61, 1969.

33. M. A. Lieberman, I. D. Yalom, and M. B. Miles, *Encounter Groups: First Facts* (New York: Basic Books, 1973).

34. Rogers, "The T-group Comes of Age."

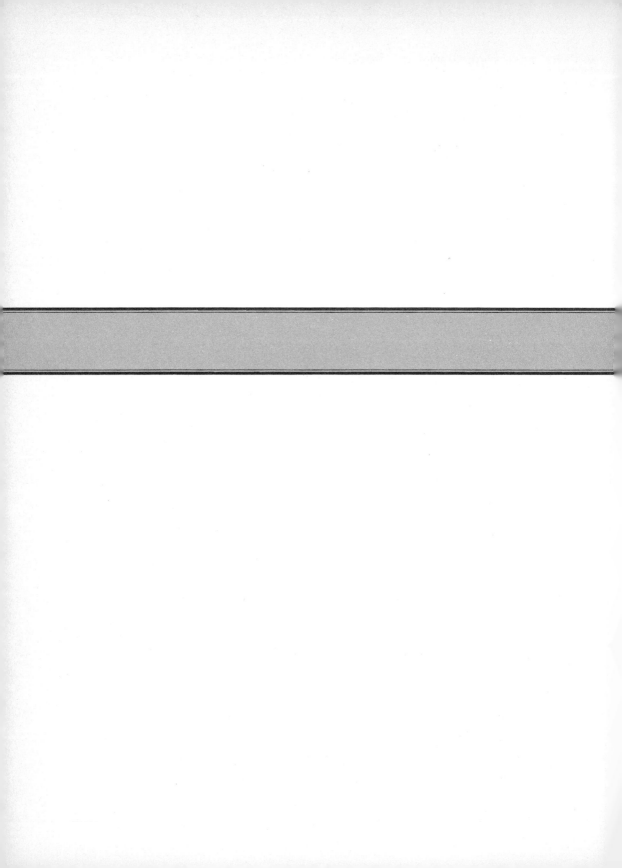

ALCOHOL AND TOBACCO

chapter eight

Sometimes it seems that the things that are most pleasurable contain an element of danger. The consumption of alcoholic beverages and smoking appear to be enjoyable to many persons; they are also deleterious to the health and happiness of millions of people in the world. There are those in society who believe that pleasure for pleasure's sake has an element of immorality in it. There are others who think that hazards should be avoided if at all possible. There are many who ascribe to a philosophy of life that allows any behavior that results in minimal harm to themselves or their community. What is done about the use of alcohol and tobacco depends on one's system of values, which is determined by what one observes his family and friends doing, what pleasures one believes can be derived from these practices, and what untoward results he thinks can or cannot accrue from using alcoholic beverages and from smoking.

ALCOHOL

Alcoholic beverages are used in some form or another by all societies. Even in cultures in which drinking is forbidden by religious beliefs, alcohol is consumed. All countries have rules and traditions about alcohol that are primarily to control its misuse. Why is a compound that is potentially dangerous so widely used?

Why Do People Drink?

Alcohol produces pleasurable sensations of relaxation and well-being. It provides a relief from the tensions and cares of daily living. Its use for these purposes is an accepted tradition by many, many people. It is relatively inexpensive in one form or another and is readily available.

Drinking has been and is a part of ritualistic ceremonies in most civilizations. It is used to pledge loyalty and friendship and to celebrate events such as engagements, marriages, births, deaths, religious rites, and business contracts.

The ability to drink is also associated with the attainment of manhood and maturity. To some it is a sign of weakness not to be able to drink. The ability to "hold one's liquor" is an admired accomplishment in our society. To many young people being able to drink is equated with adulthood.

There are many misconceptions about the use and abuse of alcohol. Which of the following statements are true or false?

1. Most, if not all, chronic alcoholics cannot learn to drink like the non-alcoholic.
2. An alcoholic is one who is continuously drunk.
3. Alcoholism is not inherited.
4. The so-called "skid-row population" is comprised mainly of alcoholics.
5. Many of the physiological changes seen in the alcoholic are due to avitaminosis.
6. The alcoholic usually drinks because he likes the taste.
7. Some alcoholics drink only beer.
8. The alcoholic needs only to exert his will power to stop drinking.
9. Diluting alcohol with a carbonated mix speeds up absorption.
10. There is a good margin of safety between acute intoxication and alcoholic coma and death.
11. The toxic effects of alcohol on the body are one of the leading causes of death by poisoning.
12. Having a "blackout" is a common phenomenon among social drinkers.
13. Abstinence will prevent alcoholism.

FOUNDATIONS OF HEALTH SCIENCE

Figure 8.1 The use of Alcoholic Beverages—A Social Custom. (Photo by Norman Wexler, courtesy Los Angeles County.)

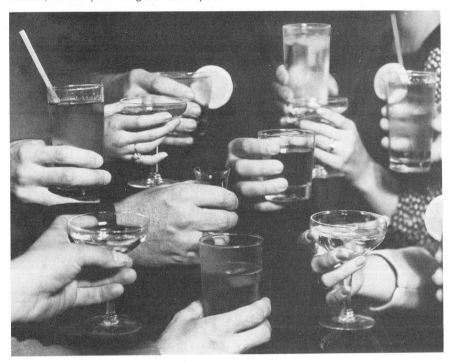

14. Keeping active will increase the rate of oxidation of alcohol so one can drink more without feeling it.
15. Chronic alcoholics have abnormal electroencephalograms.
16. Moderate drinking shortens the life span.
17. The alcoholic absorbs alcohol into the blood stream more rapidly than the nonalcoholic.
18. Alcoholism is a more socially accepted term for drunkenness.
19. It takes more alcohol to produce the same "effect or feeling" in the frequent drinker than in the rare drinker.
20. Alcohol in moderate amounts is a physiological stimulant.
21. Alcoholism produces impotence.
22. Alcohol increases perceptual ability.
23. Alcohol is an anesthetic.
23. A good way to prevent alcoholism is never to drink alone.
(All the even-numbered questions are false.)

PROBLEMS RELATED TO THE
USE OF ALCOHOL

There are a number of problems arising out of the use of alcohol as a beverage. Plaut claims that any controversy or disagreement about the use or nonuse of alcohol is a problem including "both the difficulties that persons get into by drinking and society's efforts to cope with these difficulties."[1] There is controversy and disagreement about: (1) whether or not alcohol should be available for use as a beverage since a sizeable number of people do not drink—about 30 percent—and religious groups differ in their positions regarding the moral aspects of drinking; (2) what constitutes appropriate drinking behavior; (3) how old one should be to purchase alcohol; (4) how youth should be prepared to participate in a society that drinks; (5) what the specific role of the school is in educating about alcohol; (6) how accidental injuries and deaths due to drinking can be reduced; (7) whether alcoholism is a condition or state, a disease, an illness, or a moral deficiency, and what the social, medical, and legal ramifications of labeling it one or the other of these terms are; and (8) how people with alcohol problems can be helped, plus who is going to pay for such help.

These facts are reported by the National Council on Alcoholism, Inc:

There are some 100 million persons over the age of 15 in this country who drink. Of these an estimated 9 million are alcoholics or have drinking problems.

The average alcoholic is a man or woman in the middle thirties with a good job, good home, and a family. Less than 5 percent of alcoholics are found on Skid Row.

Alcoholism ranks among the major national health threats along with cancer, mental illness, and heart disease.

Some 6.5 million employed workers are alcoholics.

Fifty percent of all fatal accidents occurring on the roads involve alcohol. Of these fatal accidents, an alcoholic is involved 50 percent of the time.

Forty percent of all male admissions to state mental hospitals suffer from alcoholism.

Problems in the use of alcohol and/or alcoholism account directly or indirectly for 40 percent of the problems brought to family courts.

Thirty-one percent of those who commit suicide are alcoholics. Their suicide rate is 58 times that of non-alcoholics.[2]

Chafetz reports, also, that problems associated with the misuse of alcohol affects almost every component of the economic and social system. Well over two and a half million arrests are related to alcohol misuse yearly, and the total economic loss to the nation from alcohol problems is over fifteen billion dollars annually.[3]

However, most people with problems related to drinking are not derelicts or down-at-the-heels–appearing bums. The National Institute on Alcohol Abuse and Alcoholism states that at least 95 percent of the population having problems with alcohol

> . . . consists of employed or employable, family-centered individuals. It has been estimated that more than 70 percent of them reside in respectable neighborhoods, live with their husbands or wives, try to send their children to college, belong to a country club, attend church, pay taxes, and continue to perform more or less effectively as bank presidents, housewives, farmers, salesmen, machinists, stenographers, teachers, clergymen, and physicians.[4]

Physiological Effects of Alcohol

Alcohol is rapidly absorbed into the circulatory system by simple diffusion. It can be detected in the blood within two minutes. The actual rate at which alcohol is diffused and the behavioral results depend upon a number of variables. Table 8.1 gives the effects of alcoholic beverages.

Kind of beverage. In all of the alcoholic beverages the major ingredient is ethyl alcohol, or ethanol. The percentage varies with the beverage.

Beverage	Percent Alcohol
Beer	3.5 (U.S.A.)
Wines	17–20
Liqueurs	22–50
Distilled Spirits	40–50 (80–100 proof)

There are other ingredients present, too, that alter the rate of absorption. These are known as cogeners. They may come from the initial substance fermented to produce alcohol, result from the fermenting process, or be added for flavor or coloring purposes. Cogeners interfere with absorption, oxidation, and metabolism of alcohol. Beer and wines have greater percentages of cogeners that reduce the rate of absorption. Diluting alcohol with water and juices slows down diffusion; carbonated mixes increase the rate, though.

Effects of food. The presence of food in the stomach, especially fats and proteins, slows down the rate of absorption of alcohol. If the alcohol is taken with a meal, the person's peak blood concentration may be reduced by as much as 50 percent.

Table 8.1 Effects of Alcoholic Beverages

Amount of Beverage	Concentration of Alcohol Attained in the Blood	Effects (Intensity of feelings vary with individual to some extent)	Time Required for All Alcohol to Leave the Body
1 highball (1½ oz. whiskey) or 1 cocktail (1½ oz. whiskey) or 3½ oz. fortified wine or 5½ oz. ordinary wine or 2 bottles (24 oz.) beer	0.02 to 0.03%	Some changes in feeling. Slight dizziness. Sense of warmth. Mild throbbing of back of head. Slight feeling of physical well-being and relaxation.	2 hours
2 highballs or 2 cocktails or 7 oz. fortified wine or 11 oz. ordinary wine or 4 bottles beer	0.05 to 0.06%	Feeling of warmth— mental relaxation, decrease of fine skills, less concern with minor irritations and restraints.	4 hours
3 highballs or 3 cocktails or 10½ oz. fortified wine or 15½ oz. (1 pt.) ordinary wine or 6 bottles beer	0.09 to 0.10%	Buoyancy, exaggerated emotion and behavior, talkativeness, noisiness, or moroseness, impulsiveness, may stagger. Chemical diagnosis of drunkenness.	6 hours
4 highballs or 4 cocktails or 14 oz. fortified wine or 22 oz. ordinary wine or 8 bottles (3 qts.) beer	0.12%	Drowsiness, impairment of fine coordination, clumsiness, slight to moderate unsteadiness in standing or walking.	8 hours
5 highballs or 5 cocktails or 17½ oz. fortified wine or 27½ oz. ordinary wine or ½ pt. whiskey	0.15%	Intoxication, unmistakable abnormality of gross bodily functions and mental faculties.	10 hours

Based on a person of "average" size (150 pounds). For those weighing considerably more or less, the amounts would have to be correspondingly more or less to produce the same results. The effects indicated at each stage will diminish as the concentration of alcohol in the blood is reduced by being oxidized and eliminated. Levels of .3% produce stupor, .4% deep anesthesia, and .5% fatality.

FOUNDATIONS OF HEALTH SCIENCE

Weight and body chemistry. The larger person who weighs more (not fat but muscle tissue) will show the effects of alcohol less quickly than the smaller person. In some people the stomach empties more quickly than in others, so they will have higher blood concentrations sooner. Also, emotions may affect the rate at which the stomach empties. Absorption may be quickened or lessened by anger, fear, stress, fatigue, or illness. People who have been drinking for a long time develop a tolerance and may require more alcohol to produce the same effects that occurred when they first started drinking.[5]

Metabolism. Certainly anything that delays absorption of alcohol retards intoxication. When a person does become intoxicated, however, how quickly the alcohol is oxidized, or metabolized, determines how soon the person becomes sober. The liver is the main organ of oxidation. As the alcohol reaches this organ it is changed first to acetaldehyde, which is an extremely toxic chemical. Acetaldehyde is rapidly changed to acetate, which ultimately is broken down to carbon dioxide and water. This process occurs at the rate of about one-third ounce per hour. This rate is *not* influenced by exercising, drinking black coffee, taking a cold shower, breathing pure oxygen, drinking fructose, or any other action. Sitting quietly in a warm room with little circulation of air in itself produces relaxation and a feeling of sleepiness. If the anesthetizing effect of alcohol is superimposed on this state, the victim more quickly is aware of dizziness, a buzzing sound, numbness and tingling sensations, and warmth. He literally does feel "tipsy or drunk more quickly."

Hangovers. Unfortunately, there is little one can do to prevent the "morning after" effects of too much alcohol. The commonly occurring results of fatigue, nausea, upset stomach, anxiety, and headache are unpleasant but not dangerous.

> Although the hangover has been blamed on mixing drinks, it can be produced by any alcoholic beverage alone, or by pure alcohol. There is inadequate evidence to support beliefs that it is caused by vitamin deficiencies, dehydration, fusel oils (nonalcoholic components of alcoholic beverages which are relatively toxic, but present in clinically insignificant amounts), or any other nonalcoholic components.[6]

None of these popularly believed remedies for a hangover are supported by scientific evidence: coffee, raw eggs, alkalizers, vitamin preparations, pep pills, insulin, or barbiturates. The best treatment is still aspirin, bed rest, and solid food.

Circulatory system. For a few minutes after ingestion of alcohol the heart beat may increase, causing the blood vessels near the surface of the skin to dilate, which creates a feeling of warmth. The specific physiological reaction is that blood vessels relax and dilate, which produces a drop in blood pressure. Recent evidence indicates that alcohol can produce heart disease (without presence of liver damage). Alcohol is apparently directly toxic to the heart and lungs. It is not particularly damaging to the kidneys even though it increases urinary output.

The brain and central nervous system. Probably the most serious consequences of alcohol, both immediate and long-term, occur in the central nervous system. The immediate results of alcohol circulating to the brain are impaired reasoning and motor coordination. This is why drinking contributes to accidents. The alcohol impairs reasoning, and "we just think we perform well." After some fifteen to twenty years of heavy drinking, alcoholic psychosis may develop. Some of the mental illnesses in which alcohol use is a factor are incurable.

The most frequent of these serious consequences is *delirium tremens* (D.T.'s). Each psychotic episode lasts for several days and is characterized by hallucinations with extreme fear and violent excitement; disorientation; trembling of hands, legs, and tongue to the point of exhaustion; and profuse sweating. Sleep eventually terminates the attack. The mortality rate is between 4 and 5 percent, even with the proper medical treatment of intravenous glucose to reduce swelling of cerebral tissue, sedatives, vitamin B-complex injections, and insulin.

Less frequent but more serious is *Korsakoff's disease*. Patients with that disease have severe memory defects that may persist for weeks, months, or for life. They are disoriented, have amnesia, and may feel euphoric and appear quite serene. The characteristic symptom is confabulation (falsification of memory).

Alcoholic personality deterioration is the ultimate fate of many years of prolonged immoderate drinking. Experimental work indicates that alcohol interferes with the action of thiamine, which is necessary for oxidative metabolism of the brain. The symptoms begin with loss of emotional control; if the disease is not arrested (the patient maintains sobriety), the end result is dementia. Victims become progressively more impulsive, untruthful and unreliable, irresponsible, irritable, critical, surly, and brutal, and in the end they have impaired memory and delusions.

Peripheral neuropathy consists of pains and paresthesias in the feet and hands, weakness of the extremities, dryness, swelling, and discoloration of the skin of legs and feet; tenderness of muscles, particularly the gastrocnemius; and loss of sensation in the feet and hands. Sometimes the afflicted is unable to walk easily or cannot walk at all.

The gastrointestinal system. Alcohol causes physical alterations in the

FOUNDATIONS OF HEALTH SCIENCE

stomach and liver. Its prolonged use produces inflammatory changes in the gastric mucosa, resulting in chronic gastritis. There may be no free acid or enzymes in the stomach, and both are necessary for digestion. Approximately 50 percent of alcoholics are so affected. Liver damage and cirrhosis are commonly associated with drinking. Three-fourths of habitual inebriates have some malfunction, and almost 10 percent have cirrhosis. Less than 1 percent of moderate or nondrinkers have this serious condition. In all probability, liver damage is due to nutritional disturbances rather than to the direct action of alcohol. In advanced cirrhosis, there is a slight fever; nausea, vomiting, and abdominal pain; emaciation; foul breath; jaundice, nodular scarred liver; ascites and edema; and mental stupor. The fatality rate is about 50 percent, and the major immediate causes of death are hemorrhage (because of weakened abdominal and esophageal veins), coma, and pneumonia.

Nutritional deficiencies result from less food eaten due to lack of interest and loss of appetite, interference with the absorption and utilization of food, and additional needs for vitamin B, the requirement for which is increased when the ratio of carbohydrate foods is considerably greater than fatty foods. Alcohol is pure carbohydrate. The symptoms of thiamine and niacin deficiencies appear to be the most common nutritional disturbances connected with alcohol.

ATTITUDES AND DRINKING PATTERNS

All cultures do not have the same difficulties with the use of alcohol. The differences are attributed to the function of alcohol in specific cultures and to the attitudes that the members hold toward alcohol. The rates of drinking, or drunkenness, of problem drinkers, and of alcoholism appear to be dependent upon the social attitudes toward the use of alcohol as a beverage. Americans from the same ethnic and cultural groups tend to have the same attitudinal sets, although variations are great.

The Italians

The use of alcohol as a beverage is widespread among Italians. Few abstain from its use, and less than 5 percent consume wine exclusively. American-Italians drink socially as well as with meals, and one purpose is for "effect." Children are given wine early in life. Italians may tolerate drunkenness, but they *do not condone it.* In Italy, alcohol is used for health and custom. Wine is the customary beverage. Intoxication is rare.

The French

In Northern France, the people consume large quantities of wine, primarily with meals. The rates of alcoholism are high in comparison with other Western countries. The attitude toward wine is that it is nourishing and strengthening, but distilled beverages are harmful. The lower classes consume greater quantities than the upper classes and do so between meals as well as with meals. In addition to consuming greater quantities of alcohol than the Italians do, the French tolerate inebriation to a greater extent.[7]

The Irish

According to Bales, the Irish-Americans have the highest rates of drunkenness and alcoholism. In addition, they do a great deal of more moderate drinking. Sociability and hospitality are associated with the serving of whiskey, not in conjunction with food. Attitudes favor "having plenty of the best quality." Alcohol is used as a means of avoiding or "drowning" unpleasant issues and situations. Being able to consume large amounts is also equated with manliness. It is an accepted practice to become drunk intentionally. Children use alcohol at early ages and see much inebriation. There is much tolerance for the drunken person.[8]

The Chinese

Among the Chinese there is little drunkenness and alcoholism. Drinking is widespread and takes place in the family setting and for purposes of celebration and festive gatherings. Intoxication is not condoned, and the associated "loss of face" is sufficient to deter repeated practice.

The Jews

The Jewish people have almost no alcoholism. Their drinking practices are similar to those of the Chinese. The use of alcohol is a part of normal living. Social sanctions demand moderation and sobriety, and drunkenness and loss of control is taboo.

The American

The results of a national survey indicated that in the United States about 70 percent of the population used alcoholic beverages and the percentage of users rose with increased education and income. According to Mulford, about 10 percent of the population were so-called heavy drinkers by an index of three or more drinks at a time, two or more times per week. Men outnumbered women, and the Protestant (excluding Methodists and Baptists), well-educated, well-to-do, high-ranking professional was the heaviest drinker.[9]

The College Student

The attitudes and practices of college students relative to alcohol are similar to those of Americans as a whole. Milt states that a study of drinking behavior among sixteen thousand students in twenty-seven different colleges revealed that 74 percent of the students reported some drinking, less than half drank more than once a month, and less than a fifth of the men and a tenth of the women drank more often than once a week. Among this study group there were no alcoholics, but among the heavy drinkers there were many problem drinkers. A substantial portion of the problem drinkers were already evidencing the beginning signs of alcoholism. For 6 percent of the drinkers alcohol usage was producing complications such as loss of friends, failure to meet obligations, and injury. Thirteen percent of the young men and 3 percent of the young women drinkers stated they had become drunk while drinking alone several times, and 11 percent of the men said they had behaved aggressively, destructively, or maliciously while intoxicated.[10]

Attitudes and Problems of Drinking

It would appear, then, that how one behaves in reference to the use of alcohol is determined by attitudes and that drinking practices are learned. Certain attitudes and practices are more apt to produce problem drinkers and alcoholics. According to Milt, if a person uses alcohol as a means of reducing psychic distress and he

> . . . happens to be living in a culture which condones and encourages the use of alcohol, in general, and especially as a way of dealing with anxiety or frustration, or other forms of mental distress, or of attaining pleasure, he will fall into the pattern and accept drinking as a part of his way of life. If on the other hand, he lives in a culture which frowns on heavy drinking, intoxication and drunkenness, and which favors other methods for dealing with psychic distress . . . he is less likely to make repeated use of alcohol for this purpose. However, even in such cultures, there will be some who either defy the norms, or are unable to find other ways of handling their psychic needs; or who lack the ego strength to utilize other alternatives.[11]

Drinking Patterns

Cross describes each of the drinking patterns present in the United States and problems about drinking that may arise.[12]

The nondrinkers. This group includes those people who never or at least very rarely drink, or the abstainers. Such persons may have such strong feelings about the use of alcohol that they are unable to accept drinking among their families, friends, and business associates. Some abstainers become overtly hostile and aggressive. In addition, they may not be accepted in groups where drinking is socially accepted.

The social drinker. The social drinkers comprise the majority of people who use alcohol. They maintain volition and control over the frequency and amounts of liquor they consume. *Rarely do they ever exhibit behavior that is unacceptable to their peers.* The criterion is social acceptability, not amounts, frequency, or place. Drinking may be light, moderate, and heavy. Within the context of social drinking, problems do arise, however. Criticism is provoked if drinking takes place at inappropriate times or occasions, such as before driving, when engaging in complex skills, or while working. Certain roles are conceived to require abstinence—physicians, ministers, teachers, policemen, and youth.

Intoxication is disapproved in varying degrees. The extent of disapproval depends upon the type of behavior and the group in which it takes place. For example, acting silly is all right at a party but not during a religious ceremony. Intoxication is culturally defined to some extent. The term is applicable to one who displays overt signs of behavior considered inappropriate by the group. The depressant action of alcohol on the central nervous system reduces sensitivity to "cues" so the drinker may be unaware of disapproval.

The episodic-excessive drinker. The episodic-excessive drinker exceeds social bounds. Periodically he loses control and drinks enough to become intoxicated, and exhibit socially unacceptable behavior. Episodes do not become more frequent. Such drinkers may be more prone to develop cirrhosis and are certainly subject to accidents during their "drinking sprees." Problems include group rejection, legal infraction due to drunk and disorderly conduct and assault and battery, plus driving while intoxicated. Medical care may be needed during acute intoxication. Acute alcoholic poisoning may occur.

Progressive-excessive drinkers. These people not only drink to an excess but do so for progressively longer periods of time with shorter and shorter intervals between each bout. They tend to drink to the point of intoxication whenever they have a chance. Such people are apt to become alcoholics if treatment is not obtained. As Cross says, "The drinker may experience physical difficulties such as acute gastritis, hangover, liver damage, and vitamin deficiency disorder. He also may find himself in difficulties with his business associates, friends, family and law enforcement agencies because his actions while drinking are socially unacceptable."[13]

Chronic alcoholics. The chronic alcoholic has developed physiological and psychological dependence on alcohol. He has lost control over when, where, and how much he drinks. His social and economic relationships are affected and he may have physical disabilities related to alcohol abuse. Alcoholism is discussed in greater detail later in this chapter.

Problem Drinking

Of the many people who drink, most manage to imbibe moderately; they suffer no apparent effects themselves and cause no problems for others. Another percentage of drinkers consume enough of one or more alcoholic beverages to become drunk or inebriated. The degrees of inebriation range from being unable to think clearly and control social and physical actions to being so anesthetized that unconsciousness, or passing out, occurs. Occasionally, so much alcohol is consumed that coma, or acute alcoholic intoxication, ensues. The victim is actually poisoned and without skilled medical care may die. Inebriation may result once in a while or every time liquor is consumed. A continual state of inebriation is typical of the "skid-row bum" who, like his associates, tries to maintain himself in a constant alcoholic fog through which problems and discomforts appear less real. Removed from the skid-row culture, this inadequate personality can live without experiencing a compulsive desire to drink. This is not true of alcoholics, who comprise less than 10 percent of the skid-row population.

When is drinking moderate and when is it excessive? The moderate, or social, drinker consumes alcoholic beverages in the amounts and frequencies that comply with the customary usages of the community and his peers. He does not have problems because of alcohol. Moderation, then, is a qualitative concept that can vary from group to group, class to class, culture to culture. Excessive drinking is that which exceeds social custom, and the results of a debauch provoke self-criticism as well as peer criticism. Among all users of alcohol, approximately 10 percent are so-called heavy drinkers. Within this group are most of the people who have serious problems because of alcohol: (1) personal and social disruptions, (2) physical disabilities, such as gastric ulcers, cirrhosis, or acute alcoholic poisoning, and (3) alcoholism.

Causes of Problem Drinking

Plaut defines problem drinking as a "repetitive use of beverage alcohol causing physical, psychological, or social harm to the drinker or to others."[14] Although the condition of alcoholism is not precluded by this definition, the alcoholic "has lost control over his alcohol intake in the sense that he is consistently unable to refrain from drinking or to stop drinking before getting intoxicated."[15] Problem drinkers do not always become intoxicated, and heavy drinking does not always end in drunkenness. Heavy drinkers who have no economic, social, family, or physical difficulties because of alcohol are not problem drinkers. Moderate drinkers who have an alcohol-induced illness, marital or social discord, or occupational difficulties because of alcohol are problem drinkers.

Characteristics of problem drinkers. Although it is not possible to predict who will have alcohol problems, there are certain characteristics common among those who have difficulties. The problem drinker:

1. Experiences difficulty in tolerating frustration and controlling impulses
2. Lacks skill in developing close and meaningful interpersonal relationships
3. Has much stress and deprivation in his life
4. Is a member of a group or culture in which there is pressure to drink but poorly defined standards of appropriate drinking patterns.

ALCOHOLISM

There are differences among drinkers, drunkenness, acute alcoholic poisoning, and alcoholism, and the approximately nine million alcoholics out of 70-some percent of the adult population that drink would say that there is a great deal of difference among these conditions. An additional five people who are family or close associates of each alcoholic also will bear witness to the differences. In the United States, 4 percent of the population have the problem of alcoholism. It appears that the nation has a very high incidence, and the states of California and New York have the dubious distinction of being in first place with the greatest numbers.

It is not improbable that an early alcoholic would rationalize that "to

FOUNDATIONS OF HEALTH SCIENCE

avoid this disease, all I have to do is live elsewhere and there will be no problem." In his thinking, the last thing he wants to admit is that he has a problem with drinking; it is much easier for him to believe that his difficulties are due to everything or anything else. The difference between the alcoholic and other problem drinkers is that the alcoholic cannot manage personal tension without drinking. He is (1) unable to abstain and (2) unable to stop drinking once he starts.

Wortis, in the *Cecil-Loeb Textbook of Medicine*, gives this widely accepted definition of alcoholism:

> Alcoholics are those excessive drinkers whose dependence upon alcohol has attained such a degree that it shows a noticeable interference with their physical and mental health, their interpersonal relations and their smooth social and economic function. The various medical and neuropsychiatric syndromes resulting from the ingestion of alcohol . . . are grouped together under the general term of alcoholism.[16]

In the development of this problem, the drinker seems to follow a pattern that may develop quickly or may take many years. The following, "A Profile of a Problem Drinker," is published in chart form by the *Industrial Relations News*.[17]

The Pre-Alcoholic Stage

The first steps toward alcoholism begin when drinking is no longer social but psychological—a release from tension and inhibition. Though still in reasonable control of drinking, the problem drinker begins to show a definite behavior pattern. These PRE-ALCOHOLIC symptoms include:

1. **Gross drinking behavior:** The individual begins to drink more heavily and more often with his friends. "Getting Tight" becomes a habit. When drunk he may develop a "Big-Shot" complex, throw his money around, make pointless long-distance telephone calls, and so on.

2. **Blackouts:** The individual starts to forget what happened "the night before." These blackouts are not the result of passing out, but a sort of amnesia. They sometimes happen to ordinary drinkers, but in people moving toward alcoholism they tend to develop into a pattern.

3. **Gulping and sneaking drinks:** More and more dependent on the pampering effects of alcohol, he tends to "toss off" his drinks, rather than sip them. He sneaks extra drinks, or has a couple before the party. He feels guilty, and avoids talking about drinking.

4. **Chronic hangover:** As he becomes more and more reliant on alcohol to cushion the shocks of daily living, the "morning after" becomes increasingly uncomfortable and more frequent. This is the final danger signal; NEXT STEP—ALCOHOLISM.

Figure 8.2 Alcoholism (Photo by Norman Wexler, courtesy of Los Angeles County.)

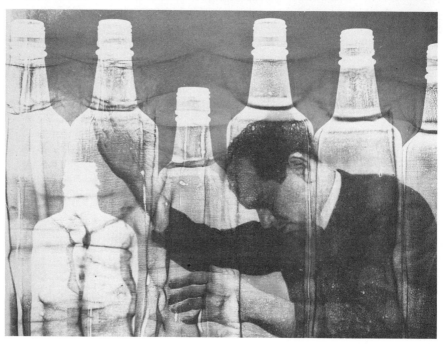

Early-Stage Alcoholism

Until now, the problem drinker has been drinking heavily, but not always conspicuously. More important, he has been able to stop drinking when he chooses. But beyond this point, he will develop the symptoms of early-stage alcoholism with increasing rapidity:

5. **Loss of control:** This is the mark of the alcoholic. In this phase, he can refuse to start drinking, but can't stop drinking once he starts. A single drink is likely to trigger a chain reaction and he will drink himself into complete intoxication.

6. **Alibi system:** He is guilty and defensive about his lack of control. He therefore erects an elaborate system of "reasons" for drinking, partly to answer family and associates, but mostly to reassure himself.

7. **Eye-openers:** Now the individual needs a drink in the morning to "start the day right." This "medicinal" drink helps kill the effects of increasingly painful hangovers: feelings of guilt, remorse, and depression. He cannot face the day without it.

8. **Changing the pattern:** Under pressure from family or employer, he tries to break the hold alcohol has upon him. He may "go on the

wagon" for a while. But one drop of alcohol can start the chain reaction again.

9. **Anti-social behavior:** The problem drinker comes to prefer drinking alone, or with other alcoholics no matter what their social level. He broods over imagined wrongs. He thinks people are staring at or talking about him. He is highly critical of others. He may become destructive or violent.

10. **Loss of jobs and friends:** His continuing antisocial behavior causes him to be dropped from jobs, and leads his friends to turn away from him. As a defensive measure, he may quit before he can be fired, and drop his friends first.

11. **Seeking aid:** Physical and mental erosion caused by his uncontrolled drinking leads him to make the rounds of hospitals, doctors, and psychiatrists. But he seldom receives lasting benefit because he refuses to cooperate or admit the extent of his drinking. He may also seek pastoral counseling at this time in hopes of learning how to drink without getting drunk. He still does not want to stop.

Late-Stage Alcoholism

Until he reached this point, the Alcoholic had a choice: To drink, or not to drink; though once he began, he had no control of his drinking. In the later stages of alcoholism, there is no choice: The problem drinker must drink however and whenever he can. The symptoms of this stage are:

12. **Benders:** The individual now drinks for days at a time, getting blindly and helplessly drunk. He utterly disregards everything—family, job, even food and shelter. These periodic escapes into oblivion mark the beginning of the final, chronic phase of alcoholism: drinking to escape problems caused by drinking.

13. **Tremors:** The Alcoholic develops "The Shakes"; a serious nervous condition. The Alcoholic diseases (acute alcoholic hallucinosis, Delirium Tremens, Korsakoff's Syndrome which is marked by the forgetting of recent events, the telling of lies to cover up amnesia, disorientation in time and space, and emotional instability) often begin at this time. After these attacks he swears off, but cannot stay away from alcohol for very long.

14. **Protecting the supply:** Having a supply of alcohol available is the most important thing in his life. He will do or sell anything to get it, and will hide his bottles to protect them for future needs.

15. **Unreasonable resentments:** In the late stages of alcoholism, the problem drinker shows hostility toward others, both as possible threats to his precious liquor supply and as a turning outward of the unconscious desire to punish himself.

16. **Nameless fears and anxieties:** Now the problem drinker is constantly afraid of something which he cannot pin down or even put into words. He feels a sense of impending doom and destruction. Nervous, shaky, he is utterly unable to face life without the support of alcohol.

17. **Collapse of the alibi system:** No longer able to make excuses for himself, or put the blame on others, he admits to himself that he is licked, that his drinking is beyond his ability to control. (This admission may be made in earlier stages too, and be repeated many times.)

18. **Surrender process:** If the problem drinker is to recover at this stage, he must give up the idea of ever drinking again, and must be willing to seek and accept help. This must take place with the collapse of the Alibi system. Only when they occur together is there any hope of recovery.

It is not always possible to clearly differentiate between alcoholism and other types of problem drinking. It is important to recognize that there are differences since treatment modalities and goals are different. Alcoholics do not necessarily drink every day. Some can manage without alcohol until they experience periods of stress or if they are in protected settings such as half-way houses. Neither do they always become intoxicated once they start drinking. Inability to abstain and loss of control depend on the particular psychological and social state of a person at a specific point in

Alcoholism is a family affair

My girlfriend in high school has a father who is an alcoholic. His condition has put a horrible strain on his wife, and especially the children. I would visit my girl and his presence always made the day gloomy. I could barely wait to get out of that house. His children did not really understand the problem yet, so they would make fun of him behind his back. His outlook, philosophy of life, and lack of participation in life will eventually affect his whole family in such a way that he and his family will deteriorate.

As far back as I can remember into grade school my father and I have had rather heated emotional arguments. They usually started around dinner time. They would always end the same. He would be saying how much he hated me, and I would be saying the same, only I would be crying and very hysterical. In the past two years I have tried my hardest to ignore him and really hold my tongue because I found out that even though he didn't cry, I was hurting him as much as he was hurting me by the nasty things we said to each other. I feel he tries harder now too. I realize he acted this way because he was sick (an alcoholic) and I was catching his illness by fighting back in his sick way. I have really improved—we hardly ever fight anymore.

FOUNDATIONS OF HEALTH SCIENCE

time. Some authors believe that there is danger in stereotyping people as alcoholics. This tends to lead to oversimplification of the problem. There are many types of alcoholics and they require different methods of treatment.[18]

Physiological Foundations of Alcoholism

There are many theories about the causes of alcoholism. In all probability there is more than one cause, and the causes are not only interrelated, but more than one may be required for alcoholism to develop. There is still insufficient evidence that physiological dysfunction causes alcoholism. Dysfunctions are apparent in chronic alcoholics, but it is unknown which preceded which. Studies have been made about endocrine pathology, nutritional deficiencies, genetic abnormalities leading to a lack of certain enzymes, and disturbed metabolism. Investigations of the role of heredity have disclosed that although this may have some influence, primary causes appear to be environmental in nature.

Psychological Foundations of Alcoholism

Isolating psychological factors in the etiology of alcoholism is an extremely complicated task. The background of alcoholics, like that of other individuals, cannot be divided into discrete categories. Sociological and biological factors, along with psychological ones, constitute a portion of the causitive background of every individual's behavior. These factors overlap and are interactive. In addition to these complicating factors, alcoholism is not confined to any particular age, sex, culture, or national origin group. Alcoholism may occur during any life period from early childhood through old age. In our culture, however, alcoholism is rare before late adolescence. The average age for alcoholics is about forty-five. The fact that alcoholic consumption is an approved adult behavior and not a culturally approved childhood behavior is no doubt a factor in the increased frequency of alcohol use in the late adolescent and early adult years. The imitation of the behavior of adults and the late adolescent's striving for adult status may produce alcoholic consumption as objective proof of adulthood.

More men than women are found among alcoholics. This discrepancy may be accounted for in part by society's tendency to condemn socially women drinkers more severely than men drinkers. The risks of sexual assault during periods of intoxication for women are great, and the role of motherhood is less compatible with excessive drinking than that of fatherhood.

Alcoholism is found among people all over the world, but its incidence appears to be much greater among certain groups of people than among others. The excessive use of alcohol is contrary to strong social tradition among the Jews; this may account for the low incidence of alcoholism among them. The Italians also have a low incidence of alcoholism, which is probably not accountable for by the same factors. The Irish and the French have a relatively high rate of alcoholism, and cultural approval of alcohol consumption has become traditional among them. However, cultural approval may be the result of alcohol consumption as common practice rather than a cause of it.

Excessive drinking is but one of many possible ways in which a person may respond to personal and social stresses of one kind or another. The ready availability of alcohol and society's approval of its use make it a handy temporary remedy for real or imagined problems of adjustment. All people suffer stresses and strains, but some individuals do not consume alcohol at all, others drink in moderation, and still others drink excessively. This phenomenon raises the question, "Is there an alcoholic personality?" That is, is there a particular personality organization that predisposes the person to use alcohol in his attempts to cope with his environment? This question has been investigated extensively without discovery of any personality characteristics peculiar to alcoholics. Alcoholics are poorly adjusted, but many inadequately adjusted persons drink without becoming alcoholic. Although studies have failed to indicate an alcoholic personality, many investigators consider alcoholics to be immature, passive dependent persons. Again, there are many immature, passive dependent persons who do not drink or who drink only in moderation. Individuals in alcoholic clinics may show antisocial characteristics, but these characteristics of lack of responsibility and low moral standards may well be the result of prolonged alcohol consumption rather than causitive of it.

Tamerin and Neumann believe that we too often describe alcoholics in terms of the behavioral consequences of their drinking rather than what they are like in their sober state. They found that

> ... rather than being uncontrolled, reckless, and unashamed, sober alcoholic people are generally cautious and careful; indeed they are often overcontrolled and inhibited. In contrast to the stereotype of the alcoholic individual as irresponsible, negligent, disorderly, and indifferent, when sober he is usually highly responsible, conscientious, orderly, cautious, and often a perfectionist, placing inordinately high performance demands upon himself. Contrary to folklore that an alcoholic person is self-centered, opinionated, and insensitive to the feelings of others, the sober alcoholic person's dedication to others in need often reflects a high degree of altruism and selflessness.[19]

FOUNDATIONS OF HEALTH SCIENCE

The alcoholic person may drink because this may be the only way he knows how to escape from the psychic prison in which he lives. He may be a self-driven, overly conscientious, overcontrolled perfectionist who may be chronically dissatisfied with himself and who experiences feelings of guilt and worthlessness.[20]

Social-Psychological Factors

Stages in the development of alcoholism are described in earlier pages of this chapter. An inspection of these patterns of behavior indicate a strong social learning factor in the early stages of the development of this condition. There are some social-psychological factors involved in the use of alcohol that should be given consideration.

The consumption of alcoholic beverages has become commonplace among young people, and the adult cocktail party has become a national institution. Drinking of alcoholic beverages is culturally acceptable and in many cases is the "in" thing to do. Alcohol is a part of our culture, it is easily obtainable, and social and moral sanctions against its use are limited. The fear-, anxiety-, and guilt-reducing properties of alcohol are rather great. The anxiety-reducing effects of alcohol serve as reinforcers for its consumption. Many researchers consider both anxiety and guilt to be basically fear responses, anxiety being fear with a future referent, and guilt being considered as fear over moral transgressions. The fear-reducing properties of alcohol have been demonstrated in the research laboratory, and it is highly probable that the "sociability" effects of alcohol consumption result from the diminution of social fears.

People who have been drinking are not expected to perform in the usual adult manner relative to responsibility. Many irresponsible social acts are excused because the offender has been drinking. Thus, drinking can be used as an excuse for the avoidance of the ordinary adult social responsibilities. Even asocial and antisocial behavior is frequently rationalized in our culture on the basis that "He would not have done so had he not been drinking." *Alcohol can be used as an excuse for the avoidance of adult responsibility as well as a reason for antisocial or even criminal behavior.*

The social acceptability of alcohol consumption and its fear-, anxiety-, and guilt-reducing qualities, combined with the social rationalizations for irresponsible behavior while drinking, make alcohol a fairly attractive beverage for a great number of people. If the nonalcoholic world of the person is grossly less attractive than is his alcohol-consuming one, he is probably a good candidate to start through the stages of alcoholism previously described.

Rehabilitation of the Alcoholic

The treatment of alcoholism can initially be carried out best in a hospital setting. A first step is deintoxification. Typically the patient is in a bad state of physical health. His system must be cleared of alcohol, and he must be maintained on an alcohol-free diet. Tranquilizing drugs such as chlorpromazine have been found to be most effective in alleviating nausea, motor excitement, vomiting, and anxiety that accompany acute alcoholic intoxication. This permits the patient to regain a normal physiological state with a minimum of withdrawal complications.

The treatment of alcoholism following the period of deintoxification is much less effective than the early phase. Typically the patient must learn to live without the use of alcohol both in the hospital and outside of it. It has been reported that once a drinker has lost his tolerance for alcohol, as does the alcoholic, he does not regain it even though he remains sober for a great length of time. In a long-range follow-up study (seven to eleven years) of ninety-three treated alcoholic patients discharged from Maudsley Hospital in London, only seven were capable of drinking alcoholic beverages in a controlled fashion.[21] The alcoholic can rarely return to social drinking without losing control, and therefore total abstinence is generally considered essential.

There are many ways of helping a patient maintain sobriety and avoid alcoholic beverages. One of these is the administration or prescription of drugs (e.g., antabuse) that produce an episode of acute illness upon the subsequent consumption of alcohol. Knowledge that drinking will produce acute illness acts as a strong deterrent to drinking. A variation on this theme is administering to the patient an alcoholic beverage to which has been added some type of emetic. The patient response to this is, of course, retching and vomiting. If this is repeated a number of times, a conditioned avoidance response develops. This kind of treatment may be accompanied by other varieties of psychotherapy, or may be used as the principal treatment technique.

One of the newer modalities of treatment is megavitamin therapy. With massive doses of B-3 and Vitamin C, some alcoholics feel better, have improved records of sobriety, and recover more quickly.

Most usually, some other form of psychotherapy is given along with deterrent therapy. Individual and group psychotherapy can be utilized to help the patient develop insight into his behavior and deal with his own life situation more effectively. Counseling of the patient's spouse or family is frequently instituted. This is designed to help the patient to make a readjustment in the community setting. It may be extremely difficult for him to return to the same situation in which his alcoholism developed and not reacquire the same drinking pattern that produced the illness. In recognition of this difficulty, a number of "half-way houses" have been established. These houses provide temporary residence for the discharged patient. While there, he can gradually get used to the community, get a job, and take important steps toward rehabilitation before returning to live in the community as a full-time participating member.

Alcoholics Anonymous is an organization of former alcoholics dedicated to treatment and rehabilitation. There are chapters accessible to most people in the country. The meetings of Alcoholics Anonymous are partly devoted to social activities and partly devoted to discussions of the problems of the alcoholic. It is a form of group therapy and provides the personally and socially isolated alcoholic with a nucleus of friends dedicated to maintaining sobriety and to helping him maintain it. The organization has had a tremendous growth over the past forty-some years and has been of great value to many alcoholics.

Medical, psychological, and social treatment of the alcoholic patient has made a great deal of progress. When these treatments are combined in an all-out effort, about 60 to 80 percent of alcoholics can be helped to achieve permanent sobriety. A stumbling block to the treatment of some alcoholics is that they do not want to get well. Their life situation is so intolerable that they would rather escape by using alcohol excessively. Many alcoholics' families, financial statuses, and job situations have deteriorated markedly during their period of alcoholism, and they have lost stature in the community. When this is the case, treatment programs are difficult and prognosis is not so good. Much drinking behavior may be partially determined by the social-cultural situation rather than by the personality of the patient. Personality change during psychotherapy, as measured by personality tests, does not necessarily correlate highly with changes in drinking behavior.[22]

Is this statement valid: "You can't help an alcoholic until he is ready for help"? The growing belief is that the statement is not true. Professionals as well as the lay population too often assume that the alcoholic must really want to quit drinking or he will be unable to do so. Chafetz maintains that the main force motivating alcoholics to recover could lie within the caretaking community. Whenever stumbling blocks to therapy are present, and when therapists underrate their role in stimulating the alcoholic to become rehabilitated, they are reinforcing the belief of the alcoholic that he is unable to stop drinking.[23]

The prevention of alcoholism is of major import. The recovery rate of 60 to 80 percent reflects the number of alcoholics who maintain sobriety. It does not indicate the general state of their health. If they were alcoholic for some period of time, they may have done irreparable damage to their bodies. They may have contracted diseases or suffered vitamin and dietary deficiencies resulting in serious physical impairment that may shorten their lives by a decade or more. Young adults should evaluate carefully the role they wish alcohol to play in their lives. Its potential dangers must be considered along with its pleasure-giving, anxiety- and tension-reducing effects.

The Decision to Drink

The decision whether or not to use alcohol beverages is nearly always made during the teen years. Young adults, whether or not they are in college, are frequently pressured to imbibe, since, after all, this is a social custom of a sizeable portion of the adult population. The consequences of drinking should be considered in making the decision.

Even though drinking is accepted by society as a whole, it is not necessarily approved or disapproved by all members or groups in society. How will one's behavior in this respect be viewed by family, friends, peers, and associates? Will one's drinking or abstaining behavior be a factor vocationally or professionally?

Because of the depressant action of alcohol, it is effective in producing relaxation and relief from anxiety, tensions, and fears. It also reduces the ability to perform mentally and physically. The unfortunate consequences of the latter effects are foolish, silly, or dangerous behavior, sexual promiscuity and venereal disease, and accidents. And there is always the very real danger of alcoholism that occurs among 10 percent of those who drink.

Chafetz summarizes these principles relative to the use of alcohol as a beverage:

> It is not essential to drink. An individual, youth or adult, who decides to abstain from alcohol for moral, medical, economic, or any other reason should not be placed under pressure to drink by other members of his society.
>
> Uncontrolled drinking, or alcoholism, is an illness. Children, including the children of alcoholic parents, should be aware that alcoholism is not perversity, not necessarily a character defect, and not even the direct result of drinking. They should know that an alcoholic, like a victim of diabetes or tuberculosis, is a sick person who can and should be helped.

Safe drinking depends on specific physiological as well as psychological factors. These factors include,

a. Early development of healthy attitudes toward drinking within a strong family environment.

b. Prevention of high intoxication levels by restricting beverage consumption to small amounts, in appropriate dilution, and preferably in combination with food.

c. Recognition that drinking is dangerous when used in an effort to solve emotional problems.

d. Universal agreement that drunkenness will not be sanctioned by the group. Most effective is to engender a public attitude that drinking to the point of intoxication is socially unacceptable.[24]

Persons who decide to drink probably do not intend to have problems. Their goal is to use alcoholic beverages either occasionally or moderately. They will find, if they are not potential alcoholics, that they will be less apt to suffer undesirable consequences if they drink noncarbonated beverages slowly and space the amount of alcohol consumption to one ounce per hour; drink after eating or eat while drinking; and choose as drinking companions people whom they respect and who have similar values.

SMOKING

People no longer question the relationship between smoking and some illnesses. In a study of more than 400,000 male subjects matched by race, height, nativity, residence, occupation, education, marital status, consumption of alcohol, plus eleven other criteria, it was found that after three years of follow-up:

1. Twice as many of the smokers had died as nonsmokers—1,385 against 662.

2. There were 110 cases of lung cancer deaths among the cigarette smokers, contrasted with only 12 among nonsmokers.

3. There were 654 smokers who had died of coronary heart diseases as compared with 314 nonsmokers.

4. There were other differences in death rates, too, from emphysema, cancers of the mouth, pharynx, larynx, esophagus, pancreas, and bladder.[25]

The consequences of using tobacco depend on the number of cigarettes smoked per day. The American Cancer Society says that "For groups of men smoking fewer than 10 cigarettes per day, the death rate is about 35 percent higher than for nonsmokers; between 10 and 19 cigarettes per day, the death rate is 95 percent higher; and for those who smoke more than 40 cigarettes a day, the death rate is 125 percent higher than for nonsmokers."[26]

Table 8.2 Mortality Ratios of Smokers to Nonsmokers

Disease	Ratio of Smokers to Nonsmokers
Cancer of lungs	10.8
Bronchitis and emphysema	6.1
Cancer of larynx	5.4
Cancer of oral cavity and pharynx	4.1
Cancer of esophagus	3.4
Ulcers of stomach and duodenum	2.8
Other circulatory cancers	2.6
Cirrhosis of liver	2.2
Cancer of bladder	1.9
Coronary artery disease	1.7
Other heart disease	1.7
Hypertensive heart disease	1.5
Generalized arteriosclerosis	1.5
Cancer of kidney	1.5

Adapted from Herbert Meehan, "Cigarette Smoking—The Hazard in Man," *Morbidity and Mortality Reportable Diseases* (Los Angeles: Los Angeles County Health Department, 5th Report, Week ending February 5, 1966), p. 1.

The varying mortality ratios between smokers and nonsmokers and the difference in death rates for selected causes are shown in Table 8.2 and Table 8.3.

Public agencies have instigated federal and state legislative action on a number of regulations to control the use of tobacco, cigarettes especially. The Public Health Cigarette Smoking Act of 1970 requires the statement that "Cigarette Smoking Is Dangerous to Your Health" in all advertising and on cigarette packages. Since 1971 the electronic communications systems (TV), under the jurisdiction of the Federal Communications Commission, have been prohibited from advertising cigarettes.[27] Smoking is being banned increasingly in public places. All in all, more than 30,000,000 adults have quit smoking. But, the percentage of smokers among youth and young adults is rising!

Chemical Components in Tobacco Smoke

Tobacco smoke is comprised of a number of chemicals that are toxic to man. The percentage of each varies with the type of tobacco and the way it is smoked. The following compounds are those deemed especially harmful to health.

FOUNDATIONS OF HEALTH SCIENCE

Table 8.3 Death Rate of Smokers Versus Nonsmokers.

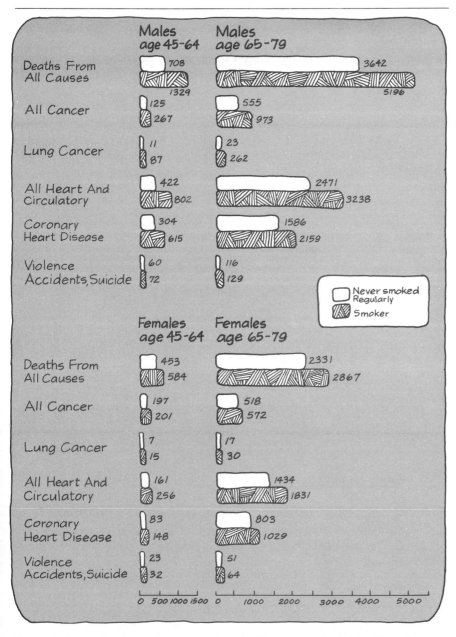

National Cancer Institute, Monograph No. 19 (Hammond Study) in *Chart Book on Smoking, Tobacco and Health*, Public Health Service Publication No. 1937 (Washington, D.C.: Superintendent of Documents, June, 1969), p. 11.

Carbon monoxide. Cigarette smoke contains sufficient carbon monoxide to interfere with physiological processes. CO, which has a greater affinity for hemoglobin than does CO_2, reduces the capacity of the red blood cells to carry oxygen. In an average smoker, 2 to 6 percent of the hemoglobin is inactivated, and in a heavy smoker the rate may be as much as 8 percent. The result is shortness of breath on exertion and inability to perform strenuously.

Hydrocarbons. Tobacco smoke contains hydrocarbons, or tar products, that are carcinogenic. Such compounds have been proven, repeatedly, to produce cancer in controlled experimentation with animals. Other chemicals are also present, such as the co-carcinogens. These do not produce cancer directly, but enhance the ability of other chemicals to produce abnormal cell growth.

Nicotine. Nicotine content of smoke ranges between one-half to two milligrams per cigarette. In concentrated doses of 70 milligrams it is a deadly poison. Nicotine causes dizziness; faintness; rapid pulse; cold, clammy skin; and sometimes nausea, vomiting, and diarrhea, not only in a beginning smoker, but sometimes in the habitual one. This is the chemical that produces that desired effect of transient stimulation. It causes a discharge of epinephrine from the adrenal glands. This in turn stimulates the nervous system and other endocrine glands and causes the release of glycogen (sugar) from the liver. The result is a feeling of stimulation or "kick" and relief from fatigue. This, however, is transient and is followed by depression and further fatigue.

The chemicals in tobacco smoke have pronounced effects on several body systems.

Physiological Effects of Smoking

Digestive tract. Tobacco smoke irritates the digestive system, which can produce inflammation and ulcers of the stomach and duodenum, as well as cancer. The number of cases of peptic ulcer reported in the 1967 illness survey was almost 100 percent higher for male smokers and more than 50 percent higher for female smokers as compared to the number of cases among those who never smoked.[28]

Respiratory tract. In the respiratory tract the mucous membranes are irritated. The cilia lining the bronchi and bronchioles are first inhibited in their function of sweeping away foreign material, and secondly may actually be destroyed. When the person stops smoking, this function is

FOUNDATIONS OF HEALTH SCIENCE

Figure 8.3 Bronchial Cilia. This important part of the body's filtering mechanism is immobilized by continued cigarette smoking. At top, the arrow points to the normal appearance of cilia, or tiny hair-like structures that serve to keep foreign particles from entering the lungs. With cilia weakened (bottom drawing), the bronchus has difficulty in getting rid of mucus that builds up. This produces the well-known "smoker's cough" as the bronchus is forced to exert unusual effort in order to expel the mucus. As long as cancer has not actually developed, as soon as smoking is stopped, the body will begin to repair the damage. (From the film "The Time to Stop is Now." Courtesy of the American Cancer Society.)

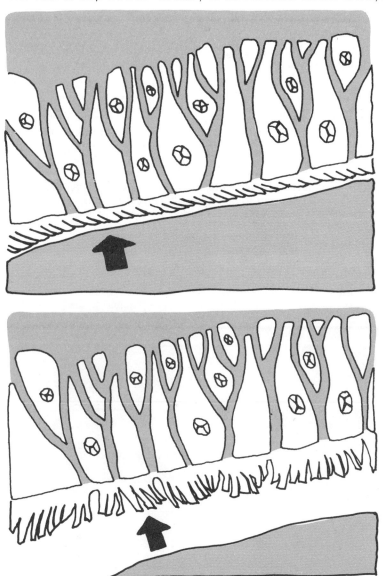

restored. The consequences of cilia immobilization and destruction are coughing, hoarseness, bronchitis, and increased respiratory infections. Persistent irritation and respiratory infections can precipitate chronic obstructive pulmonary diseases, such as chronic bronchitis, and are related to the development of emphysema.

Ninety percent more smokers than nonsmokers have cells with atypical nuclei in the esophagus as well as other epithelial lesions. Some of the lung changes resulting from smoking are reversible. Epithelial tissue will return to normal and cough symptoms can disappear. However, such abnormal changes as pulmonary fibrosis, rupturing of alveolar septums, and thickening of the walls of the arteries are not reversible, and shortness of breath lessens very slowly when smoking is stopped.[29]

The very great rise in the incidence of lung cancer is directly attributable to hydrocarbon in tobacco smoke. Lung cancer, even when detected early, is fatal more than 90 percent of the time. Cigarettes, when compared to pipes and cigars, are by far the greater villain. The risk is dependent on how much and for how long one has smoked, but the risk decreases

Figure 8.4 The Effect of Heavy Smoking on Lung Tissue. (1) Normal lung tissue, in which air sacs are too fine to be visible. (2) Lung tissue of heavy smoker, showing abundance of greatly enlarged air sacs. (Courtesy of the American Cancer Society.)

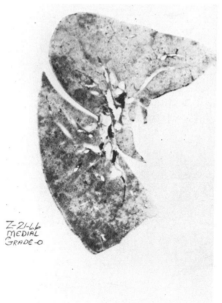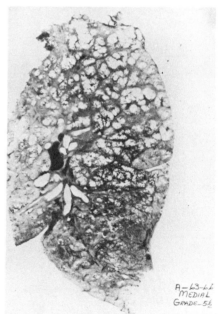

among those able to stop using tobacco. Smoking *habits* directly affect the incidence of lung cancer, too. The American Cancer Society reports that "The rate is especially high among smokers who droop the cigarette from their lips, take more puffs, smoke a cigarette faster, relight half smoked butts, and inhale more."[30]

Circulatory system. Changes in the cardiovascular system are evident immediately after smoking. These occur in the noninhaler as well as in the inhaler since some absorption of nicotine occurs through the mucous membranes of the mouth. The pulse rate may be increased as much as twenty beats per minute and the blood pressure rises. The arterioles contract, which cuts down on blood circulation, particularly in the extremities. Evidence indicates that smokers have electrocardiographic changes and increased clotting time. In addition, smokers tend to have higher levels of cholesterol. Research indicates that nicotine increases the demand for oxygen by the heart, but at the same time the carbon monoxide level in the blood of smokers decreases the capability of the red cells to transport oxygen. Autopsy studies have revealed more advanced coronary arteriosclerosis among smokers than among nonsmokers.

Pregnancy, birth, and the infant. Women who smoke not only have a significantly higher number of stillbirths and miscarriages, but have more premature, underweight babies and more infants that die during the first months of life than do nonsmokers. Since smoking increases the amount of carbon monoxide and correspondingly reduces the amount of oxygen available for fetal circulation, fetal tissue can be injured. Infants of below normal birth weight (under five and one-half pounds) are less able to withstand the rigors of birth and are more prone to disease.

Smokers do die of cancer; it may be someone in your family

About three weeks ago my Aunt had an operation where part of her lung and two ribs were removed because of cancer. Before the operation, the doctors didn't really know how bad the cancer really was. But afterwards, the doctors told my uncle that it was pretty bad and she would probably live only six months to three years. My aunt is only forty-seven years old but she had smoked ever since she was a teenager, and the doctors say this is what caused her cancer. For treatment, my aunt is taking medicine and also she is receiving cobalt.

THE FACTS ABOUT SECOND HAND
CIGARETTE SMOKE

Nonsmokers are in the majority since among the general population, only one in four smoke. *Nonsmokers, are, however, affected by tobacco smoke in their environment!* Researchers have found that 68 percent of the smoke from a burning cigarette goes directly into the surrounding atmosphere. Spewed forth, then, are appreciable amounts of tar, nicotine, carbon monoxide, cadmium, nitrogen dioxide, ammonia, benzene, formal-dehyde, and hydrogen sulphide.

Sidestream Smoke

Two types of smoke from cigarettes, cigars, or pipes gets into the atmosphere: *mainstream smoke,* which the smoker has taken in and then exhaled, and *sidestream smoke,* which goes into the air from the burning end. A cigarette burns on the average about twelve minutes. Sidestream smoke contains much more of the harmful chemicals listed above than does the mainstream smoke inhaled by the smoker. Some studies show twice as much tar and nicotine, three times as much benzpyrene (possible cancer causing agent), and five times as much carbon monoxide.[31]

Carbon Monoxide

Carbon monoxide in the blood interferes with oxygenation. After thirty minutes in a smoke-filled room, the nonsmoker may be exposed to as much as 90 parts per million (ppm), which is almost twice the maximum set for industry. Within an hour, the level of carbon monoxide in the non-smoker's blood stream will double. This amount is sufficient to cause physiological stress in heart disease patients and in other people can trigger asthma attacks.[32]

PSYCHOLOGICAL ASPECTS
OF SMOKING

Is it possible to stop smoking once the habit has become established? Evidence indicates that breaking this habit is difficult and impossible for many people. Hochbaum states that in the heavy smoker (more than one pack per day), the habit has become tied up with many needs and events that keep the habit alive and strengthen it as they occur. Breaking the habit then means developing many new patterns of behavior to replace those associated with smoking, which in turn requires a radical change in a way of life.[33]

The adolescent may begin smoking as a symbolic striving for adult status, as a rebellion against adult authority, or because of pressures from his peers. When he reaches adulthood, these forces no longer are important, but by then his smoking is linked with many other acts and conditions: drinking, eating, social activities, tension, relaxation, concentration, self-assurance; each need or activity in itself calls forth the urge to light up. When this smoker tries to stop, Hochbaum says it is

> . . . often difficult for him to concentrate on any tasks. It is exactly these conditions which he may have learned over many years to alleviate by smoking. Yet, they are intensified and made still more demanding by the very fact that he has deprived himself of his habituated means of coping with them.[34]

There are multiple reasons why people smoke and why they continue to smoke. No one method or means is satisfactory for eliminating this habit, and none of the methods in use are really effective. Currently more than seven out of ten heavy smokers are unable to stop.

Studies now in progress are attempting to discover methods of helping the confirmed smoker to "break the habit." Tomkins distinguishes four different types of smoking behavior that he believes require different treatment.[35]

Habitual smoking. In habitual smoking, the act of smoking is so automatic that the smoker is unaware of what he is doing. Treatment requires methods first of making the smoker aware so that he can again *choose* whether or not to "light up."

Positive affect smoking. The positive affect smoker is deriving either stimulation or relaxing effects. He tends to smoke under circumstances that are stimulating or relaxing in nature. He may derive sensory pleasure from the act itself and smokes when everything is going well. He needs to substitute a less dangerous act.

Negative affect smoking. The negative affect smoker is primarily trying to reduce feelings of distress or fear. The desired result is one of sedation rather than relaxation. This person resorts to cigarettes when things go badly rather than well. He needs to solve his problems or to learn other ways of making himself feel better.

Addictive smoking. The addictive smoker uses this habit for both positive and negative affects. He knows what he is doing and suffers when he cannot smoke. He believes that nothing else will substitute. The intensity of his "desire to smoke" becomes so great with time that he eventually "gives in." This whole process of trying and failing to quit only confirms what he knew already: "I can't quit smoking so why try." An effective method of assisting the smoking addict is helping him to see that he can succeed. Methods used in treating alcohol and drug dependency are being used with addicted smokers.

TESTED WAYS TO QUIT SMOKING

Willpower seems to to be a decisive factor in giving up cigarettes. To some people, the sense that they can manage their own lives is of great importance. Unfortunately, the majority of people who have tried to stop smoking—even those who are successful in controlling many aspects of their lives—have found that willpower is not enough. They try to stop, they aren't successful, and then they feel guilty about being so weak and failing. They quit trying, which is a mistake since many smokers who fail in their first, second, even their fifth attempts, finally succeed. Instead of worrying about repeated failures, people who are trying to stop smoking should concentrate on learning new behavior patterns.

An important first step in the process of quitting for many smokers is to set a date and, as it approaches, to cut down gradually on the number of cigarettes smoked. For example, you might decide to halve the number of cigarettes smoked each week, which would allow you four weeks to quitting day. Another system is to smoke only once an hour, or you might stop smoking every other hour and then extend the nonsmoking time by half an hour, an hour, and two hours.

A matter of appropriate motivation

For the past three years I've tried to quit smoking. I tried cold turkey and also gradually cutting down. I cut down, but I never quit till I started doing my self-improvement paper for this class. It wasn't because of the paper. I quit because my boyfriend pushed me along and had faith in me and I knew that it hurt him as much as me when I cheated by smoking. I have finally accomplished this task and every time I feel like I want a cigarette I just think of him and I don't want one anymore.

FOUNDATIONS OF HEALTH SCIENCE

Some smokers do not realize how many times they actually "light up." If you are one of these, try these tactics: If you always carry your pack of cigarettes in one pocket, put it in another so that you will have to fumble for it. If you always use your right hand to bring your cigarette to your mouth, use your left hand instead. Shift from cigarettes you like to a brand you don't like. Before you light up, decide whether you really want this cigarette. Can you put off smoking for half an hour or even an hour?

Cigarette smoking is a habit that is usually very well learned. You may help yourself to become aware of the nature and frequency of your smoking behavior by keeping a log of every time you light a cigarette. You can then try to change the behavior by using such aids as planning activities for periods of time during which you can't smoke (sit in nonsmoking sections of the theater, for example), associating with people who do not smoke, and removing ashtrays from your home or work surroundings and from your automobile.

Another aid some smokers find of value involves writing down the reasons why they smoke in one column and the reasons for not smoking in another. Concentration on the reasons for giving up smoking can be a factor in successfully changing behavior.

What can you do when you really want a cigarette? Try drinking water; eating fruit, celery, or other low caloric foods; chewing gum; or sucking a piece of hard candy (the sugarless kind). Try a mouth wash after meals instead of a cigarette, or spend a minute or two doing isotonic or isometric exercises to reduce muscular tension.

Changed patterns of living can be effective. Start while on a vacation. If you follow a specific routine, change it. For example, if after breakfast you always read the paper, drink coffee, and have a cigarette, don't sit at the table after you've finished eating; get up and do something else.[36] Then, treat yourself by keeping track of the money you don't spend on cigarettes and using it for something you otherwise could not have afforded.

There are numerous smoking clinics—maybe there is one on your campus—where people analyze their reasons for smoking and give each other supportive help while going through the first stages of withdrawal. You might enlist the aid of a friend whom you could phone whenever the desire to smoke seems uncontrollable.

All in all, Tomkins's descriptions of the four different types of smoking behavior—habitual smoking, positive affect smoking, negative affect smoking, and addictive smoking—that we cited earlier can aid you in determining why you smoke and can suggest courses of action to take to break the habit. You can succeed in quitting—over thirty million people have! Better yet, if you haven't started smoking, don't.

IN CONCLUSION

Alcohol and tobacco both have the potential for producing serious problems for the people who use them.

Alcohol

What people do about the use of alcohol in both an individual and a societal context depends upon their attitudes, beliefs, and knowledge about alcohol and the problems arising out of its use and abuse. There is little agreement about the amount of drinking that is acceptable, how to behave if drinking, the nature of alcoholism, what to do about the problem drinkers, whose responsibility it is to provide assistance to this kind of drinker, just what this assistance should be, and how to prevent problems related to alcohol.

We have finally recognized that all types of drinking do not produce problems. This realization "allows for more discrimination, more effective planning and policy-making—in education, legislation, and personal decision-making."[37]

Smoking

As more and more people are successful in ceasing to smoke, as more and more pressures are put on people not to smoke by making them feel socially unacceptable and uncomfortable when they do, and as more and more youths decide that smoking is a habit not worth starting, the social climate will become less and less conducive to the cigarette habit and will in itself serve to reduce substantially the number of smokers. Advertising about cigarettes already is markedly reduced, and "no smoking" signs are appearing in public places. The smoker *is* beginning to feel socially unaccepted, and per capita cigarette consumption is finally decreasing among adults.

Notes

1. Cooperative Commission on the Study of Alcoholism, *Alcohol Problems: A Report to the Nation.* Prepared by Thomas F. A. Plaut (New York: Oxford University Press, 1967), p. 4.

2. *Facts on Alcoholism* (New York: National Council on Alcoholism, Inc., 1973), n.p.

3. Morris E. Chafetz, "New Federal Legislation on Alcoholism—Opportunities and Problems," *American Journal of Public Health,* 63:206, March, 1973.

276   FOUNDATIONS OF HEALTH SCIENCE

4. *Alcohol and Alcoholism,* DHEW Publication No. HSM 72–9127 (Rockville, Md.: National Institute of Mental Health–National Institute on Alcohol Abuse and Alcoholism, 1972), p. 2.

5. Ibid., pp. 4–7.

6. Ibid., p. 6.

7. Harry Milt, *Basic Handbook on Alcoholism* (Fair Haven, N.J.: Scientific Aids Publications, 1967), pp. 13–14.

8. R. F. Bales, "Cultural Differences in Rates of Alcoholism," *Quarterly Journal of Studies on Alcohol,* 6:480–499, 1946.

9. H. A. Mulford, "Drinking and Deviant Drinking in the U.S.A.," *Quarterly Journal of Studies on Alcohol,* 25:634–650, 1964.

10. Milt, *Basic Handbook,* p. 2.

11. Ibid., p. 39.

12. Jay N. Cross, *A Guide to the Community Control of Alcoholism* (New York: The American Public Health Association, 1968), pp. 38–41.

13. Ibid., p. 40.

14. Cooperative Commission on the Study of Alcohol, *Alcohol Problems,* p. 38.

15. Ibid., p. 39.

16. Paul B. Beeson and Walsh McDermott (eds.), *Cecil-Loeb Textbook of Medicine* (Philadelphia: W. B. Saunders Company, 1963), p. 1728.

17. "A Profile of a Problem Drinker," *Industrial Relations News,* 1954. (A Chart.)

18. Cooperative Commission on the Study of Alcohol, *Alcohol Problems,* pp. 42–43.

19. John S. Tamerin and Charles P. Neumann, "Psychological Aspects of Treating Alcoholism," *Alcohol Health and Research World,* Spring, 1974, p. 14.

20. Ibid., p. 15.

21. D. L. Davies, "Normal Drinking in Recovered Alcohol Addicts," *Quarterly Journal of Studies on Alcohol,* 23:94–104, 1962.

22. M. P. Sikes, G. Faibish, and J. Valles, "Evaluation of an Intensive Alcoholic Treatment Program," *Proceedings of the 73rd Annual Convention of the American Psychological Association,* 1965, pp. 275–276.

23. John F. Mueller, "Treatment for the Alcoholic: Cursing or Nursing," *American Journal of Nursing,* 74:245, 1974.

24. Morris E. Chafetz, "Problems of Reaching Youth," *Journal of School Health,* 43:43–44, 1973.

25. *The Dangers of Smoking, The Benefits of Quitting* (New York: The American Cancer Society, 1972), p. 10.

26. Ibid., p. 15.

27. Ibid., p. 18.

28. *The Facts: Smoking and Health,* DHEW Publication CDC No. 75–8717 (Washington, D.C.: Superintendent of Documents, 1971), p. 8.

29. E. Cuyler Hammond, "Evidence on the Effects of Giving Up Cigarette Smoking," *American Journal of Public Health,* 55:690–691, May, 1965.

30. *The Dangers of Smoking, The Benefits of Quitting,* pp. 22–25.

31. Nancy C. Doyle, "The Facts About Second-Hand Cigarette Smoke," *American Lung Association Bulletin,* 60:13–15, June, 1974.

32. Ibid., p. 15.

33. Godfrey M. Hochbaum, "Psychosocial Aspects of Smoking with Special Reference to Cessation," *American Journal of Public Health,* 55:692–698, May, 1965.

34. Ibid., p. 694.

35. Silvan S. Tomkins, "Psychological Model for Smoking Behavior," in *Epidemiology to Ecology—A Panel Discussion: Smoking and Health in Transition,* pp. 17–20, Supplement to *American Journal of Public Health,* 56, December, 1966.

36. "Want to Quit Smoking? Here Are Tested Ways," *Today's Health,* 47:84, May, 1969.

37. Cooperative Commission on the Study of Alcohol, *Alcohol Problems,* p. 16.

FOUNDATIONS OF HEALTH SCIENCE

CHILDREN OF ALCOHOLICS ARE CHILDREN AT RISK

Murray Hecht

current issues

Alcoholism ranks as the fourth most important public health problem in the United States. Ruth Fox, former director of the National Council on Alcoholism, said in 1967, "One out of every 13 male adults over 20 years of age is an alcoholic"(1). Current estimates are that for every 2.6 male alcoholics there is 1 female alcoholic. This represents an increase from 10 male alcoholics to 1 female alcoholic which was the estimate about a decade ago(2).

Additionally, for every alcoholic there are five or six persons related by family or business who are also adversely affected by the problem of alcoholism. In numbers alone, alcoholism may be our worst national mental health and health problem.

Like other conditions, alcoholism has social consequences which are difficult to calculate. Current estimates are that up to 20 percent of all applications to social agencies, child guidance clinics, and public assistance departments come about because of a drinking problem within a family(3). In most instances, the presenting problem is not the alcoholism. It usually concerns marital and financial problems and conflicts of other members of the family with such social or community institutions as schools or the police. Seldom does alcoholism itself precipitate the referral for help.

Murray Hecht, "Children of Alcoholics are Children at Risk," *American Journal of Nursing*, 73:1764–1768, October, 1973. Copyright by the American Journal of Nursing Company and reproduced with the Company's permission.

279

The most common questions raised about alcoholism are these: "Is it inherited?" and "What are the effects of a parent's alcoholism on children?" Many wives of alcoholics say that not only are their husbands alcoholic, but the husbands have alcoholic brothers, or have had alcoholic fathers. Husbands of wives who are alcoholic are equally concerned, perhaps because children are more exposed. Both are troubled by the family pattern of alcoholism and immediately this is thought of as being hereditary.

There has been considerable debate as to whether alcoholism represents a genetic biochemical problem or a psychological problem. But it appears to me that the genetic problem basically is not very important, even if it exists. If there is a genetic reaction or inherited tolerance to alcohol, it would still remain that an alcoholic, victimized by his genetic makeup, could refrain from continuing on this course unless psychological factors made him pursue this self-destructive path. After all, a person who has been burned by fire learns either to handle it quite differently or leave it alone. It would appear, therefore, that an alcoholic is a person who, regardless of his genetic capacities for tolerating alcohol, continues to drink despite the fact that drinking has begun to interfere with his social or occupational functioning or domestic life. The question then remains. "Why are there so many persons with a drinking problem within a particular family?"

Educators, psychologists, and anthropologists agree, in general, that the primary mode of passing on learning about social behavior and social norms is through the family. It is here that a child learns how people relate to each other, how they share and do not share, how they compromise or do not compromise, how they communicate or do not communicate. The family forms the basic matrix of the child's education. From the interaction of various family members with each other a child forms ideas and ideals of control, relationships, and responsibility.

WAYS OF LEARNING WITHIN THE FAMILY

A child learns principally through identification. Within his living situation, he observes and absorbs his family's feelings, attitudes, and methods of dealing with others. His learning occurs consciously and unconsciously and takes place principally through *communication and role playing.*

Communication is not only what is said, but also what is unsaid. It includes not only the spoken word but the gesture, grimace, and shrug of the shoulder. These often are more meaningful than the spoken word. In the home of a person who is alcoholic, communication frequently is in half-truths and white lies, because the nonalcoholic parent needs to protect the children from the truth about the drinking parent.

Children, however, soon begin to perceive that parents don't always mean what they say and don't always say what they mean. They learn that certain kinds of communication precipitate quarrels, anger, and irritability. They learn the use of sarcasm and cutting, biting words. They are victimized by a desire to believe in their parents, particularly the one who is alcoholic, and by continued broken promises. They begin to place no reliance on verbal communications and begin to depend only upon actions and deeds.

Children in these situations are cut adrift from ordinary access to relationships within the family because words fail to carry much meaning. They learn to act out their impulses, following the model of the alcoholic parent. They learn to rely on themselves and may not develop a trust in others.

Another medium of learning within the family is *role playing*. Role playing gives a child an understanding of the responsibilities, rights, and privileges of each family member. His role is defined by the respect and power given to him by other members of the family. It is important for a young child to see his parents working in partnership, with each parent having the right and responsibility to make certain kinds of decisions in the home. However, in an alcoholic home, this is almost the last thing that is seen.

For the boy who needs to identify with a masculine personality, there are difficulties if the father is alcoholic. The alcoholic father is often passive, uninvolved in family decisions, and often violent and impulsive. Because of the vacuum created by the father's lack of responsibility, the mother begins to assume complete responsibility.

Kimmel and Spears have pointed out in their study of adolescents with alcoholic fathers that the father in the home is often relegated to the role of another child. A typical remark they quote is a 17-year-old boy's, "My father is either away from home working, drinking, or at home sleeping off a hangover"(4). The role of the father, thus, is relegated to that of a person with no responsibility, generally a failure, if not in business at least at home, and a subject for derision and humiliation by his spouse, sometimes by neighbors, and sometimes by other people in the community.

There are similar hazards for the girl whose mother is an alcoholic, but the problem is somewhat different from the boy's. First, the alcoholic housewife can conceal her drinking problem from herself as well as her family for a longer period than a husband can. She doesn't have to consume as much alcohol as possible in a short span of time. She can sip constantly throughout the day and maintain a pleasant glow without ever becoming drunk. Of course, as time goes by and the problem worsens, there is a gradual slide into less and less control. But for a long time a woman alcoholic can evade responsibility. As a result, everyone in the family becomes used to [her] concealing the drinking. The oldest daughter is usually made responsible for younger children or for part of the household chores, particularly preparing dinner.

At other times, because the mother wants to be alone so she can drink undetected, she allows the children an excess of freedom. During sober periods, she feels guilty about her behavior and often takes total responsibility again for all the household chores but, at the same time, allows the children less freedom. As a result, these youngsters are caught in a constant shift between the mother's varying moods and begin to resent her and her inconsistencies and then begin to reject the chores she has asked them to do.

RESULTS OF INCONSISTENCY

There are other problems that contribute to the general disorganization of these children. Consistency of structure and limit setting are important if children are to grow securely. Children need to know that there are rules and regulations within the family, although these need not be rigid. Children have to learn that there are causes and effects for actions. Unfortunately, in the family of an alcoholic, consistency is difficult to achieve.

When the alcoholic is the husband, his wife is so involved with him and his problems that she may fail to see some of the problems that are developing in her children, or fail to handle minor infractions as they occur. Her need is to concentrate all of her energy and being in rescuing or handling the alcoholic. It is not uncommon in our child guidance clinic, for example, to see parents becoming concerned about their children when the alcoholic parent begins to improve. I recall seeing parents who were concerned about their child's poor school work. The interesting thing was the problem had existed for years. However, because of the family's great preoccupation with the father's alcoholic problem, they were unaware or relatively less concerned about the boy's school problem. Only when the father's alcoholism was arrested, were they able to become aware of the son's problem and take steps toward handling it.

The problem is more aggravated when the alcoholic is a woman, because here the father has a double problem. He must work to maintain the family financially. Unless he has an older child at home on whom he can rely he has little effective control as to what happens with the children throughout the day. He cannot set down rules and regulations and hope that his wife will enforce them. An older child who takes over the mother's role is in the unfortunate position of having to mother her own mother and trying to control younger siblings who will still consider her just a sister. It is no wonder that a girl placed in this position tends to marry early in order to escape from a most uncomfortable household.

Alcoholics are tremendously moody people. They present models of tremendous inconsistency for children. Depending upon an alcoholic's need, he can be either quite strict or quite open and liberal, quite accepting of particular behavior, or quite rejecting. As a result, a child is never sure what reaction his behavior will evoke. He is, therefore, bound to push the limits because he doesn't know where the limits really lie. Generally, children do not persist in behavior which is unrewarding and unprofitable in terms of achieving their goals, consciously or unconsciously. However, because of the alcoholic's inconsistency and, therefore, the family's inconsistency, there are no clearcut rules and regulations in the homes of most alcoholics.

Children want the affection of their parents. It is rare, no matter how badly a child has been abused, to hear that child say he wants to leave home or that he hates his parents, and really mean it. He may be angry, resentful, and rebellious but, in spite

FOUNDATIONS OF HEALTH SCIENCE

of this, he has a tremendous need for his parents. This creates an additional handicap. He is disgusted at the alcoholic's behavior, disappointed with the drinking, and builds tremendous feelings of anger toward the alcoholic parent. This anger cannot be tolerated and is turned into feelings which he handles through various means. One is self-punishment, which is often achieved through provoking people or such institutions around him as the school or police to punish him, re-identifying with the behavior of the alcoholic parent, or becoming alcoholic himself. It is as if he must pay a costly price for the feelings of anger that have been generated in him. Further, he lives in constant fear that his home will disappear and not remain intact.

When a child in a family with an alcoholic member grows older and meets children from other families, he begins to see the contrast between his family and theirs. He develops feelings of shame regarding his family and these often become feelings of anger, resentment, and disgust, which he handles by becoming rebellious and impulsive, following the adult model already laid down for him. He tends to be unable to persevere because his model of identification is with an alcoholic parent who is full of excuses, promises, and broken promises. Repeated studies of children have shown that children of alcoholics are more prone than other children to delinquency, anxiety neurosis, depression, hostility, and sexual confusion(5,6,7).

For children who do not follow these paths and seem to have made a better adjustment, there are also difficulties. These children often develop rigid, moralistic codes of behavior. They are often driving, energetic, and demanding. They have difficulty in accepting limitations and failure. They need to dominate in order to defend themselves against internal signs of weakness or passivity.

A SYSTEMS APPROACH

It is important to view the child as growing up in the matrix of a family system, the emphasis being on system. According to general systems theory and practitioners of systemic family therapy, a system is a collection of elements in interaction; what affects one element affects each element, if somewhat differently.

The child in the family of an alcoholic is caught up in a system where usual relationships between the elements have broken down. For example, the mother cannot obtain gratification from her spouse. She then looks elsewhere within the system, namely to the children. Thus, children in the alcoholic family system are forced to play roles and meet parental needs that children in other families do not. It is not uncommon, for example, in the family of the male alcoholic for one child to be called upon to be the confidante of the mother. Nor is it unusual for one child to substitute in the parental role for the alcoholic mother. Children in these systems, like all children, need love, gratification, and acceptance. Only through these unusual roles in the family can they insure that their own needs will be met. Unfortunately, they often carry these unusual role templates into relationships outside the family(8).

The point is that the child is forced into a series of relationships and interactions within the family as each family member seeks to obtain gratification from the others and trades off and compensates for those areas that the alcoholic is not able to give. Thus, role playing and learning that take place for the children within this family are not simply vis-à-vis the alcoholic but with each element of the family system.

The social and human consequences of alcoholism are difficult to prevent because general knowledge on the subject is lacking and because families need to protect themselves by refusing to admit a problem exists.

There are no easy solutions, but there are some sound ways of preventing some of the consequences. Mental health professionals must try to help spouses of alcoholics seek help for the sake of themselves and their children before these problems become too devastating. The wife of an alcoholic must be helped to understand that her husband's drinking habit cannot be changed by nagging or verbal abuse; he will only use this as a further excuse to continue drinking. Likewise, the man whose wife drinks cannot accomplish anything by berating and humiliating her; he only intensifies her depression and guilt, and she then seeks more alcohol to blur and assuage her feelings.

The nonalcoholic spouse must be helped to concentrate energy on rescuing himself and the children from the effects of the alcoholic situation. The nonalcoholic parent also must learn to be more patient and more consistent with the children, must involve the spouse as much as possible, must avoid assigning tasks to the children that they are not ready to undertake, and avoid directing toward them the anger the nonalcoholic parent feels toward the alcoholic.

The mates of alcoholics should be guided to seek professional help for their children while they are young and before they have manifested aberrant behavior. They should also get help for themselves through a professional agency, a group such as Al Anon, or preferably both. Only when an alcoholic's mate has begun to understand himself and control his own reactions, can he begin to understand the nature of the drinking problem and make progress in helping the alcoholic to help himself.

References

1. FOX, RUTH. A multidisciplinary approach to the treatment of alcoholism. *Am.J.Psychiatry* 123:769–778, Jan. 1967.
2. HABERMAN, P. W. and SHEINBERG, J. Implicative drinking reported in a household survey: a corroborative note on subgroup differences. *Quar.J. Stud.Alcohol.* 28:538–543, Sept. 1967.
3. BAILEY, M. B. Family agency's role in treating the wife of an alcoholic. *Soc. CaseWork* 44:273–279, May 1963.
4. KRIMMEL, H. D., and SPEARS, H. R. *The Effects of Alcoholism on Delinquent Adolescents.* Paper presented at the National Conference of Social Welfare held at Los Angeles, Calif., May 1964.
5. NYLANDER, I. Children of alcoholic fathers. *Acta Paediatr. (Upps)* 49 (Suppl.121):1–134, Mar. 1960.
6. HOLDEN, M. Treatability of children of alcoholic parents. *SmithColl. StudiesSoc.Work* 16:44–61, 1945.
7. McKAY, J. R. and OTHERS. Juvenile delinquency and drinking behavior. *J. HealthHum.Behav.* 4:276–282, Winter 1963.

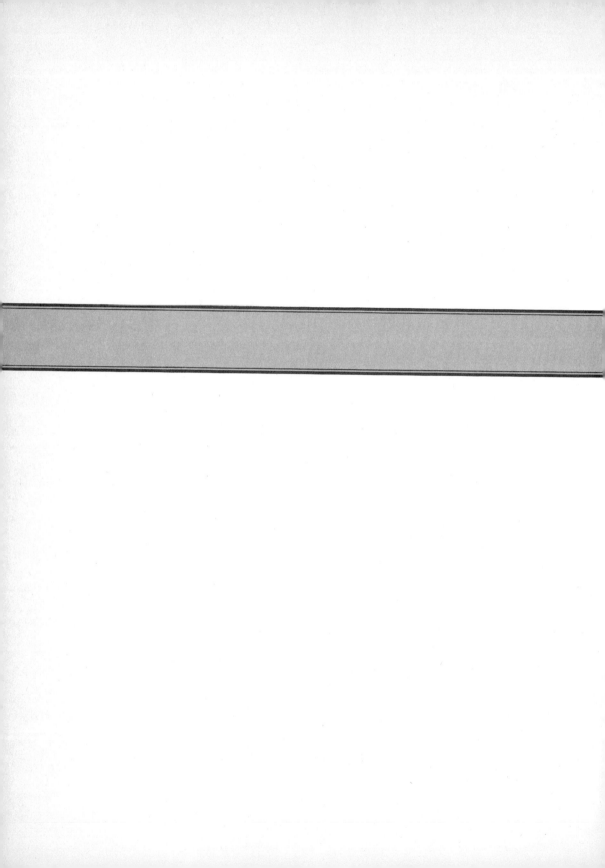

DRUG MISUSE
AND ABUSE

chapter nine

From as far back as we have records of man, we know that he has always believed in secret potions and magic charms to ward off evil spirits and to cure illness. A belief in such magic is prevalent today in the form of our expectations of the miracles that can be accomplished by drugs and medicines. Historically, each period of time seems to have had its own fads. In the early 1900's, for example, all-purpose types of medicines that were thought to cure innumerable conditions were popular. Many of these, however, were patent medicines in which the key ingredient was alcohol.

Currently the use of chemicals to alter the physical and emotional state of being is a generally accepted practice in the United States. The mass media contain numerous advertisements propounding the self-prescribing of drugs and medicines for various ailments and states of being ranging from the common cold, arthritis, obesity, constipation, and infection, to tension headaches, irritability, depression, and insomnia. Innumerable kinds of drugs, both of the prescription and nonprescription types, are readily available to treat such conditions.

Children see their parents and other adults utilize different chemical substances in many settings. Most parents also give medicines to their children: often vitamins, sometimes pain killers or sedatives during teething, and frequently aspirin for numerous mild childhood upsets. Not only do parents constantly dose children, but they select medicines in a variety of pleasant-tasting forms: candies, gums, and sugary syrups.

The home medicine cabinet nearly always contains one or more analgesics and sedatives—such as aspirin and sleeping pills—and not infrequently the very powerful tranquilizers and cortisone drugs. The latter, like other potent medicines, cannot be used indiscriminately whenever one decides to "dose himself."

Estimates indicate that between 85 to 90 percent of the population use drugs at one time or another. Among these are people we might label *drug faddists,* or those who are eager to experiment with new cures and will use anything that is receiving widespread publicity. The advances in the development of medicines, both the prescription and nonprescription varieties, by the pharmaceutical industry have aided and abetted the drug faddist.

Society is currently concerned with problems arising out of the accessibility of dangerous chemical compounds. Ever present are hazardous side effects of some medicines even when used under a physician's supervision. The toxicity of all compounds is not known, for example, as evidenced by controversies over birth control pills prescribed for women. Many nonprescription medicines are dangerous when used under certain circumstances: aspirin during the early months of pregnancy, cold tablets for those with high blood pressure, and sleeping pills taken in combination with alcohol.

The safest way to use medicines is to let a physician make the decision about what is needed. Constipation and insomnia are commonplace disorders, but if persistent, may be symptoms of serious illness, and the doctor should decide on treatment!

Many people conceive of the physician as primarily a dispenser of drugs. When they go to his office, they have already decided what they need. If he doesn't give them the treatment they desire, they go to someone else. An example of this type of person is the one who demands antibiotics at any sign of infection, such as a cold, for which the use of such drugs is useless and possibly harmful.

THE MISUSE OF COMMONLY AVAILABLE MEDICINES

Many medicines that are readily available and commonly found in the home medicine cabinet are potentially harmful. Some of the most common are aspirin, bromides, sleeping pills, tranquilizers, cold medicines, amphetamines, antidepressants, and antibiotics.

Aspirin

Aspirin, or acetylsalicylic acid, is the most widely used "over-the-counter" (available without prescription) preparation. Because of its slight sedative effect, a stimulant such as caffeine is commonly included in some brands. Since aspirin can be irritating to the gastric mucosa, a "buffer" also may be added.

This drug, invaluable as it is, can be misused. Because of carelessness, approximately two hundred deaths occur yearly. Most of these are among children under six years of age and most involve the flavored type of aspirin. Pathologically, aspirin causes minute hemorrhages in the central nervous system and viscera. Symptoms of aspirin poisoning are headache, dizziness, ringing in the ears and loss of hearing, nausea, vomiting, gastric hemorrhage, mental confusion, and in some instances, convulsions, delirium, and coma. Severe cases are difficult to treat and require very specialized medical care and laboratory examinations.

Bromides

Another readily available, over-the-counter compound is bromide, which contains the chemical bromine. The compound is used as an analgesic in several different commercial products sometimes called "nerve tonics." The bromides are not as universally effective as the aspirin compounds, and they are more dangerous. Their continual use can result in bromine poisoning. They tend to accumulate in the tissues, and the resulting toxic effects in order of frequency are: headache, irritability, emotional instability, weakness, lethargy, slurred and irrelevant speech, disorientation, hallucinations, and loss of memory. Bromide rash is found in almost 25 percent of cases of bromism. Persons who have arteriosclerosis, alcoholism, or other disorders may be more susceptible to the toxic effects of the bromides than the well person.

Prescribed Sleeping Pills

The sedatives, or hypnotics, are available only on prescription, as a rule. The most popular ones prescribed by physicians are derivatives of barbituric acid. Some preparations act quickly and others more slowly. There is danger inherent in their use even when taken legitimately by order of a physician. First, because they are so frequently dispensed, and so many homes have a supply in the family medicine cabinet, barbiturates, along with aspirin, are one of the two leading causes of poison deaths among children. Second, because of their hypnotic or sedative effects, these drugs cause mental confusion, and it is not uncommon for the "victim," while mentally confused, to take more pills than the number prescribed. No more than the maximum number allowed per day by the physician should be kept where they are easily accessible. Alcohol, tranquilizers, or other similar depressants may enhance the pharmacological action of barbiturates, and a very small dose may become dangerous when taken in combination with alcohol or these other medications.

Tranquilizers

During the 1950s depressants, known as tranquilizers, were perfected. These produce psychological changes without extensive physiological effects. When used as directed by physicians, tranquilizers are invaluable in treating emotionally disturbed patients. Popular varieties include Librium, Miltown, Equanil, Thorazine, Reserpine, and Compazine. In addition to treating psychosomatic disorders, neuroses, and psychoses, they are used to control anxiety, tension, and vomiting. Tranquilizers such as meprobamate (Equinal and Miltown) like the barbiturates, can be dangerous when taken in combination with other medicines or with alcohol.

Cold Remedies

Reportedly, Americans spend at least $300 million each year on nonprescription products that are claimed to relieve cold symptoms. Another $70 million is spent on advertising these products. Practically all the products contain at least two of three basic ingredients: a pain reliever, a decongestant, and an antihistamine. The pain reliever is aspirin, which is much cheaper when purchased separately. The amounts of the other two ingredients, the decongestant and the antihistamine, are not very effective because either too little is present or the product is not taken frequently enough (timed-release capsules).

Antihistamines are widely used to alleviate the symptoms of sneezing, runny nose, itching, and skin conditions as well as to prevent motion sickness. The larger, more effective doses require medical prescription, but to some people the small amount in a cold remedy can be dangerous. Antihistamines are contraindicated, for example, for people with high blood pressure or hypertension. Undesirable effects include restlessness, excitation, and convulsions.

Numerous brands of cough syrups are available. A number may have small amounts of codeine to help suppress the cough reflex. Cough syrups can cause impaired judgment and poor coordination as well as drowsiness. The label on the bottle will frequently state: "Persons with a high fever or persistent cough should not use this preparation unless directed by a physician. This preparation may cause drowsiness. Do not drive or operate machinery while taking this medication. If relief does not occur within three days, discontinue use and consult a physician." How many read the fine print on the label?

Amphetamines

The amphetamines were legitimately used in the past to control appetite and were an adjunct to weight-reducing diets. Currently, their proper use is to treat narcolepsy (seizures and uncontrollable and paroxysmal sleep) and some childhood behavioral disorders, which might include the hyperkinetic child. No longer is it good medical practice to use amphetamines to suppress the appetite because of the dangerous potential of the user's developing a physical dependency. The undesirable and serious consequences of abuse are delusions, hallucinations, and psychosis.

Antidepressants

Antidepressants are such medicines as Tofranil and Ritalin. As the name implies, they are used to treat different degrees of depression, not necessarily serious mental illness. The average person would not suspect that they produce drowsiness as well as mouth dryness, tremors, blurred vision, skin rash, and jaundice.

Antibiotics

Antibiotics are available only on prescription. But, people do not always use all the amount prescribed, and they too frequently "self-dose" themselves or their children with what is left over from a previous illness. Antibiotics are specific for particular pathogens, or disease-causing microorganisms. Even the so-called broad spectrum types do not affect all germs. The dosage is most important since insufficient amounts may produce resistance in the pathogen causing the infection, which, consequently, negates the usefulness of the drug. In addition, even when taken under the doctor's supervision, some people build up a sensitivity to antibiotics. This sensitivity can result in various allergic reactions such as rashes, sneezing and other respiratory symptoms, nausea, vomiting, and diarrhea.

More serious consequences of adverse reactions include nerve damage, deafness, kidney disease, and anemia. Table 9.1 contains a description of some of the readily available medicines.

Overdoses

All of us are apt to take, foolishly or inadvertently, too much of a medicine. We may think because a little is good, more is better. We have taken more than is recommended on the label before, so why worry this time. We may feel that the directions on the bottle are not too important; if the medicine were really dangerous, we couldn't get it without a prescription! We may not know what happens when we combine medicines such as cough syrup, a cold tablet, and a pain pill such as Darvon. Even physicians are not necessarily knowledgeable about how different combinations of medicines act when taken together.

In administering medicines to children, we may not be aware that dosage is based on body weight and age. Both the very young and the aged may be more sensitive to specific chemicals than are adults. Many nonprescription medicines explicitly state "Do not give to children under six years of age unless prescribed by a physician."

Despite good intentions, accidents happen. While waiting for medical advice, the suggestions in Table 9.2—*Counterdoses*—may help you save a life.

ABUSE OF PSYCHOACTIVE DRUGS

A number of drugs and medicines used to alleviate discomfort can also produce feelings of well-being or pleasure and alter perceptions. They are known as psychoactive drugs. Since some of man's drives include the avoidance of unpleasantness and the search for pleasure, it is no wonder that the readily available chemicals are being used increasingly for this purpose. The use of chemicals, nonmedically, for the sole purpose of pleasure, euphoria, and other desired states of being is labelled as *drug abuse*. Abuse is not an accepted pattern of behavior by the majority of people, and it is considered immoral to some degree by many. Even the abusers and drug dependents impose social sanctions on drug abuse.

The use of drugs for their euphoric and perceptual effects is not solely a "private act" as some would have us believe. Society is concerned about crime relating to drug abuse and rates of mental illness prevalent among a number of drug abusers. Even more detrimental to social ends is the

FOUNDATIONS OF HEALTH SCIENCE

Table 9.1 Drug Reference Chart: Readily Available Medicines

Name of Substance	Slang and Related Terms	Method of Taking	Dependency Potential	Usual Dosage	Duration of Action	Medical Uses	Possible Effects When Abused	Legal Controls
ANTIDEPRESSANTS Dibenzapines (Tofranil, Elairl) Nardil Parnate Ritalin		Orally (pills or capsules).	Psychological dependence; no physical dependence or tolerance.	10–25 mg. 10–15 mg. 10–15 mg. 10 mg.	4–6 hours	Treatment of different degrees of depression.	Mouth dryness, tremors, blurred vision, drowsiness, skin rash, jaundice.	Controlled by Drug Abuse Control Amendments.
ANTIHISTAMINES		Orally (pills or capsules).	Psychological dependence; no physical dependence or tolerance.	25–50 mg.	2 hours	Alleviating allergies—sneezing, runny nose, itching, skin conditions. Preventing motion sickness.	Restlessness, excitation, convulsions, side-effects.	Require medical prescription.
CHLORAL HYDRATE	Trichloro-acetaladehyde Mickey Finn	Orally (often mixed with alcohol).	Physical and psychological dependence and tolerance.	500 mg.	4–6 hours	None.	Acute intoxications, coma.	Subject to Drug Abuse Control Amendments of 1965.
COUGH SYRUPS Cheracol Hycodan Robitussin A-C Romilar		Orally (liquid).	Psychological and physical dependence and tolerance in opium derivative products only.	2–4 oz.	4 hours	To suppress coughs.	Impairment of judgment and coordination.	Over-the-counter or by ordinary medical prescription.
TRANQUILIZERS Chlordiazepoxide Meprobamate Phenothiazine Reserpine	Librium Equanil Miltown Chloro-promazine Compazine Stelazine Thorazine Rauwolfia	Orally (pills or capsules).	Psychological dependency; may have physical dependence and tolerance.	5–10 mg. 400 mg. 2–25 mg. 1 mg.	4–6 hours	Treatment of anxiety, tension, neuroses, psychoses, vomiting, alcoholism, psychosomatic disorders.	Drowsiness, tremors, blurred vision, dryness of mouth, skin rash, jaundice, death.	Controlled by Drug Abuse Control Amendments.

apathy and drug-induced loss of motivation that accrues. This is the focus of considerable attention. Compare the contributions to self, family, and society of the non–drug dependent to those of the drug dependent person who "tunes out" of this world rather than "tunes in."

It is impossible to do more than estimate the number of drug abusers. Some evidence indicates that the incidence is decreasing, especially in the

Table 9.2   Counterdoses

Steps to follow in the event of overdose:
1. Call your physician. Phone number _____.
2. Keep patient warm.
3. Give counterdose (see below).
4. *Do not* force liquids on unconscious person.
5. *Do not* induce vomiting if person is having a convulsion.
6. To induce vomiting:
    a. place finger down patient's throat
    b. give teaspoonful of mustard in half glass of water.

Overdose	Counterdose
Alcohol	Give glass of milk; induce vomiting; give tablespoon of bicarbonate of soda in a quart of warm water.
Amphetamine	Give glass of milk, *or* 1 tablespoonful of activated charcoal mixed with a little water; induce vomiting.
Aspirin	Give glass of milk; induce vomiting; give tablespoon of bicarbonate of soda in quart of warm water.
Barbiturates	Give activated charcoal in water; induce vomiting; give 2 tablespoons of epsom salt in 2 glasses of water.
Bromides	Induce vomiting; give 2 tablespoons of epsom salt in 2 glasses of water—except in cases where diarrhea is severe.
Codeine	Induce vomiting if patient is conscious; give glass of milk, *or* activated charcoal in water; give 2 tablespoons of epsom salt in 2 glasses of water; keep patient awake.
Headache Pills	Give glass of milk; induce vomiting; give tablespoon of bicarbonate of soda in a quart of warm water.
Cold Remedies	Give glass of milk; induce vomiting; give tablespoon of bicarbonate of soda in a quart of warm water.
Iron Compounds	Induce vomiting; give 2 teaspoons of bicarbonate of soda in a glass of warm water; give glass of milk.
Morphine-Demerol	Induce vomiting if patient is conscious; give glass of milk, *or* activated charcoal in water; give 2 tablespoons of epsom salt in 2 glasses of water; keep patient awake.
Paregoric	Induce vomiting if patient is conscious; give glass of milk, *or* activated charcoal in water; 2 tablespoons of epsom salt in 2 glasses of water; keep patient awake.
Sleeping Pills	Give activated charcoal in water; induce vomiting; give 2 tablespoons of epsom salt in 2 glasses of water.
Tranquilizers	Give activated charcoal in water; induce vomiting; give 2 tablespoons of epsom salt in 2 glasses of water.

use of hard narcotics. The problems are the greatest in the metropolitan centers, especially New York, Los Angeles, Chicago, and Philadelphia. However, the incidence of abuse of psychoactive drugs is present in suburban and rural areas and in all levels of society. The majority of those arrested for abusing such drugs are in their late teens and early twenties, and the problem is found in elementary schools as well as on secondary and college campuses.

In discussing abuse of psychoactive drugs the terms *narcotics* and *dangerous drugs* are used. Of course, any drug can be dangerous if it is improperly used. Literally, a substance is classified as a drug when it is used as a medicine. By definition, a medicine prevents or ameliorates disease and alters the structure or function of the body.

Narcotic is a term reserved for the group of drugs that produce stupor, insensibility, or sound sleep. In medical practice they are used to relieve pain as well as to produce sleep. *Hard narcotics* refer to opium derivatives and synthetics that have a dependency-forming or sustaining liability similar to morphine. *Dangerous drugs* commonly mean drugs abused by being nonmedically used for stimulant, euphoric, or hallucinogenic effects. The most common of these are the barbiturates, psychedelics, and the amphetamines, each of which produces changes in the way we feel, perceive, and react.

Abuse of drugs is not a private matter

My brother was involved with drugs with respect to dealing heavily with LSD, cocaine, pot, and hashish. He was busted by the FBI and the Federal Bureau of Narcotics and Dangerous Drugs. The situation turned into an indictment by the Federal Grand Jury for him with a possible sentence of fifteen years in a federal prison. For our family it was a very embarrassing and emotionally disturbing situation. His lawyer advised my parents to get psychiatric help for him in order to straighten him out and to show the court that he was making an attempt to better himself with respect to his involvement of the community and with his own self. This problem really messed up my family for a while and we sold our old home and moved to another neighborhood because the neighbors wouldn't let their children play with my younger brothers and sisters any more. Also some of the neighbors said some pretty nasty things to us, even though the same thing could have happened in their family. My brother went to court and got five years federal probation after verdict and was given a second chance in life to make something of himself. He has moved home now and has a job and is more helpful to my parents around the house. I hope he stays straight.

Drug Dependency

A consequence in the use of psychoactive drugs is the factor of "dependency." Drug dependency exists when a person periodically requires a specific drug to function "normally" psychologically and/or physiologically. To be considered dependency producing, a drug must fulfill three criteria: *emotional dependency* must develop in that the user must compulsively take the drug to meet psychological needs; *tolerance* must develop in that the user's body requires larger and larger doses to maintain physiological equilibrium; and *physical dependency* must be evident in that deprivation of the drug results in withdrawal symptoms of discomfort or suffering.

According to Bloomquist, probably too much emphasis has been placed on the importance of withdrawal symptoms in the abuse of drugs. "The single feature which is of vital importance in the abuse of any drug is the creation of psychological dependence."[1] Physiological dependence is relatively easy to control. Psychological dependency has not been amenable to therapy with any degree of success.

Psychological Bases of Drug Abuse

No single psychological picture is descriptive of all drug dependents. Dependency is a part of a larger pattern of cultural, social, and personality maladjustment. Understanding of the social learning factors involved in the abuse of drugs is rather limited. Immature, inadequate personalities gain important satisfactions by means of escape from unpleasant reality through the use of drugs. However, not all who are immature and frustrated resort to drug abuse as a means of coping with unpleasant reality.

Social pressures to conform have been indicated as a strong component of initial drug usage among gang members and among those on the fringes of actual gang membership. Ausubel reports that immature individuals with deep-seated personality problems who are peripheral rather than active members of a drug-using group use psychoactive substances more for their adjustive value than for "kicks." Such users, he indicates, are likely to continue drug usage and to retreat further and further from normal adult adjustment. These young people tend to feel isolated and inadequate in meeting the demands of adulthood, and they lack masculine identification. Drug usage represents a means of revolution against constituted values and authority as well as a means of reducing anxieties and tensions. Other users he has classified as reactive users who are often week-end "joy-poppers." These persons tend to follow the group mores, but typically do not take drugs often enough or in sufficient quan-

FOUNDATIONS OF HEALTH SCIENCE

tity to become dependent. They tend to drop their group affiliations and their drug usage when they mature. They become successfully identified with the adult roles of society.[2]

The President's Advisory Commission on Narcotic and Drug Abuse states:

> Some use drugs to seek relief from the tedium of their jobs and their lives. Some talented, even brilliant, individuals take to drugs to escape the fear of failure, or the knowledge that they have not fulfilled their potential. Some become "hooked" accidentally when they find themselves unable to give up the drug after undergoing medical treatment with one or more of these drugs to relieve pain. A larger number take to certain drugs to offset fatigue, and this group includes truckdrivers, theatrical people, and even doctors and nurses facing the letdown that follows long hours of tension. A very much larger group try psychotoxic drugs for "kicks," out of curiosity or bravado.[3]

Thornburg categorizes drug abusers in the following groupings: (1) the experimental user, (2) the periodic or recreational user, (3) the compulsive user, and (4) the ritualistic user. The experimental user is primarily curious and may be conforming to group pressure. The periodic or recreational user may also abuse drugs for fun and the excitement of it. However, he is past the experimental stage and through regular use has developed a pattern of drug abuse behavior. Like the social drinker, he may and often does overindulge. The compulsive user, like the alcoholic, has developed a physical and/or psychological dependence on a drug. The fourth category, the ritualistic user, will use drugs because he believes they will give him some spiritual or religious experience. The drug users in this group probably should not be considered drug abusers.[4]

In a study of 2,634 youths between the ages of fourteen and eighteen, these conclusions were derived. Of various hypotheses tested, experimentation was the single most important motive contributing to the use of drugs by high school youth. Considerable use of tobacco, alcohol, marijuana, and hallucinogens was promoted by social facilitation and/or social pressure and was instigated by a search for altered states of consciousness and/or release from inhibitions.[5]

There are a number of theories about the reasons for the present levels of abuse of drugs among those in their early teens. Some of the changes in society and in social values are often espoused as being factors. The generation gap is frequently given as one reason. Just what is this gap? The older generation favors competition and independence, but youth and young adults may feel that it is better to take care of each other and to worry less about one's own accomplishments. While the older generation values technology, the younger feel victimized by it. They are concerned with the rapid expansion of government and business with an accompanying bureaucracy. To many the difficulty of getting things done, the red tape, and the innumerable regulations are seemingly insurmountable.[6]

Superimposed upon this generation gap is the view that young people, and particularly their ideas about drugs, are the products of the times. According to Ewing, the older generation has brought up the younger generation "into an age of 'instant pleasure' tranquilization, and escape through medication. The older generation has given a horrible example . . . with its medicine cabinets overflowing and its denial that anxiety, worry, and depression are often the 'normal' feelings for mankind as he struggles with his environment."[7]

Taintor believes, in addition, that "the older generation's emphasis is on *doing and thinking* and the younger generation's emphasis is on *being and feeling*."[8] Is it so illogical, then, to find youths turning to drugs to relieve anxiety, worry, and depression? Is it illogical to find them using drugs to alter "being and feeling"? Is this harmful? For most, probably not. But for some, definitely yes. The consequences of drug abuse—primarily to produce feelings of euphoria and pleasure—are dependent upon the physical and psychological make-up of the user, the motivation for taking the drug, and the type of drug or drugs being used.

PSYCHOACTIVE DRUGS

Using psychoactive drugs is both an old and a new practice. Such drugs as peyote, or mescaline, have been used by American Indians for generations in the performance of religious rituals. Under such circumstances, drug usage does not seem to be any great danger to society or the user. The purpose of much present usage, though, is to gain "new aesthetic experiences," outside religious or ritualistic settings. This type of motivation can pose problems for the drug user and for society.

Marijuana

Marijuana is a drug of ancient origin that is used throughout the world for its psychic effects. It may be smoked, chewed, swallowed, or snuffed. The Arabs call it hashish, the Hindus call it bhang, and Americans call it grass, but the generic name of the plant from which the drug is derived is *Cannabis sativa*.

According to every indication, marijuana use is widespread and increasing among teenage and young adult groups. The greatest number of users are found in the western part of the United States. The psychologically disturbed or socially unstable are more likely to make regular, heavy use of marijuana. Heavier marijuana use is associated with taking other drugs. The groups using it the least are those in the service and protective professions.[9]

Kinds of marijuana. An understanding of some of the conflicting reports about the hazards of marijuana requires knowledge about the plant itself. *Cannabis sativa* is a single species of plant with a number of varieties that differ in quantity and strength of the resin they produce. However, the variety appears to be determined by the geological conditions under which the plant grows. *Cannabis indica,* or hashish, is grown in India and *Cannabis mexicana* and *Cannabis americana* grow in North America.

Cannabis, or hemp, is a plant that is quite useful. It is the source of an oil used in paints, varnishes, and linoleum. The fibers may be manufactured into twine, rope, clothing, and paper. For greatest commercial value, the plant requires a cold or temperate region with abundant rain. The amount of resin, which produces the psychotoxic effects, is greater when cannabis is grown in hot, dry areas. The resin contains more than one psychotoxin, but the most potent are the tetrahydrocannabinols, commonly known as THC.

Cannabis goes by many names in different countries. In India, common names are charas, bhang, ganja, or hashish. In Mexico, it is called mota, moto, Mo-tul, and manteca. In Africa, it may be known as mbanzhe, mata, kwane, and daga. In the United States the more common terms are grass, weed, pot, hemp, tea, and Mary Jane. According to Bloomquist, five kinds of Cannabis might be used in the United States. Bhang, an Indian smoking mixture, is not especially potent. Ganja, considerably more potent, is used for smoking and in beverages and sweet-meats. Charas is pure resin from plants grown for ganja and is referred to by Americans as hashish or resin. Hashish is from five to six times stronger than marijuana that is derived from *Cannabis mexicana*. The mild form is the kind most commonly used in this country.[10]

Psychochemical reactions. Little is known yet about the specific mode of action of cannabis. Its original constituents are transformed in the body into metabolites that persist for several days. Experienced users metabolize the drug more rapidly.

Subjective effects, which are highly variable, partly depend on the user's expectations and the setting in which he consumes the marijuana. Most effects are pleasant, but one in five users in one study experienced temporary overwhelming negative feelings. Commonly reported feelings are enhanced sensations of touch, taste, smell; awareness of subtlety of meaning in sight and sound; vividness of experience; and alteration of time perception (a slowing down of time sense).[11]

The physiological effects include an increase in pulse rate, reddening of eyes, and decreases in intraocular pressure. Neurological effects seem to be minimal. While we have no good evidence of brain atrophy, we do have some data showing decreased levels of testosterone, the male sex hormone, among heavy users.

Acute marijuana intoxication causes a deterioration in intellectual and psychomotor performance. The effects on short-term memory are probably due to the fact that the drug reduces the ability to concentrate while intoxicated.[12]

Acute toxic physical reactions are relatively rare. Chronic effects resulting from frequent heavy use in the United States are common. One study of American military personnel using *Heavy Hashish* did show more bronchitis, asthma, and nose and throat irritations that were cleared up when use of hashish ceased.[13]

Technically, we have little evidence of marijuana's causing chromosomal abnormalities or birth defects. We do know that THC can cross the placental barrier in animals and can enter the fetal circulation. Consequently, since the potential for birth defects is unknown, use during pregnancy is unwise.[14]

Psychological effects of marijuana. Marijuana is much like alcohol in its effects, except that marijuana is more euphoriogenic. It acts by reducing conscious controls on behavior. Under its influence, judgment and inhibitions are impaired. Bloomquist describes these possible psychological reactions to the kind of marijuana used frequently in the United States.

> The more common reaction to smoking cannabis is the rapid onset of a feeling of "inner joy" that is totally out of proportion to apparent motivation. The user soon finds himself dreaming, relaxing, lolling in the delicious state of effortless nothingness produced by the drug. It is inaccurate, however, to assume that this is always the case, for some people become quite agitated during the early stages of the cannabis trip. This reaction, however, is not seen in the majority of users . . . .
>
> The use of cannabis promotes a feeling of self-confidence that is usually, if not always, unwarranted. The user acquires a feeling of exultation and omnipotence, but such a sensation can quickly dissipate as a result of some negative factor and be replaced by feelings of anxiety and paranoia. Such feelings and the trip they occur on are referred to as a "bring down" and a "bummer". . . .[15]

Experienced marijuana smokers who smoke two or three cigarettes customarily report a feeling of being "high." According to Thomas, Smith, and Knotts, "They also exhibit a slight decrease in intellectual efficiency, increased jocularity, and a slight loosening of associations."[16]

The *Report to Congress* states that high doses of cannabis can produce hallucinations and delusions though these reactions are more common

FOUNDATIONS OF HEALTH SCIENCE

among inexperienced users. Evidence is unclear as to the role of marijuana in mental illness. Studies suggest that pre-existing pathology is the major factor, not cannabis use. The question of loss of motivation due to cannabis is another issue that is still not resolved.[17]

Facts and fiction. Some things said about marijuana usage are true; some are false. Proponents of smoking "pot" acclaim that legalizing marijuana would reduce the consumption of alcohol and ultimately the incidence of alcohol problems. Would it? In fact, users of marijuana consume alcohol more frequently and in larger amounts than those who do not experiment with marijuana.[18]

Marijuana has been attributed with having aphrodisiac properties. We have no scientific evidence to substantiate this—only that "thinking makes it so." Neither do we have evidence that marijuana precipitates sexual behavior; such behavior would have taken place without its use.

The use of "pot" does not lead to the use of heroin. About 85 percent of heroin addicts have previously smoked marijuana, but 90 percent or more had used alcohol. Less than 1 percent of the cannabis users, it is estimated, go on to heroin or other hard narcotics.[19] The National Clearinghouse for Drug Abuse Information, which is operated by the National Institutes of Mental Health, says "... that the person who becomes seriously overinvolved with any drug is likely to have the emotional need to seek out other kinds of drugs and try them repetitively."[20] Thus the emotional need and serious involvement of a drug user are the factors leading to further use, not any special property of a specific drug, such as marijuana.

How dangerous is the chronic use of marijuana? Ewing says we don't really know yet. Current studies suggest that in some subjects marijuana may interfere with the thinking processes. Such interference could

> ... lead to personality changes developing over a few years. These include diminished drive, lessened ambition, decreased motivation, apathy, shortened attention span, distractability, poor judgment, impaired communication skills, a peculiar fragmentation in the flow of thought, habit deterioration, and progressive loss of insight.[21]

However, other studies show no long-range effects. *The Report to Congress* contains these conclusions:

> As our knowledge of the properties of marihuana and related materials has expanded so has our awareness of the many questions that require answers in assessing the health implications of their use. The overall questions of what dosages, frequency and duration of use are clearly likely to be injurious to health in various groups remain unresolved.
>
> Because the material in its natural state is quite variable, more needs

to be learned about it since the implications of use for different types of marihuana may not be the same. The mode of action of the drug and its many components needs to be elucidated. Little, for example, is presently known about the effects of marihuana on the biochemistry of the brain.

The whole question of interaction between marihuana use and that of other drugs is an important one. Some of the reports of adverse effects may be the consequence of multiple drug use in which one or more other psychoactive drugs in combination with cannabis are more injurious in combination than alone.[22]

Table 9.3 contains a summation of the common effects of marijuana usage.

Psychedelics

By definition psychedelic means mind expanding. The effects are determined more by the expectation of the user and his surroundings than is the case in other psychoactive substances, though.

> For many users, these drugs switch on a deep mental state akin to dreaming or meditation, in which thoughts drift toward "ultimate" concerns and unexpected connections between ideas. Psychedelics also change the sensations of seeing, hearing, and touching and intensify perception of colors and shapes.[23]

Fort notes that "psychedelics can also intensify emotions, making the pretty seem beautiful and the unpleasant revolting."[24]

Lysergic Acid Diethylamide, LSD, is taken orally in liquid or capsule form. The effects take about forty-five minutes to appear and last for approximately eight to twelve hours. Psilocybin is a psychedelic very similar to LSD. Another type is DMT, or dimethyltryptamine. This drug is derived from a Haitian plant and is used in Haiti in religious rites. DMT, which is taken by injection or inhalation, produces hallucinatory visions in ten minutes or so. Its effects wear off more quickly than those of LSD.

It is now apparent from medical and legal records that these drugs produce serious disorders and are far from being safe and without side effects. In 1966, federal law made it a felony to use, possess, sell, or manufacture these substances without permission. LSD–25 ingestion by normal persons can produce changes in brain-wave patterns similar to those found in schizophrenics.[25]

LSD, which is colorless and tasteless, has few objective symptoms of usage, and observation cannot detect whether or not a person is under its influence. Physical changes in blood pressure and appetite are transient. The pupils may be dilated and the eyes sensitive to light. Although no two people have exactly the same effects, users tend to be flooded

FOUNDATIONS OF HEALTH SCIENCE

Table 9.3 Drug Reference Chart: Marijuana

Name of Substance	Slang and Related Terms	Method of Taking	Dependency Potential	Usual Dosage	Duration of Action	Medical Uses	Possible Effects When Abused	Legal Controls
MARIJUANA Cannabis sativa	Grass, hash, hemp, joint, Mary Jane, muggles, pot, reefers, stuff, tea, weed (THC–liquid)	Smoked or orally.	Psychological dependency, no tolerance or physical dependency.	Variable 1 cigarette or pipe; in India, 1 drink or cake.	4 hours	None—some evidence of use for depression, loss of appetite, tension, high blood pressure, glaucoma	Dilated eye pupils, excitability or drowsiness, talkativeness, laughter, hallucination, increased appetite, impairment of judgment and coordination, panic reactions.	Under Marijuana Tax Act of 1937. Also legislation involving drug with narcotics.

with sensations, hear sounds, and have mystical experiences. Although the claim of users is that LSD expands consciousness, actually consciousness or awareness is diminished, since thoughts are directed inward and the perception of external stimuli is diminished.

Some of the adverse effects that physicians are called up to treat have led them to the conclusions that LSD may produce:

1. **Totally unpredictable results.** Careful prescreening of users does not eliminate bad experiences, and these might occur the first time or the one hundredth time of use.

2. **Recurrence of bad experiences without usage.** Undesirable and frightening effects reoccur as long as a year after usage. The effects are similar to those first experienced, have the same intensity, and the episode is unrelated to presence or lack of stress. Reoccurrence is unpredictable.

3. **Unpreventable bad trips.** Users erroneously believe that they won't have a bad trip, or experience, if they have the right attitude, setting, and a guide and if the tranquilizer thorazine is available.

4. **Decreased performance.** Carefully designed studies indicate that the subject loses his ability to function as efficiently as usual even though he "feels subjectively" that he does better.

5. **Changed behavior patterns.** Users become indrawn or autistic rather than outgoing and loving of mankind. The change in their value systems is noticeable, and their interest in work decreases. There is great preoccupation with the use of psychedelics to the point of forming LSD groups, writings, music, and paintings.

Potentially serious hazards exist, then, in the unsupervised and uncontrolled use of such drugs. Since the experience can be terrifying and the user emotionally labile and consequently susceptible to suggestion, the setting must be supportive. Cohen emphasizes that many should not experiment with LSD. Who should not use it? The immature who may remain

A tragic prank

A friend of mine, male, age about twenty-one, flipped out on something that was put in his drink one evening at a summer beach area. No one knew what was happening although the results were quite horrifying. He became very paranoid and fearful of the people around him. He went off into a corner and began thinking someone was out to kill him. With this idea in his head, he refused to let anyone come near him. As the drug wore off he got better, but his family had to put him in the state hospital.

unstuck; the one out of one hundred persons who is a borderline psychotic; the schizophrenic; the potential paranoid (the person who is overly suspicious and overly egotistical or who feels overly persecuted); the depressed; and the highly anxious are questionable candidates.[26] Cohen states that the

> ... ideal candidate for LSD is one who is mature, intelligent, and stable, who is fairly well acquainted with himself, and whose life has been a sort of preparation for this remarkable experience ... he has survived defeats, frustrations, and losses and has learned from them ....
>
> It is evident that many poorly adjusted people "get away" with LSD-taking. This they do by never encountering themselves and dealing with their inadequacies. When they eventually come face to face with themselves, they "freak out" or "flip."[27]

Table 9.4 contains a summary of the effects of psychedelic drugs.

STIMULANTS

Stimulants are compounds that are adrenalin-like in their action. They affect the nervous system and act upon the sensory areas of the brain. They enhance alertness, elevate mood, suppress appetite, reduce awareness of fatigue, and, in large doses, cause confusion and hallucinations. Physiologically, physical activity is increased, blood pressure is elevated, heart action is quickened, sweating becomes more profuse, and the user is restless, nervous, and unable to sleep. These drugs are useful in medical treatment and are prescribed to treat depression and narcolepsy. Stimulants also induce a feeling of heightened sensitivity, euphoria, exhilaration, or escape.

The most commonly abused stimulants in the United States are the amphetamines, taken orally, and the methamphetamines (speed), administered by injection. Cocaine, a stimulant with locally depressing effects, is sometimes used. Betel nuts are chewed in the East Indies and coca leaves in South America. Caffeine is a stimulant found in coffee, tea, and cola drinks.

One of two ways in which abuse of stimulants is effected is in their use to assure wakefulness. Amphetamines such as "bennies" and "dexies" may be used for this purpose by travelers, truck drivers, students (especially during exam periods), night workers, or anyone desiring to remain awake for long periods of time. "To another group of abusers, the use of stimulants may represent a thrill, a spree, a 'kick,' a feeling of heightened sensitivity to surroundings, a state of euphoria, exhilaration, or escape from depression," according to Knotts.[28]

When powerful stimulants such as the amphetamines are used to

Table 9.4 Drug Reference Chart: Psychedelics

Name of Substance	Slang and Related Terms	Method of Taking	Dependency Potential	Usual Dosage	Duration of Action	Medical Uses	Possible Effects When Abused	Legal Controls
MESCALINE (peyote)	Cactus Devils root	Orally (chewing).	Psychological dependency and tolerance; no physical dependency.	350 mg. (12 buttons)	8–12 hours	Experimental study.	Excitation, hallucination, rambling speech, change in color perception.	Under Drug Abuse Control Amendments, September, 1966 (Native American Church approval).
PSILOCYBIN	Mushrooms Psilocin	Orally.	Psychological dependency and tolerance; no physical dependency.	25 mg.	6–8 hours	Experimental study.	Excitation, hallucinations, rambling speech, imagery.	Under Drug Abuse Control Amendments, September, 1966.
SYNTHETICS DMT	Dimethyltryptamine	Orally.	Psychological dependency and tolerance; no physical dependency.		3–5 hours	Research only: alcoholism, mental illness.	Visual and auditory imagery, anxiety, nausea, impaired co-ordination, precipitates psychosis, panic reaction.	Brought under control of Drug Abuse Amendments of 1965.
LSD	Acid, trip			100–50 micrograms	8–12 hours			
STP	DOM			5 mg.	6–24 hours			
OTHERS Asarone Bufotenine Catnip Fly agaric Morning glory seeds Nutmeg Ostoluiqui	Flagroot, Rat-root Toad skins Toadstools Myristicin	Orally or sniffed.	Psychological dependency, tolerance unknown; no physical dependency.	Variable	2–4 hours	None.	Impaired judgment and coordination, hallucinations.	None.

306

combat fatigue, the user may continue to the point of exhaustion. When the effects of the drug wear off, elation often is replaced by depression and weakness. Physiological dependency does not occur, but in chronic habituation the user exhibits increased tolerance and paranoid delusions, aggressiveness, and assaultive behavior. Hallucinations are a common phenomenon. Schizophrenic episodes are found among some abusers.

The following is a summary of the effects of stimulants:

A. *Psychochemical Reactions*
   1. Increased blood pressure, pulse, peristalsis, sweating, and dyspnea
   2. Depressed appetite
   3. Allayed feelings of fatigue
   4. Exhilaration
   5. Supersensitivity to sight and sound
   6. Incessant talking, bizarre ideation
B. *Psychosocial Aspects*
   1. Used primarily by younger people in their teens and early twenties
   2. Taken by those who desire to speed up, act, and accomplish
   3. Taken by many to overcome depression and allay symptoms of fatigue
C. *Hazards of Usage*
   1. Rapid psychological dependence
   2. Exhaustion, collapse, and circulatory damage resulting from unusual expenditure of energy due to the masking of signs of fatigue
   3. Argumentative behavior
   4. Confusion
   5. Loss of inhibitions, unpredictable and irrational behavior, and violence
   6. Aggravation of existing heart disease, stroke (in susceptible persons), and possible shock and death
   7. Paranoia, hallucinations, and perseveration
   8. Possibility of deep depression and suicide resulting from sudden withdrawal

Table 9.5 contains a summary of the commonly used stimulants.

DEPRESSANTS

Depressants are compounds that decrease alertness and psychological activity, sometimes to the point of stupor and coma. Respiration is slowed,

Table 9.5 Drug Reference Chart: Stimulants

Name of Substance	Slang and Related Terms	Method of Taking	Dependency Potential	Usual Dosage	Duration of Action	Medical Uses	Possible Effects When Abused	Legal Controls
AMPHETAMINES Benzedrine Dexedrine Methedrine	Pep pills, uppers Bennies Cartwheels Dexies, Xmas trees Crystal, Meth, Speed	Orally or by injection.	Psychological dependency and tolerance; no physical dependence.	2–5 mg	4 hours	Anti-appetite, mild depression, narcolepsy, fatigue.	Dilated eye pupils, tremors, excitation, talkativeness, hallucinations, loss of appetite, insomnia, toxic psychosis, restlessness, irritability.	Controlled under Drug Abuse Control Amendments of 1965. Methamphetamine added in 1966. By prescription only.
CAFFEINE APC Coca-Cola Coffee No-Doz Tea	Coke Java	Orally.	Tolerance, moderate psychological dependency; no physical dependency.	5 mg. 1 bottle 1–2 Cups 5 mg. 1–2 Cups	2–4 hours	Mild stimulant, treatment of some forms of coma, reduction of fatigue.	Insomnia, restlessness, gastric irritation.	No regulations in any manner.
COCAINE	Coke, Snow	Sniffed or by injection.	Psychological dependency; no tolerance or physical dependency.	Variable		Local anesthetic in past.	Extreme excitation, tremors, hallucinations, elation, chronic insomnia, loss of appetite, nausea, paranoid delusions, convulsions.	Under Harrison Narcotic Act of 1914.

FOUNDATIONS OF HEALTH SCIENCE

cardiac output lessened, and blood pressure decreased. All body functions slow down. The change in psychological activity can interfere with conscious controls that inhibit certain behaviors. While in a depressed state because of the drug, the user may act "high" or do silly things he would not do normally.

Barbiturates

Barbiturates are being increasingly misused to produce alterations in mood. Sometimes a combination of opiates and barbiturates are taken. Barbiturates are easily obtained in the form of sleeping pills, millions of which are prescribed yearly. The fast-acting varieties such as pentobarbital, secobarbital, and amobarbital give the kind of "kick" the user wants. The slower-acting compounds such as phenobarbital and barbital are not used for kicks by choice.

Medically, the barbiturates are prescribed to produce sedation, induce sleep, inhibit convulsions, and cause surgical anesthesia. Physioligically, they depress respiration, but have a minimal effect on the circulatory system, metabolism, and renal functions. They are usually taken in pill or capsule form. The results vary depending on the user's emotional state and on whether or not his stomach is empty.

We have no evidence that these drugs, when used in the prescribed manner, cause tissue damage. When they are taken for a prolonged period of time in very large doses, however, tissue damage and inevitable personality changes occur. The psychological damage may be more difficult to treat than the tissue damage. When the barbiturates are used with opiates or with alcohol, their effects are intensified due to potentiation. Withdrawal from barbiturates is more dangerous than from opiates. Patients cannot sleep; they vomit, have twitching and writhing movements of their arms and legs; and they may have severe convulsions. Eventually some users experience hallucinations, are disoriented, and may even become psychotic.

Methaqualone

Methaqualone is a sedative drug prescribed for the relief of anxiety, tension, and insomnia. Some of the trade names include Sopor, Parest, Optimil, Somnavac, and Tuazole. It is known on the "street" as soprs, sopes, quacks, or ludes.

Methaqualone has the same potential for abuse as the barbiturates. When it is used in combination with alcohol, it is particularly dangerous.

Dependency can be both psychological and physiological, and withdrawal symptoms include headache, loss of appetite, nausea, abdominal cramps, and sometimes convulsions.

Methaqualone, which comes in tablet or capsule form, is inexpensive. It is attractive to drug users because its effects are rapid and long lasting and it may be taken to potentiate the effects of other drugs. Methaqualone's value to drug users has been described by Distasio and Mawrot: It lowers "inhibitions for those seeking successful social encounters, and a perpetual state of sedation can be maintained by taking a pill whenever life's pressures are felt."[29]

Inhalants

A number of volatile chemicals act as depressants or intoxicants on the human body when their fumes are inhaled. These include airplane glue, cleaning solvents, paint thinner, gasoline, and a variety of other substances. Glue sniffing, sometimes called "flashing," was first reported in the United States in 1955 and rapidly expanded as a practice into the next decade. Lingeman described some of the deliriant effects of the fumes of model-airplane glue (containing toluol) as follows:

> These induce, in the first stage, a feeling of hazy euphoria something like that from alcohol. Soon follows a disordering of perception: double vision, ringing in the ears, and even hallucinations. The user's speech becomes slurred, and he staggers around with poor coordination, as if he were drunk. After thirty-five to forty minutes he falls into a state of drowsiness or stupor lasting an hour, during which he is unable to recall what he was doing.
>
> Occasionally sniffers erupt into violence or have delusions of grandeur, during which they think they can fly, or lie on railroad tracks; such impairment of judgment has resulted in serious or fatal accidents. Overinhalation can result in kidney damage or even death, though such occurrences are rare.[30]

Table 9.6 contains a summary of the effects of depressants.

NARCOTICS—OPIATES

In the past, when the term *addict* was used, we envisioned a "hype" or user of narcotics—opiates and their synthetic counterparts. These drug dependents are a small group when compared to the numbers now using marijuana, stimulants, and other depressants. They do create, however, serious problems of a medical, legal, and social nature.

Table 9.6 Drug Reference Chart: Depressants

Name of Substance	Slang and Related Terms	Method of Taking	Dependency Potential	Usual Dosage	Duration of Action	Medical Uses	Possible Effects When Abused	Legal Controls
BARBITURATES Amobarbital Nembutal Phenobarbital Pentobarbital Secobarbital	Barbs, Blue Devils, Dolls, Goofers, Phennies, Red Devils, Yellow Jackets	Swallowing pills or capsules.	Physical and psychological dependency and tolerance (tendency to increase dosage).	50 to 100 mg.	4 hours	Sedation, sleep-producing, epilepsy, high blood pressure, insomnia, tension, anesthesia.	Drowsiness, staggering, slurred speech, euphoria, impaired judgment and reaction time, irritability, weight loss.	Controlled in accordance with 1965 Drug Abuse Control Amendments (medical prescription).
METHAQUALONE Sopor Parest Optimil Somnavac Tuazole	Soprs, Sopes, Quacks, Ludes	Pills, capsules.	Physical and psychological dependency and tolerance.	300 mg.	4 hours	Anxiety, tension, insomnia.	Headache, nausea, cramps, convulsions, dizziness, shakiness.	Controlled in accord with 1965 Drug Abuse Control Amendments (prescription).
VOLATILE SUBSTANCES Cleaning fluid Glue Lighter fluid Paint thinner	Flashing	Inhalation of fumes.	Psychological dependency and tolerance; physical dependency unknown.	Increases as tolerance develops.	2 hours	None.	Stupor, drowsiness, slurred speech, staggering, euphoria, impaired judgment and coordination, liver, brain, and kidney damage.	No federal controls. Glue sales restricted in some states.

(Continued on next page)

Table 9.6 (Continued)

MEPERIDINE	Demerol, pethidine	Orally or by injection.	Physical and psychological dependency and tolerance.	50 to 200 mg.	2–4 hours	To relieve pain.	Similar to morphine; higher doses produce excitation, tremors and convulsions.	Since 1944 included under Harrison Act.
METHADONE	Dolly	Orally or by injection.	Physical and psychological dependency and tolerance.	7 to 10 mg.	3–5 hours	To relieve pain, maintenance therapy with addicts.	Same as Morphine.	Since 1953 included under Harrison Act.
OPIATES Codeine Dilaudid Heroin Morphine Opium Paregoric	Methylmorphine Hydromorphine H, Horse, Junk, Smack M, Morph O, Op PG	Orally or by injection in muscle or vein. Opium by smoking (inhalation).	Physical and psychological dependency and tolerance.	C–30–50 mg. D–2 mg. H–4 mg. M–5–10 mg. O–pipe P–mixture	1–6 hours	To relieve pain, codeine for coughs, paregoric for sedation and diarrhea control.	Drowsiness, stupor, euphoria, pinpoint eye pupils, panic reactions, alteration of time perception, impairment of judgment and coordination.	Federal control provided under 1914 Harrison Narcotic Act (medical prescription, except for heroin).

Ausubel states that unlimited use of narcotics by dependents is socially and personally harmful.

> ...it has been unequivocally established by systematic observation under controlled conditions that when an addict is permitted to use as much drug as he wants, he characteristically becomes lethargic, slovenly, undependable, and devoid of ambition. The drug-satiated addict loses all desire for socially productive work and exhibits little interest in food, sex, companionship, family ties, or recreation. The so-called push which he attributes to the influence of the drug becomes evident only when he becomes concerned about the source of his next dose. His belief that he can work more efficiently under the influence of drugs is merely an illusion created by the euphoria he experiences with drug usage. Objective tests actually demonstrate deceleration in speed of tapping and learning and in verbal and motor reaction time. The typical addict uses as high a dose of the drug as he can afford or obtain, and almost invariably more than he requires to remain free of the uncomfortable symptoms he experiences upon withdrawal of the drug.[31]

Ausubel goes on to say that the existence of outstanding physicians, philosophers, or any other men of learning who supposedly limit themselves to a small periodic dose of an opiate to calm their nerves and to make their intellectual abilities more acute is mostly a myth.

The dependent on hard narcotics is usually a passive-aggressive person who acts in an immature, irresponsible, and impulsive manner. He not only has difficulty in withstanding frustration; he tries to avoid it. He is primarily self-centered and is more concerned with satisfying immediate desires than in working toward goals. This pattern of personal behavior frequently derives from an inadequate family background characterized by poor social and familial relationships.

Opium

Opium as such is not widely misused in the United States today. It is customarily smoked in a special opium pipe. The "milk" from the unripe seed pod of the poppy *Papaver somniferum* or *album De Candolle* is collected, mixed with glycerine and water, and boiled into a very heavy syrup, and then formed into small pellets. When these pellets are burned they give off an unmistakable, sickeningly sweet odor. The active principle in opium is morphine, which is given off in the smoke and thus inhaled.

Continuous use of opium in any manner leads to dependency. Since it is not as potent as some of its derivatives, the development of physical dependency and the abstinence syndrome may take longer. It is a fallacy that the Chinese, who smoked this drug for many years, did not become physically and psychologically dependent upon it. Some historians surmise that the decline in the advancement of the Far East nations is in part related to this once widespread practice.

Morphine

Morphine is used medically to relieve pain. Tolerance for this drug builds up quite quickly. The physician prescribes doses of one-quarter to one-half grain, but the dependent may take as much as ten grains per day to support his habit. This drug is not extensively used illegally except among members of the medical or nursing professions and other para-medical groups.

Heroin

Heroin is manufactured from morphine, and its use for any purpose is against the law in the United States. Of the opiates, it is the drug of choice for most dependents since it seems to produce the greatest degree of euphoria. Because of the rapid development of tolerance and its very powerful depressant effect on the respiratory system, it is not medically valuable. The illegal source of this narcotic on the West Coast is usually Mexico, and on the East Coast, the Orient or the Near East.

The drug is nearly always administered by injection. At first the user tends to inject it into fleshy parts of the arms and legs, but as the "need for the effect" grows greater, it is eventually injected into the veins (the mainline), where its action can be felt within a matter of seconds. Eventually, the large veins become sclerotic (hardened) and any reachable vein (on the backs of the hands, between the fingers or toes, and under the tongue) is used. The scars resulting from these injections, some of which have been infected, are so distinctive that their presence is accepted as legal proof of dependency.

The injection "kit" consists of a spoon in which the narcotic is dissolved by adding a little water and then heating with a match; a small wad of cotton to strain the mixture; an eye dropper (more easily obtained than a hypodermic syringe); a hypodermic needle; and something to use as a tourniquet. If a needle is not available, any sharp instrument such as a razor blade or pin may be used to make an incision and the eye dropper is inserted directly into the vein. Very seldom is any of this done under aseptic conditions. If the "kit" is used by more than one "hype" it may transmit syphilis, serum hepatitis, and other diseases.

FOUNDATIONS OF HEALTH SCIENCE

When heroin is first used, it is often snuffed through the nose. Then it is usually taken intermittently, "joypopping." In time, the user becomes familiar with the effect and will take a shot more often. The initial reactions, which are rather unpleasant, include nausea and vomiting, itching, flushing, and a semisomnolent state from which the victim can be aroused easily.

The opiates do not produce a deep sleep or coma unless they are taken in amounts sufficient to be dangerous to life. The user who has developed a high degree of tolerance can take amounts of narcotics that would be lethal to anyone else. Even they occasionally die of overdoses since they are never sure of the exact strength of illegally purchased heroin. By the time the dependent buys the heroin, it has been cut or mixed several different times with milk sugar. Quinine is usually added to provide the bitter taste of heroin. Measuring is quite inaccurate, and the conditions of mixing are not aseptic.

When opiates, or similar synthetic drugs, are abruptly withdrawn from one who is physically dependent, a characteristic syndrome develops. Within twenty-four hours—the exact amount of time depends on the particular opiate—the victim becomes restless, nervous, and jittery; soon lacrimation, a runny nose, excessive perspiration, and yawning occur (these become progressively more acute and are followed by chills and muscular cramps). The victim is unable to remain still and he twitches his arms, legs, and feet; first he feels too hot and then too cold; eventually retching, vomiting, and diarrhea incapacitate him. As these subside, after several days, he develops nervousness, insomnia, and weakness which may last from several weeks to several months. The severity of these reactions depends on the amount of drug he was using. Withdrawal from heroin, dilaudid, and demerol is usually more intense than from morphine but less intense than from methadone.

Under the effects of these drugs, the abuser has impairment of intellectual functioning, confusion, poor judgment, depression, melancholia, and psychic regression. He may also have ataxia, tremors, and nystagmus, and may be dirty and unkempt.

The following is a summary of the effects of narcotics:

A. *Psychochemical Reactions*
   1. Pain relief, depressant
   2. Sedation, drowsiness, and lassitude
   3. Pinpoint pupils
   4. Constipation, depressed sexual drive
   5. Craving for sweets
   6. Euphoria and sense of well-being

B. *Psychosocial Aspects*
1. Dependents usually live in large urban centers.
2. Dependents are usually under 30 years of age (one study of 7,200 dependents showed that the majority stopped using heroin at 35 years of age and by 47 years, 87 percent had stopped).
3. Dependents who start usage in the United States usually have a history of delinquent behavior before heroin usage, which is not necessarily true of armed forces personnel from Vietnam.
4. Criminal offenses are associated with getting funds to support the habit, usually by shoplifting, burglary, and prostitution.
5. Over one-half of the dependents are from minority groups of black, Puerto Rican, and Mexican extraction.
6. Opiate users seem to have unusual needs for drug-produced feelings of tranquility.
7. Dependents usually exhibit a preference for using avoidance to resolve anxieties related to pain, sexuality, and expressions of aggression that provoke them.
8. Dependents are usually passive, immature, narcissistic persons who feel insecure and inferior and who have little interest in sex.
9. Opiate users are usually dependent personalities with overprotective mothers.

C. *Hazards of Usage*
1. Rapid physiological dependency
2. Infections following injections that may produce abscesses, emboli
3. Syphilis, tetanus, and hepatitis from contaminated needles
4. Dermatitis
5. Hypoglycemia (low blood sugar)
6. "Heroin longevity sign"—in a dependent of two or more years duration, carious or absent front teeth (etiology unknown)[32]

DRUG CONTROL

The prevention of drug dependency is in part assisting people to find less destructive means of adjusting to the stresses and strains of daily living. For those who turn to drugs for help in meeting their problems, the "long road back" is difficult and not readily achieved. Drug control requires measures that reduce the availability of drugs for illegal purposes, which is primarily a law-enforcement problem. One aspect of enforcement is regulating the dispensing of narcotics and dangerous drugs; a second aspect is control of the dependents.

Government Regulations for Dispensing Narcotics

The federal government regulates the dispensing of narcotics and dangerous drugs and works with the individual states, which may impose additional restrictions. *The Harrison Act,* enacted in 1914, mandates that anyone who imports, manufactures, sells, deals in, dispenses, or otherwise distributes narcotics must register with the Secretary of the Treasury. A tax is imposed on drugs produced or imported for sale purposes, and a special form is required to transfer drugs. Only the physician and pharmacist dispensing narcotics to the patient are exempt from obtaining such a form.

In 1922 the *Narcotic Drugs Import and Export Act* was passed, which authorizes the Secretary of the Treasury to regulate the importing of crude opium and cocaine for medical and scientific use. It prohibits the manufacturing of heroin and opium for smoking and provides for regulations about the export of narcotic drugs so that they are used only for medical and scientific reasons.

Since additional controls seemed needed, the *Marijuana Tax Act* in 1937 restricted the production and sale of marijuana, and the *Narcotic Control Act of 1956* provided for stringent fines, imprisonment, and certain minimum mandatory sentences for violations of the federal laws. In 1960 the *Narcotic Manufacturing Act* required licensing of all manufacturers and established quotas limiting the amount of natural and synthetic drugs produced. In 1965 Congress passed one more group of regulations. *The Drug Abuse and Control Act,* which makes it a violation to possess and sell certain stimulants and depressants illegally and requires that manufacturers, retailers, and distributors keep an inventory of all these drugs they receive and dispense. The specific requirements are:

1. That all wholesalers, jobbers and manufacturers of controlled drugs must register annually with the Food and Drug Administration and keep records of controlled drugs.
2. That pharmacists, hospitals, and doctors who regularly dispense and charge for controlled drugs must keep records of all transactions.

In addition, the act prohibits:

1. Refilling a prescription for one of these drugs more than five times or later than six months after it was originally written.

2. Manufacturing, processing and compounding the designated drugs, except by registered drug firms.
3. Distributing the designated drugs to persons not authorized to receive them by federal or state law.[33]

The *Comprehensive Drug Abuse Prevention and Control Act* was passed by Congress in 1970. The Act divides drugs into five classes with different penalties for the illegal manufacture, distribution, possession, and possession for sale established for each class. Class I drugs have no medical use in the United States, and the penalties for this group are the most severe: from three to thirty years imprisonment and $15,000 to $50,000 in fines. Drugs in the remaining four classes are used medically, but the illegal use of these results in less years of imprisonment and lesser fines.

These acts and controls are administered at the federal level of government under the Bureau of Narcotics and Dangerous Drugs in the Justice Department.

Control of the Abuser

The dependent obtains, usually, the drugs he needs illegally. Consequently, it is difficult to separate dependency from infractions of the law. Many programs of rehabilitation are connected with law-enforcement agencies, which in itself makes it hard to consider the problems involved in rehabilitation entirely medically. The law-enforcement approach, which is not always satisfactory, consists of several alternatives. The most stringent alternative is to provide the death penalty. Nations have not found this penalty too effective as a deterrent. In the United States, provisions in the Boggs Act permit this penalty under certain circumstances. A second alternative is incarceration. However, when the user returns to the community, he frequently resumes the use of narcotics.

In an attempt to keep former users "straight," some law-enforcement agencies require as a condition of parole that they be tested periodically. In several studies, 38 percent of those on such a program seemed to stay drug free; others used smaller amounts of narcotics so that they could more easily finance their habit without commiting felonies.

A third alternative is compulsory hospitalization. Are dependents able to accomplish rehabilitation outside of an institution and without supervision? Present evidence indicates that many cannot. Those who voluntarily commit themselves can nearly always voluntarily release themselves before the recommended rehabilitation period of from six to twelve months elapses. They relapse much sooner and oftener. Dependents who return to the community without supervision, especially compulsory supervision, also relapse sooner and more frequently.

FOUNDATIONS OF HEALTH SCIENCE

The drug dependent is typically in poor condition both physically and psychologically. A program of treatment designed to build the patient up physically is usually instituted immediately. The program involves, among other things, breaking the physiological dependence on the drugs. Dependency on opiates and barbiturates requires a special withdrawal treatment that is primarily a medical matter. Withdrawal and withdrawal treatment may be feared by the patient even though the process takes a relatively short time, and physiological dependence is shortly terminated. Withdrawal symptoms, described earlier in this chapter, can be alleviated by the administration of synthetic drugs. Withdrawal even with synthetic drugs is far from pleasant. At best, it has been described as rarely being worse than a case of influenza.

The medical task of withdrawing the drug and breaking physiological dependence is much easier than the psychological and social tasks of bringing about more adaptive ways of responding and adjusting to life and the community. Hospital treatment designed to break physiological dependence and re-establish physical health starts the patient back toward recovery, but it does not prove adequate for establishing lifetime freedom from drug dependency. In addition to medical treatment, it would appear that long-range psychotherapy and social assistance are essential if the patient is to make an adequate recovery. Adequate recovery means not only abstinence from drug usage, but learning to face the problems of social living realistically, finding an acceptable adult role, and becoming a contributing member of the community.

The prognosis for rehabilitating the narcotic dependent is still considered unfavorable. Statistics are misleading since the criteria for "cure" are so variable. These can include comparisons of employment records, number of arrests, incidents of repeated drug abuse, or pursuit of education; and, each of these criteria might be compared for different periods of time—three, six, twelve, or sixty months. According to Phillipson there does not seem to be any one most effective treatment program since "addicts differ in their needs and in the kinds of therapy which are most helpful to them.[34]

Institutional Treatment

A number of modalities or types of treatment and therapy are used in rehabilitation programs. In traditional institutional treatment the dependent is removed from his community to a closed setting. The cost to retrain and re-educate him is higher than in community-based programs. For many years the primary treatment institutions were the two federal hospitals, one in Fort Worth, Texas, and the second in Lexington, Kentucky. These hospitals are now primarily research centers.

Today many states have inaugurated their own institutional treatment types of programs that include compulsory therapy in rehabilitation centers and enrollment in outpatient groups. In one state, over 90 percent are committed to the rehabilitation center involuntarily. During the average six month's to two-and-one-half years' stay at the center, group therapy and vocational education are provided to help the dependent become better prepared to cope with life "on the street." Before he is released on recommendations of an evaluation committee, a job has been secured, living arrangements have been made, and a parole agent has been assigned. Some parolees stay in one of several half-way houses available in the nearby metropolitan area. The patient is checked weekly by the parole agent, he attends weekly outpatient group sessions, and he is required to have frequent medical examinations to make sure that he is "clean," or not reusing narcotics. In a study of a sample of 2,300 of these outpatient parolees, one out of three had remained drug free for one to three years. Two out of the three had remained clean for part of a year. After three years of abstaining from the abuse of narcotics, 239 were released from the program. Only one of these is known to have reverted. These are much better results than those obtained in past federal programs.[35]

Outpatient Clinics

Outpatient clinics are most effective when their use is combined with other treatment modalities. In these clinics intensive counseling is provided both individually and in groups, specialized medical care is given, and training and job placement are available.

Probation-Parole

Probation-parole has been demonstrated to be of value in reducing recidivism among drug abusers. One of the major problems is the availability of a sufficient number of parole officers to give the parolees the supportive aid and supervision they require.

Crisis Centers

Crisis centers have been rapidly expanding in size and number. Here are utilized such intervention techniques as crash pads, rap houses, hot lines, and store-front walk-in clinics. These have special appeal for youths in the early stages of drug involvement.

Methadone Maintenance

Methadone maintenance is the substitution of a synthetic opiate for heroin. The abuser becomes dependent on methadone instead of heroin, but his anti-social behavior is reduced. This program is not less expensive nor has it proven to be more effective than other types of treatment. New drugs that act like methadone are currently being tested; because of their longer lasting effects, the patient would not be required to come into the clinic as frequently and could thus live a more normal life.

The Therapeutic Community

The therapeutic community is a live-in-treatment environment staffed primarily by ex-dependents. Encounter and confrontation in an authoritarian setting are the primary means of rehabilitation. The communities are of two types. In one, the dependent is expected to stay for a year or so, but the ultimate goal is to reintegrate him into society. In the second type, he is expected to remain in this closed setting and be part of the community continuously. Synanon is of the second type.

IN CONCLUSION

Bowen aptly summarizes the drug abuse picture in this nation.

> Reliance on drugs by the people of our present generation is unequaled in the history of mankind. For many, life depends on drugs. There are pills to calm us and pills for pep; pills to help gain weight and pills to lose it; pills to avoid conception and more pills to help it.
>
> Drugs are, however, two-edged swords. They may save lives as well as wreck lives. It all depends on the prescriber and the user. Some of our most dangerous and habituating drugs are very useful under proper circumstances and in proper hands.
>
> The abuse of drugs today poses a major health problem and creates a real social danger.[36]

The effects of the long-term abuse of stimulants, depressants, and psychedelics are not as fully understood as they might be. This we do know: withdrawal, alienation, and unconcern for the future do not contribute to an effective society. The use of chemical compounds that reduce behavioral controls is detrimental to society. The abuse of drugs is not a "private act," it does interfere with the rights of others.

The serious personal and social consequences of drug dependency strongly indicate that further knowledge of the means of preventing abuse is imperative. The recovery of those who become dependent is slow and none too certain. Societal acceptance of drug dependency as a result of inappropriate personal-social learning rather than as a sign of moral degeneracy would be a notable step toward improved treatment.

Notes

1. E. R. Bloomquist, *Marijuana* (Toronto: Glencoe Press, 1968), p. 13.

2. D. P. Ausubel, "Causes and Types of Narcotic Addiction: A Psychological View," *Psychiatric Quarterly*, 35:523–531, 1961.

3. The President's Advisory Commission on Narcotic and Drug Abuse, *A Report to the Nation* (Washington, D.C.: Superintendent of Documents, 1963), p. 4.

4. Hershel Thornburg, "The Adolescent and Drugs: An Overview," *The Journal of School Health*, 43:643–645, 1973.

5. Morris Weitman, Robert O. Scheble, and Kit G. Johnson, "Survey of Adolescent Drug Use," *American Journal of Public Health,* 64:420, 1974.

6. Zebulon Taintor, "The 'Why' of Youthful Drug Abuse," *The Journal of School Health*, 44:27, 1974.

7. John A. Ewing, "Students, Sex, and Marijuana," *Medical Aspects of Human Sexuality*, 6:115, 1972.

8. Taintor, "The 'Why' of Youthful Drug Abuse," p. 27.

9. DHEW, *Marihuana and Health, Second Annual Report to Congress* (Washington, D.C.: Government Printing Office, 1972), pp. 11, 13.

10. Bloomquist, *Marijuana*, p. 10.

11. DHEW, *Marihuana and Health*, pp. 16–18.

12. Ibid., p. 29.

13. Ibid., pp. 21–22.

14. Ibid., p. 23.

15. Bloomquist, *Marijuana*, p. 102.

16. John A. Thomas, Michael T. Smith, and Glenn R. Knotts, "Current Assessment of Marijuana," *The Journal of School Health*, 42:383, 1972.

17. DHEW, *Marihuana and Health*, pp. 25–26.

18. Ewing, "Students, Sex, and Marijuana," pp. 114, 115.

19. Dorothy V. Whipple and Dodi Schultz, "Answers to the Most Controversial Questions About Drugs," *Today's Health*, 50:16–20, 60, 61, 1972.

20. Ibid.

21. Ewing, "Students, Sex, and Marijuana," pp. 114, 115.

22. DHEW, *Marihuana and Health*, p. 28.

23. Joel Fort, *American Drugstore* (Boston: Educational Associates, 1975), p. 37.

24. Ibid.

25. Carl C. Pfeiffer et al., "Time-series, Frequency Analysis, and Electrogenesis of the EEG's of Normals and Psychotics Before and After Drugs," *The American Journal of Psychiatry*, 121:1147–1156, 1965.

26. Richard Alpert, Sidney Cohen, and Lawrence Schiller, *LSD* (New York: The New American Library, 1966), pp. 70, 71.

27. Ibid., p. 71.

28. Glenn R. Knotts, "The Central Nervous System Stimulants in Drug Abuse," *Journal of School Health,* 39:353–354, 1969.

29. Carol Distasio and Marcia Mawrot, "Methaqualone," *American Journal of Nursing,* 73:1922, 1973.

30. Richard R. Lingeman, *Drugs from A to Z* (New York: McGraw-Hill Book Co., 1969), p. 83.

31. D. P. Ausubel, *Drug Addiction* (New York: Random House, 1965), p. 13.

32. George Pillar and June Narus, "Physical Effects of Heroin Addiction," *American Journal of Nursing,* 73:2105–2109, 1973.

33. John H. Kesling, "Drug Addiction—A Pharmacist's Viewpoint," *Journal of School Health,* 39:178, 1969.

34. Richard Phillipson, "Drug Abuse Treatment," *Journal of School Health,* 42:627, 1972.

35. Otis R. Bowen, "Medico-Legal Conflict in Drug Usage," *Journal of School Health,* 39:168, March, 1969.

36. Ibid., p. 165.

MARIJUANA:
The Health Questions
Is marijuana as damaging as recent reports make it appear?

Edward M. Brecher and the
Editors of Consumer Reports

current issues

Over the past year the news media have carried many stories warning that smoking marijuana produces severely damaging effects on the human body. CU has followed these news accounts with great interest. In our special publication, "Licit and Illicit Drugs," published in 1972, we presented an exhaustive study of the scientific, social, and legal evidence through the end of 1971. Based on the evidence then available, we recommended that marijuana should be regulated rather than prohibited, that all persons currently imprisoned for marijuana possession or for sharing marijuana with friends should be released, and that past offenses of these kinds should be erased from the legal records. The time has come to take a fresh look at the alleged dangers of marijuana.

THE SCIENTIFIC CASE AGAINST MARIJUANA

Many of the recent allegations concerning the effects of marijuana

Edward M. Brecher, an award-winning science writer and investigative reporter, has been a frequent contributor to *Consumer Reports* since 1938. He was a principal collaborator on "The Consumers Union Report on Smoking and the Public Interest" (1963), which foreshadowed the U.S. Surgeon General's report of 1964; and he was the senior author of "Licit and Illicit Drugs," the CU report cited by the American Library Association as one of 43 books "of outstanding merit" in 1972.

325

on health have appeared in reputable scientific journals. Here, in summary, is the case against marijuana recently presented to the public.

1. Smoking marijuana damages the brain irreversibly and ages it prematurely.

In December 1971, the late Dr. A. M. G. Campbell and his associates reported in a leading British medical journal, *The Lancet,* on X-ray studies of the brains of 10 chronic marijuana smokers. Compared to a group of nonsmokers of the same age, the marijuana group reportedly showed "evidence of cerebral atrophy"—that is, a wasting away of brain tissue.

Such X-ray studies, called air encephalograms, can be painful and hazardous, and no other research group has yet ventured to repeat the Campbell study. Several studies involving other techniques, however, are often cited in support of Dr. Campbell's findings. At the Tulane University School of Medicine, for example, Dr. Robert G. Heath implanted electrodes deep in the brains of six rhesus monkeys and recorded the monkeys' brain waves before, during, and after heavy exposure to marijuana smoke. In monkeys, as in humans, temporary changes in brain-wave patterns are normal with almost any change in the body or its environment. But persistent changes are cause for concern. Dr. Heath reported that after his monkeys were subjected to marijuana smoke in large doses daily for months, the changes became persistent; they could be observed as long as five days after marijuana ex-

posure was discontinued. Further, an autopsy report on two of Dr. Heath's monkeys indicated "structural alteration of cells in the septal region of the brain." The alterations were said to be "minimal," visible only under a microscope. "Our previous experience with similar conditions," Dr. Heath stated, "would lead us to assume that this chronic smoking of marijuana has probably produced irreversible changes in brain function."

Dr. Campbell's 10 patients and Dr. Heath's two monkeys provide the only direct evidence of possible brain damage to date. Indirect evidence, however, comes from Drs. Harold Kolansky and William Moore, psychiatrists at the University of Pennsylvania School of Medicine and the Institute of the Philadelphia Association for Psychoanalysis. Drs. Kolansky and Moore are convinced, on the basis of their observations of marijuana-smoking patients, that chronic smoking produces "a specific and separate clinical syndrome," or pattern of behavior, which has been called "the amotivational syndrome." The hallmarks of this syndrome are said to be "disturbed awareness of the self, apathy, confusion, and poor reality testing." Other signs are sleep disturbances, memory defects, and impairment of the time sense.

"Many of those we examined," Dr. Kolansky said, "were physically thin and often appeared so tired that they simulated the weariness and resignation of some of the aged. All appeared older than their chronological age...." These observations, the Philadelphia psychiatrists concluded, "seemed to imply some form of organic change" in the brains of chronic marijuana smokers.

2. Smoking marijuana lowers the body's resistance to infectious diseases and cancer.

The human body has several defenses against infectious diseases, foreign protein substances, and possibly even against some types of cancer. One of these immunological defenses is provided by the "T-lymphocytes"—certain white blood cells derived from the thymus gland. When viruses or some other foreign substances invade the body, the T-lymphocytes multiply very rapidly and attack the invaders. This is an important aspect of the "immune response."

Dr. Gabriel G. Nahas and his associates at Columbia University's College of Physicians and Surgeons reported in *Science* in February 1974 that the immune response of marijuana smokers is impaired. The Nahas group based its conclusion on a complex series of laboratory procedures. They removed some T-lymphocytes from the blood of 34 marijuana smokers, allowed the cells to multiply in laboratory cultures for 72 hours, and then exposed them to pooled donor lymphocytes or to a specific chemical —either of which normally evokes the immune response in those cells.

Under these circumstances, the T-lymphocytes of the marijuana smokers assimilated less thymidine (an important cell building block) from the culture solution than did those of the nonsmokers. This result suggested that the cells from the smokers were not multiplying normally.

Dr. Nahas interprets this finding to mean that the immune response of the T-lymphocytes of marijuana smokers is impaired. In this respect, he states, they resemble the T-lymphocytes of some patients with cancer or kidney disease. He concludes that marijuana smokers lack an essential means of defense against infectious diseases and cancer.

In October 1974, Dr. Sudhir Gupta and his associates at Roosevelt and St. Luke's Hospitals in New York City reported related findings in *The New England Journal of Medicine*. Using a procedure that tests the response of T-lymphocytes to sheep red blood cells, they observed that the reaction of T-lymphocytes from marijuana smokers was weaker than the reaction of T-lymphocytes from nonsmokers. They concluded that marijuana might induce a reduction of T-lymphocyte function in man.

3. Smoking marijuana increases the likelihood of birth defects and of hereditary diseases.

Most normal human cells have 46 chromosomes. Each chromosome carries numerous genes, or units of DNA (deoxyribonucleic acid), which govern the manufacture of proteins within the cell and regulate many of the cell's other functions. Sperm cells and ova each contain only 23 chromosomes; these are of particular importance, for they carry DNA "genetic code" from parents to offspring.

Back in 1967, reports began to appear alleging that the drug LSD damages chromosomes. Subsequent careful studies failed to confirm this allegation, and the earlier reports are now generally discredited.

Among those who reported that

LSD does not damage chromosomes was Dr. Morton Stenchever of the University of Utah College of Medicine. In January 1974, however, Dr. Stenchever and his associates reported in the *American Journal of Obstetrics and Gynecology* that they had found a somewhat elevated proportion of damaged chromosomes in the lymphocytes of 49 marijuana smokers, including some who smoked marijuana only twice a week or less.

Another chromosome study, not published at this writing, was described at hearings of the U.S. Senate Subcommittee on Internal Security last May. Dr. Akira Morishima, an associate of Dr. Nahas, told the subcommittee that he had compared 956 lymphocytes from marijuana smokers with 954 from nonsmokers. More than 30 percent of the lymphocytes from smokers contained fewer than 31 chromosomes instead of the usual 46. Among lymphocytes from nonsmokers, only about 10 percent contained so few chromosomes.

"Since lymphocytes constitute an essential component of cellular immunity and chromosomes are basic units of inheritance at the cellular level," Dr. Morishima told the Senate subcommittee, "it seems logical to anticipate potential danger in [the] immune defense system, development of cancer . . . , genetic mutation and birth defects."

In the Nahas experiment, it will be recalled, T-lymphocytes failed to multiply rapidly when challenged with foreign substances. The *reason* they failed to multiply, Dr. Nahas declares, was that they could not manufacture enough DNA. Dr. Morishima similarly attributes his finding of too few chromosomes to a defect in DNA manufacture.

4. Smoking marijuana causes precancerous changes in the lung cells and other lung damage.

Damage to lung cells from marijuana smoke has been reported by Drs. Cecile and Rudolph Leuchtenberger of Switzerland and also by Dr. Forest S. Tennant, whose studies were performed while he was a medical officer stationed with the U.S. Armed Forces in Europe. In addition, some clinical studies suggest that those who smoke large amounts of marijuana for long periods may be more likely to develop chronic bronchitis or other conditions indicating lung-cell damage than those who do not.

Dr. Cecile Leuchtenberger's work, however, goes far beyond lung-cell damage. She grew lung cells of human origin in her laboratory and subjected them to repeated whiffs of marijuana smoke. Under these conditions, she found damage to chromosomes, changes in the number of chromosomes, and changes in DNA manufacture—which she interpreted as suggesting precancerous changes. She also reported abnormal sperm cells in mice exposed to marijuana. Thus, Dr. Leuchtenberger alleges five different kinds of marijuana damage—more than any other scientist to date.

5. Smoking marijuana may lead to sterility, impotence, or both, among men.

Testosterone is the most potent male sex hormone. The concentration of testosterone in the blood of a human male can be readily measured. In April 1974, Dr. Robert C. Kolodny and his associates at the Reproductive Biology Research Foundation in St. Louis (the Masters-Johnson sex research center) reported in *The New England Journal of Medicine* that they had studied testosterone blood levels of 20 frequent marijuana smokers and 20 nonsmokers. The levels in the marijuana smokers, though within normal limits, were lower than the levels in the nonsmokers. And the levels in subjects who smoked 10 or more marijuana cigarettes per week were lower than the levels of those who smoked only five to nine per week.

Six marijuana smokers had relatively low sperm counts and two complained of impotence; such effects might (or might not) be related to low testosterone levels. When one of the men who complained of impotence stopped smoking marijuana, he reported his potency had been restored.

SENATOR EASTLAND'S CONCLUSIONS

Many of the findings reviewed above were nationally publicized last spring at hearings of the Senate Internal Security Subcommittee, chaired by Senator James O. Eastland of Mississippi. Senator Eastland drew these personal conclusions from the testimony:

"(1) If the cannabis [marijuana] epidemic continues to spread . . . we may find ourselves saddled with a large population of semi-zombies— of young people acutely afflicted by the amotivational syndrome. . . .

"(2) We may also find ourselves saddled with a partial generation of young people—people in their teens and early twenties—suffering from irreversible brain damage. . . .

"(3) The millions of junior high school and grade school children who are today using marijuana may produce another partial generation of teen-agers who have never matured, either intellectually or physically, because of hormonal deficiency and a deficiency in cell-production during the critical period of puberty. . . . We may witness the phenomenon of a generation of young people who have begun to grow old before they have even matured.

"(4) . . . There is the possibility . . . that we may develop a large population of youthful respiratory cripples. And there is the possibility —which can only be confirmed by epidemiological studies—that marijuana smokers are producing far more than their quota of malformed and genetically damaged children. . . ."

If the scientific reports of adverse marijuana effects are well-founded, there can of course be no possible objection to their then being widely publicized through Congressional hearings, news accounts, or other means. The truth about marijuana should be known. But if the reports are poorly founded, that fact needs to be reported, too. For such misinformation serves only to frighten the public unnecessarily, especially the millions of marijuana smokers, former smokers, and their families— many of whom may now be waiting in dread for brain damage, cancer, and other predicted disasters to strike themselves or their loved ones. Accordingly, it may prove useful for

CU to review recent medical evidence overlooked—or ignored—by the Eastland subcommittee and by the press that covered the hearings.

THE JAMAICA STUDY

Back in 1970, when CU's "Licit and Illicit Drugs" was still in the research stage, a different but almost equally horrifying collection of marijuana hazards was being publicized. Yet many marijuana smokers appeared to remain in good health and in good spirits, just as they do today. Perhaps, we reasoned, it is too early to gauge the true effects of marijuana smoking in the United States or Canada.

But what of other countries where marijuana has been a daily custom for generations? If dire adverse effects existed, they would surely be readily visible there, observable without air encephalograms, implanted electrodes, or other sophisticated laboratory procedures. Scientists dispatched to such countries would not have to *predict* the long-term consequences of marijuana use; they could readily see and measure those effects.

The same idea, of course, occurred to others, including administrators at the National Institute of Mental Health. They commissioned the Research Institute for the Study of Man to study marijuana effects on the island of Jamaica. For decades, Jamaicans have smoked marijuana much stronger than that smoked in the United States.

Although the Jamaica report was completed nearly three years ago, it has still not been published in the United States. Indeed, CU was unable to obtain a copy from the Government agencies concerned. An edition in English was finally scheduled to be published last month (February) by Mouton, a Dutch firm in The Hague. The report, titled "Ganja in Jamaica," is by Drs. Vera Rubin and Lambros Comitas, director and associate director, respectively, of the Research Institute for the Study of Man.

In Jamaica, the report explains, marijuana is called "ganja" and is used in many ways. It is smoked, brewed as a tea, chewed, and used in cooking. In rural areas especially, it is an important element of folk medicine and superstitution. "Children are introduced to ganja quite early," the Jamaica report notes, "first as a medicament in 'bush tea' or in a crude method of vaporizing, where adults blow smoke at an infant with respiratory congestion." Increasing doses of marijuana tea throughout infancy are recommended as a prophylaxis against disease. Schoolboys are urged to smoke marijuana to "help them study," to "improve memory," and to "help pass examinations." This widespread use of marijuana is found both among farmers and villagers and among residents of the slums of Kingston, Jamaica's capital.

The Jamaica study was launched in June 1970, when six anthropologists were sent into the field—five into rural districts and the sixth into an urban slum neighborhood. They found heavy ganja smoking common among the poor, despite severe legal penalties (not less than eighteen months' imprisonment with hard labor for a first offense).

One of the anthropologists, Dr. Joseph H. Schaeffer, studied the effects of marijuana on ability and willingness to work. He recorded in

330

detail how much work both smokers and nonsmokers did in a sample week and how much metabolic energy they expended while at work. In general, Dr. Schaeffer found that field laborers actually performed more motions and expended more energy after smoking marijuana than before. But they appeared to accomplish less when on marijuana—weeding a smaller patch of crops in an hour, for example. Dr. Schaeffer also reported, however, that marijuana use in group labor situations tended to increase the social cohesiveness of the workers. While it may have decreased overall efficiency, it appeared to make the prospect of long hours in the field more palatable and increase the laborers' willingness to work.

The Jamaica report calls this the "motivational syndrome"—as distinguished from the "amotivational syndrome" described by other psychiatrists.

Following this and other field studies, the Jamaica research team brought 30 male marijuana smokers and 30 nonsmokers to University Hospital at the University of the West Indies for six days of intensive medical examinations. The 60 subjects ranged in age from 23 to 53; the average age was 34. All but one of the marijuana smokers had first smoked before the age of 20; they had been smoking marijuana for 17.5 years, on the average (the range was from 7 to 37 years). They did not smoke marijuana while in the hospital.

But it was the frequency with which they smoked that will startle American readers. To qualify as a "heavy" smoker in the Jamaica study, one had to smoke at least eight "spliffs" (ganja cigarettes) a day. In the U.S., a "heavy" smoker is often defined as one who smokes more than seven marijuana cigarettes a *week*. And the typical Jamaican spliff is more potent than the typical North American marijuana "joint." Thus, Jamaicans smoke considerably heavier doses than their American counterparts, even though the latter tend to inhale more deeply than Jamaicans.

The 30 control subjects were matched with the ganja smokers for age and socio-economic status. It was, however, impossible to enlist enough working class males in the right age bracket who had never once used marijuana. Accordingly, the control group was composed of 12 men who had never smoked ganja plus 18 confirmed nonsmokers who had smoked only occasionally in the past. All but three of the ganja smokers and all but 11 of the controls also smoked tobacco cigarettes. (Tobacco is also sometimes mixed with ganja in spliffs to make a "better smoke.")

Summarizing the examination findings, the Jamaica report notes "no significant physical abnormality" in any of the controls or in 28 of the 30 ganja smokers. One ganja smoker had a long history of asthma; another had a little-understood nervous condition known as "Jamaican neuropathy," suspected of being an atypical form of neurosyphilis. "There is nothing to suggest that these disabilities were in any way related to the use of cannabis," the report states.

The marijuana smokers and controls were well matched in height as well as age, but the smokers weighed seven pounds less on the average—a difference, the report noted, that "might indicate that the chronic use of cannabis causes some suppression of appetite."

X-rays of the lungs were normal in both groups except for some scarring of the lungs in one of the subjects who did *not* smoke marijuana. Since smoking tobacco cigarettes impairs lung function, it was also necessary to discount that effect when gauging the effects of marijuana. At worst, the Jamaica findings suggest, impaired lung function is produced by inhaling smoke, whether tobacco or marijuana.

Since the marijuana smokers in the Jamaica study were also in many cases the children and grandchildren of persons who smoked marijuana, and since many of them were probably exposed to marijuana before birth as well as during infancy, childhood, adolescence, and adult life, the study of their chromosomes by Dr. Marigold J. Thorburn of the University of the West Indies is of no small interest. Briefly, the chromosomes of the marijuana smokers were in good condition. In fact, they showed slightly fewer abnormalities than were found in the control group, though the difference was not statistically significant.

In addition to these and other studies of physical health, both ganja smokers and controls were given thorough psychiatric examinations by Drs. Michael H. Beaubrun and Frank Knight, both psychiatrists. Only one ganja smoker and one control reported a history of past mental illness. Four ganja smokers and three controls had had alcohol problems sufficiently acute to interfere with work or social functioning. Two ganja smokers, however, "reported that they had been able to reduce their alcohol intake, and seemed to relate this to ganja use."

On the Eysenck personality test, the "extroversion scores" were identical for ganja smokers and controls. The only man suffering from depression, as gauged by the Hamilton Ratings Scale for Depression, was not a marijuana smoker. Not a single smoker or control appeared to be schizophrenic on either of two rating scales.

The brain-wave recordings of both ganja smokers and controls were also compared. Significant differences were not found.

A battery of 19 psychological tests designed to compare ganja smokers and nonsmokers on 47 measures, including 11 measures of intelligence, was administered in the Jamaica study. Smokers had not smoked marijuana for two days before the tests and did not smoke on the test day. The marijuana smokers scored better on 29 of the 47 measures—a statistically insignificant finding.

Drs. Beaubrun and Knight summed up as follows: "The data clearly indicate that the long-term marijuana use by these men did not produce demonstrable intellectual or ability deficits when they were without the drug for three days. There is no evidence in the results to suggest brain damage."

The psychiatrists also asked about regularity and continuity of employment and frequency and nature of job changes. No significant differences were found between marijuana smokers and controls. Thus, careful psychiatric examination showed no evidence that these Jamaicans were "semi-zombies" after having smoked very large quantities of very strong marijuana for an average of 17.5 years.

CONFLICT OF EVIDENCE

By far the greatest conflict of evidence on marijuana exists between the Jamaica study and the studies cited earlier. But there are also notable conflicts among the latter studies themselves. Here are some examples.

1. Brain damage. The Campbell report, it will be recalled, found evidence of brain damage in a group of marijuana smokers. But was the damage present before the patients started to smoke marijuana? If not, was it caused by marijuana, by some other drug, or by some nondrug factor, such as a blow on the head? Here is what Dr. Kolodny—the scientist who believes marijuana smoking lowers testosterone levels—had to say about the Campbell report:

> Research in cannabis effects on humans has not always been performed or presented with objectivity. Many studies have been severely limited by indiscriminately including multiple drug users, thus frequently raising more questions than providing useful information. As an example of such research, I would like to comment briefly on the [Campbell] study entitled "Cerebral Atrophy in Young Cannabis Smokers. . . ." In the 10 cases reported, all 10 men had used LSD —many of them over 20 times— as well as cannabis, and 8 of the 10 had used amphetamines. One subject had a previous history of convulsions, four had significant head injuries, and a number had used sedatives, barbiturates, heroin,

or morphine. On the basis of these facts, speculative connection between cannabis use and brain damage is highly suspect. Unfortunately, this type of report is typical of much of the research done in this field.

Next, consider this comment on the work of Dr. Heath, who reported brain-wave changes in rhesus monkeys exposed to marijuana smoke, by Dr. Julius Axelrod, who won a 1970 Nobel Prize for two studies, one of them concerned with the effects of drugs on the brain. Dr. Axelrod appeared as a witness before the Eastland subcommittee to warn against marijuana. Asked at the subcommittee hearings about Dr. Heath's experiments, Dr. Axelrod replied:

> . . . One of the fundamental principles in pharmacology is the amount of a compound or drug that enters the body. You could take the most poisonous compound, and if you take too little, there is no effect. One may take a very supposedly safe compound, and if you give enough of it, it will cause toxic effects. This, I think, all pharmacologists recognize. I respect Dr. Heath; he is a fine neurologist; but the doses he has given for the acute effect, for example, would be equivalent to smoking 100 marijuana cigarettes, a very heavy dose of marijuana. And the amount he has given for the chronic effect represents smoking 30 marijuana cigarettes three times a day for a period of six months. [Even the heavy ganja smokers in the Jamaica study smoked only a fraction of this.] The results indicate that marijuana causes an irreversible damage to the brain. But the amounts used are so large that one wonders

whether it's due to the large toxic amounts Dr. Heath has given. I think it would be a better experiment if he had done what is done in pharmacology, a dose-response [curve]: smaller amounts equivalent to that used by an occasional marijuana smoker and larger amounts used by a chronic smoker [would be given] to see what levels would produce these irreversible effects. I hope that this will be done.

Dr. Lester Grinspoon of the Harvard Medical School similarly points out that the monkeys in the Heath study did not smoke marijuana voluntarily but had the heavy doses forced into their lungs. Since the monkey lung is about 1/15th the size of a human lung, the concentration of marijuana in the monkey lung may have been 15 times as high as that of a comparable dose in the human lung. Allowing for this and other dosage disparities, Dr. Grinspoon notes, it is possible that Dr. Heath's monkeys were exposed to marijuana concentrations vastly greater than those experienced by the usual human smoker.

Nor have the brain-damage allegations of Drs. Kolansky and Moore gone unchallenged. At the University of Pennsylvania (with which Drs. Kolansky and Moore are associated), another team of researchers headed by Dr. Igor Grant administered a neurological examination to 29 marijuana smokers and 29 nonsmoking controls, all of them medical students. In addition to the neurological functions usually tested, six measures specifically designed to reveal brain damage were used. The examiners did not know which examinees were marijuana smokers and which were nonsmokers. No difference was found between the two groups.

In addition, the Grant team administered a battery of neuropsychological tests designed to reveal brain damage. "We found no difference between marijuana smokers and nonsmokers on seven out of eight measures," Dr. Grant and his associates reported. "Marijuana smokers did not perform quite as well as nonsmokers . . . on one of the three subtests of the Tactual Performance Test." The team added, however, that "the absence of confirmatory findings in the other tests has led us to conclude that this one finding did not indicate a neuropsychological deficit among marijuana smokers." They summed up their findings in these terms:

A battery of the most sensitive neuropsychological tests now available could demonstrate essentially no difference between moderate users and nonusers of marijuana. These results agree with those of Mendelson and Meyer who employed similar tests with 10 casual and 10 heavy users.

Finally, the allegations of an "amotivational syndrome" and of brain damage are challenged by the findings of Dr. Norman Q. Brill and his associates at the University of California at Los Angeles School of Medicine. This group checked the college grades of 1,380 UCLA undergraduates in 1970, then followed up on the same sample in 1971 (1,133 students) and 1972 (901 students). Many of those who left college as well as those who stayed on were followed up.

Six groups of students could be discriminated during this study: those who had never smoked marijuana; those who began smoking during the study; those who increased use during the study; those whose usage remained stable throughout the study; those who decreased use; and those who quit marijuana altogether.

All six groups showed a steady improvement in college grades from year to year. The nonsmokers had the highest grades as freshmen but the lowest grades as seniors and graduate students; the differences were not statistically significant. Neither college grades nor other factors checked by the UCLA scientists supplied any evidence of brain damage or of an amotivational syndrome. "So far as we have been able to determine by this longitudinal study," the Brill group concluded, "the dire consequences that were predicted have not materialized."

2. Lowered resistance to disease. Dr. Nahas, it will be recalled, grew T-lymphocytes from marijuana smokers in laboratory cultures and then challenged them with foreign substances. He interpreted his results as indicating an impairment of the immune response among marijuana smokers—an impairment similar to that found in some cancer patients.

Among those alarmed by the Nahas findings were Dr. Melvin J. Silverstein and his associate, Ms. Phyllis J. Lessin, at the University of California at Los Angeles. Patients with this kind of defect in immunity, they noted in a recent issue of *Science*, "develop cancer at rates at least 80 times that of the general population." But was Dr. Nahas right in interpreting his results to mean a loss of immune response?

To check on the Nahas claim, Dr. Silverstein and Ms. Lessin took an approach that determines the immune response in the human body itself instead of in a test tube. They challenged chronic marijuana smokers with a foreign substance called DNCB (2,4-dinitrochlorobenzene). A small amount of DNCB was first rubbed on the skin to sensitize it; two weeks later, small doses of DNCB were injected into the skin. Under these circumstances, 96 percent of all adults develop an immune reaction—a reddening of the skin around the test area and sometimes more severe skin changes. These changes can be graded from 1-plus (a minimum reaction) to 4-plus (a very severe reaction, including blistering).

When this test was run on 22 marijuana smokers, the results clearly indicated that their immune responses were intact and vigorous. All 22 showed a response to even a small (50-microgram) dose of DNCB, and in 21 of the 22 the response was severe (3-plus or 4-plus). Even with only a 25-microgram dose, 21 of the 22 showed an immune reaction, and 14 of the reactions were 3-plus or 4-plus. No resemblance was found to the immune reactions of a control group of cancer patients. Tests with other foreign substances confirmed this finding of a normal immune response in marijuana smokers.

". . . There is no clinical or epidemiologic evidence to suggest that chronic marijuana users might be more prone to the development of neoplastic [cancerous] or infectious processes," Dr. Silverstein and Ms. Lessin noted. "Since responses were normal in the chronic marijuana users we tested, it would appear that chronic marijuana smoking does not produce a gross cellular immune defect that can be detected by skin testing."

3. Birth defects and hereditary disease. The Stenchever report that marijuana damages chromosomes, like earlier claims that LSD damages chromosomes, is being heavily challenged by contradictory evidence.

At the Institute for Medical Research in Camden, N.J., for example, Dr. Warren W. Nichols and his associates performed a well-controlled study of marijuana effects on chromosomes. They first checked the chromosomes of 24 occasional marijuana smokers and found them to be in good condition. They then gave their 24 subjects measured doses of marijuana daily for five or 12 days and checked their chromosomes again. No damage was detected.

Other investigators who have failed to find marijuana damage to chromosomes include Dr. Thorburn of the University of the West Indies (in the Jamaica study), Dr. Henry B. Pace and his associates at the University of Mississippi, and Dr. Richard L. Neu of the Upstate Medical Center, State University of New York. Animal studies have also failed to provide evidence of chromosome damage.

As for the Morishima report that the lymphocytes of marijuana smokers have *fewer* than the normal number of chromosomes, two difficulties should be noted.

First, all of the lymphocytes studied by Dr. Morishima and reported by him to the Eastland subcommittee came from just three marijuana smokers and three nonsmokers; this is an extremely modest base from which to anticipate, in Dr. Morishima's words, "potential danger in [the] immune defense system, development of cancer . . . genetic mutation and birth defects."

The second difficulty: if more than 30 percent of the lymphocytes of chronic marijuana smokers con-tain fewer than 31 chromosomes instead of the normal 46, how could this gross lack of chromosomes have escaped the attention of Drs. Nichols, Stenchever, Thorburn, Pace, Neu, and others who have been intensively examining lymphocytes for chromosome breaks and other minor abnormalities?

4. Lung damage. Though the evidence to date is far from decisive, there is no reason to doubt that marijuana smoke, like tobacco smoke and other kinds of smoke, may damage human lung cells. *How much* damage remains an unanswered question. But the extent of damage is probably more closely related to the amount of smoke inhaled than to the type of smoke. Thus, it is hardly plausible at this stage of scientific knowledge to worry that someone who is smoking a pack of tobacco cigarettes a day— 140 a week—may experience further lung damage by adding two or three marijuana cigarettes a week.

For very heavy users who smoke many marijuana cigarettes a week, of course, the risk of lung damage may be serious. Dr. David E. Smith of the University of California at San Francisco Medical School, who is also medical director of the Haight-Ashbury Free Clinic, has accordingly suggested that such users switch from marijuana smoking to other forms of marijuana consumption—such as drinking marijuana tea—to protect their lungs from smoke.

5. Sterility and impotence. Back in 1971, Dr. Kolodny and his associates at the Masters-Johnson sex research center in St. Louis reported that male homosexuals have lower testosterone levels than male heterosexuals. That report, like the Kolodny report on low testosterone levels in marijuana smokers, was widely circulated by the mass media. Within two or three years, however, three efforts to replicate the Kolodny finding failed, and it is now generally agreed that no significant difference exists between homosexual and heterosexual testosterone levels. The Kolodny report on testosterone levels and marijuana is now experiencing a similar challenge.

In November 1974, Dr. Jack H. Mendelson and his associates at the Alcohol and Drug Abuse Research Center, Harvard Medical School-McLean Hospital, reported a carefully controlled study of marijuana effects on testosterone. Like the Kolodny study, the Mendelson study was published in *The New England Journal of Medicine*.

The Mendelson group selected for its study 27 young male marijuana smokers, some of them casual smokers and others heavy smokers who had consumed more than one marijuana cigarette a day for the past year and who had been smoking marijuana for an average of 5.6 years (range, three to nine years). All subjects were requested to refrain from marijuana smoking for two weeks and were then admitted for a 31-day stay in a locked hospital ward, where access to marijuana and other drugs was rigorously controlled.

During the first six days of the experiment, no marijuana was permitted. Testosterone levels were measured each morning. The average levels were in "the upper range of normal adult male levels." The heavy smokers had somewhat higher levels than the casual smokers, but the difference was not statistically significant.

During the next 21 days, the subjects were allowed to "earn"

marijuana by performing a simple manual task. They were required to smoke this marijuana under observation to make sure it was really consumed. As the days rolled by, both the casual and the heavy marijuana smokers gradually increased their consumption, some of them to very high levels. Their testosterone levels did not fall. Under these carefully controlled conditions, the Mendelson group concluded, "high-dosage marijuana intake was not associated with suppression of testosterone levels. . . ."

THE PATTERN OF EVIDENCE

Out of all of these many studies (and others not reviewed here), a general pattern is beginning to emerge. When a research finding can be readily checked—either by repeating the experiment or by devising a better one—an allegation of adverse marijuana effects is relatively short-lived. No damage is found—and after a time the allegation is dropped (often to be replaced by allegations of some other kind of damage due to marijuana).

If the test procedure is difficult —like the air encephalograms that Dr. Campbell employed, or like Dr. Heath's work with electrodes implanted deep in the brain—independent repeat studies are not run in other laboratories. So these allegations of damage continue to be cited in the scientific literature and in the lay press. Then they, too, are eventually replaced by fresh allegations of marijuana damage.

After reviewing the voluminous evidence available up to January

1972, CU did not conclude in "Licit and Illicit Drugs" that marijuana was "harmless." On the contrary, we then pointed out, "no drug is safe or harmless to all people at all dosage levels or under all conditions of use." We see no need to withdraw or modify that conclusion.

We do, however, see a need to comment on the adverse legal and social consequences of misinformation about the health effects of marijuana. We shall do so next month.

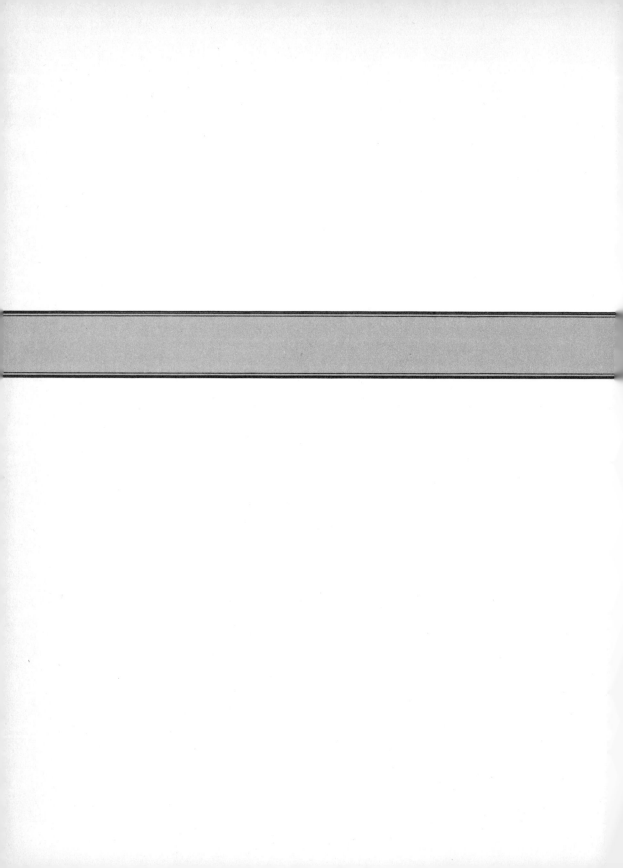

SEXUALITY AND MARRIAGE

chapter ten

The man-woman relationship is one of the most vital ones in our culture. Dating, courtship, love, marriage, sex, family relations, and child rearing are of great personal, social, literary, and academic concern. The satisfactions deriving from man-woman relationships are many and varied; so, too, are the problems. This short treatment of the male-female relationship cannot deal with all the ramifications involved, nor can satisfactory solutions to problems be prescriptively offered. Some of the significant aspects of man-woman relationships are presented and examined in the hope that a clearer understanding of them may evolve.

EARLY AMERICAN FAMILY AND TRADITIONS

To comprehend better some of the attitudes and practices in contemporary marriage, a brief look at the background from which it emerged is in order.

The early American family was a rural one with an agricultural economic base. The family was very largely self-sufficient and cooperative. It was both an economic and a social unit. The family had to work together in cooperative effort to insure the survival of its members, and all had to perform tasks that were important for the family as a unit. The work day was long, and the required tasks were demanding of time, energy, and strength. The family provided a great share of its own recreation, amusement, and socialization and met its own physical wants for food, clothing, and shelter. If the family was to survive, it *had* to fulfill most of its own needs, and adequate fulfillment of these needs required the active participation and full cooperation of all members.

Marriage itself was frequently an economic arrangement. Mate selection was centered about such practical concerns as having good physical stamina, good habits of work, and ability to perform household duties. These qualities were sought in a marriage partner. Love and regard for the affectional quality of the marriage relationship often were secondary concerns in the economically motivated marriage.

The early American family expected its members to forego individual interests and pursuits in favor of the interests and welfare of the whole family. The family, not the individual member, was really the important unit. Each person was but a member of this important unit and was expected to subjugate his own interests. Individuality was suppressed in favor of the goals of the family group.

One family member, typically but not always the father, made the decisions and passed judgments. Compliance with the decisions of the authority was expected, and little in the way of individual freedom was allowed. This authority-dominated family amounted to an association of unequals. Youths and male adults were favored; women and children fared less well. Family members were valued not so much for their intrinsic worth as human beings but for their abilities to contribute to the family's economic well-being. The tradition was to have large families. Children could provide much needed labor in an economy where there was little mechanization.

Perhaps the first real change in the American family came with the expansion westward. Young people could break away and move to the frontiers. This pattern broke the authoritarian domination by a "family head," and new or different behavior was required by the family members.

The urbanization and industrialization of the nation brought about further changes in the structure of the family. The rural-to-urban shift in population was accompanied by a continuing decline in self-sufficiency of the family, a change in its authoritarian structure, and changes in attitude toward it as a unit. Some of the functions of homemaking became institutionalized. Protection, medicine, recreation, and education were largely taken over by specialized agencies and services outside the home. Even food, clothing, and shelter began to come under outside control. Many of the household tasks became less burdensome as a result of technological advances. The family was freed from many chores that previously had been necessary for survival. More time and energy remained for the development of individual interests and pursuits.

Authoritarian management of family affairs was difficult to maintain when the members ventured away from the household for purposes of work, socialization, and recreation. They became exposed to new and different social patterns, and the family no longer served as the sole source of values, ideals, and mores. In turn the roles of the various members, including the husband and the wife, were altered; greater concern for the individual member and his welfare developed.

CHANGING ROLES AND THE FAMILY

Some people and groups have a tendency to view any change with alarm. The "emancipation" of women has been held responsible for what is viewed as the "deterioration" of the American family. This view, of course, makes two assumptions of a highly questionable nature. It assumes that women have been emancipated and that the family is deteriorating.

Although the treatment of women has changed markedly over the past years, they have not been freed from much of the prejudice and discrimination of which they have been victims. Women occupy few key places in either elective or appointive offices in government, for example, which is not solely a result of their lack of interest or of male support. Women still suffer from prejudices of their own sex as well as from those of men.

Sex Roles and Motivations

Any discussion of sex role must consider the differences between the sexes that exist in many areas besides the obvious ones of anatomical and biological structure. To claim superiority of one sex over the other is quite another matter. Arguments about equality or inequality of the sexes are characterized by more emotion than relevant data. Although men and women differ, the differences can hardly be used as a basis for claims of the superiority of one over the other. The data relative to sex differences do not support the concept of equality of men and women, nor do they support the inequality of the sexes. The fact that there are major differences should be understood, but the words "equal" and "unequal" are inappropriate when applied to male or female capacities and abilities. For success and happiness in modern marriage, men and women must discard long-outmoded ideas about the superiority or inferiority of either sex.

Sex roles have changed, are changing, and will continue to change. Attempts are being made constantly to redefine appropriate masculine-feminine behavior in our society. Adjustments are inevitable in order to meet the changing demands of modern life. The roles of men and women now overlap in many areas and are no longer as distinctly different or separate as they were in the past.

Conventional definitions of "man's work" and "woman's work" are no longer functional for our culture or for most modern households. Since the roles of modern man and modern woman are in a state of flux, conventional sex role definitions and role expectancies must be flexible. Much is made of the changed and changing role of women, but men's role in the culture is also being rapidly altered. Attempts to cling to the concepts of masculinity and femininity of a half-century or more ago will not meet the requirements of effective living in a modern society. The role requirements for men as husbands and fathers are quite different now than they were then. What women are expected to be and do is much talked and written about; too little is mentioned that what men are expected to be and do has also changed.

Differences in motivations vary from culture to culture and from generation to generation as well as with age and the two sexes. Women's motivations are in a state of great change currently, and their motivation toward achievement has received particular investigative attention from Matina Horner.[1] Horner has advanced the concept that one of their motivations is to avoid success. Moreover, she has theorized that such a motive is characteristic of bright women involved in achievement-oriented situations. She contends that such women worry not only about being failures but about avoiding becoming "too successful." This motive to avoid success is considered to operate when women fail to aspire to high-level positions within an achievement hierarchy. While this interesting theory that has been developed and reported may have considerable validity and may hold considerable explanatory power, Horner, in her research, has used fantasy-based measures in assessing the motive she postulates.

The use of fantasy-based measures of achievement motivation have been severely criticized, and some researchers have considerable doubt that these measures are of sufficient validity or reliability for such research purposes.[2] Preliminary data, gathered in a rather extensive investigation using an inventory in assessment, indicate that the motive to avoid success may be as common among employed men as it is among employed women,[3] which makes some sense when one looks at the world of employment and tries to arrange positions within an area of employment in a hierarchical fashion. The investigator's hierarchy need not

FOUNDATIONS OF HEALTH SCIENCE

coincide with that of the employed person. The investigator may consider a shop foreman as higher on the hierarchy (he is paid better) than a machinist. But many good machinists have no desire to become shop foremen and thus would have a motive to avoid success. The same general state of affairs may hold for college professors. Although most assistant professors work to attain full professorship and are achievement-oriented to that extent, they do not strive to become chairmen of their departments or to become deans, presidents, and so forth. If we judge these latter positions to be closer to the top of the hierarchy (they pay better) than the professorship, then we could say these assistant professors possess a motive to avoid success. Actually, satisfaction in one's job or with one's status in life might, thus, be interpreted as reflecting a motive to avoid success, when in reality it may be symptomatic of good emotional adjustment and realistic life goals. It should be interesting to follow the research on the motive to avoid success over the next few years. Until more data are available, however, healthy skepticism would seem to be in order.[4]

Sex Role and Sexuality

Much of the change in roles of the sexes is attributable to the changing social organization. Young adults began to break with tradition in many ways following World War I. Long-accepted standards of behavior that were challenged gave way to a freer way of living. Women gained the right to vote and to hold public office. Smoking and drinking spread from the world of men to the world of women. "Sex" became an acceptable word and gradually became an acceptable area for conversation. Women moved from their secluded and controlled existence under masculine domination and began to seek greater participation in all areas of life. They moved from a position of subservience to men to one of companionship with them in a short period of time.

Many social changes had occurred by World War II. At this time the lives and activities of both men and women underwent profound changes. There was a scarcity of workers and it became a patriotic duty for women to work outside of the home even if they were married and had children. When the war was over, the rising cost of living dictated that many women continue to be employed outside the home. Many couples got used to the idea of two family paychecks and accepted a wife's working as a necessity. Some women continued working for the personal and social satisfactions they derived from work other than homemaking. Many husbands found that life was better with a working wife.

Young people today know and enjoy a type of family life in which there are no well-defined and exclusive areas of work for either men or women. Happiness and success are based on compatibility, cooperation, and adaptability. The traditional ideas of man's and woman's work disappear in the face of modern household appliances and abundances of goods and services that are available commercially. The disappearance of precisely defined roles for men and women has created ambiguity. The roles of both have broadened, and a great diversity of patterns are found. Some boys have never seen their fathers cook a meal or dust a floor while others take it for granted that a father may do these things.

Patterns of authority differ from family to family as greatly as do the divisions of labor. In some families, the father is the autocratic head and the mother assumes a subservient and passive role. In others, the situation is reversed and the father is more or less a figurehead. In still a third pattern, clearly defined and compartmentalized areas of authority and responsibility are shared between husband and wife. A variant of this is a fourth type of family configuration, in which all members share responsibility, and authority stems from the responsibilities assumed. This latter pattern is more compatible with the democratic philosophy of living. A certain kind of maturity is required, since satisfactions are gained from the achievements of other individual members, rather than one's own. Self-esteem is enhanced rather than threatened by the accomplishments of a spouse or children.

The American family has changed and is changing. It serves some of its old functions and also serves some quite different ones. The modern family is probably serving its purposes as well in the current culture as families in the past have served theirs, and the emerging concept of family life, with its more democratic and loose organization, could possibly contribute more to the happiness, welfare, creativity, independence, and individuality of its members than earlier families did.

Currently, group marriages, rearing of children by unmarried couples, single-parent adoptions, communal living, and a variety of other life styles are contributing to the impossibility of depicting the "typical" American family. The "typical family" is a myth. Which family life style is best has not been determined. Indeed, little agreement exists as to what the criteria for an appropriate family life style should be.

Sexuality. Acquisition of sex role is a part of the social-learning processes that are continuous in the life of the individual. Little boys soon learn that they are little *boys* and little girls soon learn that they are *girls*. Boys are treated as "masculine" in the culture of the family and girls are treated as "feminine" in the family culture. If learning proceeds as the culture intends, boys should grow to manhood confident of themselves as men and pleased that they are male. Girls should grow to maturity confident in their womanhood and pleased that they are female. Certain attitudes and behaviors are characteristic of each sex, and their attitudes and behaviors should be reflected by the adult personality. An integral part of personality is sexuality.

Enticement and attraction are a part of the sexual behaviors of both men and women. Males and females learn which behaviors are appropriate to their own sex and which are rewarded. Some behaviors and some attitudes of the sexes are changing rather rapidly in the United States. Aggressiveness and assertiveness, in the past, have been characteristics of the male role and were considered manly and attractive in him. This attitude still prevails but is also to be found as a changing part of femininity. No longer is the timid, reticent female considered to be the acme of femininity. Greater aggressiveness, assertiveness, and social participation are becoming characteristics of attractive females. Nevertheless, adequate differentiating characteristics (physiological as well as attitudinal) of males and females still exist so that under ordinary conditions little confusion in sex role identification should occur.

Attitudes toward sex and sexuality are changing constantly. Over the past several years, people have lost much of the shame associated with their bodies. The body used to be considered as a kind of necessary evil that should be concealed and for which one should apologize. Polite society denied both body and body functioning, including sex. A recent attitude has been that of acceptance of the body and bodily functions as a part of life and living, and still more recently has been the development of pride in the possession of physical (sexually attractive) attributes that are revered by our culture. No longer are gross attempts made at overconcealment in dress, and as a matter of fact, sexuality is emphasized in fashion and manner. Nudity and semi-nudity have gained a greater acceptance as more affirmative attitudes have developed toward the body. Largely rejected are the older notions of the evils of physical functions including those of sex; as a result, people are open in their attitudes toward sexuality. "Sexual satisfaction is an obvious and entirely legitimate goal which most individuals in our society seek. . . . it remains a goal worth deliberate thought through most of adult life.[5]

Although attitudes toward physical aspects of humanity have changed rather markedly, it is questionable that overt sex relations have increased as a result and that great promiscuity is occurring. Although each college generation looks upon itself as more sexually liberated than the one before, we have little evidence of any greater overt sexual activity. People are currently more capable of discussing and studying sex and the role of sex in personality development and social living, but sexual behavior patterns may not have changed as drastically as is usually believed. College couples have been living together for years, and their relations have tended to be relatively stable rather than promiscuous. Promiscuity and variety of sex partners are probably not any more commonplace than they were a generation ago. A college junior may have summed this issue up rather well when, in response to a question relative to sex on the campus, he said: "Sex on campus is mostly talk, talk, talk, talk, talk! I *talk* a lot, too."

Sexual intercourse used to be dealt with as the primitive expression of base instincts and it was therefore a private matter and subject to rejection and denial. A healthier attitude is the current one that sees sex relations as part of the expression of affection, trust, acceptance, and mutual concern between men and women. With increased efficiency of birth control methods, greater freedom of sexual enjoyment has developed and decision making about sexual behavior in or out of marriage may be more difficult.

An aspect of sexual involvement that may have served as a deterrent to sexual activity in the past is that of conception. With current methods of contraception, however, fears of pregnancy can be largely removed, and sexual decisions must be made on other bases. The responsibility for contraception has probably shifted from the male to the female because of the "pill." If this is true, even more than previously, decision making relative to sex becomes a female responsibility.

Homosexuality

Homosexuality is the most common of the sexual variations and is also the most controversial. The term *homosexual* is usually reserved for males and the term *lesbian* for females. A number of homosexuals and lesbians prefer to be called "gay." In 1973 Sorensen reported that about three-fourths of adolescents regard homosexual acts as abnormal or unnatural, but 40 percent believe that if one wants to have sexual relations with someone of the same sex it is all right. Weinberg and Williams in a 1974 study found that 71 percent in a public opinion survey viewed homosexuality as an illness, while 29 percent viewed it as either a crime, a sin, or a preference.[6] Another survey showed two-thirds of the adult U.S. population considered homosexual behavior to be obscene or vulgar, but the majority also considered it a curable illness.[7] So, homosexuality is still not widely accepted as being normal or natural.

The vast majority of homosexuals believe that homosexuality is completely beyond one's control, but the homosexuals disagree widely on the issue of whether or not one is born homosexual or heterosexual.[8]

Cause. Henderson says:

> Traditionally, medical science has placed all homosexuals in the same diagnostic basket. Today many investigators have concluded that there may

be a variety of circumstances that can influence a person toward homosexuality, only some of which are related to childhood.

Moreover, studies have confirmed that homosexuals, just as other persons, must make many adjustments in life that have nothing to do with sex. In the past, the total existence of the homosexual had been interpreted through the prism of his or her sexual object choice. What has become evident is that homosexuals must solve all the problems of daily living that heterosexuals do. Like the heterosexual, the homosexual is apt to be concerned with work, leisure, friendship, relations with parents, religion, and other concerns of day-to-day life. In this process, sexual object choice often takes a decidedly second place.[9]

Most members of the medical profession no longer assume that homosexuality is an emotional illness. By far, the majority of homosexuals, as is true of heterosexuals, cope with the demands of life without a psychological breakdown. Data from a number of studies show that homosexuals have the same range of emotional and social adjustments as do their heterosexual counterparts.[10]

Authorities do not agree on the origins, or a cause, for this sexual variation; some believe that there might be an endocrine basis, but few regard the evidence as convincing. Administering testosterone to male homosexuals does not affect the orientation of their sexual drives.[11] The most widely accepted theory is that homosexuals have not been able to establish a clear sense of personal sexual identity because of inadequate relationships and models within the family unit. A high percentage of such individuals have close-binding, intimate mothers and emotionally detached or hostile fathers.[12] Other possible causative factors, says Hooker, include:

> inappropriate identifications with the opposite sexed parent; fear or hostility to either parent; reversal of masculine and feminine roles in parents; cultural overemphasis on the sterotype of "masculinity," which produces feelings of inadequacy in males who are not able to fulfill this expectation; rigid dichotomy of male and female social roles, with failure to allow for individuals who do not fit easily into either of these; and easier access to sexual gratification with members of one's own sex in adolescence, resulting in habit patterns which persist.[13]

Life styles. Homosexuals, like the heterosexuals, have many life styles. Some are conventionally married and only once in awhile engage in secretive affairs. Some live openly as homosexual couples; some "hide their sexual preferences" because it may affect their jobs (teaching, for example); while others, such as those in the arts, become more prominent and publicly acknowledge their sexual preferences. Homosexuals are found in all socioeconomic levels and in all occupations. About 2 percent of the male population of the United States participate exclusively in homosexual relationships. A larger group, about another 3 percent, use homosexual relationships as but one of several sexual outlets.

Behavior, among the males especially, is influenced by harassment, censure, and persecution by society. Only in some large cities can Gays live in relative freedom. For the most part, they live psychologically isolated from others, depend on themselves for sexual expression, and live by a concealed system of social relations. The covert (hidden) homosexual pass for heterosexual most of the time. They may lead a double life. The overt (open) individuals comprise a much smaller group. They rely on the homosexual community for gratification of their psychosocial needs including those that are sexual. This group may have their own churches, clinics, and social clubs; many of them are defiant of the "straight" world. The covert and the overt groups tend to shun each other.

Male stereotyping. It is not necessarily true that male homosexuals are effeminate "swishes," "faggots," or "fairies." Some are, but many are body-building enthusiasts, and by far the majority exhibit the same continuum of behavior found in heterosexuals. Also a myth is that in a couple arrangement one is passive and the other active (one the husband and the other the wife). Relative to sexual behavior, there is nothing that the heterosexual does that male homosexuals do not do except have vaginal intercourse. The relationships tend to be short term. Most live alone, and approximately two-thirds never have a relationship that lasts more than a year.[14]

Lesbians. Possibly one-half to one percent of the female population of the United States are lesbian. Individually they are indistinguishable from the general population. Lesbians tend to form more lasting ties and operate in less differentiated subcultures than do male homosexuals, possibly because they are less detected and harassed. More of them pair off and live together as couples than do the males, too. Roles seem to be more defined with one assuming "head-of-the-family" responsibility. However, along with the blending of masculine and feminine roles among the heterosexuals is the blending of roles among lesbians. It is a myth that one is always a "butch"—acts and dresses like a man—and the other a "femme."

The causes of lesbianism are presumed to be the same as those for male homosexuals. There is an element in the history of many lesbians of early sexual experience leading to the preference for a member of the same sex.[15]

Latent homosexuality. The possibility of being a latent homosexual causes much concern among the general population. Many of us have fleeting homosexual thoughts, but these are not diagnostic of our being homo-

FOUNDATIONS OF HEALTH SCIENCE

sexual. Numbers of early adolescents, pairs of both boys and girls, have participated in mutual sexual exploration, such as masturbation or auto-stimulation, which in itself is not evidence of their homosexuality. Hett-linger says most aptly:

> If men and women know that some homosexual attraction is common among heterosexuals, they are less likely to be disturbed when they discover a homosexual element in themselves. If they are liberated from a sense of obligation to play stereotyped sex roles they will not fear that deviation from the expectations of the peer group necessarily implies homosexuality. Men with less than average interest in sexual adventure on campus will cease to be haunted by anxieties about their masculinity. Women who become deeply involved in women's lib and find themselves exclusively intimate with members of their own sex will not be misled into supposing that they are necessarily lesbians.[16]

DATING

Dating is a social practice that has developed in the United States with the decline of arranged marriages. The freedom to select one's own mate, and other changes in the social milieu that have provided more individual freedom, necessitated that means of meeting and getting to know other people outside the sponsorship of the family be developed. But dating, as practiced in the United States, serves other functions than that of mate selection. It has become a part of the culture and provides a means of acquiring social competence, increasing self-understanding, and getting to know and understand others. It is a method for discovering others' conceptions of sex role and a way to learn about others' values, ideals, goals, and purposes. Dating has become an institution that provides an opportunity for social maturation and growth and is a preliminary to mate selection.

Dating Patterns

Dating begins relatively early in life in the United States. Studies indicate that the first date is likely to be between the ages of thirteen and fifteen. An inspection of census findings indicates that 40 percent of all girls in the United States marry before they are twenty and that one-half are married before they are twenty-one. Half of the boys marry by the time they are twenty-three. College-educated people tend to marry at a somewhat later age, but they begin dating as early as the rest of the population.[17]

In that boys are somewhat older than girls at the time of marriage, the dating period of life lasts longer for boys than for girls. Girls date more frequently than boys of the same age, and girls tend to date boys somewhat older than themselves. The earlier people begin to date, the more frequently they date. In general, people with higher socioeconomic and educational backgrounds start dating earlier, date more people before going steady, and after steady dating for a while, again start dating the field.

Steady dating is an expression that has no universally accepted definition. Among some ages and social groups, going steady represents social success and ensures a date for recognized social functions. Many high-school-age couples go steady but do not intend to become engaged or married to each other. College students are more likely to date the field until they have found someone to whom they feel they could become seriously attached. This couple then dates steadily and may become "pinned" where this is the custom. Some young people go steady with one person for a length of time, and then the relationship is dissolved and a series of dates is initiated with another person. For others, casual or occasional dating may occur with a variety of people over an extended period of time.

Steady dating has received much attention and much criticism over the past decade or so. Many adults fear that limiting the number of persons one dates will curtail the opportunities for social learning and development. Parents may encourage steady dating because it is socially acceptable and represents social success for their offspring, but they may also discourage the practice because they fear that early involvement with one person will encourage sexual exploration and activity that can lead to difficulty. The studies of steady dating indicate that the percentage of people dating steadily and the number of persons dated has probably not changed significantly over the past thirty years or so.[18]

The number of different persons one dates is related, of course, to the number of persons with whom one is associated. Those who reside in relatively congested areas such as fraternities, sororities, dormitories, or boardinghouses have a more expanded sphere of acquaintances than do those who reside at home. The probability of dating larger numbers of people and having more frequent dates is greater for most resident college students than it is for those who live at home and commute to college.

Dating and Physical Involvement

A serious problem in dating has to do with how far one should go in terms of physical involvement with the dating partner. Unfortunately, there are no strict guidelines for such behavior during dating. Holding

FOUNDATIONS OF HEALTH SCIENCE

hands or sharing a good-night kiss may have been considered improper in the past, but this is certainly not true in most contemporary dating. The kinds of involvement that are considered appropriate vary from group to group and individual to individual and depend upon the previous training, moral judgment, and ethical considerations of the partners.

Restraints on physical involvement long have been exercised because of the presumed socially or personally deleterious effects of early or casual sex relations. A generally held belief is that familiarity leads to further familiarities and exploration leads to further explorations, and thus the dangers arising from feelings of guilt for having gone too far, the lack of readiness to cope with intimacy, the lack of maturity essential for marriage, and the possibility of pregnancy all militate against involvements that lead to premarital intercourse. Many forms of physical contact have frequently been frowned upon because they might be preliminaries to sexual intercourse.

Physical involvement in dating has been treated as a continuum of intimacy, with necking at one end and premarital sexual intercourse on the

Love requires self-understanding and maturity

A girlfriend of mine, age nineteen, is having trouble with her boyfriend who is twenty-one. She is an only child and has been a loner most of her life. She's never really dated someone for as long as she's been dating her boyfriend now. She has been going with him for over a year. The trouble she is having is caused by the fact that she is too possessive and he wants more freedom than she is willing to give. Also, she likes men to be romantic and he is not romantic by nature so she nags him pretty much. The fact that his mother is a big nag doesn't help either. This couple fights a lot and are frequently on the verge of breaking up. She is confused. She loves him yet she may even hate him, too. She tries to talk things over with him, but he seldom talks seriously. She has given in to him very much lately and things are going more smoothly, but I don't think she loves him as much as she used to and I think she is repressing a lot of her feelings into her subconscious.

I was really getting too involved with not just one guy but many guys at the same time when I first came on this campus. I got too emotionally involved and my mind was getting all mixed up. I improved this by not seeing all these guys and started seeing a counselor to help me find the reason why I carried on like that. It seemed that I just had to be popular with everyone. I think I am beginning to understand myself better and see that I don't "have to" run around with everyone just to be popular.

other. Petting is placed between these two. Should people on dates engage in necking? Necking usually refers to kissing, light embracing, and other such contacts above the shoulders. Current questions deal not with whether or not to neck, but when and where to neck. Should it be on the first, second, or third date, and so forth? Is it a so-expected behavior that it occurs with any or all dates? Is it done when the couple is alone, in a group, or in public? Is it normal not to neck? Indeed, more may be wrong with not engaging in these behaviors than in engaging in them, for the person who is so frightened of personal involvement that no physical contact can take place probably has some serious adjustment problems that would make him or her unsatisfactory as a date or a mate. Clearly defining when necking becomes "heavy" necking is impossible, but the latter term usually includes prolonged and intense kissing and embracing.

Petting involves more intimate behavior that includes fondling of the breasts and genitalia. Such activity occurs among some dating partners but is not as open or as much discussed as is necking. Some petting may occur out of curiosity in young couples engaging in a kind of sexual exploratory behavior. It may also occur as an exercise in determining where the limits of physical involvement are going to be established and which partner establishes them. Petting, in addition, is overt preparation for sexual intercourse. A wit once defined petting as necking with extraterritorial privileges.

Although college students' attitudes toward an engagement in premarital sexual activities have been investigated rather extensively, most of the investigations are of historical rather than present interest. Early studies reported that a little over half of the college men and a bit over one-third of the college women had had premarital sexual relationships. Studies conducted over the years of the 1950s and 1960s generally showed that about two-thirds of college men and one-half of college women reported premarital intercourse. These same findings have tended to persist in the current decade.

We have no current research findings to indicate whether sex relations before marriage are becoming more commonplace with engaged couples. We do know that couples are no longer so reticent about discussing such relationships. Most young people plan to defer the experience of sexual intercourse until after they are married. However, couples who are engaged frequently find it difficult to keep love-making within the limits they have agreed upon and may have sex relations even when they have planned not to. The principal deterrents to premarital sex relations have to do more with the partners' sense of morality than with fear of pregnancy. With increased individual freedom, the morality of refraining from premarital sexual intercourse may be changing, although research findings on premarital sex activity show few differences during the last several decades.

PREMARITAL SEX EXPERIENCE

Prohibitions against premarital sex may be decreasing in our culture. The great increase in sexual knowledge and its dissemination over the past decade or so, the liberation of women, the modernization of the family organization, the "pill," and a host of other factors contribute to this changing attitude. Premarital sexual intercourse for all age levels appears to be regarded by many people as a matter of personal choice. Open promiscuity is not as acceptable as our sex-oriented magazines would have us believe, but it is certainly true that sex with commitment and love among unmarried couples in a variety of circumstances has been gaining in acceptance.[19]

However, our culture in general has taught sexual abstinence before marriage and this lesson has been an important part of our general morality. Parents who may be acceptant of intercourse among unmarried adults are not as acceptant of intercourse among their unmarried children, especially those of college age or younger.

Familial training is a powerful influence on behavior and on attitudes toward behavior. Many young people can indulge in premarital sexual intercourse only with considerable emotional conflict. Young people are quite conscious of the attitudes of their parents and families toward their sex behavior and cannot find much satisfaction in premarital relationships that they fear may be discovered or that would tend to bring sorrow and shame to their families. The awareness of society's standards and expectations, religion, and family attitudes and teaching all may act as deterrents to premarital sex relations. Fear of venereal disease or pregnancy with its consequent social ostracism probably still exerts some pressure, but the social deterrents and the basic idealism of young people appear to be the major factors in determining whether or not they will have premarital sex.

In some areas and within limited circumstances, cohabitation between unwed couples is acceptable. As many as 33 percent of college students have indicated that they have been involved with a member of the opposite sex in cohabitation. Some of these alliances result in marriage, while others are dissolved at graduation. Usually the couple living together have a commitment to each other's welfare that goes beyond "each doing his own thing." Parental concerns about the students' grades being negatively affected by cohabitation or the concerns about their suffering emotional trauma have not been borne out.[20]

Some couples arrange to live together for a time-limited period that is often extended or shortened at the pleasure of one or both partners; they may agree to marry later on. Other couples may decide to live together with an agreement that the arrangement is not to lead to marriage and may be terminated by either without prejudice. Couples agree to live together during the period of their engagement. Couples agree they will live together and perhaps rear a family but will not marry.

Unless such arrangements are approved, or not strongly disapproved, by their immediate community, sexual activity of unmarried persons usually must be carried out secretively and furtively. The physical surroundings are not always what they should be for most satisfactory relations, and feelings of guilt for having behaved contrary to familial and cultural mores are likely to develop. If sex relations are carried out under conditions where the danger of detection is considerable and the surroundings unsatisfactory, negative feelings of guilt and inadequacy may develop and be carried forward into the marital relationship. Some experts think marital sex satisfactions may be inhibited by guilt about premarital sexual behavior.[21] Conducting investigations to determine whether premarital sex relations are a hindrance or a help in subsequent marital adjustments is very difficult. Studies by Masters and Johnson on sexual inadequacy indicate that such relations can be hazardous.[22]

Does the fact, if it is found to be true, that those who engage in premarital sex have more difficult marital adjustments prove a causal relationship? Possibly those who do have premarital sex relations are those who would have difficulty in adjusting to marriage even if they had not had such sex relations. Conversely, if those who have premarital experience are found to make better adjustments in marriage, they may have done so whether or not they had had previous sex relations.

The problem of sexual compatibility is sometimes viewed as one that can be solved by experimentation before marriage. Such experimentation can only inform people that they are physically capable of mating—a finding that should come as no surprise because only a very small percentage of couples are not biologically equipped to mate with each other. The problems of sex adjustment in marriage are basically psychological rather than biological. Psychological adjustments relative to sex behavior require time and patience if happy and mutually satisfying sexual relations are to be achieved. Premarital sexual activity can be a source of frustration and dissatisfaction. Although a study of 1,000 engaged couples (505 of whom later married) indicated that no difference existed between the sex adjustments of those couples who had had premarital sex relations and those who married as virgins, more of the engaged couples in the study who were having premarital intercourse eventually broke their engagements.[23] Learning to enjoy sex together in marriage is not frought with the difficulties of guilt and possible social ostracism because of premarital pregnancy that surround premarital sex. Two people who are psychologically compatible can expect to be able to create together in marriage a sex relationship that is a happy and successful one, which is most difficult to do outside of marriage.[24]

FOUNDATIONS OF HEALTH SCIENCE

Sex: Casual vs. Committed

Casual sex can be described as engaging in sexual intercourse with an individual to whom one has little or no commitment—that is, by having sex relations with a casual date, having sex relations for commercial reasons, having sex for the release of personal tensions without particular concern for the sex partner. Such sexual relations are generally considered in our culture to be rather base and more animal-like than human. The enjoyment that derives is purely self-centered and sensual. It really amounts to a sensual experience of short duration provided by a person of little concern. Sex activity of this nature cannot compete with sex relations between committed partners. Committed persons are genuinely concerned for each other's well-being as well as enjoyment. The relationship is one of love, tenderness, care, and sharing. The response in sexual relations is then a deep emotional, personally and mutually enjoyed behavior. The satisfactions do not stem solely from the performance and the sensual stimuli deriving from the act as in casual sex.

Sex with commitment is more enjoyable, satisfying, and complete. By its very nature it is not an act of temporary or fleeting engagement. It is, rather, an expression of love, concern, and commitment. The partners are dedicated to each other's welfare, and their lives are developing together. The sex life is a part of this developmental process.

The average male can more frequently achieve sexual gratification independent of love than can the average female. For many women sexual intercourse is inseparable from love. Married men rate sexual intercourse with the woman for whom they feel affection as the most important feature of their marriage.[25] College-educated men are more concerned with

We can't ignore the consequences of guilt. We are not always as 'free' as we would like to believe

A female friend, age 16, went through a terrible ordeal after having sex for the first time with her boyfriend. Her boyfriend disappeared after that and left her feeling guilty and afraid. Her guilt lasted for some time but by talking to her friends about the situation she eventually could deal with things (her feelings and fears). A year later when the guy started coming around again she became friends with him and through talking with him was better able to understand the situation as it was. She never renewed the relationship because of the painful memory she still feels when reminded of that time in her life, but she has become able to speak to the guy. I think both of them have changed and grown up since then.

mutual sexual gratification than are those with less education.[26] This concern probably extends from the sense of commitment and mutuality accompanying the relationship as well as an increased knowledge of female sexuality.

Making the Decision

The decision as to whether or not to have sex either casually or committedly is of concern to most, if not all, college students. Some may wonder what they would do, others must decide. The article at the end of this chapter, "Sexual Pressures: How to Make the Right Decisions for You," gives some points to consider. Although the authors direct their comments to women, the points made can be helpful to men. In our culture, one of the criteria of manliness or masculinity has been, and still is for most, sexual performance. For the younger male, emphasis is often given to frequency and number of "conquests" rather than quality and caring. Like his feminine counterpart, he may not be ready for sexual intercourse and he knows it. But he may feel, like his counterpart, he must conform to social pressures to maintain status with his peers.

MATE SELECTION

The choice of a partner for marriage is a matter of great personal importance, but in spite of this fact, attempts to improve the methods of selection are much resisted. Selection has become even more important in modern marriage than ever before. Modern marriage is one of companionship. Marriage is no longer exclusively an arrangement for economic, protective, and procreative purposes. Persons today usually want to marry someone with whom they can share interests and activities; whom they like, trust, and respect; and whom they can love and who will return that love. For these ends to be served, the task of selecting a mate can hardly be viewed as other than complex and demanding the closest attention.

Love

Most people generally concede that one should be in love with the person one intends to marry. Love thus becomes a basis for modern marriage and, in some instances, an excuse for it. The question frequently is raised whether love is a sufficient basis for marriage. The whole concept of

FOUNDATIONS OF HEALTH SCIENCE

love is difficult to describe and discuss because of our exposure to the romantic superstitions of our culture. Love is not a violent, uncontrollable, unpredictable emotion. It is not a form of compulsion that holds two people together.

Love is the concern of two people for each other. You love a person if his or her happiness and well-being matter as much to you as your own. Love is not something that comes full blown, or that one "falls" into. Rather, it is a positive feeling that develops out of a relationship and contributes an important element to the richness of that relationship. People who accept and respect themselves as individuals can give acceptance and respect to another person. Mutual acceptance and respect form the cornerstones of the concept of love. Love is not a one-sided game. It takes two people to be in love; mutuality of feelings and concerns is essential.

In the love relationship the two people feel secure and confident. They have no need for control or domination of one by the other and no fear of losing the love of the other. They can enjoy cooperative efforts and still retain their individuality, for they are in love with each other and not with the relationship. Love does not guarantee that all will be sweetness and light and that agreement in all phases of life will be attained. It does mean that those who love each other will maintain supportive rather than destructive attitudes toward each other even in the face of adversity. They can be generous in their judgments of each other and tolerant of their differences. Acceptance, understanding, companionship, and sexual attraction are all components of love. Love, conceived of in such a fashion, is a prerequisite for happy marriage.

Some Romantic Ideas

The concept of *love at first sight* is an interesting phenomenon. Its occurrence is attested to by a number of people. However, if love is a relationship that grows upon cooperation and companionship, we cannot but wonder about the reality of love at first sight.

While a person might see in another of the opposite sex outward characteristics of the sort that are sexually attractive, this sexual attraction may or may not be related to underlying qualities that would elicit love. Emotional excitement engendered by an attractive sex object can be mistaken for love. Of course, such initial physical attraction may develop into a love relationship, but the instantaneous existence of a love relationship is unlikely.

The idea that a person can love and be happy with *one and only one* other person is a notion that has been used in romantic literature. This superstition is even less well-founded than is the "love-at-first-sight" phenomenon. The idea that two persons should be "perfectly" matched in all respects before love can develop has little to support it. Many people who say that they never married because "the right one just never came along" may be using this idea to conceal their lack of interest in or capacity for the establishment of close, long-lasting relationships with members of the opposite sex. The establishment of unrealistically high standards for themselves and for others as the result of early training and subsequent experience may also lead one to choose not to become involved with anyone seriously enough to allow love to develop.

The romantic assertions that *love conquers all* or *love will find a way* are sometimes used as rationalizations devised to ignore problems, or they may derive from naïvete. Love will not solve problems related to continued education, parents, finances, or religion. Assumptions that such facets of life are unimportant when one is "in love" are extremely unrealistic.

People who love each other obviously do so in a romantic manner. Feelings of loneliness when deprived of each other's companionship, exhilaration when together, and a mutual concern for each other's well-being and happiness are a part of genuine love as well as a part of the romantic attachment. Tremendous feelings of elation, depression, and anxiety that characterize romantic love are probably more a reflection of emotional instability than they are of the depth of the relationship. Romantic love, wherein unrealistic excitement and attachments occur, may have difficulty in developing into a dependable love relationship and by itself is not a sufficient basis for marriage. The few people who demonstrate ecstatic affectional involvement may be momentarily envied by their acquaintances, but this involvement may be reflective of instability and immaturity that does not make for long-lasting and happy relationships.

Companionability

In the quest for a mate, many young people take for granted that in our culture marriages are based on love. As just stated, love is a relationship that develops and grows under proper nourishment. Are there other requisites for marriage?

People today marry at a relatively early age and expect that the marriage arrangement will be a permanent one. Life expectancy being what it is, most married couples, then, will spend nearly fifty years together and the wife will live as a widow for a few additional years. People who intend to spend such a large portion of their lives together will be deeply affected by a great variety of personal characteristics, attitudes, beliefs, aspirations, and ideals of their prospective mates.

When asked to rate eighteen factors in order of importance in mate selection, both college men and women put "dependable character" first. This attribute was followed in order by emotional stability and maturity, pleasing disposition, mutual love and attraction, and good health. Such things as favorable social status, good financial prospect, and similar political background were at the lower end of the ranking. Engaged men and women rated compatibility and common interests much higher as factors making for success in marriage than either love or sex as such.

One proposal is that couples should seek in each other characteristics that will complement their own personalities. The thesis that the need pattern of each spouse should be complementary rather than similar to the need pattern of the other spouse (opposites attract) has not received much empirical support. While it is true that some marriages are made on this basis, they are probably a small proportion of the total. Investigations indicate that greatest happiness in marriage is achieved when "like marries like."[27] Couples who have the most in common, particularly in general social characteristics, tend to get along better in marriage. Similarity in interests, age, race, religious background, education, and socioeconomic status all tend to be important in the success of marriage. The factors that they have in common probably tend to enhance the general compatibility of the couple and enhance the marriage relationship.

Computer-arranged mate selection has become a lucrative business. Advertisements in nearly every college newspaper urge "scientific" selection of mates. No doubt the probability of finding a companionable mate is enhanced by computerized matching persons of common interests, hobbies, and values, but such services can provide only a start and should not become substitutes for courtship, dating, and the chance for couples to get to know each other in the give and take of social interaction.

Personality Factors

A great variety of personalities can be married to each other successfully. The person with dating experience is well aware that some personalities do not get along well together. Personalities may "clash." In the marriage relationship, the personalities of the pair should have sufficient characteristics in common, in terms of general temperament and disposition, that they can have a number of similar attitudes and appreciations. The social life of a pair composed of one who is highly socially oriented and one who is shy and withdrawn may suffer a number of handicaps.

Personality test results interpreted by a good counselor can often be helpful in assisting people to understand themselves and their prospective mates. Skilled counseling and personality test results, though, cannot replace the more personal means of getting to know and understand each other. An extended period of dating and going steady and a reasonable period of engagement are probably the best available ways to test people's compatibility. Only after a considerable length of time do some dating couples or people going steady begin to let their real personalities show. The early part of dating is a period when both are on their best behavior; it takes some time and familiarity before they can really get to know each other.

Some factors of compatibility that you should explore carefully during courtship are listed here. Any area in which you make a negative response should be explored. Several negative responses require careful reexamination and evaluation of your relationship with your dating partner.

	Yes	No
1. Is considerate of me	—	—
2. Is considerate of most others	—	—
3. Is at ease with me	—	—
4. Is at ease with most others	—	—
5. Enjoys being with me	—	—
6. Likes most of the things I do	—	—
7. Likes my friends	—	—
8. Shares my religious attitudes	—	—
9. His/her family culture is about like mine	—	—
10. My parents both like him/her	—	—
11. His/her parents both like me	—	—
12. Feels that we are equal	—	—
13. Treats me as an equal	—	—
14. Has interests and activities I share	—	—
15. Has sexual attitudes like mine	—	—
16. Is emotionally stable	—	—
17. Has energy and health as good as mine	—	—
18. Feels the sexes are equal	—	—
19. Is not unhappy if he/she doesn't win or excel in most things	—	—
20. Thinks of sex as a wholesome part of living	—	—

Marriage of persons who are emotionally immature or personally maladjusted are likely to be unhappy ones. Marriage relationships are for mature, responsible people. No one is in perfect psychological health, but problems involving large deviations from what might be termed reasonable mental health should be resolved before marriage is undertaken.

FOUNDATIONS OF HEALTH SCIENCE

Marriage is not a cure for emotional disturbance; neither does it produce significant changes in ideals and attitudes.

Physical Health and Biological Considerations

The physical examination is a part of good general health practice. It is particularly desirable that a thorough physical examination be had before marriage. The medical examination can serve to identify any conditions in need of treatment and can alleviate any apprehensions that one might have about general health conditions. A premarital medical examination includes a thorough check of the genitalia and for women a pelvic examination. Any irregularities or physical conditions that might be aggravated by or cause difficulty in sex relations for the couple can be detected and remedied before marriage. Psychological and social adjustive demands make initial sexual adjustments in marriage difficult enough for many people without the additional burden of possible physiological impediments.

The physician can be of considerable help in supplying information and service relative to family planning and birth control, which is described in Chapter 11. The engaged couple should have previously discussed and agreed upon whether they wish children, what size family they propose to have, when the children will be wanted, and what means of controlling family size they would like to use. Decisions on those issues should be made in joint consultation with the physician.

For most couples there will be little concern about possible unfortunate consequences to offspring that can result from adverse genetic conditions. A history of conditions that have resulted in mental retardation, disease, or physical impairment in either or both families does become a serious area for consideration. Genetic clinics, located in most major cities, should be utilized if the couple has doubts as to whether inheritable disorders are likely in the proposed family. Many people are now advocating that couples considering marriage should contact genetic clinics as routinely as they currently do medical clinics.

ADJUSTMENT IN MARRIAGE

Initial and Early Adjustment

Marriage is a different way of life, and adjustment to it must be made by both parties. Sufficient planning should take place before the marriage so that as few problems and frustrations as possible will arise within the first few days or weeks. Such planning means that not only the details of the marriage ceremony itself should be adequately taken care of but that the first few days should require little in the way of decision making by the couple. The well-planned honeymoon provides a time when the couple can be together, uninterrupted by well-meaning friends and relatives. They can enjoy each other and engage in marital sexual intimacy with less feelings of embarrassment and self-consciousness than if they had to interact with family and friends during these early days of marriage. The honeymoon is a valuable marital experience and should probably not be foregone except under the most unusual of circumstances.

For some couples taking the honeymoons under physical conditions that are foreign to them is likely to be a mistake. A honeymoon in an exceptionally luxurious and elite establishment when the partners are used to more humble surroundings may just provide more new and different things to add to their feelings of self-consciousness in their new relationship. A period of time is essential for adjustments to being married, but it is doubtful that overextending the finances of the couple in order to have an elaborate honeymoon is a worthy emotional or financial investment.

Sexual adjustments in the first few days may not be as satisfactory as the couple would like to have them be. Adequate sexual adjustment takes time, patience, and practice. Most couples will share reasonably satisfactory early sex relations that gradually develop into more complete fulfillment for both partners. As people begin to understand each other better by learning more about their partners, their lives together become more and more comfortable and sex becomes a part of living together effectively.

The couple should have a place of their own to return to following their honeymoon. Preferably, living accommodations should have been obtained and equipped in advance of the wedding.

Major Problems

Marriage offers a world of companionship, affection, and satisfactions to its successful participants. Also, it presents problems to be solved, obstacles to be overcome, and frustrations to be tolerated. Some of the major problems of living as man and wife have to do with sex relations, financial matters, religion, social life and recreation, in-laws, and the training and disciplining of children. Many of these problems are readily solved by people who love and respect each other if they develop and maintain habits of communication. General agreement on money matters and religion should be and frequently are worked out before marriage.

FOUNDATIONS OF HEALTH SCIENCE

In the event that such general agreements have not been made, they should be made early in marriage before they begin to present unsurmountable problems.

Developing the practice of discussing differences and problem areas freely and openly goes a long way toward preventing problems. Communication is of vital importance in marital relationships, and both partners should try to see that habits of conversation and communication are adequately developed. If each knows what the other is thinking and how he or she feels about important problems, much can be done to prevent differences from arising or to reconcile them when they do occur.

Minor Problems

Living together as husband and wife is a very intimate relationship in which each discovers many things about the other. Many of these discoveries add to the enjoyment of each other, but as each learns little details of the other's behavior, each is bound to find some things to be irritating. Little routine habits or mannerisms that would go unnoticed in a friend or casual acquaintance may become annoying when they are constantly encountered in the wife or husband. Such little things as squeezing the toothpaste from the wrong end of the tube, leaving a ring on the bathtub, failing to hang clothing in the closet, not replacing a magazine in the rack, being slow about coming to the dinner table, taking too long to get dressed, or talking while the TV is on can become so irritating to a spouse that an explosion results. These trivial things that often cause friction in marriage out of all proportion to their real importance have been called "tremendous trifles." Discussion and efforts to be understanding on the part of both parties is likely to provide the best resolution of such conflicts. Learning what little things are sources of annoyance and trying to minimize their occurrence can help. Lifelong habits and mannerisms are difficult to modify and overt attempts by one partner to make over the behavior of another may lead to more serious problems. Even when each tries to avoid a behavior that may aggravate the other, it is bound to occur. When it does, humor and acceptance probably provide as effective a way of coping with the situation as any.

Working Mothers

The working mother is becoming more and more common, for reasons of choice as well as economics. Douvan and Adelson report little relation between a mother's employment and her adolescent son's activities and psychological characteristics.[28] Daughters of working mothers were more likely to share home responsibilities and participated in fewer leisure activities. Adolescent daughters of working mothers tended to admire and respect their mothers more than did the daughters of nonworking mothers.

The employed mothers have been popularly considered to provide less supervision of children, which in turn leads to delinquency. In an extensive study of delinquent boys, where five hundred delinquent boys were matched with an equal number of nondelinquents on age, ethnic background, and general intelligence, Glueck and Glueck observed no difference in the proportion of delinquents and nondelinquents whose mothers were regularly employed.[29] Most studies have shown that working mothers have a more favorable attitude toward children than those not employed outside the home.[30]

In a study of fifth-grade children of lower-class working mothers, it was found that children of mothers who were employed full time away from home achieved better social adjustment and intelligence scores than those whose mothers worked part time or worked at home.[31]

Several studies have found that children of working mothers develop in much the same fashion as children whose mothers remain at home. A mother's outside employment apparently is not likely, in itself, to have unfavorable effects. When children of working mothers do have difficulties, these are likely to arise from factors that also have effect on the children of home-bound mothers (factors such as poverty, marital discord, a broken home).

Sexual Adjustment in Marriage

Mutually satisfactory sex relations constitute an important factor in marital happiness. Sexual gratification is an important aspect of marriage, but it is not the basic and all-important factor that many couples think it will be. Sexual relations may become the focal point of various disturbances and conflicts in the marriage because they are the most intimately cooperative activity in which the couple engages. One partner may be sufficiently unhappy so as to resist sexual intercourse and thus produce deeper conflicts and resentments. Couples can agree to disagree about politics or they can tolerate differences over how money is to be spent, but they must cope more directly with the problem of sex, since disagreements and differences are often taken as personal rejections.

Young married couples are frequently concerned about matters related to their enjoyment of sexual activity. How frequently should they engage in intercourse? The data that are available suggest that frequency is almost exclusively a matter for individual couples to work out for themselves. Sexual desires are extremely variable from person to person, and any pattern of frequency from which the couple obtains mutual pleasure would seem to be appropriate. Young newly married couples may enjoy sex relations daily, or more often, until the novelty of sexual freedom wears off. Following this period, they may gradually settle into a frequency that is satisfactory to both. The rate will vary for individual couples; each couple must determine for themselves what is "normal" for them.

Recent findings indicate that in the last several decades changes have occurred regarding marital intercourse practices. Katchadourian and Lunde state "Married people are currently engaging in intercourse more frequently, spend more time doing it, rely on more variations, and obtain greater satisfaction from it."[32] They also report that the weekly median times of sexual intercourse for different age groups is:[33]

18–24 years	3.25 times per week
25–34 "	2.55 " " "
35–44 "	2.00 " " "
45 and over	1.00 " " "

The variety of sexual stimulation employed by couples in sex foreplay is also extremely great. Here again the amount and nature of sexual stimulation and exploration that a couple desires is a highly individual matter. Any kind of stimulation that is a source of mutual arousal and enjoyment by the partners and is not physically or psychologically damaging to either would seem to be appropriate. Human beings are capable of coitus in a variety of postures and positions and under a great number of circumstances. Mutuality of stimulation and enjoyment of sexual relations has come to replace older conceptions of women's passive role in sex activity. Enjoyment of sexual activity is a learnable phenomenon and much of our sexual enjoyment is conditionable.[34] In recent years sex clinics have become popular, but many of these are said by authorities to be bilking the public.[35]

Maintaining Attractiveness

Maintaining personal attractiveness can help sustain the happiness of marriage. The woman who was well groomed, neat, and attractive during her days of dating and engagement sometimes becomes careless about her appearance after she is married. She may find herself occupied with maintaining a household, perhaps also working outside the home, or caring for children, and neglect to pay adequate attention to her own appearance. She may also allow herself to get out of touch with current events and with her husband's interests.

The same general factors are operative with husbands. Before marriage, part of a man's attractiveness may have been the fact that he was healthy, vigorous, considerate, and well groomed. The husband may allow himself to become lethargic, forget about small considerations, and become careless about grooming and appearance. If his wife does not seem to be as interested in him as a person as she once was, possibly it is because he is not as attractive as he once was.

A little time and energy devoted to the maintenance of reasonable health, considerateness, knowledge of what is going on in the world, and personal appearance is repaid many times over by the creation and preservation of a vital marriage relationship.

COPING WITH PROBLEMS

When differences arise that two married people cannot seem to overcome, they can consult numerous agencies for professional help. Marriage counselors, psychiatrists, psychologists, social workers, ministers, and many others now are trained in the area of human relations and can frequently be of considerable assistance in reconciling differences and in establishing happier marital relationships. Assistance in selecting reputable professional help can be obtained through family service agencies, medical associations, psychological and psychiatric associations, and various social ministerial associations.

Most people now recognize that outside help may be necessary for many couples in order for them to build successful marriages. Couples who are mature enough to seek outside assistance when things develop that they cannot cope with by themselves have an excellent chance of resolving their difficulties.

Divorce must be looked upon as a drastic means of problem solution. When happiness is recognized as a goal of marriage, divorce must be recognized as one way out of an unhappy situation. Divorce is a form of adjustment that should be resorted to only after other avenues of adjustment have been explored unsuccessfully. It represents the failure of two people in a highly personalized situation. Failure experiences of most kinds can be damaging to a person, and failure in such a personal venture as marriage can leave psychological scars that are difficult to heal.

Divorce has become more and more common in the United States over the past several decades. It is no longer looked upon by most people as sinful, and the general public, including religious bodies, is more tolerant of divorce than in the past. This new attitude is in recognition of the fact that social forces make modern marriage quite a different institution from what it once was. The bonds of the modern family are mutual love and respect, rather than ties of common property, work, and large families. If these bonds of love and respect are lost, there remains little to salvage by sustaining an unhappy marriage.

Tracing the effects of divorce on offspring is difficult since divorce is usually an outgrowth of a complicated family situation. Divorce may come as a shattering experience for the children. It may represent a formality, legally acknowledging the dissolution of a marriage in which the partners have, psychologically, been divorced for some time. For the parents, then, it may come as a great relief.

Over a thousand parents participated in a study by Burchinal of the effects of divorce on children of adolescent age.[36] The findings indicated that children in homes broken by divorce do not fall into a class by themselves with certain common characteristics that distinguish them from other children. As a group, adolescents from broken homes showed less delinquent behavior, less psychosomatic illness, and better adjustment to parents than those from unhappy, unbroken homes.[37] Family conflict has a pronounced effect on children of various ages and social class.[38]

Since remarriage is a frequent sequel to divorce, many children must adapt themselves to step-parents. As with other adjustments, children can be expected to respond to a step-parent in their own individual ways.[39]

Remarriage of divorced persons is rather common, but the data indicate that as far as permanence of marriage is concerned, second marriages are about 50 percent more risky than first marriages. This figure may be reflective of inability or unwillingness of divorced persons to work out solutions to problems of personal and marital adjustment. In such cases, divorce is not a solution to the real problems of personal adjustment and happiness.

IN CONCLUSION

Modern marriage is one of love and companionship. Persons today usually wish to marry someone with whom they can share interests and activities; someone whom they like, trust, and respect; and someone whom they can love and who will return that love. Fulfilling this wish requires considered deliberations. Even then, in the best of marriages, minor frictions and occasional disagreements are bound to occur. These problems can usually be solved by mature adults who have learned to discuss their problems and are reasonably flexible individuals.

Notes

1. M. S. Horner, "A Psychological Barrier to the Achievement of Women: The Motive to Avoid Success," in I. C. McClelland and R. S. Steel, eds., *Human Motivation* (Morristown, N.J.: General Learning Press, 1973).

2. D. R. Entwisle, "To Dispel Fantasies About Fantasy-based Measures of Achievement Motivation," *Psychological Bulletin,* 77:377–391, 1972.

3. M. Forsberg, "Do Women Show More Motive to Avoid Success than Men in Male Dominated Career Fields, Unpublished Research Paper, San Jose State University, San Jose, California, 1974.

4. J. M. Sawrey and C. W. Telford, *Adjustment and Personality* (Boston: Allyn & Bacon, 1975).

5. Willard Dalrymple, *Sex is for Real: Human Sexuality and Sexual Responsibility* (New York: McGraw Hill, 1969), p. 57.

6. R. C. Sorensen, *Adolescent Sexuality in Contemporary America* (New York: World Publishing, 1973), pp. 294–295.

7. M. S. Weinberg and C. J. Williams, *Male Homosexuals: Their Problems and Adaptations* (New York: Oxford University Press, 1974), pp. 93–96, 147.

8. Ibid., p. 113.

9. Bruce Henderson (writer) and John Gagnon (issue editor), *Human Sexuality* (Boston: Little, Brown & Company, 1975), p. 52.

10. Richard F. Hettlinger. *Human Sexuality* (Belmont, Calif.: Wadsworth Publishing Company, 1975), pp. 168, 169.

11. Ibid., p. 171.

12. Ibid.

13. Evelyn Hooker, "The Adjustment of the Male Overt Homosexual," *The Problem of Homosexuality in Modern Society* (New York: E. P. Dutton and Co., 1963), pp. 171, 172.

14. Weinberg and Williams, *Male Homosexuals*, pp. 99, 236.

15. Hettlinger, *Human Sexuality,* p. 171.

16. Ibid., p. 165.

17. Landis and M. G. Landis, *Building a Successful Marriage* (Englewood Cliffs, N.J.: Prentice-Hall, 1968), p. 48.

18. Ibid., p. 51.

19. E. S. Morrison and V. Borosage, *Human Sexuality: Contemporary Perspective* (Palo Alto, Calif.: National Press Books, 1973).

20. E. D. Macklin, "Going Very Steady," *Psychology Today,* 8:53–58, 1974.

21. E. Hamilton, *Sex Before Marriage* (New York: Meredith Press, 1969), Chapter 3, "Premarital Intercourse—Pro and Con," pp. 33–44.

22. William H. Masters and Virginia E. Johnson, *Human Sexual Inadequacy* (Boston: Little, Brown, & Co., 1970).

23. E. W. Burgess and T. Wallin, *Engagement and Marriage* (Philadelphia: J. B. Lippincott, 1953), pp. 367–371.

24. A. Fromme, *The Ability to Love* (New York: Pocket Books, 1966), Chapter 11, "Love and Loneliness."

25. B. A. Kogan, *Human Sexual Expression* (New York: Harcourt, Brace, & Jovanovich, 1973).

26. W. H. Masters and V. E. Johnson, *Human Sexual Response* (Boston: Little, Brown & Co., 1966), p. 202.

27. P. H. Landis, *Making the Most of Marriage,* 3rd ed. (New York: Appleton-Century-Crofts, 1965), p. 265.

28. E. Douvan and J. Adelson, *The Adolescent Experience* (New York: John Wiley and Sons, 1966).

29. E. Glueck and S. Glueck, "Working Mothers and Delinquency," *Mental Hygiene,* 41:327–352, 1957.

30. F. I. Nye, "Marital Interaction," In F. I. Nye and L. W. Hoffman, eds., *The Employed Mother in America* (Chicago: Rand McNally, 1965).

31. M. B. Woods, "The Unsupervised Child of the Working Mother," *Developmental Psychology,* 6:14–25, 1972; and B. M. Lester, M. Katelchuck, E. Spelke, M. J. Sellers, and R. E. Klein, "Separation Protest in Guatemalan Infants: Cross-Cultural and Cognitive Findings," *Developmental Psychology,* 10:79–85, 1974.

32. Herant A. Katchadourian and Donald T. Lunde, *Fundamentals of Human Sexuality.* (New York: Rinehart and Winston, 1975), pp. 309 and 310.

33. Ibid.

34. H. K. Klemer, *Marriage and Family Relationships* (New York: Harper & Row, Publishers, 1970), pp. 227–235.

35. *Medical World News,* 15:17–18, May 10, 1974.

36. L. G. Burchinal, "Characteristics of Adolescents from Unbroken and Reconstituted Families," *Journal of Marriage and the Family,* 26:44–51, 1964.

37. F. I. Nye, "Child Adjustment in Broken and in Unhappy Unbroken Homes," *Marriage and Family Living,* 19:356–361, 1957.

38. T. Jacob, "Patterns of Family Conflict and Dominance as a Function of Child Age and Social Class," *Developmental Psychology,* 10:1–12, 1974.

39. A. T. Jersild, C. W. Telford, and J. M. Sawrey, *Child Psychology* (Englewood Cliffs, N.J.: Prentice-Hall, 1975).

SEXUAL PRESSURES:
How to make the right decisions for you

Loma J. Sarrel and
Philip M. Sarrel

There is a tendency today to think of sex as so natural that anyone who is not hung-up can do anything and everything sexual very easily, very well, almost instantly. This is very misleading, particularly to the young. This September, about four million young women will enter college in the United States with thoughts, wishes and fantasies about meeting men, dating, going to parties, perhaps falling in love, but not so many we suspect will think specifically about sex. But sex will be a major issue throughout their next four years. The sum total of their experiences with sex in this period will have lifelong impact, for this is a time of sexual un-

Loma J. Sarrel and Philip M. Sarrel, "Sexual Pressures," *Glamour*, 71:58, 74, 80, 86, August, 1974. Copyright © 1974 by The Condé Nast Publications Inc.

folding, a gradual learning about their own sexuality through a variety of life experiences. Many will be transformed from girls to women, and the unfolding of that part of personality which we call sexuality will play a major role in the transformation. Sadly, some women will be more confused, uncertain and disturbed as a result of these years.

The entering college student is actually less sexually experienced than her peers who do not go on to college. Whereas almost 50 percent of all female high school students have had intercourse, only 25 percent entering college are nonvirgins. By the time of college graduation, approximately 50 to 60 percent will have had intercourse.

The decision to have or not to have intercourse for the first time is a

373

serious decision, faced by almost every young woman today. Many students and student couples ask our advice about having intercourse. We always say to them, no one can tell you whether you should or not, but perhaps we can help you think it through by suggesting these questions to ask yourself.

1. Do you know why your parents and/or religion have taught that intercourse should wait until marriage? Do you accept these ideas? If so, then you would be creating a lot of inner turmoil to go against your own beliefs.

2. If you do not accept these beliefs you were taught, is it only at their intellectual level? Do you feel really comfortable and firm in your own beliefs? Try to imagine how you would feel about losing your virginity. Would it make you feel less valuable, less lovable, less good? If so, it is a bad "bargain." This is not to say that an emotional reaction to first intercourse is a sign of trouble. On the contrary, it is a very important moment and an outpouring of feelings can be expected—feelings of joy and sadness, pleasure and disappointment.

3. Have you said no to intercourse not out of moral consideration but out of fear? Many women have fears about sex, especially first intercourse. Do you fear pain and/or bleeding? Do you think there is some reason you would have an unusually difficult time? Are you afraid you would be unable to respond sexually? Are you afraid your parents would find out? A moral decision made out of fear or ignorance is not really moral. You must understand your own feelings and try to find someone (perhaps a doctor) who can hear your

concerns and help answer your questions.

4. Are you yielding to group pressure from your friends against what you feel is right for you? Don't dismiss this question lightly. Most people don't recognize the full extent of the influence exerted on them by peers. It is easy to feel you are "hung up" or abnormal when your way is against most of the people around you. Remember also that some friends may be giving the impression they are more sexually experienced than they actually are.

5. Are you expecting too much from intercourse? If you believe that intercourse will transport you to the stars, make you overnight into a "real" woman or other overblown fantasy, it won't. Try to get your expectations down to earth before you decide.

6. What does intercourse mean to you—permanent commitment for life? Fidelity for both partners? Love?

7. However you answer question 6, does your current relationship meet these criteria? Does he understand what it means to you and do you understand his feelings?

8. Would you feel comfortable being naked with a man, touching his penis and having him touch your genitals, seeing him ejaculate, allowing yourself to respond sexually with him? If not, slow down and go through the stages of physical intimacy at a pace that feels right to you before having intercourse.

9. Is your current relationship emotionally intimate and open? Could you tell him if you were scared or if something hurt? Could he tell you he never had intercourse before and was really nervous? You are much more likely to have a satisfying

experience if the relationship is at this level before you have intercourse.

10. Can you and/or he get effective contraception and will you both use it faithfully and correctly?

11. Are you prepared to face a pregnancy should your contraception fail?

12. Do you and/or he have the opportunity for uninterrupted privacy, free from the fear of being heard or intruded upon?

If, after asking yourself these questions, you still feel confusion and doubt, try to find a trusted person with whom you can talk it out—a religious counselor whose ideas you respect, an older sister, a woman you are close to or a doctor who cares enough to spend time talking with you.

When a young woman enters college she encounters a new environment. For some, there is a drastic change of values and attitudes she senses all around her. Perhaps she comes from a small midwestern town where she and all her close friends simply assumed that most nice girls managed to be virgins until marriage. Sex was not very openly discussed and girls were somewhat guilty and embarrassed if they felt they were going further sexually than their peers. At some colleges or universities she may well encounter a very different atmosphere. Her two roommates may already be on the Pill and display the fact openly—even proudly. Girls may have conversations with new friends which include detail of sexual interactions or concerns about contraception. The peer pressure often goes unrecognized, the girl only knows that she is beginning to change her ideas, sometimes drastically and suddenly. One sopho-

more felt that pressures to be sexually sophisticated were so enormous that she rather cold-bloodedly looked around for a guy to sleep with. She never admitted to him or any of her friends that she was a virgin because, as she put it, "virginity is socially embarrassing."

There does, however, seem to be a ripple of a counter-trend characterized by a respect for virginity, not because this is Mom and Dad's value system, but because postponing intercourse, at least for the time being, makes sense to the individual. We have even heard of one campus which had a "virginity club." It may be that a club is needed to give support to those who want to resist the prevailing trend.

Just about every adolescent or young adult has fears, anxieties and inhibitions to overcome in the process of unfolding sexually. In addition to anxieties and inhibitions, the average college student must also overcome ignorance. The degree of ignorance is sometimes astounding.

Last year, we asked a class of three hundred college students to write a definition of sexual intercourse. We received at least sixteen different definitions, ranging from "any social exchange between two people" to "intimate touching" to "true intercourse is when ejaculation occurs within the woman's vagina at the same time as she is having an orgasm."

Our definition: "Intercourse is the presence of the penis within the vagina." Intercourse does not necessarily include ejaculation, female orgasm, pain or bleeding. None of these qualifications is necessary to complete the definition.

A surprisingly large number of

students are ignorant about the location and nature of the hymen. More than half think it is located deep inside the vagina, near the cervix. This has led to a potentially dangerous situation in several instances. A couple had assumed that they did not have "real" intercourse because the penetration was not very deep and there was no resistance by a closed membrane (their understanding of the hymen). In one instance, this had occurred right at mid-cycle. The male did ejaculate, but the couple did not think about getting the morning-after pill because they had assumed the hymen would keep the sperm from getting to the uterus. The facts about the hymen are as follows: it is a band of tissue near the opening to the vagina (about one-quarter inch inside) which has a hole in it. This hole is often large enough for insertion of the penis without any pain or bleeding. The hymen does not provide any protection against pregnancy.

By the time females enter college, approximately 25 to 30 percent have masturbated. There is evidence to show that in the last two or three years the number of young women who do masturbate is rising sharply. This is not surprising, considering the mass media's focus on female sexuality and more specifically, the widespread mention of female masturbation not only as an acceptable practice but as a healthy step in evolving one's sensual and sexual capacities. Here again some women feel pressured into trying something because it is the thing to do. When they find they cannot respond to self-stimulation, they assume there is something wrong with them—that they are hung-up, neurotic. We would like to emphasize that masturbation is not a prerequisite to being sexually responsive. Masturbation is in no way harmful. It is perfectly normal. But it is also perfectly normal *not* to masturbate.

The young woman who doesn't masturbate and who has not experienced orgasm in some other way may find herself curious about this well-publicized part of female sex response. Many respected authorities have written that any person who says, "I'm not sure whether I've experienced orgasm" has *not* experienced it. They say this because the feelings associated with orgasm are usually distinct and quite intense. While it is true that most people who have orgasm know it, we have spoken with many young women who, we are convinced, were having orgasms without realizing it.

This can happen for several reasons. First, there is the common misconception about orgasm; for example, that it can only happen during intercourse, or that only clitoral stimulation can cause orgasm. Thus, an orgasm caused in some other way is dismissed as "just a nice feeling." This is especially true of orgasms which occur in "unexpected" situations, such as while climbing a rope in gym class, or riding a horse, or awakening from a dream. Second, some people have overly romantic ideas about orgasm gleaned from literature. They expect the earth to move and the stars to burst. When their exaggerated fantasy doesn't occur, they assume they haven't felt "the real thing." Third, a few people in this day and age of a clinical approach to human sex response look for particular bodily changes which they have read about that supposedly signify orgasm. If this particular sign is absent, they, too, assume they are not having an orgasm.

Do college men care about this question of female orgasm? Most of them do—but it goes well beyond simple curiosity and the desire to give pleasure into the male tendency to ego-trip his sexual prowess (or, conversely, his tendency to feel inadequate if he can't "give" his partner an orgasm). The whole subject of sex has become contaminated with the values of our postindustrial, work-ethic society. The pleasures of touching, sharing, communicating and just plain feeling good in a sexual exchange have been buried somewhere under the pressures to achieve a goal, to prove something about one's adequacy and, for the very achievement-oriented college student, to get an A in sex.

It is difficult enough to navigate the waters of sexual unfolding during adolescence and young adulthood without the added burden of performance pressures. They are felt by male and female alike and lead to deep and lasting feelings of self-doubt in many young people who are perfectly adequate.

Sex is a natural function in the sense that the physiologic capacity to experience sexual response is present in all healthy persons. From birth baby boys have erections every eighty to ninety minutes, while baby girls exhibit the female counterpart of erection, vaginal lubrication, with the same periodicity. We continue to exhibit these natural functions in sleep every eighty to ninety minutes throughout our lives.

If sex were entirely biological, or if our society promoted the full and healthy development of sexuality in each of us, then sex would be as simple as eating. But sex is socio-psycho-biological. Our culture, our families and our heads play an enormous role in our sexuality and sexual response. One woman in her junior year at Yale said it beautifully: "When I was a freshman, I thought sex was simple. Now I know it's incredibly complicated."

One added "complication"—bisexuality—is becoming an ever more open issue for young people. Recent articles in popular magazines leave one with the impression that bisexuality is the "in" thing. Some branches of gay activist and women's liberation groups are proselytizing homosexuality and/or bisexuality. Some young men and women will undoubtedly feel these pressures and some may have sexual experiences with their own sex which they might not have had in a different atmosphere. Some, perhaps, will "choose" to consider themselves homosexual or bisexual.

To ask whether this is good or bad opens a hornets' nest. So much depends on one's personal views about homosexuality—whether it is an illness or a lifestyle, a sin or perfectly natural, an affront to society and a menace to young children or simply the private expression of one form of sexuality. As counselors of college and graduate students, our concern about the current "vogue" for bisexuality is the possibility of adding one more *outside* pressure for a particular kind of sexual experience.

Not everyone can integrate this kind of experience psychologically. At age thirteen, fourteen, fifteen, many girls feel very uncertain of their own sexual identity. When asked to draw a picture of "a person," girls this age often draw a figure without a definite sex, and label the picture "neuter" or "it." This reflects their own indefinite self-image as a female. By college age the sense of femaleness is becoming more solidified. But for many it is still a shaky part of their self-image. A homosexual encounter can shake these none-too-sturdy foundations in a way that is painful and disrupting.

The pendulum has swung so far that the new sexual freedom has become just another form of tyranny—a new prescription for "normal" behavior. What is needed, in fact, is an awareness of and tolerance for individual differences. No two people are exactly alike in terms of what will promote their sexual and emotional health. Each person must struggle to understand her- or himself—what she or he believes, feels, what kind of sexual exchange in what kind of relationship will be right.

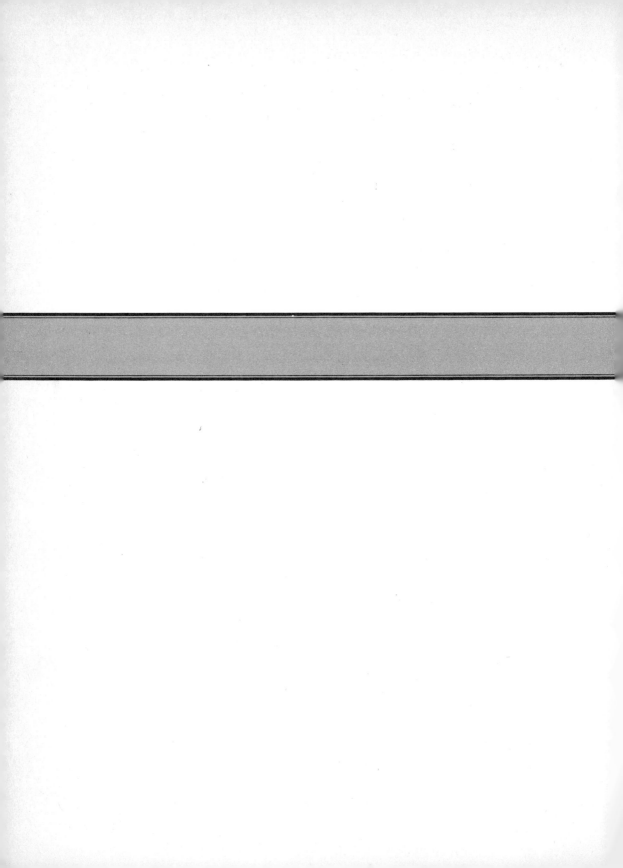

REPRODUCTION
AND FAMILY
PLANNING

chapter eleven

Human sexuality is comprised of many components: our perceptions of our sexual roles, our abilities to establish close relationships with others and to communicate with them, and our capabilities for having sexual relationships (including the most intimate of all relationships, coitus or intercourse) and for making decisions about whether or not to have children—that is, about responsible parenthood. Functioning adequately in these areas and making decisions about our behavior requires understanding of the reproductive system and its care, the nature of coitus, and conception.

PHYSIOLOGY AND ANATOMY OF THE REPRODUCTIVE SYSTEMS

In addition to learning about the physical characteristics of the reproductive systems, we should know how they function. In this chapter, we discuss the male and female reproductive system as well as the problems peculiar to the nature of each.

Hormones and Reproduction

Hormone action commences before birth and affects the personality of either the male or female fetus. By the time birth occurs, the differences between the sexes, other than the more obvious ones of external appearance, that will affect behavior have been established. Differences in behavior between the two sexes are also reinforced by social expectations. Exactly how much is due to hormones and how much to the influence of society no one has determined. At the time of adolescence the sex hormones are excreted in greater amounts and produce additional changes that in turn alter behavior. Again, we cannot say which has the greater influence on maturation and development during the adolescent years, nature or nurture.

Some of the reproductive hormones are produced in the gonads (testes or ovaries), and some by other endocrine glands, namely the anterior lobe of the pituitary and the hypothalamus. These latter hormones are called gonadotropic (acting on the gonads). The gonadotropic hormones act similarly in the male and female with this exception: Beginning in puberty, men are continuously fertile while women are fertile only for short, periodic times, usually once a month. The male continues to have some degree of fertility for the remainder of his life, but the female stops being fertile during her late forties or early fifties. The sex hormones of the male may also be called androgens. Table 11.1 contains a description of the sex hormones.

Parenthood is not everyone's bag

I don't know what to do. Tom and I have the good life now. We both graduated from college and have good paying jobs. For the first time in four years we don't have to worry about money. We're free to come and go as we please. The thing we enjoy the most is the spontaneity of our lives. We can do what ever we want, when we want it, be it sex, a movie or a week-end trip. We always said we wanted children but we love the life we lead now. Who says having children makes a true, fulfilled marriage. I know our whole life will change if we have a baby. I'm happy doing what I'm doing now. I love this freedom. As much as I think I would enjoy a child I don't think I'm ready to give up my way of life. At this time I see a child as an end to myself as a person. Tom and I can never be happier than we are now. I have one life to live. I want to live it to the fullest, and at this time—and possibly forever—it does not include children.

FOUNDATIONS OF HEALTH SCIENCE

Table 11.1 The Sex Hormones

Hormone	Source	Effects
Follicle Stimulating Hormone (FSH)	Anterior lobe of pituitary	*Female:* follicle growth and estrogen production *Male:* sperm production
Luteinizing Hormone (LH)	Anterior lobe of pituitary	*Female:* corpus luteum formation and secretion *Male:* testosterone secretion
Releasing factors	Hypothalamus	*Female:* stimulates pituitary secretion *Male:* stimulates pituitary secretion
Testosterone	Testis	*Male:* male characteristics, inhibits LH secretion
Estrogens	Follicle of ovary	*Female:* uterine growth, female characteristics, inhibits FSH secretions, stimulates LH secretions
Progesterone	Corpus luteum of ovary	*Female:* uterine maintenance, inhibits LH secretion

The Male Reproductive System

The gonads in the male are the two testes located outside the body in the scrotal sac. Inside the testes there are numerous seminiferous tubes that contain several levels of cells called *spermatogonia.* At the time of puberty, these begin to grow large and form primary *spermatocytes.* The spermatocytes, after several changes, develop into mature sperm containing twenty-three unpaired chromosomes, one of which is a sex determinant. Chromosome *X* is female and *Y* is male. If the *X*-bearing sperm fertilizes the female gamete, the baby will be a girl; and if the *Y*-bearing sperm is the fertilizing agent, it will be a boy. The female egg carries *X* chromosones only. The male germ cell, then, determines the sex of a child. The 30,000 genes in each sperm can pair in almost infinite combinations with the 30,000 genes in the ovum. The seminiferous tubes in each testis empty into a much larger tube known as the *epididymis.* While in the epididymis, the sperm attain maturity.

The mechanism of excreting sperm is called *ejaculation.* This takes place in two stages. Although a small quantity of sperm may be stored in the *epididymis,* most are stored in the *vas deferens (ductus deferens).* Peristaltic contractions of the duct walls propel the mixture of sperm and nutrients along. Now, the *seminal vesicles,* which are two glands that secrete a mucous substance containing additional nutrients, empty into the ducts and as the ducts pass through the *prostate gland,* the latter adds a thin alkaline fluid that enables the sperm to stay alive and remain motile.

The ducts, joining together, empty these secretions and sperm now, called *semen,* into the urethra.[1] The motile, fertile sperm can travel at a rate of about 4 mm. per minute, and they tend to move in a straight line. A slightly alkaline environment increases their activity, and a slightly acid one destroys them. Outside the body, sperm survive between twenty-four to seventy-two hours.

The second stage of ejaculation is the propulsion of semen out through the urethra. This results from a rhythmical throbbing caused by the surging and resurging of blood in the erectile tissue surrounding the urethra. Erectile tissue is comprised of large cavern-like veins that are normally collapsed like an empty balloon. During sexual excitement, these caverns, or sinuses, become distended with blood and make the penis firm, elongated, and erect. Either psychological or physical stimuli can cause an erection. Some semen can possibly be excreted prior to ejaculation, but the clear fluid that seeps out first during sexual arousal is usually

Figure 11.1 Reproductive Organs of the Male. (From Arthur C. Guyton, *Textbook of Medical Physiology* [Philadelphia: W. B. Saunders Company, 1961], pp. 1067, 1068, adapted from Maximow and Bloom, *Textbook of Histology.*)

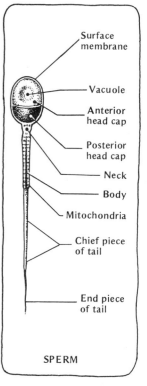

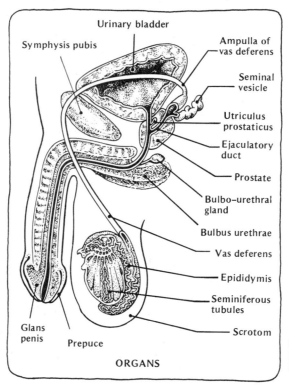

Urinary bladder
Symphysis pubis
Ampulla of vas deferens
Seminal vesicle
Utriculus prostaticus
Ejaculatory duct
Prostate
Bulbo–urethral gland
Bulbus urethrae
Vas deferens
Epididymis
Seminiferous tubules
Scrotom
Glans penis
Prepuce
ORGANS

Surface membrane
Vacuole
Anterior head cap
Posterior head cap
Neck
Body
Mitochondria
Chief piece of tail
End piece of tail
SPERM

FOUNDATIONS OF HEALTH SCIENCE

from the *Cowper's glands,* which empty into the urethra. Cowper's secretions provide a certain amount of lubrication for the sexual act and neutralize the acidity of the urethral canal and the vagina of the female. Figure 11.1 shows the male reproductive organ and a typical sperm.

The normal male, particularly in adolescence, may ejaculate as the result of erotic thoughts or dreams. These emissions, usually at night (nocturnal), range in occurrence from several times per week to several times per month during the teen years. In young adulthood they decrease, and after a regular pattern of sexual relations is established, they are infrequent. Nocturnal emissions are a normal physiological reaction, which does not cause sterility or impotence. Well over 90 percent of all males precipitate ejaculation by manual stimulation of the penis—masturbation or auto-stimulation—which too is more common in the pubertal period. Some males (and females, too) use auto-stimulation or mutual stimulation to relieve sexual tensions in preference to premarital or extramarital intercourse. Such stimulation is not harmful physiologically. If psychic trauma results, it is probably due to attitudes about the practice, not the practice itself.

Hygiene of the male. The *glans,* or end of the penis, is covered with a foreskin, or *prepuce.* Between the glans and the prepuce are small organs that secrete a waxy-like material called *smegma.* Accumulations of smegma and urine are irritating, so the foreskin should be pulled back each day and the glans or head of the penis washed thoroughly. Many males have a portion of the prepuce removed surgically (circumcision), which is preferably done during infancy. Although this practice makes cleanliness easier, it is not a requisite for good hygiene. Improperly performed circumcisions may cause more problems than they are purported to prevent.

Puberty in the male. Collectively, male hormones are known as *androgens.* The primary androgen is *testosterone.* The testes produce most of this hormone, though small amounts are synthesized in the adrenals. At approximately ten years of age, just before the onset of puberty, testosterone production increases rapidly and continues at a high level until about forty years of age, when the level gradually begins to decline. By eighty or so years, the amount is negligible. During the ages of ten to twenty, this increase is responsible for the growth of the penis, scrotum, and testes, as well as the development of masculine hair distribution, the typical bass voice of the male, thickening of skin over the entire body, a tendency to perspire, increased musculature and thickness of the bones, and greater metabolic rate. The sex hormones also cause additional secretions by the sebaceous glands, and while the body is acclimating itself to these changes, oversecretion may result in acne. During puberty, sperm begin to mature and the seminal vessicles and prostate gland begin to secrete.

These changes occur gradually over this ten-year period and progress more rapidly in some boys than in others. If changes have not started during the latter part of the teens, medical studies should be made. Virility (ability to procreate) can not be measured by the degree of male characteristics. Neither is the size of the developed male genitalia an indication of degree of virility. Heredity influences the disposition of the body hair, ruggedness of physique, and quality of voice and skin. Although variations may exist in the size of the scrotum and flaccid penis, upon erection the penis is usually about six inches long and one and one-half inches in diameter. Masculinity is a composite of physical characteristics and personality traits. The latter are influenced by environment and culture. The male *learns* how to act masculine, and the female *learns* how to act feminine.

As the level of testosterone production begins to decrease, during the late forties and fifties, the male will begin to experience some lessening in sexual function, but he will continue to produce sperm throughout his life. Usually this change occurs slowly and the man will not be conscious of any particular symptoms of discomfort from a male climacteric. Masters and Johnson report that males can have satisfactory sexual relations well into their eighties.[2]

The Female Reproductive System

The gonads in the female are the two *ovaries* located in the lower portion of the abdominal cavity. At birth, thousands of immature germ cells, or *ova*, are present in the ovaries. At puberty some of these start maturing. Under the influence of hormones, one of these usually matures and leaves the ovary during the middle of each menstrual cycle. The changes that occur to make implantation and growth of the fertilized ovum possible are described in the section below on the menstrual cycle.

The *Fallopian tubes* are passageways analogous to the male vas deferens. They are approximately four inches long and about the size of a pencil. The open end is trumpet-like in shape and surrounds an ovary. The other end is connected to and opens into the upper body of the uterus. The walls of these tubes or oviducts are made up of muscle tissue and a lining of mucous membranes containing cilia. The peristaltic action of the walls and the wave-like motion of the cilia suck the ovum into the tube and propel it toward the uterine cavity. The ovum is fertilized in the Fallopian duct, although in rare instances sperm have traveled out through the trumpet end of the duct and fertilized an egg in the abdominal cavity or even in the opposite tube.

The *uterus,* or womb, is a hollow muscular organ. In the nonpregnant state, it is about the shape and size of a pear and might hold about a teaspoon or so of liquid. The top, broad portion is called the *fundus* and the narrow neck-like opening at the bottom, the *cervix.* It lies low in the abdominal cavity between the urinary bladder and the rectum. The uterus is suspended by strong ligaments attached to the pelvic bones and is supported by heavy muscles beneath. The functions of the womb are to nourish the fertilized ovum until it is sufficiently mature to live on its own and then at the time of birth to forcibly push the baby through the birth canal and out of the body of the mother. Not only is the heavy musculature of its walls powerful enough to push the child out (it can exert 25 to 30 pounds of pressure) but it is so elastic that during prenatal growth the uterus stretches to the size of a large pumpkin. It, also, is lined with mucous membrane, called *endometrium.*

The *cervix,* or mouth of the uterus, is almost one-inch long and the inner passage is about one-eighth inch in diameter. The endometrium lining the cervix secretes much more mucus than that in the body of the uterus. The cervix is very insensitive to pain. During childbirth, it must stretch to permit the passage of the child. Because of this insensitivity, the female may have little if any discomfort when the cervix is diseased.

The cervix opens into the upper end of the *vagina,* or birth canal. The vaginal tract is between four and five inches in length, and its mucous-covered walls are arranged in thick folds. The walls are capable of being greatly stretched with little discomfort. The vagina is kept moist by secretions excreted from the uterus and the cervix. The *Bartholin glands* are located near the outer edge or orifice. These, like the Cowper's glands in the male, excrete secretions during sexual excitement. However, these excretions appear only after prolonged sexual stimulation. The major source of lubricating fluid is vaginal, and it makes its appearance within a few seconds of sexual arousal.

The external genitalia consist of two pairs of skin folds or *labia* that act to protect the birth canal against dirt and infection. These join at the upper margin to form the *clitoris,* which becomes engorged and swollen during sexual excitement. It is composed of the same type of erectile tissue as is found in the penis. Between the labia and above the vaginal orifice or opening is the small opening of the urethra, which in the female, is between one and two inches long and serves exclusively for the passage of urine. The lower edge of the orifice is rimmed by a fold of skin called the *hymen.* In some women, this membrane partly occludes the opening; in the rare instances when it completely covers the entrance to the vagina,

Figure 11.2 Reproductive Organs of the Female. (Courtesy of M. Edward Davis and Reva Rubin, *De Lee's Obstetrics for Nurses* [Philadelphia: W. B. Saunders Company, 1962], p. 16.)

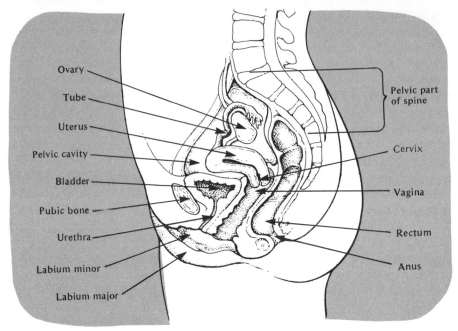

medical treatment is necessary. How extensively the hymen covers the vaginal opening or the ease by which it can be stretched during intercourse are not indexes of virginity. As is true in other individual differences, there is great variation among women. Figure 11.2 shows the female reproductive organs.

Hygiene of the female. Because of the continuous slight secretions from the vaginal tract and glands as well as the periodic menstrual flow, women may be concerned about the need for special hygiene care. Is it necessary to do more than cleanse the external genitalia daily with soap and water? Douching is irrigating and cleansing the vagina with some type of liquid. Physicians disagree as to whether or not it is a desirable practice. The normal vaginal secretions are bacteriostatic. Removing these secretions by irrigation can predispose to infection, and some douching materials may be irritating. Little if any odor exists within the healthy vaginal tract; odors are the result of external secretions. Many physicians agree that although not necessary, douching after intercourse and after the menstrual period is probably not harmful, and the safest solution to use is lukewarm tap water.

FOUNDATIONS OF HEALTH SCIENCE

Nuisance disorders. Because of the nature of the woman's reproductive system, she may suffer from several "nuisance" disorders. Friction and irritation from sexual intercourse occasionally affects internal and external organs adversely, as can persistent unresolved sexual arousal. The female urethra is short and close to the vaginal opening. Sometimes it becomes inflamed and bacteria enter, travel up to the bladder, and produce a condition known as *cystitis*. The symptoms are burning and difficulty on urination. This condition is sometimes referred to as "bride's disease." The Bartholin glands also may be inflamed from sexual irritation. If their ducts become irritated and blocked, secretions accumulate and the glands become very swollen and painful. These conditions are correctable and frequently can be prevented by adequate lubrication, including the use of jellies or creams, during sexual play and intercourse.

Repeated sexual play and stimulation not followed by orgasmic release may also have an adverse affect on either sex. During sexual arousal, the genital area becomes congested and swollen. Tension builds up. In the male, in addition to increased blood supply in the genitals, there is an increase in prostatic fluid. After prolonged petting sessions the male may suffer from low back pain, a mild urethral discharge, and pain in the testes. In the female, the repeated sexual arousal without orgasm or release may produce pelvic pain and vaginal discharge.

Ovulation. Ovulation is the periodic release of a mature ovum. The ovum is the largest of all human cells and is about 6/1000 of an inch in diameter. A tablespoon could hold about two million ova. In addition to the cellular materials necessary to recreate life, the ovum contains small amounts of nutrients, sugars, and proteins to keep the egg alive for about eight days until, if fertilized, it implants itself on the uterine wall and then obtains support from the mother. Normally, one egg is produced per cycle from either ovary. The nonfertilized ovum lives possibly twenty-four hours but is considered most viable for six to ten hours.

A woman with one ovary can produce an egg every month. Although thousands of immature eggs are present at birth, only four hundred to five hundred will ripen during the period between puberty and menopause. The evidence is not clear that preventing ovulation will extend the number of years that a woman remains fertile.

As the ovum matures, several changes can be observed. A small sac containing the ovum fills with fluid and swells to about the size of a marble. This sac, called a follicle, rises to the surface of the ovary. It bursts, freeing the egg, which is then usually sucked into the nearby Fallopian tube. The follicle cells then change, or luteinize, by filling with lipoid materials. This new mass is known as the *corpus luteum*. Under influence of the pituitary gland, the corpus luteum secretes for several weeks large amounts of progesterone and estrogen that regulate the maintenance and growth of the endometrial lining of the uterus.

The menstrual cycle. There is only a short period of a few hours each month when the female is able to conceive. Her normal reproductive function is characterized by monthly rhythmical changes in the secretion of sex hormones, which create alterations in the generative organs. These monthly changes are called the *menstrual cycle.* The two female hormones, estrogen and progesterone, are produced primarily by the ovaries in the nonpregnant woman. For the first years of her life, the level of secretion is low. At about seven years of age, the ovaries begin to grow and gradually secrete additional amounts of both estrogen and progesterone. By the time a girl is approximately twelve years of age, the level is sufficiently high to produce secondary sexual characteristics. The most eventful change is the beginning of menstruation, called the *menarche.* As in males, maturation may commence anywhere between ages ten and twenty years. However, a girl who has not started her "periods" by sixteen years of age should receive a medical examination.

As an egg in one of the ovaries begins to mature, hormones cause a thickening of the endometrium of the uterus, and the rich supply of blood vessels increase in size. The proliferative, or estrogen, phase of the endometrial cycle occurs prior to ovulation. After ovulation, large quantities of both estrogen and progesterone are secreted. Under their influence, there is considerable swelling of the uterine lining, and the glands in the lining increase and secrete small quantities of endometrial fluid. The whole purpose of these changes is to produce nutrients for the implantation of a fertilized ovum. If fertilization does not take place, the ovum disintegrates in a matter of hours, and about twelve days later the secretion of ovarian hormone level drops markedly. The enlarged blood vessels constrict and cut down circulation to the lining, which causes death or necrosis of the endometrium. The dead tissue falls or sloughs off and the underlying vessels hemorrhage. The accumulation of this debris in the uterine cavity causes muscular contractions and expulsion of the contents. The sloughed tissue and bleeding is called the menstrual flow. Because of the amount of fibrinolysin present, the menstrual fluid is nonclotting, and because of a great increase in the number of leukocytes, the uterus is resistant to infection.

The most regular characteristic about menstruation is that it occurs fourteen days after ovulation. Some women tend to be "regular," or vary only a day or two; others may have as much as several weeks difference between cycles. Average cycles range between three to six weeks, and the menstrual flow lasts about three to six days. Figure 11.3 depicts how hormones from the pituitary gland in the brain influence ovulation

Figure 11.3 Menstrual Changes. (From Kenneth N. Anderson, "Is the 'Pill' the Answer?" *Today's Health,* 43:33, June, 1965, published by the American Medical Association.)

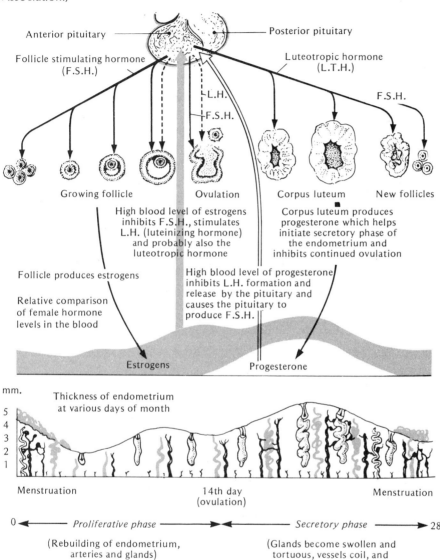

Anterior pituitary — Posterior pituitary

Follicle stimulating hormone (F.S.H.)

Luteotropic hormone (L.T.H.)

L.H.

F.S.H.

F.S.H.

Growing follicle   Ovulation   Corpus luteum   New follicles

High blood level of estrogens inhibits F.S.H., stimulates L.H. (luteinizing hormone) and probably also the luteotropic hormone

Corpus luteum produces progesterone which helps initiate secretory phase of the endometrium and inhibits continued ovulation

Follicle produces estrogens

Relative comparison of female hormone levels in the blood

High blood level of progesterone inhibits L.H. formation and release by the pituitary and causes the pituitary to produce F.S.H.

Estrogens   Progesterone

mm.

Thickness of endometrium at various days of month

5
4
3
2
1

Menstruation   14th day (ovulation)   Menstruation

0 ◄——— *Proliferative phase* ———►◄——— *Secretory phase* ———► 28

(Rebuilding of endometrium, arteries and glands)

(Glands become swollen and tortuous, vessels coil, and blood supply increases) and in turn how the development of the ovum and the corpus luteum influence changes in the uterus.

Menstruation is much misunderstood. It is a normal process that should be accompanied by little or no pain. Of the 15 percent who are quite uncomfortable, medical treatment can assist most. A close relationship exists between discomfort and attitude. The woman who expects to feel "sick," is resentful of the additional care she must take of her body during this period and does not routinely attend to the day-in-and-day-out regimen for healthful living such as proper diet, exercise, and sleep will have more discomfort. Common sense calls for avoiding undue or unusual physical stress, chilling, and fatigue at this time. The physiological changes taking place can cause some discomfort. A number of women become depressed and irritable, develop skin blemishes, notice a gain in weight of several pounds and an increase in the size of the abdomen, feel chilly or too warm, and are nauseated. Medication can alleviate many of these annoyances. Abnormal symptoms that should be checked are periods that occur consistently less than three weeks or more than seven or eight weeks apart, bleeding that lasts more than a week, large clots, a foul odor, and severe cramps or pains. The following are fallacies about menstruation.

1. *"Stopping" or "shortening" a period is bad, because the poisons cannot get out. False!*

    It is extremely unlikely that a woman could stop her period by certain activities, and medical evidence does not indicate that altering a period is physically harmful.

    Many people erroneously believe the following activities could "stop a period."
    a. Bathing, either in a tub or shower, or by using a basin of water.
    b. Swimming.
    c. Consuming iced foods or drinks.
    d. Shampooing or having permanents.
    e. Eating certain kinds of foods such as strawberries, pickles, or watermelon.

2. *Women are unclean during menstruation and should keep to themselves. False!*

    Nothing about the blood and tissue that comprise the menstrual flow is unclean. It does not contain poisons or germs. When exposed to the air, these excretions will decompose and an undesirable odor is apparent.

3. *Sexual relations during menstruation are harmful. False!*

    No physiological reasons support this belief. If this practice is

FOUNDATIONS OF HEALTH SCIENCE

aesthetically undesirable to one or both, or if relations produce any discomfort in the female, abstinence is desirable.

During the period of menstrual flow, a woman will feel more comfortable if she bathes frequently. We have no scientific evidence that sitting in warm water will stop or start a period or will cause infection. The type of protection used is a matter of individual choice. The active modern girl and woman may prefer to use tampons rather than sanitary napkins, if not for the whole time, at least during the waning days. These are more comfortable and produce less odor. They do not cause cancer or impair virginity.

When a girl first begins to menstruate (menarche) and when a woman reaches menopause the periods are apt to be irregular and scanty. Rarely does a girl, during the menarche (beginning), start menstruating regularly every three to five weeks. During menopause, which starts in most women between forty and fifty years of age, the same type of pattern is usual. Because of the rapid decrease in the amount of female hormones produced, some women experience symptoms such as irritability and hot flashes. These, too, can be aided by medical care.

PLANNING CONCEPTION

Planning conception is having children by choice instead of by chance. Such planning is not new, but the techniques available to accomplish it have been greatly improved during the last twenty years, and information about them is being widely disseminated throughout the world.

No one method of contraception is right for every woman all of the time. A method that works for one woman may not be suitable for another. Also, what may work well during one period of time, may not be the best for another period of time. While almost any method is better than nothing, all are not equally effective. *Effectiveness is pretty much dependent upon the user.* A couple must be careful to use a specific method properly and be equally careful to use it regularly if they are to attain any degree of success in planning to conceive or not to conceive. Any method that is unpleasant, uncomfortable, embarrassing, or disagreeable in any way to either partner is not a good method for them.

Effectiveness of contraceptive devices is based on the number of unplanned pregnancies that occur among a group using that device for a specific period of time. The less effective a method is, the greater the number of women in any group who will become pregnant.

The basis of all methods of family planning is the prevention of the union between the egg and the sperm. The methods, each having varying degrees of success, fall into four categories: avoidance of insemination, erection of mechanical barriers between the sperm and the egg, prevention of ovulation or spermatogenesis, and inhibition of implantation.

Coitus Interruptus

Coitus interruptus is one of the oldest—and still widely used—methods of avoiding insemination. The male withdraws before the sexual act is completed. Since sperm may be present in the secretions prior to ejaculation, fertilization occasionally occurs. Ejaculation sometimes is so precipitous that the man may fail to interrupt the sexual act in time. Psychologically, this practice is considered undesirable since it may leave either or both sexual partners unsatisfied.

Rhythm

Abstinence during the fertile period is called the *rhythm method*. It is one of the less effective methods for most women because of the difficulty in determining the safe days during the menstrual cycle. These are the physiological facts upon which rhythm is based: Normally only one egg is produced during each menstrual cycle, the active life of the egg is about twenty-four hours, and the sperm lives for about forty-eight hours after being deposited in the vagina. Therefore, abstinence for two days before ovulation and one day afterward should prevent pregnancy. The success of this method depends on the accurate prediction of the time of ovulation.

Ovulation usually takes place twelve to sixteen days *before the next menstrual period, not two weeks after the last period.* The woman must know just how much variation there is in the length of her menstrual cycles. This requires maintaining a written record of variations for one year. Secondly, a daily record of body temperature should also be made for one year. A woman takes her temperature rectally on awakening every morning—before getting out of bed. Usually a slight dip in temperature below the level that has been constant for a week or ten days provides the signal that ovulation has begun; this dip in temperature is then followed by a rise of $1/2°$ to $3/4°$F. over a period of twenty-four to seventy-two hours. Illness or activity may cause fluctuations in daily temperature that have nothing to do with the time of ovulation.

The calendar rhythm method is based on the length of the woman's shortest and longest menstrual cycles. She first must record the length of eight menstrual cycles from the first day of bleeding of one period until

FOUNDATIONS OF HEALTH SCIENCE

the first day of bleeding of the next period. She then calculates the fertile period of the ninth cycle as follows: subtract eighteen from the length of the shortest cycle to find the first fertile day; next, subtract eleven from the longest cycle to find the last fertile day. Recording of each cycle must be continuous since each month's unfertile and fertile periods are based on the preceding eight cycles.[3] Figure 11.4 and Figure 11.5 are examples of such calculations.

The calendar and temperature methods restrict the total number of days in which a woman can safely have intercourse to a period of about two weeks per menstrual cycle. This is unsatisfactory for many couples. In addition, 15 percent of women menstruate with too much irregularity to find these methods of any value. During the year in which records and temperature charts are being kept, during the first few months after childbirth, and when menopause is commencing, ovulation is sufficiently hard to predict that other methods of family planning should be used.

Douche

Chemical destruction of deposited sperm can also prevent fertilization. One of the oldest and still widely used of these methods is douching.

Figure 11.4 The Calendar Rhythm Method

Length of shortest period	First fertile day after start of any period	Length of longest period	Last fertile day after start of any period
21 days	3rd day	21 days	10th day
22 days	4th day	22 days	11th day
23 days	5th day	23 days	12th day
24 days	6th day	24 days	13th day
25 days	7th day	25 days	14th day
26 days	8th day	26 days	15th day
27 days	9th day	27 days	16th day
28 days	10th day	28 days	17th day
29 days	11th day	29 days	18th day
30 days	12th day	30 days	19th day
31 days	13th day	31 days	20th day
32 days	14th day	32 days	21st day
33 days	15th day	33 days	22nd day
34 days	16th day	34 days	23rd day
35 days	17th day	35 days	24th day
36 days	18th day	36 days	25th day
37 days	19th day	37 days	26th day
38 days	20th day	38 days	27th day

(From *Birth Control Handbook*, Montreal Health Press, 1973, p. 36.)

Figure 11.5 Rhythm Method Temperature Chart

First published in *Sexual Awareness,* by Gere B. Fulton. Copyright 1974, Holbrook Press, Inc. Reprinted by permission.

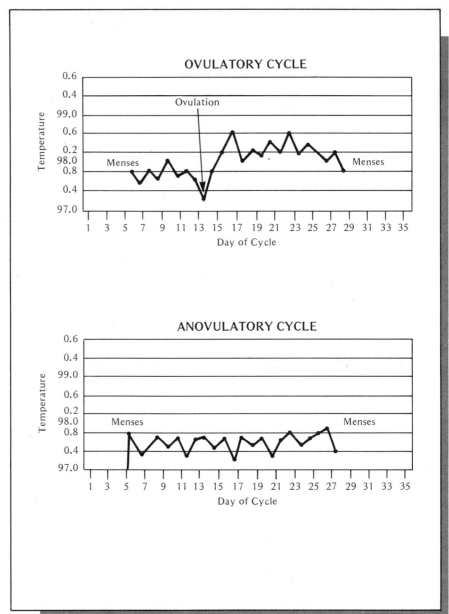

FOUNDATIONS OF HEALTH SCIENCE

Chemicals or medicines are not necessary in the douche solution, since water itself is spermicidal. Douching is not often very effective since it must be done within a few seconds after ejaculation to have any degree of success, which can interfere with sexual satisfaction.

Vaginal Spermicides

A variety of spermicides in the form of jellies, vaginal tablets, suppositories, and foams are available and can be purchased without a prescription for but a few cents. Few are very satisfactory in preventing pregnancy inasmuch as they must be used properly. They must be applied just before intercourse, and if intercourse is repeated another application of the spermicide should be made. Occasionally, the male or female may be allergic to the spermicide. Many couples find the use of these physically or psychologically undesirable.

Condom and Diaphragm

Mechanical barriers of one kind of another have been used for centuries. The most commonly applied is the rubber condom used by the male. When put on correctly, it prevents fertilization most effectively. The condom is a thin, skin-tight sheath that is pulled over the erect penis just prior to intercourse. The tip of the condom acts as a receptacle to catch the seminal fluid, thus preventing the sperm from being released into the vagina. This method may be made more effective if it is used in combination with a vaginal spermicide. The penis must be withdrawn very carefully after intercourse so that the condom does not break and permit sperm to escape into the vagina. If the penis is not removed immediately after ejaculation the sheath may slip off as the erection subsides. Too vigorous intercourse may also cause it to slip off, and it is easily punctured. Couples may find the use of the condom or sheath reduces sensation; some women whose vaginal tissues are not very moist may find it irritating unless a lubricant is used. These protective devices are available in any drugstore without prescription, and they are inexpensive. They are a valuable back-up method to provide extra protection.

The most physically and psychologically satisfactory mechanical barrier is the diaphragm, used by the female. It is available only on prescription since it must be fitted by a physician and the woman instructed in its use. The vaginal diaphragm is made of soft rubber, shaped like a bowl, with a flexible spring enclosed in the outer edge. Contraceptive cream or jelly must be used with it. When properly placed it fits securely between the rear wall of the vagina and the upper edge of the pubic bone. In this position, it completely covers the cervix, holds the contraceptive cream or jelly tightly over the cervical opening, and thus provides a chemical barrier that kills the sperm.

The diaphragm must be used whenever intercourse takes place. It can be inserted at bedtime as a matter of routine so that the woman is always prepared and it may be left in place for twenty-four hours. The diaphragm properly positioned in the vagina should cause no sensations. If the woman does feel it, either it has been inserted incorrectly or it is not the right size. If intercourse does not take place for more than six hours after insertion, or if intercourse is repeated, additional contraceptive jelly should be used (the diaphragm does not need to be removed to do this). Most women can use the diaphragm effectively, and it does not interfere with sexual enjoyment. The mechanics of insertion are distasteful to some women.

Birth Control Pills

The most successful method of temporarily preventing conception is the "birth control pill." For the 90 to 95 percent of women who experience no side effects, it is completely satisfactory. This type of oral contraceptive has the advantage of being disassociated with the sex act, so it has no psychological drawbacks. It should be used under the supervision of a physician, costs less than two dollars for a monthly supply, and must be taken at about the same time daily without exception for the prescribed number of days. Some of the common unpleasant side effects are nausea, a slight gain in weight, and occasionally intermenstrual bleeding (breakthrough bleeding). These discomforts tend to disappear if the pill is continued for several months; sometimes a change to a different brand alleviates such problems. About one-third of the couples who use birth control rely on the pill.

The pills inhibit ovulation in the following manner. Normally and naturally, after an ovum is fertilized and implanted, the human body requires that other ova not be released during the pregnancy. The progesterone and estrogen secreted by the corpus luteum in the ovary and later by the placenta signal the pituitary gland to suppress the secretion of the gonadotropic hormones that stimulate ovulation. In addition, progesterone helps maintain an enlarging uterus, keeping it a suitable place for the embryo to grow. To inhibit ovulation artificially, progesterone or estrogen is given orally to induce a pregnancy-like condition. A combination of the two hormones in one pill reduces the undesirable effects that result when either hormone is given singly. Table 11.2 shows how this type of contraceptive works (see pages 400–401).

FOUNDATIONS OF HEALTH SCIENCE

Within one to two months after discontinuance of the pill, pregnancy can take place. It may take longer. If a couple uses no type of birth control, one-fourth will conceive in the first few months after commencing coitus regularly. By the end of a year, 80 percent of the couples using no type of birth control will conceive. The remaining 20 percent may take longer to conceive, have trouble with fertility, or be sterile.

Birth control pills may have some serious side effects. Alan Guttmacher, M.D., long associated with Planned Parenthood–World Population, does not believe the side effects are sufficiently serious to prohibit use of the pill:

> They are not sufficiently serious in my judgment to make us discontinue the pill because I think the pill is a tremendous asset. There are many, many persons—particularly among the less motivated segments of our population —who would not use any birth control method except the pill. The risks they face in multiple pregnancies and labors are infinitely greater than the risks associated with the pill.[4]

Guttmacher says the overall death rate of 1 per 25,000 women might be attributed to pills, but this rate is considerably less than that from penicillin. All potent drugs do carry some risk of morbidity and mortality. He also gives these comparisons based on the studies done in Britain:[5]

Mortality Rate From Pulmonary Emboli or Cerebral Thrombosis

Ages in Years	Women on Pill	Women not on Pill
20–35	1.5/100,000	.2/100,000
35–45	3.9/100,000	.5/100,000

One of the world's most extensive study of oral contraceptives has involved 46,000 case histories submitted by 1,400 family physicians in Britain. The findings were:

1. No association between pill use and cancers, even those of the breast and cervix.
2. Some association with an increase in blood pressure, but fewer than 1 percent were affected in the first year and 95 percent did not develop hypertension after five years.
3. Significant increase in stroke and increased incidence of deep-vein thrombosis of the leg.
4. A 20 percent to 50 percent increase in vaginal infection and vaginal discharge, but a reduction in menstrual disorders.[6]

However, rising evidence indicates that the use of some kinds of estrogen is related to an increasing incidence of breast and cervical cancer. Retrospective studies made in Washington and California indicate some

Table 11.2 Bodily Changes and Day They Occur During Average (28-Day) Menstrual Cycle, Pregnancy, and Pill Cycle

Day	Usual Menstrual Cycle	Menstrual Cycle Interrupted by Pregnancy	Pill Cycle
1	Menstrual period—when bleeding occurs, accompanied by regression of endometrium (uterine lining).	Menstrual period	Menstrual period—same as in usual menstrual cycle.
5			Start taking pill—one pill taken daily for 20 consecutive days, beginning on the 5th day following the onset of menstruation; ovulation is inhibited.
6	Proliferative phase—growth of endometrium, development of Graafian follicle (sac within ovary in which ovum or egg cell matures and ripens).		Proliferative/secretory phase—similar to same phases during menstrual cycle, but brought about more rapidly and seldom fully developed.
14	Ovulation—follicle ruptures and releases egg cell.	Fertilization—occurs when ripe egg cell unites with sperm cell.	No ovulation
15	Secretory phase—development of corpus luteum which is a yellow mass of cells formed where follicle has ruptured. It produces progesterone which causes endometrium to thicken preparatory to receiving fertilized egg.	Secretory phase—same as in usual menstrual cycle.	Predecidual phase—resembling predecidual phase of usual cycle but not as completely developed. In usual cycle this at day 23.
21		Decidual phase—continuation and accentuation of predecidual development. Endometrium thickens in response to continuing progesterone secretion as a bed for the developing egg. Progesterone (secreted by the corpus luteum and later by the placenta) maintains this phase and prevents further ovulation.	

...terior development — condensation of dense cells around the small arteries of the endometrium.

24		Last day of pill (day 24). Because of earlier and more rapid development, cells in endometrium are small. Predecidua is incompletely developed.
27	Premenstrual phase—regression of corpus luteum and endometrium.	When pill is stopped, hormone support for endometrium ceases and it regresses (bleeding occurs in about two days) and . . .
1	Menstruation begins again.	Menstruation begins again.

Adapted from *Prescription for Family Planning* (New York: A. D. Searle Reference and Resource Program, 1966).

relationship.[7] It is recommended that older women, especially those over 40 use other methods of contraception.[8]

Some of the current research is aimed at developing a morning after pill; a once-a-month pill; and pills that primarily contain progestin since the estrogen appears to cause symptoms and dangerous side effects, and progestin could be taken every day rather than on a twenty-day schedule. One type of pill that is being investigated would destroy a fertilized ovum before it becomes implanted. Contraceptive injections that are being studied would protect for a three- to six-month period. Progestin could be implanted under the skin in a silastic tube and could thus prevent fertility for as long as three years.

The morning after pill. The morning after pill, stilbesterol or DES, has been approved for use only in case of rape or incest. Research has proven that stilbesterol given to pregnant women can cause vaginal cancer in a female child (this becomes evident during puberty), though the risk is small. Such data have accumulated from the several thousand women in North America who received this hormone during the 1940s and 1950s for the purpose of preventing miscarriage. Regulations in Canada and the United States forbid the use of this drug during pregnancy. Authorities in family planning recommend that women should not use the morning-after-pill unless they intend to have an abortion should the drug fail to prevent pregnancy. Studies also reveal that males exposed to DES in utero have a higher incidence of genital abnormalities and are less fertile.[9]

Intrauterine Devices

The IUD concept is not new, but the new plastic construction makes it a safe and practical contraceptive device for about 80 percent of the women who have tried it. For the other 20 percent, these devices will not stay in place or are uncomfortable. The great advantage of the IUD is that after placement by a physician, it can remain in the uterus for as long as necessary. It is inexpensive and does not require that the woman remember to take a pill or that either the man or woman prepare before intercourse or interrupt the sexual act in any way to prevent conception.

Although the IUD's effectiveness in preventing pregnancy is known, how it works is not understood. When it is in place, leukocytes and macrophages increase in the endometrial tissue. This local inflammatory reaction results in the destruction of most sperm before they reach the Fallopian tubes. Some experts also believe that this inflammation may interfere with implantation of the fertilized ovum.

Different types of devices are available. Those that are the most effective in preventing pregnancy produce the most adverse reactions, such as

FOUNDATIONS OF HEALTH SCIENCE

cramping, increased menstrual flow, or expulsion. The coil-shaped IUD results in the fewest pregnancies but has the highest rate of expulsion. It lies free in the uterine cavity with threads protruding out through the cervix so that determining whether it is still in place is easy. Two newer kinds of intrauterine devices are the Copper T and Copper-7, which contain copper as an additional contraceptive. These have the advantage of being smaller and can be inserted in a woman who has never been pregnant (nullipara). The copper IUD's appear to cause less severe cramps and bleeding and have fewer expulsions, but they must be replaced every two years or so. Long-term effects of copper are unknown.

The average pregnancy rate is from 1 to 3 percent of patients who use the Loop or Saf-T-Coil. The rate of pregnancy protection improves the longer the IUD is used. For each one hundred women who have a device inserted, about eleven will expel it in the first year, and another twelve will have it removed because of discomfort. Women over thirty years of age have much lower rates of expulsion as do women who have had several children. Those who find the IUD satisfactory tend to continue to use it more frequently than do those on pills.[10] Even though the Saf-T-Coil and Copper 7 can be used in a woman who has never been pregnant, they may be quite uncomfortable to insert.

About 2 percent of the women using IUD's have the complication of pelvic inflammatory disease. Next to pain and bleeding, this is the most common reason for removal of the IUD. Ectopic or tubal pregnancies occur six times more often among IUD users. If pregnancy occurs, the physician will usually leave the device in place, and it will be expelled during childbirth; there is no evidence that this causes fetal abnormalities, while removal might interfere with the pregnancy.

Manisoff of Planned Parenthood–World Population gives these key points in the use of intrauterine devices:

1. Insertion is usually done during the menstrual period because the uterus is softer and the cervix more easily dilated.
2. Neither patient or her sexual partner can feel an IUD since it is inside the uterus.
3. Spotting and bleeding often occur after insertion.
4. The first few periods may be heavier and be closer together.
5. After several months the menstrual cycle and flow should return to the original pattern.
6. Tampons can be used and douches taken if desired.
7. The IUD can be left in place indefinitely but physicians desire to check the woman at least once a year (every six months is better), and do a cervicle smear test.[11]

Figure 11.6 illustrates the different types of IUDs.

Figure 11.6 Intrauterine Devices

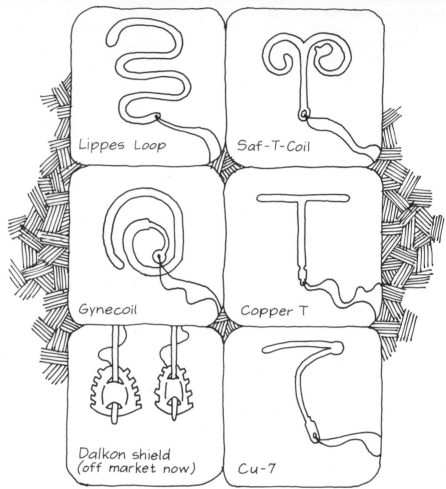

Lippes Loop

Saf-T-Coil

Gynecoil

Copper T

Dalkon shield
(off market now)

Cu-7

*In 1974, at the request of the FDA, distribution of the Dalkon Shield was suspended. Data indicated that there was a higher level of deaths and septic abortions from this type of IUD than from the others. No recommendation has been made to remove the Shield from women having no adverse effects or reactions.

Sterilization

All over the world more and more people who seek to limit the size of their families or who decide to not have children at all are choosing permanent sterility. In 1975 some 674,000 tubal ligations and as many as 639,000 vasectomies were performed.[12] Data from a 1973 survey of married couples revealed that one-quarter of all couples who practiced birth con-

FOUNDATIONS OF HEALTH SCIENCE

trol had been sterilized. Among couples of all ages who desire no more children, sterilization is used second only to the pill as a contraceptive method. A few more females than males are presently being sterilized. Sterilization is the most popular method for women 30 or older.[13]

A word of caution! Sterilization in both the male and female should be considered a permanent condition. Despite scientific reports that some procedures have been developed that can reverse tubal ligations and vasectomies, the results have not produced high levels of fertility. In males, the major percent remain infertile. Sterilization should be reserved for those older people who have had the number of children they desired, those whose health may not be conducive to pregnancy or child rearing, and those with serious, transmissable genetic defects.

Female sterilization. Female sterilization refers to all operations per-formed on a woman that permanently prevent conception. The procedure, most often, consists of cutting, tying, occluding, or removing a portion of the Fallopian tube. Such an operation has no physical effects, and the woman retains her menstrual and sexual function. The approach to the tubes may be either vaginally or abdominally. Vaginal ligation requires hospitalization for several days. No abdominal incision is made since the tubes are reached through the vagina. Some medical or physical condi-tions preclude this procedure.

The newest procedures are the endoscopic methods of laparoscopy, culdoscopy, and hysteroscopy. These do not require hospitalization. The most popular of the methods is the laparoscopy, which is sometimes re-ferred to as the "bandaid operation" since the incision or incisions are so tiny. A fiberoptic telescope and accessory instruments are inserted through a one inch incision (or two one-inch incisions) near the umbilicus. When performed by a trained surgeon, the laparoscopy has a failure rate of 0.1 percent to 2 percent. To ensure that failure is not due to an already exist-ing pregnancy, the procedure should be done immediately following menstruation. Laparoscopy is safe, inexpensive, and efficient.

Figures 11.7 and 11.8 illustrate the tubal ligation approach to female sterilization.

Vasectomy. Techniques for sterilization of males are becoming more proficient; the vasectomy is inexpensive, efficient, simple, and can be done in the physician's office. It take less than one-half hour in all to perform, and only one or two incisions may be made. The surgeon removes one-fourth to one-half inch of the vas deferens. The cut ends are then sealed in various ways. In about 50 percent of vasectomies reconnecting the tubes is possible, but less than 30 percent of these restorations result

Figure 11.7   Tubal Ligations

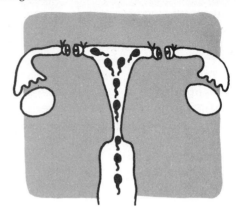

Egg and sperm prevented from meeting

in fertility. After a vasectomy, physiological changes that occur apparently interfere with ability of sperm to impregnate. This procedure to prevent conception should be considered irreversible. Currently a new micro-surgical technique is being researched that seems to produce much higher percentages of reversals and fertility.

Figure 11.9 illustrates the vasectomy approach to sterilization.

Contraceptives for Males

Chemical contraceptives for males are a possibility, though not available for use in the United States. They can cause sterility. Techniques to block the vas deferens are being tested. One is the use of a clamp that could be removed when fertility is desired, and a second is the injection of a plastic material into the vas deferens. The latter has been effective in preventing fertilization for as long as a year in animal experimentation. The effect of heat on the testes to produce temporary infertility is also in the research stage.

Effectiveness of Contraceptives

As indicated before, if couples do not practice contraception some 80 percent will conceive within the year and probably one-fourth will conceive within the first several months after establishing sexual relations on a regular basis. One of the functions of premarital counseling is to advise about the method of family planning that will be in accord with the

FOUNDATIONS OF HEALTH SCIENCE

Figure 11.8   Tubal Ligations—Ways to Reach Tubes

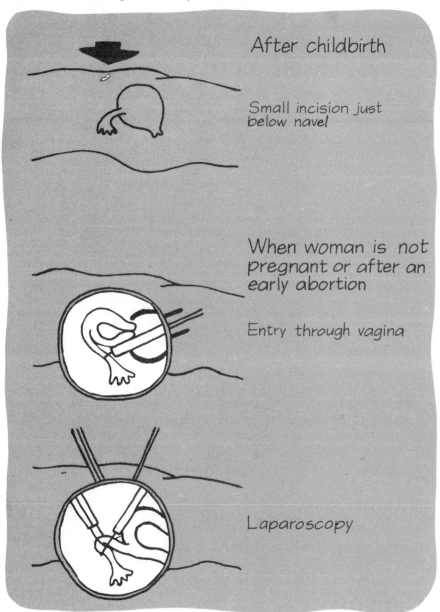

After childbirth

Small incision just below navel

When woman is not pregnant or after an early abortion

Entry through vagina

Laparoscopy

Figure 11.9 Vasectomy

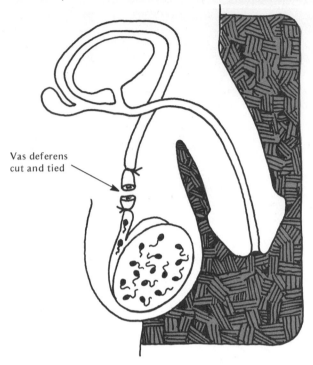

Vas deferens
cut and tied

values and beliefs, the likes and dislikes, and the convenience of both the man and woman. Some methods are more effective than others, and all have certain advantages and disadvantages. Even the best may not always work because of individual differences and human error. In addition to one's personal physician, planned parenthood centers in most communities are available for counseling. More and more college health services are assisting students in making these decisions, too. Table 11.3 gives the proportion of married women who become pregnant within twelve months while using a specific contraceptive (this failure rate includes method failure as well as use failure) and also the Table gives methods of contraception used in 1970 by married couples.

Abortion

Legalization of induced abortion has resulted in a decline in abortion deaths, a decrease in hospitalization of women with complications from abortion, lower out-of-wedlock birth rates, and improved infant and maternal health. When abortions are prohibited by law, they do occur, but the conditions under which they take place are not supervised by either medical or legal authorities. With the availability of antibiotics and blood for transfusion, and with knowledge of asepsis, nearly all deaths from induced abortion can be eliminated. According to estimates, when abortions were illegal in the United States, about one million were still performed yearly.

The motives most often given for terminating a pregnancy are: (1) economic, (2) too many other children, (3) preservation of the marriage, (4) out-of-wedlock conception, and (5) emotional inability to cope with the pregnancy. There is little danger when abortion is performed under desirable medical conditions. What are the legal and medical issues involved in the arguments for and against abortion when there seem to be valid reasons for having one?

Who may have an abortion? Any woman, unwillingly pregnant, whose doctor agrees to the decision. The Supreme Court, in its abortion decision of January, 1973, decreed that the right of privacy is broad enough to include a woman's decision whether or not to terminate her pregnancy. The following quotation from a 1975 editiorial in *Newsweek* is representative of the present views held by the public about abortion.

> As a matter of public opinion and social policy, the right to an early abortion now is firmly established and some of the nation's right-to-life groups no longer seem opposed to certain abortions, particularly those intended to save the mother's life. After last fall's elections [1974], an NBC poll found that 58 per cent of the voters questioned (and 46 per cent of the Roman Catholics) approved of laws permitting abortion during the first three months of pregnancy.[14]

Table 11.3 Effectiveness and Use of Contraceptives

Contraceptive	Use Failure* (Percent Pregnant in 12-Month Period)	Percent of Married Couples Using†
Sterilization	0.1–2.0	16.3
Pill	5	34.2
IUD	8	7.4
Diaphragm	18	5.7
Condom	19	14.2
Withdrawal	23	2.1
Rhythm	30	6.4
Foam	32	6.1
All other	33+	7.8

*Phillips Cutright, "Illegitimacy: Myths, Causes and Cures," *Family Planning Perspectives,* 3:42, 1971.

†Charles Westoff, "The Modernization of U.S. Contraceptive Practice," *Family Planning Perspectives,* 4:11, 1972.

In the United States, most states did not even pass antiabortion laws until the mid-nineteenth century, and then the motive was mainly to protect women from serious injury or death in a highly risky procedure. Similarly, protecting women from the butchery of illegal abortionists was a reason why contemporary reformers sought to have antiabortion laws overturned.[15] The Supreme Court also decreed in the 1973 decision that dangers during the second trimester of pregnancy are sufficient that the state has a right to regulate abortions; for example, by requiring that they be performed in hospitals and that in the last twelve weeks of pregnancy the state may proscribe or have laws to prevent abortion in the interest of maintaining a viable fetus except when termination of the pregnancy is necessary to preserve the life or health of the mother.[16] States vary in exercising their "right to regulate" during the second trimester of pregnancy.

The laws restricting abortion during the second trimester (or second twelve-week period) do work a hardship on women who are young, single, poor, or belong to minority groups. (Second trimester abortions account for approximately 15 percent of the total).[17] Restrictions affecting this group include such requirements as Medicaid funds cannot be used to pay for terminating a pregnancy, or physicians and hospitals cannot be forced to perform abortions against their better judgment.

Physicians can be (and some have been) prosecuted (manslaughter of a fetus), when there is a chance that the fetus is twenty-four weeks old. Since determining the precise date at which conception occurred is sometimes difficult, and since between the twelfth to sixteenth week of pregnancy abortion is not safe because of the position of the uterus, the decision of whether or not to abort during the second trimester is not easy for physicians to make.

The most frequent age for potential viability of the fetus is twenty-

Such thoughts frequently follow an abortion. They are normal.

A friend of mine, age nineteen, had an abortion when she was in high school. She really believed that the guy she liked really cared about her, but he didn't and after she got pregnant, he wanted nothing to do with her. As she was planning to have the abortion she pretended that this boy and she were still very close. Actually he wanted to get it over with and be done with her. She pretended to be going to the beach for the weekend when she actually went for the abortion. Everyone in school knew what was happening to her even though she pretended that everything was all right. Now, after the abortion, she sometimes thinks about how old the baby would be and what it might have been like if she hadn't had the abortion.

FOUNDATIONS OF HEALTH SCIENCE

eight weeks, but it may be earlier. A fetus that weighs less than 2.2 pounds has about a 20 percent chance of surviving, but because of immaturation of the nervous system, the risk of mental retardation is high. A fetus less than 1.3 pounds has practically no chance of survival. With the most advanced technology, the survival rate for infants weighing 2.2 to 2.7 pounds can be 60 percent; 1.7 to 2.2 pounds, 30 to 40 percent; and 1.2 to 1.6 pounds, possibly 2 percent.[18] Because of the variation in potential viability of the fetus, and because of inaccuracies in determining the date of conception (and consequently fetal age in weeks), many hospitals are refusing to permit abortions after sixteen weeks of pregnancy and are, in fact, then, limiting abortions to the first twelve weeks or first trimester.

Abortion procedures. Close to 25 percent of all pregnancies terminate in spontaneous abortion, which is often referred to as miscarriage or stillbirth. Most of these aborted embryos are defective. However, for another percentage of unwanted pregnancies, induced abortion is considered. Abortion should always be thought of as a *back-up method to contraceptive failure*. It should never be conceived as a method of controlling conception. Although there are less undesirable effects from a properly induced abortion than there are from pregnancy and childbirth, there are some complications. A woman who has had a number of abortions may have difficulty in carrying a pregnancy through to term if later she decides she wants a child.

The method used to terminate pregnancy depends upon how long the woman has been pregnant. Laboratory tests that confirm pregnancy are not highly accurate until the fourth to sixth week of pregnancy. Abortion is considered safest when it is performed during the first trimester, but in the second trimester, it is still legal and relatively safe.

Vacuum aspiration. The commonly used method during the first trimester is vacuum aspiration. This procedure can be done in a clinic setting wherein the woman is counseled about the procedure, anesthetized, aspirated, and observed for several hours before going home. In vacuum aspiration, the size and position of the uterus is checked, a plastic cannula or tube is inserted through the vagina and cervix into the uterus, and then the cannula is attached to a suction machine. The mouth of the cannula is then run over the wall of the uterus and vacuums up or aspirates the endometrium. The advantages of the plastic cannula is that it is flexible and will bend or turn to conform to the shape of the uterus.

Another similar procedure is *menstrual extraction*. If a woman is late in beginning her menstrual period and there is a possibility of pregnancy, she does not wait to confirm it. She will have immediate aspiration of the endometrium. This procedure takes only a few minutes. She is not faced with the decision of whether or not she is really aborting since she does not know that she is even pregnant. (Menstrual extraction is also used to shorten a menstrual period, reduce amount of flow, or ameliorate discomfort.)

Dilitation and curettage (D. & C.) The D. & C. is still in use, especially during the first trimester. It involves dilation of the cervix and insertion of a curette, or scoop-like instrument, that is used to scrape the endometrium. Although this procedure has more adverse effects than the vacuum aspiration, it is more fool proof. The D. & C. requires hospitalization.

Saline infusion. Three procedures can be used to abort during the second trimester. Hysterotomy, not as widely used as the other two, consists of surgically entering the uterus through the abdomen and manually removing the fetus. The other two ways to abort are by infusion. The preferred method, saline infusion, is an injection of salt solution into the amniotic sac. This solution terminates the life of the fetus, usually in an hour or so. The mother will then go into labor in eight to seventy-two hours. Should the solution accidentally get into the mother's blood stream, it could produce convulsions or clots. Safer is the use of prostaglandin, which is a hormone that will produce strong uterine contractions. Prostaglandin is also injected into the amniotic sac. It is safe for the mother, but may result in a viable fetus.

Table 11.4 gives the complication rates for each method of abortion. Figure 11.10 shows the techniques of abortion.

Table 11.4 Complication Rates Per 1000 Abortions by Type and Method of Termination

Type of Complication	D & C	Suction	Saline	Hysterotomy	Total
Hemorrhage	0.9*	0.5	5.1	3.0	1.1
Infection	0.7	1.0	5.3	11.9	1.5
Perforated uterus	1.6	1.1	0.2	5.9	1.2
Shock	—	—	0.1	0.6	—
Retained tissue	0.4	0.5	20.1	1.2	2.9
Failure	—	0.1	2.3	—	0.3
Lacerated cervix	0.3	0.2	0.1	0.6	0.2
Other	0.2	0.2	0.9	6.0	0.3
Total	4.3	3.7	34.2	28.5	7.7

*Rate per 1000 cases.

Adapted from Jean Pakter, Donna O'Hare, Frieda Nelson, and Martin Svigir, "Two Years Experience in New York City with the Liberalized Abortion Law—Progress and Problems," *American Journal of Public Health*, 63:532, June, 1973.

Figure 11.10 Techniques of Abortion

D & C

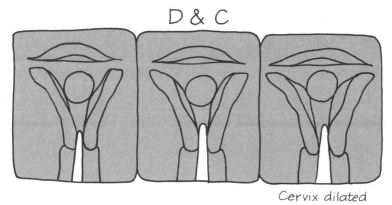

Cervix dilated

Uterine contents removed by curettage

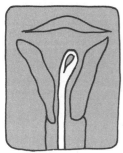 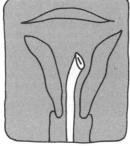

Conventional curette   Suction curette

Saline Injection

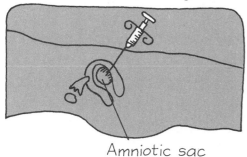

Fluid removed,
then replaced
with concentrated
salt solution.

Amniotic sac

Teenage Pregnancy

About 40 percent of all marriages in the United States involve teenagers, and more than 50 percent of high school brides are pregnant on their wedding date. Divorce rates are three times higher among this group than among marriages consummated between ages twenty-one and forty-five. "Seventeen percent of all births occur to teenagers at a time when the likelihood of adverse health and social consequences for mother and infant is much greater than if the birth were postponed to the years between twenty and thirty-five," states the Commission on Population and the American Future.[19] In addition, 27 percent of girls fifteen to nineteen years deliver out-of-wedlock.

For the very young mother, the risks that the baby will be stillborn, die soon after birth, be born prematurely, or have a serious physical or mental handicap are much higher than for women in their twenties. The increased risk of prematurity is the most important medical aspect of teenage pregancy. Prematurity is even more closely related to the trimester of pregnancy in which prenatal care begins than it is to the age of the mother. The complications of pregnancy most frequently mentioned for young mothers are toxemia, prolonged labor, and iron-deficiency anemia. Menken states, though, that ". . . the voluminous literature on the pregnant teenager overwhelmingly points toward social rather than medical [or biological problems] as the primary concern."[20] Social aspects of teenage pregnancy, in or out of wedlock, are not auspicious: permanent disruption of schooling, economic disadvantages in terms of occupation, income, and assets when compared to other couples, and higher marital dissolution rates for the premaritally pregnant.[21]

CHILDBIRTH

By using knowledge of conception, a woman today can conceive and bear children under as optimal conditions as possible. She can carry her child during the best years, which are from twenty to thirty, and can limit pregnancies to a desirable spacing of one every two or three years. In addition, the husband and wife can have a child when they feel ready emotionally and economically. Many facilities in the community are available to help them prepare for the coming birth and parental responsibilities. Despite planning for conception, when the event actually happens both the father and mother will feel doubts. It is not uncommon for couples to "wish the pregnancy hadn't happened now." Understanding what is taking place physically and emotionally can reduce such doubts and make the period of pregnancy, childbirth, and child rearing a fulfilling experience.

Conception

At the instant that one sperm penetrates the ovum in the Fallopian tube, all inherited characteristics of this new life are determined. Much of what happens during the course of pregnancy, though, can affect how this child will develop as he grows and matures after birth. The mechanism of fertilization is not completely understood. Electronic microscopes and timelapse photography have enabled scientists to record this event by placing a human ovum recovered surgically in media containing sperm. The germinal cells are not attached to the mother, and they are so small that she cannot feel conception. At this momentous instant of fertilization and the beginning of life, the parents don't *know* that it has happened. They only know it could happen.

As described previously, the ovum is viable for less than twenty-four hours and probably highly fertile for no more than six to twelve. Although sperm can live for as long as seventy-two hours in the female genital tract, they, too, are most likely highly fertile for only twelve to twenty-four hours. The female secretions in the cervix and uterus are more easily penetrated by the spermatozoa when an ovum is present, and during ovulation there seems to be something that attracts the sperm to the Fallopian tubes. Of the approximately 400 million sperm deposited, though, only a few hundred thousand travel through the cervix to start the several hours journey to the egg.

Multiple Births

An average of one out of a hundred pregnancies produces twins; this number squared, triplets; and cubed, quadruplets. One of the causes of multiple births is heredity, and the chances are greatly increased if both the mother and father carry such genes. Oriental people have fewer and blacks more multiple births than the white population. Women between thirty and thirty-five years have the greatest number.

Multiple births are of two types. When more than one ovum is present, the result is fraternal twins. These children are no more similar or dissimilar than siblings born from different pregnancies. One-egg twins have the same genetic background and are alike in all characteristics, including sex. In the case of identical twins, something causes the fertilized egg to divide into equal parts before cell differentiation takes place. Frequently, the physician is able to tell at the time of birth whether or not twins are identical or fraternal. (Obviously, if the twins are of different sex, they must be of the two-egg type.) In mammals that regularly produce more than one ovum per cycle, fertilization can be accomplished by sperm from more than one male. In humans, this is not probable though it has occurred.

"Choosing" the Baby's Sex

Theory is that the X and Y chromosome-bearing sperm are biologically different. This difference determines which type of sperm is more likely to fertilize the ovum. The X chromosome-bearing sperm is larger than the Y-bearing one, it is less susceptible to adverse environmental influences such as the pH of the vaginal tract and cervical mucus, and it lives longer. The Y-bearing sperm are smaller and move much more quickly, and many more of them are in the ejaculate of most males. At the time of ovulation, the secretions in the vagina and the cervix are most favorable to the longevity and motility of all sperm. When the female has an orgasm at the same time her partner ejaculates, the environment is even more favorable. Timing of intercourse, then, may be a factor in determining sex. Intercourse at or close to the time of ovulation is more apt to produce a boy baby, while coitus two or three days before the time of ovulation is more likely to yield a girl baby since the X-bearing sperm can survive longer. An alkaline douche prior to intercourse favors boy sperm and an acid douche favors girl sperm. In several studies, couples using this knowledge had an 80 to 85 percent success rate, in selecting the sex of their child.[22]

Amniocentesis during the second trimester can be used to determine sex. This procedure is considered a low-risk prenatal diagnostic procedure for genetic screening if it is done by an expert. However, a decision to abort solely to select sex of the expected child poses ethical questions. Abortions do, of course, involve greater risks during the second trimester.

Another experimental sex prediction procedure is an examination of cells from the endocervical canal during the first trimester. This method poses little if any risk to mother or embryo. Accuracy of gender prediction was 93.9 percent according to investigators.[23]

Embryonic and Fetal Development

A little more than a day after penetration of the egg by the sperm, cell division begins. At the end of three days, there are thirty-two cells, which look very much like a berry and are called the *morula*. During this time,

FOUNDATIONS OF HEALTH SCIENCE

the fertilized ovum is slowly traveling down the tube. Once it reaches the uterus, it is another four days before the morula attaches itself to the uterine wall. By now two layers of cells are apparent. The inner layer will develop into the embryo and the outer layer is composed of trophoblasts or feeding cells. At the point of implantation the trophoblasts burrow into the uterine lining by dissolving some of the cells of the endometrium, including small blood vessels, so that soon the morula has tiny pools of blood around it. Next, fingerlike projections, or *villi,* sprout out into the pools. Through the membranes of these villi, the exchange of nutrients and waste products occurs between the embryo and its mother. By three months, the trophoblasts rooted into the uterine wall develop into the *placenta,* which is a network of maternal and fetal blood vessels and membranes. At the end of nine months, this organ has grown to a diameter of about eight inches and weighs approximately one pound. As Figure 11.11 shows, there is no intermingling of blood per se between the embryo and the mother.

In the early stages of development, a sac forms around the embryo called the *amnion,* which secretes amniotic fluid in which the embryo is suspended. The umbilical cord also forms. It contains the two arteries and one vein through which the baby's blood flows to and from the placenta. The word "embryo" is frequently used to designate the baby from the

Figure 11.11 Placental Circulation. (From Arthur C. Guyton, *Textbook of Medical Physiology* [Philadelphia: W. B. Saunders Company, 1961], p. 1100, adapted from Gray and Gross, *Anatomy of the Human Body,* and Arey, *Developmental Anatomy.*)

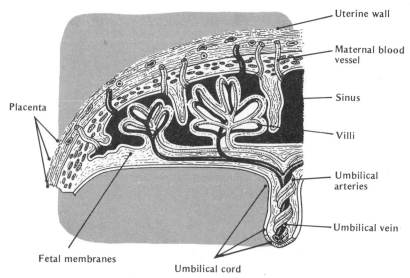

period of conception until the third month of growth, at which time it is called a *fetus*.

A woman usually considers herself one month pregnant by the time she misses a menstrual period. Actually, the embryo is only two weeks old. When the physician refers to length of pregnancy, he bases fetal age on lunar months, or four-week intervals. Beginning with conception, the fetus requires on the average ten lunar months for prenatal growth and maturation. Figure 11.12 shows the increase in size during the first twelve weeks after conception.

The first four to six weeks of embryonic development are the most crucial. Many things that happen to the mother during this time can influence proper cell growth—such as the danger of infection with the virus causing rubella. The thalidomide story is another example of interference with normal growth. Many of the tranquilizers in current use are being investigated.

No woman can be sure she is pregnant just because menstruation does not take place at the expected time. Some of the presumptive signs of pregnancy are missed menses, frequency of urination due to nervous irritability of the bladder, tingling in the breasts, and nausea and vomiting, particularly when getting up in the morning. Any of these may be due to other causes and laboratory tests must be completed by a physician to

Figure 11.12 Growth of the Embryo in Early Pregnancy. Normal fetuses, 8, 9, 10½ and 12 weeks old. (Courtesy of M. Edward Davis and Reva Rubin, *De Lee's Obstetrics for Nurses* [Philadelphia: W. B. Saunders Company, 1962], p. 48.)

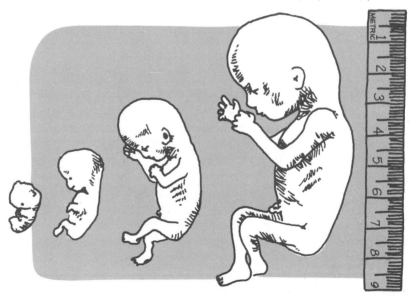

FOUNDATIONS OF HEALTH SCIENCE

determine whether a woman is actually pregnant. Definitive signs of pregnancy do not appear until the fourth to fifth month, when the baby begins to move (quickening), the fetal parts can be palpated through the abdominal wall, and the fetal heartbeart can be heard through a stethoscope.

Any woman during the child bearing years who has had intercourse without contraceptives during her fertile period should assume she is pregnant if she misses a period. If she is ill or exposed to viral infections, she should see a physician, and the doctor should be informed about a possible pregnancy whenever he prescribes medications so he can avoid using those drugs that have been shown to affect embryonic development.

Prenatal Care

Prenatal care to assure a healthy mother and baby begins with the normal birth of a girl and is continued by the maintenance of desirable health habits during childhood, adolescence, and young adulthood. The woman who has practiced the principles of good nutrition, rest, exercise, relaxation, and prevention of infection, and who has attained emotional maturity, has the best chance of going through pregnancy with minimal discomfort and giving birth to a strong, well-developed baby who is able to withstand the rigors of infancy. During the course of pregnancy, the normal changes that occur in the woman's body need to be understood; special measures should be taken to safeguard her own and her child's well-being; and the possible appearance of danger signals should alert her to the need for immediate medical care.

Nearly all pregnancies proceed without serious problems. For the very small percentage that do not, good prenatal care can lessen difficulties. The personal health habits of the mother are primarily an extension of those health practices she should have had prior to pregnancy. However, neglecting to adhere to the principles of good hygiene at this time may affect the growing baby as well as herself. As soon as conception is suspected, by the second missed period, she should get medical advice. Her first visit might be to her regular family physician, but for the best care she should obtain the services of a physician especially skilled in obstetrics. Many general practitioners are well qualified (as are licensed midwives), keep up-to-date on techniques, and deliver numerous babies. More frequently than not in the large metropolitan areas, the pregnant women will be referred to an obstetrician, one who is specially certified in this field.

Early visits to the doctor can assure:

1. Any existing health problem will be detected and treated.
2. Anatomical and physiological conditions that might interfere with the

mechanics of carrying and delivering the child can be corrected or precautions taken.

3. Maximum care is used to insure normal fetal growth.
4. The mother is advised of special nutritional needs and other required changes in daily living due to the pregnancy.
5. Constant vigilence is maintained to prevent or detect early danger signals.

Research has statistically proved a direct correlation between the number of months the mother has been under medical supervision and the percentage of successful births.

During the first six months, the doctor will want to see the mother every four weeks. Then she will be requested to come in every two weeks up until a month before the expected date of delivery. During this last period, the physician will see her weekly. The mother's body must supply nutrients and remove wastes for the baby. This places additional demands on the maternal circulatory and urinary systems so, at each visit, the physician will check heart, blood pressure, urine, and weight.

As the embryo, later the fetus, grows, certain physiological changes that take place within the body of the mother exert stresses and strains on her body and result in discomfort. During the first six weeks discomfort is due primarily to endocrine changes. The first is the suppression of menstruation, although occasionally a woman may have a small amount of bleeding at the time her period would be due for a month or so. In another three or four weeks about one-half of all fecund women have nausea and some vomiting, particularly upon arising in the morning. This condition should last only four to six weeks. The initial increase in size and change in the position of the uterus irritates the urinary bladder. This irritation produces a sensation of "fullness," and the woman feels she must urinate frequently. This, too, subsides in about a month. The expectant mother may be easily fatigued and desire a great deal of sleep. She may be very moody at times and may have apparently unprovoked emotional outbursts, which are both psychological and physiological in origin.

As pregnancy progresses, other signs appear. The increasing vascularization of the vaginal tract causes the genital area to become rather bluish in color; vaginal secretions increase; and the mucus in the cervical canal becomes quite thick and plugs or seals the opening. This plug protects the fetus from possible infection. The secretions may cause itching, and sometimes the vaginal pH level is sufficiently altered to be irritating to the woman or to the husband during intercourse. The breasts will enlarge considerably, and some women feel a tingling sensation in the nipples. The skin may darken, especially in brunettes, over the face, breasts, and abdomen. The facial discoloration will disappear after childbirth.

None of these changes are proof of pregnancy. The only 100 percent assurance is during the fourth to fifth month, when these signs are evident: fetal heart sounds, fetal movement, and outline of the fetal skeleton. Chances are, though, that a woman in good health who is ten days late or past her normal menstrual period time is pregnant. Not until this point do any of the laboratory tests have any degree of accuracy. After the second missed period, the tests are better than 95 percent correct.

After the fifth month of pregnancy, the growth of the fetus, uterus, and placenta, plus the production of amniotic fluid, place increasing amounts of pressure on and displace the internal organs, as shown in Figure 11.13. The mother may have indigestion or heartburn, shortness of breath, constipation, a reoccurrence of frequency of urination, backache from postural strain, and an interference in circulation to the lower extremities that results in swelling of the ankles, muscular cramps, and sometimes varicose veins. Competent medical care, adequate rest, and good nutrition can reduce much of the discomfort associated with these pressures.

Figure 11.13 Ninth Month of Pregnancy. Note how organs have been displaced by pressure of fetus. (Courtesy of M. Edward Davis and Reva Rubin, *De Lee's Obstetrics for Nurses* [Philadelphia: W. B. Saunders Company, 1962], p. 65.)

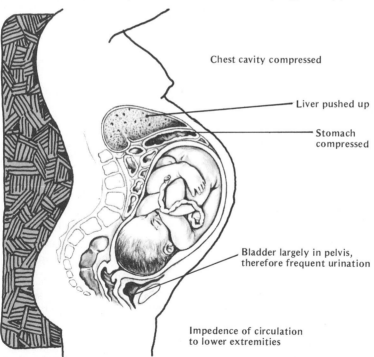

Chest cavity compressed

Liver pushed up

Stomach compressed

Bladder largely in pelvis, therefore frequent urination

Impedence of circulation to lower extremities

Excessive weight gain aggravates discomforts. Most women do not need to increase their daily caloric intake until the last several months of pregnancy, and then only a few hundred additional calories are necessary to meet the requirements of increased metabolism and fetal growth. If more food than is necessary is ingested, the excess will be converted to fat tissue. The pregnancy itself accounts for approximately fifteen pounds by delivery time. Obesity places additional strain on the heart, kidneys, and circulatory system, and it may be a contributing factor to dangerous toxemia or eclampsia. The specific cause of toxemia of pregnancy is unknown, but warning signs are: increased blood pressure, edema, albumin in the urine, convulsions, and coma. Eclampsia is the major cause of maternal death, prematurity, and neonatal death.

Other discomforts or danger signals that are not normal indicate the need for immediate medical attention if the health and life of the mother and fetus is to be maintained. These are vaginal bleeding, no matter how slight, swelling of the face or hands, severe continuous headache, dimness or blurring of vision, abdominal pain, persistent vomiting, chills and fever, and any loss of fluid from the vagina. Vaginal bleeding indicates that the placenta is separating from the uterine wall. This separation interferes with the oxygenation of the fetus. Any loss of fluid from the vagina means that the cervix is open, the amnionic sac in which the baby floats has broken, and the danger of infection is present. Abdominal pain may be a symptom of disorder in the abdominal cavity or a signal that labor is beginning. Chills and fever are associated with infection, and any severe illness has an adverse effect on pregnancy. Persistent vomiting will result in dehydration. Vomiting that is continuous and prolonged is not a normal development, even in the first few weeks after conception. The symptoms of swelling, headache, and visual disturbances are related to kidney dysfunction and toxemia.

Medications can interfere with embryonic development and fetal growth. A pregnant woman should *never* take medicines without first checking with her physician. *This rule includes everything.* For example: aspirin compounds may cause fetal bleeding; nose drops may constrict blood vessels and interfere with fetal circulation; strong laxatives may induce a miscarriage; tranquilizers and sleeping pills not only can disturb embryonic development but may interfere with oxygenation; babies can be born with narcotic dependency; excessive smoking is related to prematurity; and even vitamin and mineral supplements can be overdone.

The expectant couple will have many questions, not only about the pregnancy itself, but regarding preparations to make for the baby. Usually, attendance at expectant parent classes sponsored by health departments, hospitals, or the American National Red Cross is most helpful. Some couples find attending advantageous before a second child as well as before the first. Such classes assist the parents-to-be in understanding what is happening. The physician will usually know where classes are available. Any couple that cannot afford private obstetrical care can receive this care through the local health department and government funded hospital. Some parents are interested in one of the several techniques of natural birth, and the County Medical Society can refer them to physicians who specialize in these methods of childbirth.

Birth of the Baby

Knowledge of what is happening during childbirth can do much to allay. needless fear and minimize discomfort. About two weeks before labor begins, the baby may drop lower into the pelvic cavity. The mother will have less discomfort in breathing but may notice an increased pull on her back muscles and will need to urinate quite frequently. Labor is longer for the first baby, as a rule, and there is seldom any need to worry about getting to the hospital in time. Labor takes place in three stages. Stage I is dilation of the cervix; in Stage II the baby passes out through the vagina or birth canal; and Stage III is the expulsion of the placenta and fetal membranes.

Stage I. The first indication that Stage I is beginning is a rather steady dull ache in the low back that radiates toward the front. Next, the mother will notice abdominal cramping. Cramps or pains result when the uterus contracts and pushes the head of the baby against the cervix. In time, these contractions become harder and come at regular intervals. Eventually, as the contractions keep pushing the baby's head against the cervix, the mucous plug will be expelled. This is tinged with blood (bloody show), which the mother may or may not notice. By the time the contractions last sixty seconds or so and come every few minutes, the mother is starting the second stage of birth. In about one-third of all deliveries, the membranes will have ruptured by now and the mother will have noticed a gush of fluid. The first stage lasts anywhere from eight to twenty hours, during which period the mother can be up walking a good part of the time. When the contractions become hard enough to produce much discomfort, the physician will give the mother something to alleviate the pain.

Stage II. By the time the cervix is completely dilated, contractions will be quite hard. The second stage of labor starts as the baby begins to descend down the birth canal. It takes about an hour for the baby to make this journey. In 97 percent of all births the infant is born head first. In breech presentations (bottom first) the second stage will be longer. Disparities between the size of the fetus and the pelvic outlet can be determined prior to labor. Although vaginal birth is the safest for mother and infant, removing the baby surgically, by Caesarean section, through the abdominal wall sometimes becomes necessary. Figure 11.14 depicts the second stage of labor in the vaginal birth.

Stage III. Stage III begins as soon as the infant emerges. At first, the baby is rather bluish-looking, and the vessels in the cord are distended with blood. The baby nearly always cries immediately, and as his lungs expand, he becomes pink in color and pulsation in the cord diminishes and ceases. In about fifteen minutes, uterine contractions will resume to expel the placenta and the amniotic membranes. While waiting for the afterbirth, or placenta, to be born, the mother is able to rest, and care is taken of the infant. Mucus is aspirated from his mouth and nose; the cord is cut after the placenta is expelled; his heart and lungs are checked; medication is

Figure 11.14 Second Stage of Labor. (About one hour.) (Courtesy of M. Edward Davis and Reva Rubin, *De Lee's Obstetrics for Nurses* [Philadelphia: W. B. Saunders Company, 1962], pp. 136 and 137.)

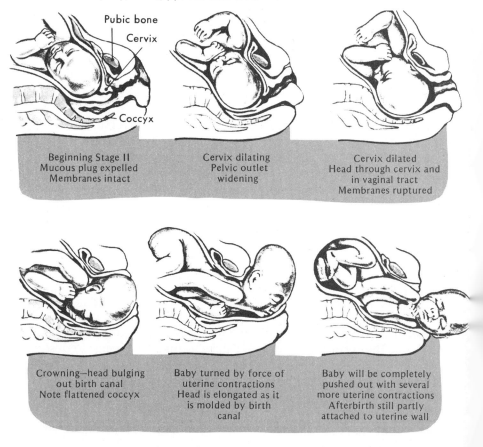

Beginning Stage II
Mucous plug expelled
Membranes intact

Cervix dilating
Pelvic outlet
widening

Cervix dilated
Head through cervix and
in vaginal tract
Membranes ruptured

Crowning—head bulging
out birth canal
Note flattened coccyx

Baby turned by force of
uterine contractions
Head is elongated as it
is molded by birth
canal

Baby will be completely
pushed out with several
more uterine contractions
Afterbirth still partly
attached to uterine wall

FOUNDATIONS OF HEALTH SCIENCE

placed in his eyes to prevent possible gonorrheal infection leading to ophthalmia neonatorum; and he is wrapped and put in a warm place. Although most mothers want to know about the baby's sex and if he is "all right," they are usually sufficiently tired that rest is uppermost in their thoughts for the first day or so.

In emergency childbirth, cutting the cord is not necessary. The danger of infection or injury to either the mother or baby is less likely if the cord is left alone. After the placenta is expelled, it can be wrapped separately and placed with the baby, with the cord left attached. If the cord was never severed, it would become hard and dry and pull away from the umbilicus in a few days.

Despite advances in scientific knowledge, the mechanism that triggers the labor process is unknown. A physician can do little *safely* to induce labor or to reduce the length of the birth time. The hazards of using drugs potent enough to stimulate strong uterine contractions are far greater than the inconvenience or discomfort of letting "nature take its course." Artificially induced labor should be reserved for those situations where it is more dangerous to allow the pregnancy to continue than to terminate it.

Pregnancy is a normal, natural process. Adequate preparation for the coming child and proper prenatal care of the mother can make it a rewarding experience for both husband and wife. When questions arise, answers should be sought from a physician or someone especially trained in the field of obstetrics. Friends and neighbors are not usually valid sources of information. Neither are couples wise to think that because

Parenthood has its ups and downs.

Larry and I were terribly happy our first four years of marriage. Don't get me wrong, we still are. We thought about having children—our in-laws bugged us enough about it —but we were afraid of the unknown. One afternoon we went to a family picnic and enjoyed watching our friends with their kids. That night, perhaps because of too much vino, we decided maybe a baby—a child couldn't be that bad. Our friends with children seemed happy enough. To make a long story short, it's been three years since that night.

At times I do resent the fact that I can't go out to dinner when I'm too tired to cook. I resent the fact that when in a group everyone goes out for pizza and beer and we have to go home because of the baby sitter. When I really think about it all, though those are just small annoyances, my life has been enriched by my child. I thought I was fulfilled before but now, now I know what enrichment and fulfillment really mean. I wouldn't trade what I have now for the past for anything. I am happy.

they have had one baby, they know all the answers. For too many years, old wives' tales have perpetuated foolish beliefs that plague the mother-to-be. A few that are still being broadcast are listed here. Did you think any of them were true?

1. You get fat during pregnancy.
2. You lose a tooth for each baby.
3. If you stretch your arms over your head, the cord will twist around the baby's neck and choke him.
4. If you look at blood, it will mark the baby.
5. You must eat twice as much since you are eating for two.
6. If you crave a certain food, you have some kind of deficiency that must be satisfied.
7. Bathing is dangerous.
8. Exercise will cause a miscarriage.
9. A shock such as a death in the family will cause a miscarriage.
10. What you think about or listen to can affect the baby.
11. Sexual relations will hurt the baby.
12. A fall or blow will bring on a miscarriage.
13. Your baby will be deformed if you sleep on your stomach.
14. Your baby will stick to your back if you sleep a lot.
15. Certain foods are harmful during pregnancy (lemons, oranges, or bananas, etc.).
16. Wine and beer are "good" for pregnant or lactating women.
17. Lactating women do not get pregnant.

PROBLEMS RELATING TO CONCEPTION

Several problems concerning conception disturb many couples. One is the inability to conceive, and another is the possibility of having a defective child.

Sterility and Infertility

Sterility is the absolute or permanent inability of the male or female to fertilize or be fertilized. Infertility, though, is a relative condition. There may be temporary periods in which conception cannot occur; or there may be a low level of fertility when it is difficult for a couple to conceive except under the most favorable conditions. Infertility is usually the result of more than one condition and is frequently caused by a combination of physiological and psychological factors. The extent of sterility and infertility is about 10 percent. The fault can be that of the man or of the woman, in a two-to-three ratio, respectively. If both happen to have a low level of fertility, remarriage to other parties may result in conception.

The major causes of either infertility or sterility are: defects in the germinal cells, obstruction in the passageways, and anatomical defects that prohibit proper deposition of the sperm. In the male, abnormalities of the sperm result from several conditions. During the uterine growth of a male child, the testes develop inside the abdominal cavity, and during the last few weeks of prenatal life, they descend through the inguinal canals into the scrotum. If this fails to happen, the germinal tissue degenerates. The physician frequently can determine abdominally located testes during the first few weeks of life. Any child with potentially undescended testicles should be periodically examined. If the testes have not descended by six or seven years of age medical treatment is necessary to help prevent sterility. This disorder, known as *cryptorchidism,* is difficult to diagnose and to correct.

Infections, especially mumps, may cause an inflammation of the testes. When this happens after puberty begins, a small percentage of males may have involvement of both testicles followed by atrophy of the germinal tissue and sterility. Malnutrition, any debilitating disease, and glandular deficiencies may result in the production of abnormal or insufficient numbers of sperm. If much less than the average number of approximately 400 million sperm are not deposited in the area of the cervix at each ejaculation, infertility is probable. Anatomical abnormalities of the penis and premature ejaculation may interfere with the mechanism of deposition.

In the female, conditions that interfere with monthly ovulation reduce fertility. Malnutrition, debilitating disease, and glandular deficiencies may result in anovulatory cycles, Anatomical and psychological factors that prevent the penetration of the penis so that sperm cannot be deposited properly reduce the chances of conception.

Some individuals are born with defects of the passageways. Frequently, infections in the seminal ducts or in the Fallopian tubes result in scar tissue and obstruction. Of the various infective agents, the gonococcus is the major pathogen producing this type of sterility. Abnormalities in the quality of seminal fluid and the structure of the uterus, position of the uterus, and the quality of the uterine lining may interfere with conception and successful implantation of the embryo.

Sterility is not easily remedied but much can be done to increase fertility. Of 10 percent of the married couples confronted with this problem, about 40 to 50 percent can be helped in fertility clinics and by specialists.

Sterility and impotence are not the same thing. Impotence is the inability to achieve or maintain an erection. The sterile or infertile male (or female) can have satisfactory sexual relations. The impotent man is not necessarily sterile, but he cannot have satisfactory relations. This latter condition is nearly always psychogenic in origin, but can be the result of diseases of the genitalia as well as systemic disorders and glandular dysfunctions.

BIRTH DEFECTS

Estimates indicate that about one-fourth million babies are born in the United States each year with some type of birth defect. Some of these are genetic—the result of defective genes—and others are congenital—the result of defective development after conception. Damage to the embryo and fetus can result from maternal exposure to drugs, other chemicals, radiation, and pathogens such as viruses and disease-producing microbes. There are a number of defects for which the cause is still unknown.

Heredity

When one sperm finally penetrates all the way into the ovum, a change takes place that causes all other sperm to be repelled. The tail of the sperm is no longer apparent and the head portion containing its twenty-three chromosomes merges with the nucleus of the ovum containing its twenty-three chromosomes derived from the mother. The arrangement of the genes as each pair of chromosomes match up determines the inherited characteristics of this new life.

It is assumed by many people that genetic contributions of parents are blended in each offspring so that what is passed on from one generation to the next is a compromise of traits from the sperm and ovum. This belief is far from true. The units of inheritance, *genes,* are arranged in a sequence like beads on a string. The string is called a *choromosome,* and it is found in the nucleus of each cell. Each gene has its own place, *locus,* on the chromosome. The purpose of the gene is to tell the cells how to replicate themselves. The genes have different sets of instructions called *alleles.* When the sets of instructions at a particular locus on the chromosome from the sperm and the chromosome from the ovum are the same, the individual is said to be homozygous for that trait. If these sets of instruction are different, he is said to heterozygous. There may be hundreds of alleles at a given locus. Some sets of alleles are dominant and some are recessive. Dominance does not mean that the dominant gene is more apt to be transmitted than a recessive gene; such genes are not more common, nor are they more

428   FOUNDATIONS OF HEALTH SCIENCE

apt to replace recessive alleles in the process of evolution, nor are they better or worse than recessive genes. It is true that sometimes recessive alleles are harmful in double doses (received from each of the sperm chromosomes and ovum chromosomes). The X chromosome contains a number of loci for genes that have nothing to do with sex, but some genes are called "sex-linked" only because they are on the X chromosome.

Characteristics determined by heredity include body proportions, stature, weight, coloring, blood types, potential intelligence, potential muscular performance, potential musical ability, and predispositions to certain diseases such as allergies, diabetes, hypertension, other cardiovascular disorders, some forms of mental illness, and possibly cancer. Several genetic disorders are of particular concern to people because of the serious effects in newborns and the developing child.

The Rh Factor. Rh disease is caused when an Rh negative mother is immunized by the red cells of her Rh positive fetus. The Rh factor is a substance found on the surface of some red blood cells. A baby with an Rh positive father and an Rh negative mother often inherits the Rh factor from its father. Sometimes during pregnancy, but more often from delivery, miscarriage, or abortion, some of the infant's Rh positive blood cells get into the mother's blood stream. Since they are foreign to the mother's blood, her body may manufacture an antibody to fight them off, which can circulate back to a fetus.

This process, anti-Rh isoimmunization, destroys the infant's red blood cells and produces anemia, heart failure, and sometimes elevated abnormal chemicals that are toxic to the brain. Such infants may receive exchange transfusions of compatible Rh negative blood, but this practice involves some risk, including edema, brain damage, and severe heart failure. About 13 percent of all women are Rh negative, and approximately 10 percent of them are sensitized in each pregnancy. Although many Rh negative mothers have three or more Rh positive infants without becoming immunized, there is an added risk with the birth of each Rh positive child. An immune globulin, $Rh_0(D)$ immune Globulin (Human) is now available. This globulin must be used at the termination of each pregnancy to prevent hemolytic disease in the next pregnancy. It works by temporarily suppressing the anti-Rh isoimmunization process that is stimulated by removal of the uterine contents during delivery, miscarriage, or abortion.

Sickle Cell Anemia. The name Sickle Cell Anemia comes from the effect this disorder has on the hemoglobin of red blood cells; it causes them to elongate and assume a sickle or crescent shape. Genetically, this condition is due to a recessive gene. Two genes, one from each parent, produce the disease. If only one defective gene is present, the person is said to be a "carrier" and can transmit the trait to any offspring. A carrier is rarely affected by symptoms of sickle disease.

In a person with sickle disease, lack of oxygen causes the red corpuscles to assume a sickle shape. These cells, then, cannot glide smoothly through the capillaries. They jam up and prevent the blood from circulating. When this blockage occurs, the person is said to have a "crisis." Crises are characterized by extreme pain and ultimately failure of major body organs. No satisfactory treatment is known for Sickle Cell Anemia, and life expectancy for those who have it is usually under thirty years of age.

Sickle Cell Anemia primarily affects those of African ancestry, and one out of every ten blacks in the United States possess the genetic trait, *but not the disease.* Unfortunately, determining whether the fetus has the disease prior to birth is impossible.

Tay-Sachs Disease. Tay-Sachs Disease is another genetically caused disorder that is ten times greater among Jews of central and eastern European ancestry. In this disease, cerebromacular degeneration and faulty metabolism of fats result in retardation. Life expectancy is three months to eighteen years of age. Fortunately, detecting this disorder is possible prenatally —soon enough for the parents to elect therapeutic abortion if so desired.

Trisomy 21. Trisomy 21 is more widely known as mongolism or Down's syndrome. If in the process of maturation of the ovum a pair of chromosomes remain stuck together, when fertilization takes place the embryo will have three of a particular chromosome—*trisomy.* Some times a chromosome is lacking; this condition is known as *monosomy.* Usually, trisomy or monosomy are fatal; the embryo does not survive. When the chromosome pair number 21 is affected, the embryo can survive and is born with a configuration of symptoms called trisomy 21, or Down's syndrome.[24] One in 2,000 women twenty-five years of age produce a mongoloid child, but the average for women over forty-five years is one in fifty.

The syndrome is characterized by short stature, slightly slanted eyes, and varying degrees of mental retardation. Usually this choromosomal error is a result of environmental influences during prenatal development, but approximately 3 percent of the time it is hereditary.

Genetic Counseling

Genetic counseling provides and interprets medical information. According to the National Foundation–March of Dimes:

Used as tools, the basic laws governing heredity, plus knowledge of the frequency of specific birth defects in the population enable the genetic counselor to predict the probability of recurrence of a given abnormality in the same family. Sophisticated new techniques are being rapidly developed and refined to translate statistical estimates into accurate forecasts, using tests before birth to determine the presence or absence of a growing list of inherited defects.

Genetic counseling is concerned with *all* factors causing birth defects. A counselor must first determine whether the defect in question is transmitted by the genes passed from parents to children or is due to infection or other influence during life in the womb. The primary aim is to prevent defects, or if that is not possible, to reverse or at least reduce their damaging effects.[25]

Although inbreeding (marrying a blood relative) can increase the chances of undesirable traits appearing, it can also increase the chances of desirable traits. If a couple is related, or if either or both sides of the family have a history of a particular disease or abnormality, they may find discussing the chance of passing on deleterious genes to their offspring with a geneticist will be helpful. Studies indicate, though, that environment is a greater force in shaping physical and emotional maturation than heredity. Environmental influences begin at the time of conception, so what happens to the child before it is born may determine its future. Research has also shown that individuals' potentials are much greater than their achievements. Modern programs can help the most "limited" human being develop to levels unknown in the past.

IN CONCLUSION

The nurturing of a child starts with conception. Heredity and the environmental influences acting upon the child before birth will have already determined to some extent what he or she will be after birth. All children are born with capacities or potentials that they rarely attain. Attainment requires that children be "wanted." The time of their birth should be planned. Parents who understand how children grow and develop can provide a family setting that will help each child to become more nearly what he or she is capable of becoming.

Notes

1. The male urethra acts as an excretory passage for both semen and urine. Only one function takes place at a time. During penile erection, pressure prohibits the flow of urine from the bladder.

2. William H. Masters and Virginia E. Johnson, *Human Sexual Response* (Boston: Little, Brown & Co., 1966), p. 266.

3. *Birth Control Handbook* (Montreal: Montreal Health Press, 1973), p. 36.

4. Alan Guttmacher, "Family Planning," *American Journal of Nursing*, 69:1332, 1969.

5. Ibid.

6. "Contraceptives, Biggest Pill Study Ever," *Medical World News*, 15:4, June 28, 1974.

7. Rose Kushner, *Breast Cancer* (New York: Harcourt, Brace & Jovanovich, 1975), pp. 126–146.

8. Libby Machol, "Birth Control: Which Way Is Best?" *Family Health*, 8:68, April, 1976.

9. Malcom Manber, "Diethy/Stilbesterol," *Medical World News*, 17:44–57, August 23, 1976.

10. Miriam T. Manisoff, "Intrauterine Devices," *American Journal of Nursing*, 73:1189, 1973.

11. Ibid., p. 1192.

12. "1.3 Million Sterilized in "75," *The Nation's Health*, 7:3, June, 1976.

13. "Contraception," *Medical World News*, 17:5, May 31, 1976.

14. "Abortion," *Newsweek*, 85:19, March 3, 1975.

15. Ibid.

16. Ibid.

17. Ibid., p. 23.

18. Ibid., p. 25.

19. Jane Menken, "The Health and Social Consequences of Teenage Childbearing," *Family Planning Perspectives*, 4:45, 1972.

20. Ibid., p. 51.

21. Ibid.

22. Benjamin A. Kogan, *Human Sexual Expression* (New York: Harcourt, Brace & Jovanovich, 1973), p. 219.

23. David N. Leff, "Boy or Girl: Now Choice, Not Chance," *Medical World News*, 16:45–57, December 1, 1975.

24. The National Foundation—March of Dimes, *Genetic Counseling* (White Plains, N.Y.: The National Foundation—March of Dimes, n.d.), pp. 10–11.

25. Ibid., p. 5.

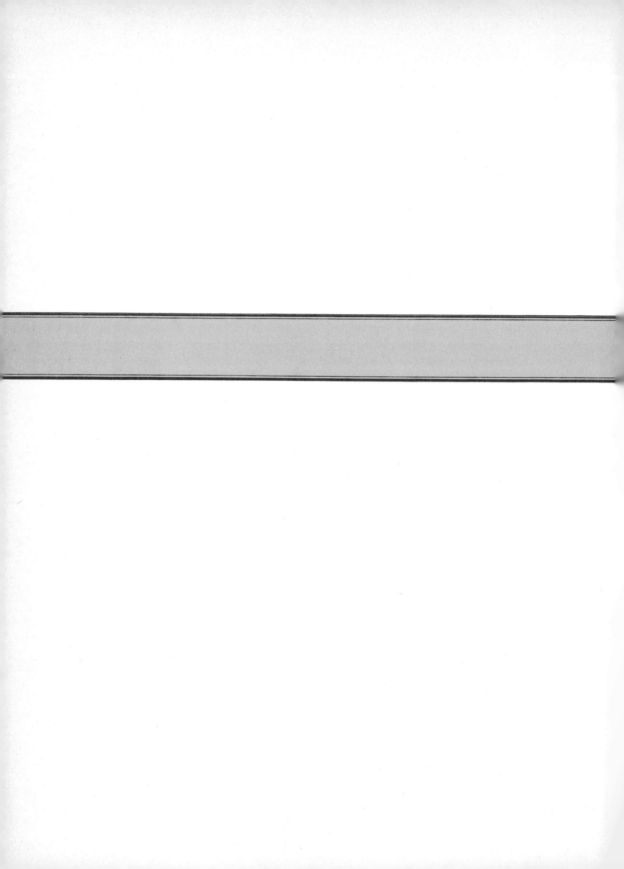

DEBILITATORS: CHRONIC AND DEGENERATIVE DISEASES

chapter twelve

Chronic and degenerative diseases are the great debilitators. They deprive many individuals of happy, productive years of life. The effects of these debilitators can be ameliorated through the application of proper health maintenance procedures described in Chapter 3. As consumers of medical services, each of us also needs to know the nature of specific chronic disorders so that we can make wise decisions about when to obtain medical care and about how to avoid the huckster who eagerly preys on those who are afflicted.

CARDIOVASCULAR DISEASES

Diseases of the cardiovascular system are the leading cause of death and one of the major causes of disability. In the United States they account for approximately one-half of the mortality in the age range of forty-five to sixty-five years. However, progress in research, a decrease in smoking, at least among older adults, and improved eating habits among the better-educated, high-risk population, plus more skilled cardiac care, have contributed to a drop in coronary mortality of about 10 percent during the last five years. Since increasing numbers of people are over sixty-five years of age, though, we can continue to expect that cardiovascular diseases will remain in first place as a cause of morbidity and mortality. Twenty-seven million Americans do have some type of heart disease and about 1.2 million die from this cause yearly.[1]

The term *cardiovascular* refers to the heart and blood vessel system comprised of arteries, smaller vessels called arterioles, capillaries, venules, and veins. Defects may be of the heart itself or of the blood vessels. Disorders of the vessels place a strain on the heart that in time can cause it to become diseased. Abnormalities of the arteries supplying the brain, kidneys, and the heart muscle can reduce the circulation in these organs to the point where the organs cannot function. Four out of five deaths due to cardiovasculorenal conditions are caused by disorders of the heart itself. However, disease of the arteries of the heart, coronary artery disease, is the most prevalent; it accounts for 90 percent of all deaths from heart disease. Figure 12.1 is a diagram of the heart.

Arteriosclerosis and Atherosclerosis

Arteriosclerosis means hardening of the arteries. The artery is made up of an outer lining called "adventitia"; a middle layer of smooth muscle cells, or "media"; and an inner lining, or "intima." As aging occurs, deposits of calcium develop in the media and make it less and less elastic.

Do you take care of yourself?

Sickness really scares me. Last August my Uncle died of cancer. Now I know, sickness can happen to anyone. You never expect it will happen to you but it does. People should really take care of themselves but even if they do they can still get sick. It is like a never ending battle and even if you try as hard as you can you may still come up the loser. When I get sick, I take care of myself but I also try to think that things could be worse. If I have a little ache or pain I try to remember that it is not the terrible agony—and I mean *agony* that I could have with something worse. I don't like to be sick because it scares me. I'm so afraid that some one close to me is going to get really sick. When some one gets sick and dies they leave the people around them sick. That is a kind of sickness that doesn't go away. I just don't understand why people don't take care of themselves. The consequences are awful. I wouldn't want to hurt my family by letting them watch me sick and dying.

FOUNDATIONS OF HEALTH SCIENCE

Figure 12.1 The Heart. The drawing on this page is a pictorial diagram to show the course taken by the blood from the body → to the heart → to the lungs → back to the heart → and to the body again. The heart is a powerful hollow organ divided, by a muscular wall, into two main divisions—a right and a left. Each side has two chambers which work together as a unit. The blood flows from the body into the right side of the heart through veins. From there it is pumped to the lungs, where it gets rid of a waste gas (carbon dioxide) collected from the body cells and picks up oxygen to carry to the body cells. After passing through the lungs the blood flows into the left side of the heart, from which it is pumped to the body through arteries. (Courtesy of the Metropolitan Life Insurance Company.)

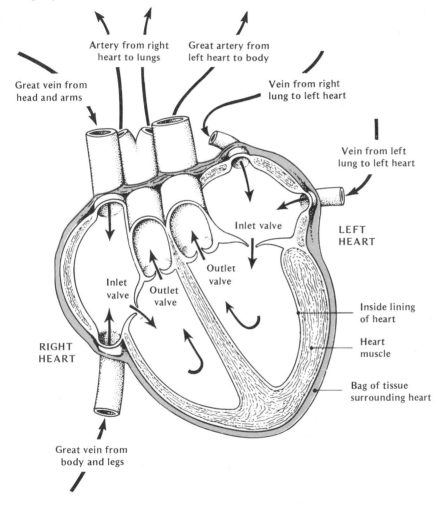

If these tubes become too rigid, circulation is impeded. The arterioles, which are between the arteries and the capillaries, have similar layers but their proportion of smooth muscle cells is greater. The immediate cause of high blood pressure is change in the muscle lining of the arterioles.

Atherosclerosis is a different kind of hardening of the arteries. Plaques of cholesterol develop in the arterial wall, but in this instance in the inner lining, the intima. These hardened spots grow out into the lumen, or passageway. Sometimes they protrude far enough into the lumen to block it, and in other instances the plaques are so rough that they injure the platelets in the blood as it flows by. When platelets are damaged, a blood clot forms. If this blood clot attaches itself to the roughened spot, it is called a *thrombus*. If it breaks away and circulates in the blood stream, it

Figure 12.2   Development of Atherosclerosis in a Coronary Artery. (From *Heart Attack,* American Heart Association. Pamphlet, 1956. © American Heart Association. Reprinted with permission.)

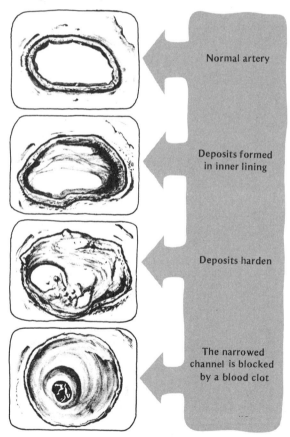

Normal artery

Deposits formed
in inner lining

Deposits harden

The narrowed
channel is blocked
by a blood clot

FOUNDATIONS OF HEALTH SCIENCE

is known as an *embolus*. When a thrombus becomes large enough, it will occlude the passage. An embolus may eventually be swept into an artery smaller than it is and cause blockage. Figure 12.2 demonstrates the development of atherosclerosis in the arteries of the heart.

Coronary Artery Disease

When there is insufficient blood to the heart muscle, *coronary insufficiency,* a typical pattern of pain ensues called *angina pectoris.* Anginal pain may result from a slowing down of circulation or actual stoppage due to an occlusion. Figure 12.3 contrasts these two causes of cardiac pain.

Angina can be a warning of an impending heart attack. When a person recognizes the pattern of this pain, he can get medical attention sufficiently early—this is a key to survival—to prevent death. Many of the 250,000 out-of-hospital deaths claimed by heart attacks in this country yearly could have been avoided.[2] All pains in the chest *do not* mean a heart attack; dull soreness or jabbing pains in the left chest are likely to be the result of tension. The illustrations in Figure 12.4 depict patterns of coronary pain signaling possible heart attack.

Coronary occlusion is the kind of heart disease that most people fear because it is apparently sudden. Actually, the symptoms of atherosclerosis and coronary artery insufficiency are present some time before any crisis. A heart attack usually refers to a sudden closing or occlusion of one of the coronary arteries by an embolus or a thrombus. When an obstruction nears the end of an artery, necrotic changes occur. The area affected is cone like in appearance and is referred to as an *infarct.* (Infarcts may occur in other organs than the heart.) Laboratory tests can show the amount of heart muscle damaged and the rate of repair that follows. Figure 12.5 illustrates coronary occlusions.

Men have an annual incidence rate of first myocardial infarction that is five times that of women. About one-third of these are fatal in forty-eight hours. Of those that survive sixty days, three-fourths are alive at least five years, and one-half live for ten years.[3] Myocardial infarction is twice as prevalent among males who smoke, who are 15 percent above average in weight, and who have low levels of physical activity. The chances that infarction in men will be fatal is also much greater among those not physically active. Figure 12.6 depicts the average annual incidence rate for these men.

Fortunately, when an occlusion or stricture in one of the large arteries takes place, small arteries will expand in time and take over the job of circulation. Sometimes new arteries grow. This process is referred to as developing *collateral circulation.* The victim may need to rest quietly

Figure 12.3 Differential Diagnosis of Stable Angina Pectoris and Pre-Infarction Angina. (Courtesy of Ives Laboratories Inc., New York.)

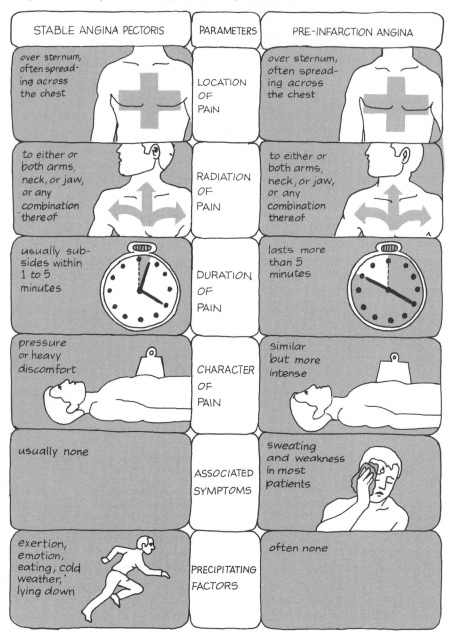

STABLE ANGINA PECTORIS	PARAMETERS	PRE-INFARCTION ANGINA
over sternum, often spreading across the chest	LOCATION OF PAIN	over sternum, often spreading across the chest
to either or both arms, neck, or jaw, or any combination thereof	RADIATION OF PAIN	to either or both arms, neck, or jaw, or any combination thereof
usually subsides within 1 to 5 minutes	DURATION OF PAIN	lasts more than 5 minutes
pressure or heavy discomfort	CHARACTER OF PAIN	similar but more intense
usually none	ASSOCIATED SYMPTOMS	sweating and weakness in most patients
exertion, emotion, eating, cold weather, lying down	PRECIPITATING FACTORS	often none

FOUNDATIONS OF HEALTH SCIENCE

Figure 12.4 Patterns of Coronary Pain. (Reprinted from "Alerting Public to Heart Attack Signs—Without a Stampede," *Medical World News* 14:18–19, March 9, 1973, and 15:14, April 6, 1973. Copyright © 1973, McGraw-Hill, Inc.)

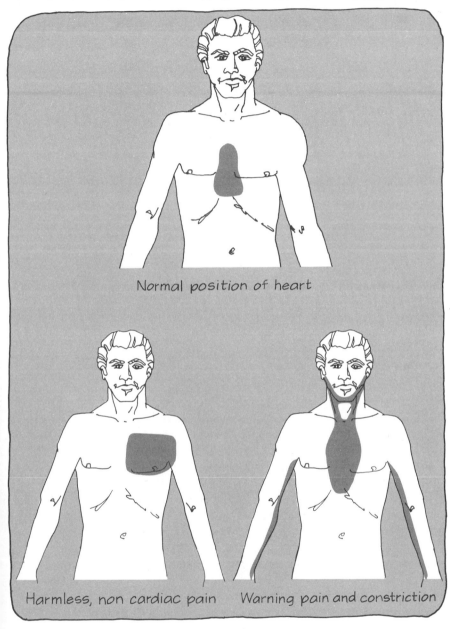

Normal position of heart

Harmless, non cardiac pain   Warning pain and constriction

Figure 12.5 Coronary Occlusion. (From *The Circulatory System,* PHS. No. 482. Washington, D.C.: Superintendent of Documents, 1963, p. 40.)

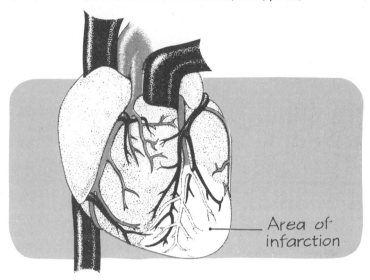

Area of infarction

while the necrotic tissue is being absorbed, and collateral circulation occurs. Medications are available that aid in dissolving clots as are vaso-dilators to relax and expand arteries.

Follow-up studies of persons who have suffered acute heart attacks show that many can resume their normal occupations or other suitable work and live for many years in reasonable health. Those people without occlusions live longer than those with. Among those without an infarct, 85 percent can survive five years and 60 percent at least ten years. Among people with an infarct, three-fourths can survive five years and one-half for ten.[4] Therefore, getting the victim to the hospital in the preinfarct stage is of vital importance in increasing longevity.

A commonly accepted view is that some personality types are more apt to have heart attacks than others. Two prominent cardiologists believe our behavior is a greater determinant of premature coronary artery disease than other factors. As quoted in *Medical World News,* these men, Friedman and Rosenman, state in their book, *Type A Behavior and Your Heart,* that 90 percent of heart attack victims are aggressive, impatient, competitive, and time conscious.[5] Possibly half of all U.S. males and a large number of females fall into this category, which they call Type A. Changing patterns of behavior can reduce coronary risk substantially. They have devised a simple self administered test that can reveal whether the person is a Type A. However, this hypothesis is not widely accepted by the medical community or by such organizations as the American Heart Association. The

FOUNDATIONS OF HEALTH SCIENCE

Figure 12.6 Average Annual Incidence of First Myocardial Infarction among Men in Relation to Over-all Physical Activity Class (Age-adjusted rates per 1,000). (From Sam Shapiro and others, "Incidence of Coronary Heart Disease in a Population Insured for Medical Care [HIP]," *American Journal of Public Health,* Supplement, Part II, 59:19, June, 1969.)

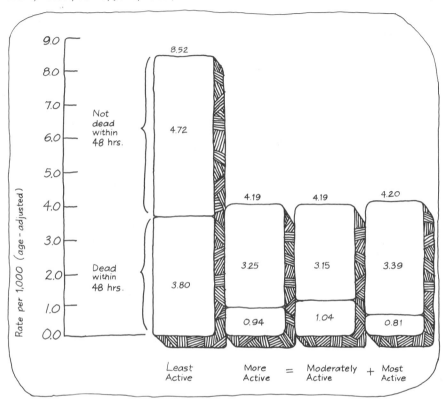

Association's present position is that Type A behavior is not the major cause, instead multiple factors influence heart attack risks. These act in varying proportions with different individuals. The roles of behavior, stress, personality, and life style have a bearing, but also do hypertension, smoking, and high serum cholesterol levels.[6] Friedman and Rosenman did not include the factors of obesity and exercise.

Congestive Heart Failure

In congestive heart failure, the heart becomes so filled with blood that it is unable to work. The left ventricle cannot empty itself, and slowly blood becomes dammed up in the atrium and pulmonary veins. The muscle wall enlarges in an attempt to increase the circulatory output, but the ventricle eventually becomes distended and inefficient. Failure occurs. The lungs also become congested and the victim has trouble breathing (cardiac asthma). If the same thing occurs on the right side of the heart, the blood backs up into the inferior vena cava, the vein bringing blood from the lower portion of the body. Congestion then takes place in the liver and other abdominal organs. When organs or systems are congested with blood, fluid seeps out of the blood vessels into the extracellular spaces and interferes with their functions.

Medical treatment is both long-range and immediate. The long-range plan is to ameliorate or reduce the causes underlying ventricle inefficiency, which include scarred valves, myocardial infarction, and chronic hypertension. Immediate action is to relieve the congestion by administering medicines such as digitalis to improve heart action and to begin regimens to reduce fluid retention in the tissues by such things as diuretics to increase kidney output and low-sodium or salt-free diets. Physical activities must be modified and kept in line with the ability of the heart to work. This disease develops slowly, but the sooner the victim is under medical supervision the less apt he is to require drastic changes in his pattern of living.

Congenital Heart Disease

Thirty to forty thousand babies are born yearly with defects of the heart or aorta. If these are minor they may cause little trouble. During fetal life, oxygenation of the blood takes place in the placenta rather than in the lungs, so that in fetal circulation most of the blood bypasses the lungs. This shunting occurs by way of a small duct between the aorta and pulmonary artery (ductus arteriosus) and an opening between the two upper chambers of the heart (foramen ovale). These normally close shortly after birth, but if they remain open (patent), the heart is not efficient. Another, and the most common, anomaly is a ventricular septal defect through which, during contractions, blood from the left ventricle can be forced into the right, thus bypassing the lung. Sometimes coarctation of the aorta occurs, in which a stricture or narrowing of the aorta prevents the passage of blood. In many cases, congenital heart conditions can be remedied surgically.

Cerebrovascular Accidents

Approximately one out of every one hundred people will suffer from a cerebrovascular accident, known as CVA, *apoplexy,* or *stroke.* This condition is the result of some interference in the circulation to the brain. Clotting or cerebral thrombosis is more common in people past sixty years of age and accounts for two-thirds of CVAs. Hemorrhage is the cause of about one-fifth of the cases and occurs after fifty years of age.

About one-third of stroke victims have such preliminary symptoms as dizziness, nausea and vomiting, transient weakness, or loss of sensation of one side of the body. However, at least three-fourths have a history of cardiovascular disorder. Possibly as many as one-third of stroke victims have *transient ischemic* attacks (TIA). A transient ischemic attack is produced by a temporary reduction or loss of blood supply to a region of the brain. This reduction may be caused by a partial or total obstruction of the carotid or vertebrobasilar system or a critical fall in blood pressure. These symptoms, which *clear in twenty-four hours,* include: slurred speech; paralysis on one side, or merely weakness or numbness; blindness in one eye; double vision; sudden falls due to weakness of the legs; staggering or incoordinated walking; and sudden movement or whirling of surrounding objects.[7]

TIA can herald an impending stroke. Estimates indicate that over a five-year period, 35 percent of patients with histories of TIA will have a major stroke. Such stroke-prone individuals may also display such symptoms as a harsh bruit (noise) in the neck (heard with a stethoscope), episodes of auricular fibrillation, cholesterol or platelet fibrin emboli observable in the retinal arterioles (eyes), elevated blood pressure, elevated fasting blood sugar, abnormal electrocardiograms, increased serum cholesterol, and a history of cardiovascular disorder.[8]

Vascular surgery is often indicated to reduce the frequency of transient ischemic attacks and to prevent a stroke. The lesions most easily removed surgically are those located in the cervical carotid artery or in the arch of the aorta. If these blood vessels are constricted, they can be bypassed by vein grafts or Dacron prostheses. If the cause is an embolus and it can not be reached surgically, anticoagulants might be used.[9] The treatment of any existing heart disease, hyperlipidemias, and diabetes reduces the probability of stroke, too.

At the time of the cerebral vascular accident, the patient may suffer headache, nausea and vomiting, convulsions, and coma. The specific symptoms depend upon where the lesion is. The most common ones are paralysis of one side of the body (hemiplegia) and speech disorders. Memory may also be affected. The signs develop suddenly and become severe within a few minutes. The outcome depends on the size and place of the damage. Unless there is extensive hemorrhage, death is rare. After two to three weeks, the paralysis tends to improve, though it may take as long as six months to know the exact extent of permanent damage. Figure 12.7 depicts how strokes occur.

The most important aspect in the treatment of stroke is rehabilitation

Figure 12.7 How Strokes Occur. (Adapted from *Facts About Strokes,* American Heart Association. Pamphlet. © American Heart Association. Reprinted with permission.)

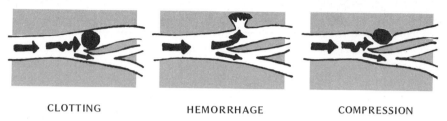

CLOTTING   HEMORRHAGE   COMPRESSION

to reduce paralysis and restore speech. Rehabilitation including speech training should begin as soon as possible. Proper positioning of limbs, massage, and exercise will restore function to some paralyzed muscles. Studies indicate that 70 to 80 percent of the patients who survive the first month after onset of a stroke can achieve self-care. Even though about one-half the victims have severe handicaps, quite a few can return to work.

Essential or Primary Hypertension

Hypertension is the most common of the diseases that affect the heart and blood vessels, and it is likely the most important affliction producing premature sickness, disability, and death in the adult population. The incidence among blacks, particularly black males, is much higher than among whites. The chance of dying, as compared to normals, is 60 percent greater among those with mild hypertension (diastolic pressure of 95 to 100), and 200 percent greater for those with severe hypertension (diastolic pressure over 105). High blood pressure not only can kill directly, but is the key contributing cause to premature heart attack and stroke deaths. Estimates are that 5 percent of the population suffer from hypertension and that yearly it causes more than a million heart attacks and strokes that either kill or make invalids of their victims. One-half of the cases of hypertension are undetected, and one-half of the known hypertensives are untreated.[10]

Physicians who care for adolescents are becoming increasingly concerned since hypertension is a significant problem among teenagers even though they have no apparent symptoms or abnormalities. Young people with elevated blood pressure readings (systolic pressures over 130) do have a higher mortality rate from coronary disease within the next twenty or thirty years than do those with lower readings.[11]

Primary hypertension is twice as common among women as among men, and the incidence is greater in the obese, diabetics, and those with a

FOUNDATIONS OF HEALTH SCIENCE

familial tendency. The average age of symptomatology is thirty-two with few new cases developing after fifty. Life expectancy is only twenty or more years after symptoms appear.

In primary or essential hypertension, the arterioles remain in a more or less constantly constricted state and produce high blood pressure. The arterioles in the kidneys, pancreas, liver, and periadrenal tissues are the ones usually affected. A diastolic pressure remaining continuously above 90 may be present for many years without other symptoms. Some people complain of periodic episodes of fatigue, nervousness, dizziness, weakness, and headaches. Eventually, they have signs of congestive heart disease, myocardial and cerebral occlusion, kidney disorder, and retinal changes in the eyes. Obesity and emotional stress will aggravate symptoms and the use of tranquilizers and drugs that reduce blood pressure are quite successful in controlling arteriole and small artery disease. Treatment cannot only lengthen the survival of patients, it can bring under control the diastolic blood pressures of nearly two-thirds of those treated, and consequently, appreciably reduce death from cerebrovascular accidents and renal complications.[12]

These are some of the things the medical profession believes everyone should know about high blood pressure or hypertension:

1. Only about 5–10 percent of all cases of high blood pressure can be traced to a specific cause.
2. In 90–95 percent of all cases of prolonged hypertension, the blood pressure increases because for some unknown reason certain small vessels (arterioles) that carry the blood become narrowed and make it harder for the heart to pump blood through the circulatory system.
3. Most people with hypertension do not feel sick or have symptoms that would alert them to the fact that their blood pressure is high.
4. High blood pressure usually cannot be cured and requires lifetime medical care. It can generally be controlled.
5. Anyone who is being treated for hypertension or who has ever been told that he has high blood pressure should have it checked regularly. There are devices available that an individual can use by himself at home to do this between medical checkups.
6. High blood pressure is a major cause of stroke, heart failure, and kidney failure. Control of hypertension reduces the possibility of these complications occurring.[13]

Prevention of Cardiovascular Diseases

In summary then, these are the characteristics of one who is a typical heart attack victim (if more than one characteristic is present, the risk is even greater for having a premature heart attack): a high level of blood cholesterol, high blood pressure, an abnormal electrocardiogram, poor respiratory functioning, a tendency toward overweight, low levels of physical activity, and excessive cigarette smoking. Physicians recommend the following measures to lessen the dangers from cardiovascular disease.

1. Obtain periodic physical examinations to detect cardiovascular changes early.
2. Follow regimens prescribed to *lower high blood pressure* and cholesterol levels.
3. Limit animal sources of fat.
4. Maintain weight at normal or even slightly below normal level.
5. Abstain from the use of tobacco, especially cigarettes.
6. Participate in vigorous physical activity of some type daily.
7. Provide for relaxation and tension-reducing activities daily.

CANCER

Even though most people know that cancer is one of the leading causes of death, many are unaware of the appearance of beginning signs of malignancy in themselves. The best means of reducing the toll taken by cancer is diagnosis during the early stages, when treatment is more successful. Too many people believe that malignancy is incurable, very painful, and most common in the aged. Almost one-half of those who die of cancer are under sixty-five, and it is the leading cause of death among women ages thirty to fifty-four years. Out of every six people who have cancer, only two will survive; yet with present techniques of treatment, three could survive, according to the American Cancer Society.

Nature of Cancer

The cells of the body are constantly multiplying, growing, sustaining injury, repairing themselves, doing their work, and eventually disintegrating. Some injuries or environmental forces produce changes that alter the genetic structure of a cell, and this change is then transmitted to new cells. Slight alterations in the genes may have no observable effect on cell function, but the accumulation of changes may eventually result in the production of a malfunctioning, abnormal cell.

In cancer, the cells stop reproducing themselves in an orderly fashion, and a disorganized proliferation of cells continues, if not stopped, until the death of the host. The exact mechanism instigating abnormal growth is not known, but it is probably the result of several different factors: endocrine imbalance, enzymatic changes, chemical compounds, irritation, radiation, and viruses. The wildly proliferating cells tend to clump together in a mass called a *neoplasm* or *tumor*. Since there is a great deal more activity in the nuclei of these cells, they divide long before they are mature and they tend to die early. Also, as the mass of cells, or neoplasm, gets larger, it extends itself beyond its capacity to obtain nourishment and circulation. This process causes cells to die (necrosis) in the center of the neoplasm, which results in ulceration and bleeding—two symptoms of cancer. The tumors eventually crowd out other body tissue and interfere with growth and function. They may press on nerves and produce pain and discomfort.

Neoplasms are benign or malignant. The physician tends to use the term *tumor* for benign growths. In these, the neoplasm is usually confined in a shell or capsule that limits its invasion of normal tissue. The malignant growth, known as cancer, is not confined in a capsule and is characterized by the breaking away of clumps of cells that spread to other parts of the body, where they continue to grow. This spread is called *metastasis*. The pathologist can determine by cytological examination of secondary growths the source of the original or primary neoplasm. The malignant neoplasms metastasize by spreading into neighboring tissue and permeating either lymph or blood vessels. Once in the circulatory system, they travel throughout the body. Those that get into the lymph system tend to localize in the lymph nodes. Those that travel through the blood often set up secondary growths in the lungs, bones, and liver. Once they invade the abdomen or chest cavities, they may spread throughout the whole cavity.

Cancers are classified into two main groups. *Carcinomas* arise from epithelial tissue, which is composed of cells covering the body surface and lining all the cavities, such as the lungs and genitourinary system, including the tubules of the kidneys. *Sarcomas* derive from connective tissues, which make up bone, cartilage, tendons, ligaments, and blood, Neoplasms may occur at any period of life, but the death rate increases markedly with age. Some kinds of tumors are more frequently found at one age than another. Figure 12.8 shows cancer incidence and deaths by site and sex.

Changing Patterns in Morbidity and Mortality

During the last several decades the age-adjusted cancer death rate has been declining slowly among women but has increased among men.

Figure 12.8 Cancer Incidence and Deaths by Site and Sex. (From *Cancer Facts and Figures,* 1976. American Cancer Society, p. 8.)

1976 ESTIMATES
CANCER INCIDENCE BY SITE AND SEX*

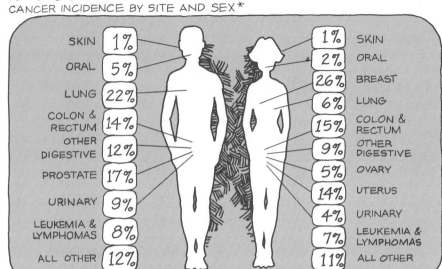

	MALE		FEMALE	
SKIN	1%		1%	SKIN
ORAL	5%		2%	ORAL
			26%	BREAST
LUNG	22%		6%	LUNG
COLON & RECTUM	14%		15%	COLON & RECTUM
OTHER DIGESTIVE	12%		9%	OTHER DIGESTIVE
			5%	OVARY
PROSTATE	17%		14%	UTERUS
URINARY	9%		4%	URINARY
LEUKEMIA & LYMPHOMAS	8%		7%	LEUKEMIA & LYMPHOMAS
ALL OTHER	12%		11%	ALL OTHER

CANCER DEATHS BY SITE AND SEX

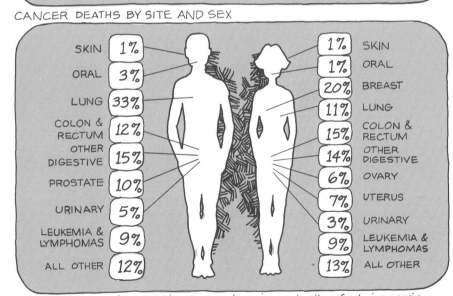

	MALE		FEMALE	
SKIN	1%		1%	SKIN
ORAL	3%		1%	ORAL
			20%	BREAST
LUNG	33%		11%	LUNG
COLON & RECTUM	12%		15%	COLON & RECTUM
OTHER DIGESTIVE	15%		14%	OTHER DIGESTIVE
			6%	OVARY
PROSTATE	10%		7%	UTERUS
URINARY	5%		3%	URINARY
LEUKEMIA & LYMPHOMAS	9%		9%	LEUKEMIA & LYMPHOMAS
ALL OTHER	12%		13%	ALL OTHER

*Excluding non-melanoma skin cancer and carcinoma-in-situ of uterine cervix.

FOUNDATIONS OF HEALTH SCIENCE

These changes are due to the early detection and treatment in females of cancer of the uterine cervix, and to the 125 percent increase since 1950 in males of lung cancer. Half of all mortality among persons over age sixty-five is due to malignancy and among women thirty to fifty-four, it is the leading cause of death while in children three to fourteen years of age more die of cancer than from any other disease.[14] (Age-adjusted rates refer to a method used to make valid statistical comparisons by assuming the same age distribution among different groups being compared).

More than one-fourth of all malignant neoplasms among women are located in the breast, and this site accounts for the heaviest cancer mortality. Each year about 15 percent of all newly diagnosed cases among both men and women are attributed to cancer of the colon and rectum combined. Cancer of the colon occurs more often in women than in men, but the reverse is true for cancer of the rectum. The incidence of stomach cancer is declining, but since it is rarely diagnosed in an early stage, the prognosis is poor. Cancer of this site is more common in men, but an estimated 6,000 deaths are expected yearly among women.[15] Although Hodgkin's disease accounts for only 1 percent of all malignancies in the United States, it is responsible for nearly 10 percent of the malignancies in the age range fifteen to thirty-four. Leukemia causes an estimated 15,000 deaths yearly; about 2,000 of these among children under fifteen years of age.[16] For the future, ". . . despite widely heralded progress in inducing remissions in childhood leukemia—some series report cure rates up to 50 percent . . . one cannot consider the disease cured. It is still a very vicious deadly cancer, and in adults it is almost uniformly fatal within a year," so reports *Medical World News.*[17]

Detection of Malignancy

The change from nonmalignant to malignant growth appears to be a gradual, continuous process. Some types of cancer grow more rapidly than others. The only way to determine accurately whether a growth is benign or malignant is by cytological or microscopic examination. Cells for this examination may be obtained by biopsy, which is the surgical removal of a piece of tissue. The procedure allows the pathologist to compare both the normal and the abnormal cells. Another technique for obtaining tissue for cytological observation is by aspirating a small number of cells from the edge of the growth with a needle. This process can be done under local anesthesia and does not require major surgery.

A third method of cytological observation is the Papanicolaou (Pap) smear. This consists of examining mucous secretions from the vagina, cervix, lungs, stomach, or any secreting organ for the presence of cast-off (exfoliated) cells that are abnormal. Special staining techniques are used to identify precancerous cells long before clinical evidence of a malignant growth exists. A "positive" test does not mean cancer, but only abnormal cells, which often can be prevented from becoming malignant. The cervical smear test for uterine cancer is well known, but the same kind of technique is used to detect early lung and stomach tumors. The practice of a yearly, or, even more desirable, a semi-annual cervical smear test is causing drastic reductions in deaths from cancer of the cervix and uterus.

A high index of suspicion on the part of everyone, including physicians, about beginning malignancy is vital to early treatment. The danger signals of cancer are listed here; any that are present longer than two weeks require medical attention:

Cancer's Seven Warning Signals

Change in bowel or bladder habits

A **sore** that does not heal

Unusual bleeding or discharge

Thickening or lump in breast or elsewhere

Indigestion or difficulty in swallowing

Obvious change in wart or mole

Nagging cough or hoarseness

Breast exam. Women should conduct monthly examinations of their breasts for lumps several days after the menstrual period terminates or, if they have ceased menstruating, at the same time each month. Most lumps are not cancerous, but should one be, early excision will almost double the chance of cure. Physicians and other trained persons can instruct

This cancer death could be prevented by preventive examinations.

At the present my grandmother has cancer. She was told this five years ago when they removed one breast. Then within a month or two the other was removed. She goes back and forth to the hospital in Columbia, Missouri. (She lives out in Mo.) Right now she's in the hospital because the cancer is just eating away at her body. The radiation treatments are just awful for her. But she keeps hanging in there. One thing that bothers me is that, "last Christmas the doctors told us she wouldn't make it." It'll be a year this Christmas. She was here this past summer and even though the weight loss is great, she looks good.

women in the technique of self-examination, and pamphlets and films are available from the local Chapter of the American Cancer Society. Figure 12.9 illustrates how to do breast self examination.

Mammography is another means of detecting breast cancer early. It is an appropriate screening procedure on a yearly basis for women past thirty-five years of age who have had previous breast cancer, a strong history of breast cancer in mother, sister, or aunt—especially on both sides of the family—and for all postmenopausal women. A good mammogram can have important diagnostic value in screening since in studies made so far 90 percent of the cancers found were picked up by mammography alone, compared with only about 60 percent by physical exam alone.[18]

Testicular cancer. Malignancy of the testes constitutes a major fraction of cancers in men between twenty and thirty-five years of age. Nearly all tumors of the testes in this age group are malignant. The average time between a man's first noticing a lump in a testis and his seeking medical help is at least six months. No one knows how soon such a lump will metastasize. The more common cancer is a seminoma, which has a cure rate of 90 percent when treated early by surgery and radiation.[19]

Figure 12.9 Self-Breast Examination. (Reprinted by permission of the American Cancer Society, Inc.)

How to examine your breasts

In the shower:

Examine your breasts during bath or shower; hands glide easier over wet skin. Fingers flat, move gently over every part of each breast. Use right hand to examine left breast, left hand for right breast. Check for any lump, hard knot or thickening.

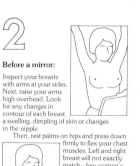

Before a mirror:

Inspect your breasts with arms at your sides. Next, raise your arms high overhead. Look for any changes in contour of each breast, a swelling, dimpling of skin or changes in the nipple.

Then, rest palms on hips and press down firmly to flex your chest muscles. Left and right breast will not exactly match—few women's breasts do.

Regular inspection shows what is normal for you and will give you confidence in your examination.

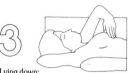

Lying down:

To examine your right breast, put a pillow or folded towel under your right shoulder. Place right hand behind your head—this distributes breast tissue more evenly on the chest. With left hand, fingers flat, press gently in small circular motions around an imaginary clock face. Begin at outermost top of your right breast for 12 o'clock, then move to 1 o'clock, and so on around the circle back to 12. A ridge of firm tissue in the lower curve of each breast is normal. Then move in an inch, toward the nipple, keep circling to examine *every part of your breast*, including nipple. This requires at least three more circles. Now slowly repeat procedure on your left breast with a pillow under your left shoulder and left hand behind head. Notice how your breast structure feels.

Finally, squeeze the nipple of each breast gently between thumb and index finger. Any discharge, clear or bloody, should be reported to your doctor immediately.

Males can easily conduct regular self-examination at least every six months. The procedure is as follows:

1. Examine after a warm shower or bath when the scrotal skin is most relaxed.
2. Feel each testicle gently between the fingers of both hands.
3. Learn what the epididymis feels like; it is a cordlike collecting structure at the back of the testicle.
4. Feeling each testicle between the fingers and thumbs of both hands, check for lumps or areas of unusual consistency.
5. An abnormality is likely to be a firm area on the front or side of the testis.[20]

In about 10 percent of cases the first sign of testicular tumor may be enlarged tender breasts; in another 10 percent the first sign may be a sudden accumulation of fluid or blood in the scrotal sac. These symptoms are readily apparent. It is the small painless lumps on the front or side of the testicles that can escape detection for a long time if not looked for actively according to urologist Ravera.[21]

Cancer of colon and rectum. The medical societies, in conjunction with the cancer societies, are promoting educational campaigns directed toward physicians as well as the general population to include proctological examinations for those over forty years as a part of their periodic physical checkups. The examination consists of manual palpation as well as the insertion of a narrow fiberoptic tube. Digital palpation, a simple finger probe of the rectum, can detect clinical prostate disease. However, only 12 percent of bowel cancers can be detected in this manner. "The risk of death from cancer of the lower bowel can be virtually eliminated by regular proctosigmoidoscopic examination, by removing all benign appearing polyps or adenomatous lesions . . . before they have an opportunity to develop further."[22]

Cancer typically begins as a local disease and the majority of cancers originate on the surface of some tissues such as on the skin, the lining of the uterus, mouth, stomach, intestines, bladder, bronchi, ducts in the breast, or prostate gland. Those that are still at the original site (in situ) are not visible to the eye. In time, these cells become invasive—they penetrate the underlying tissues. As long as they stay put, the condition is termed localized. Eventually some cells will become detached and spread through the lymph or blood vessels to other areas—metastasis, which is advanced cancer. Death is almost inevitable. Some cancers grow and spread slowly, others rapidly. About half of all cancers can be detected early enough to be cured. Figure 12.10 gives the five-year cancer survival rates for selected sites.

Figure 12.10 Five-Year Cancer Survival Rates (Adjusted for Normal Life Expectancy) for Selected Sites. (From *Cancer Facts and Figures,* 1976. American Cancer Society, p. 8.)

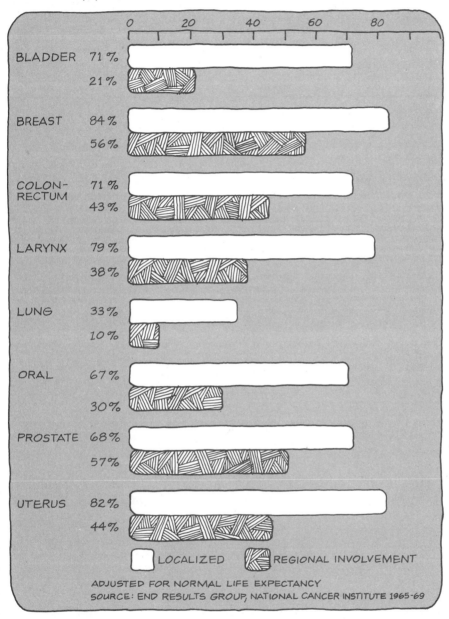

Treatment

The two major methods of curing cancer are still surgery and radiation, especially in early, nonmetastatic growths. Chemotherapy and immunotherapy tend to bring about remissions rather than cures. Cancer cure is defined as freedom from the recurrence of that growth for five years. Modern treatment nearly always consists of a combination of surgery, radiation, and chemotherapy. The team approach to treatment is best—that is, one in which the skills of the surgeon, radiologist, and chemotherapist are utilized from the beginning.

Surgery. Surgery, the most effective way of curing operable neoplastic diseases, is constantly being improved. New procedures for minimizing hemorrhage and the effects of shock, drugs that prevent infections, intravenous infusions that maintain normal body chemistry, tools such as freezing (cryosurgery), ultrasonic waves and the laser beam, and improved skills of the surgeon are enabling increasing numbers of lives to be saved.

Ionizing radiation. The nucleus in the cancer cell is especially sensitive to bombardment by ionizing radiation. The radiologists determine which source of radiation, dosage, and spacing of treatments is most effective for each specific growth. Radiation can harm normal tissues, particularly around the area treated, so radiotherapy requires a fine degree of regulation of the dose—sufficient to destroy neoplasms without greatly injuring normal tissues. Common reactions to radiation treatment are reddening of the skin, peeling, and generalized effects of malaise, nausea, vomiting, and reduction of the white and red cells. Figure 12.11 depicts an example of radiation treatment equipment.

Chemotherapy. As yet, few chemicals have been found that will cure cancer despite the fact that thousands are tested yearly. However, several are effective in causing a regression of the number of cancer cells for a period of time. Nitrogen mustard increases comfort and prolongs life for victims of cancers of the blood, such as those with acute and chronic leukemia and Hodgkin's disease. Some chemicals are of value in treating cancer of the lungs and ovaries. Most of the drugs fall into several categories. The alkylating agents disrupt the chemical organization of the cell by substituting a hydrocarbon for a hydrogen atom, and antimetabolites interfere with cell nutrition. Certain cancers of the reproductive system seem to become more prevalent when the amount of female or male hormones has decreased. Administration of sex hormones or the cortisone-like compounds that alter endocrine balance cause remissions in some cancers.

Researchers are also investigating the value of using viruses and im-

Figure 12.11 The linear accelerator, a facility for the treatment of cancer, photographed at St. Vincent's Hospital, New York City. One of the advantages of the linear accelerator is the accuracy with which the radiation fields can be defined. The equipment allows more precise definition of the dosage area so that the tumor receives a larger percentage of the dosage, with minimal effect on healthy tissues. Maximum effect of the accelerator is below the skin, whereas less penetrating types of equipment have a greater effect on the skin. (Courtesy of the American Cancer Society.)

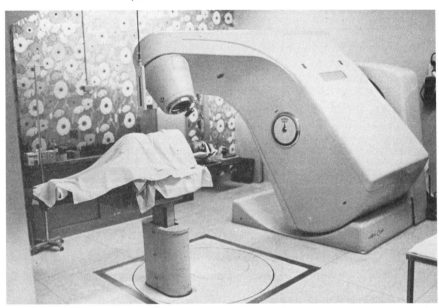

munity. Some viruses localize in and destroy different types of cells, including cancerous ones. Antibodies that are not present in others are found in cancer patients, which possibly may be the reason why more people do not have malignancies. Immunological reactions can be stimulated by injecting tumor material from one patient into another with the same type of tumor and vice versa. Within ten to twelve days, the recipient's body rejects the alien tumor material. The recipient does this by building up antibodies. The antibodies of the recipient are then injected into the donor's body and act on his cancer. This technique has resulted in partial remissions of incurable cancers in a limited number of cases.

Prevention of Cancer

Even when cancer is diagnosed early and the tools of medicine are used judiciously, numbers of people still cannot be helped. How can these diseases be prevented? Much can be done, even though the exact causes or probable causes of cancer are not known. The conditions listed below appear to be factors in the development of malignancy:

1. Tar products or hydrocarbons in cigarettes
2. Heat from pipes and cigars
3. Chronic irritation of pigmented moles by belts, straps, or shaving
4. Chronic inflammation of the cervix in women (usually from unnotice-able infections)
5. Chronic inflammation of the penis from lack of cleanliness (especially true in uncircumsized males)
6. Nonpregnancy and non–breast feeding in the female
7. Goiters from a nutritional iodine deficiency
8. Jagged teeth or ill-fitting dentures
9. Air pollution due to hydrocarbons released from incomplete combustion of gasoline, oil, and coal
10. Occupational exposure to such chemicals as tars, pitch, arsenic, benzol, asbestos, and vinyl chloride
11. Occupational exposure to ionizing radiation
12. Overexposure to sunlight.

In addition to avoiding these factors, the American Cancer Society says we should take these safeguards:

The Seven Safeguards Urged by ACS

Lung: Reduction and ultimate elimination of cigarette smoking.

Colon-Rectum: Proctoscopic exam as routine in annual checkup for those over 40.

Breast: Self-examination as monthly female practice.

Uterus: Pap test for all adult and high-risk women.

Skin: Avoidance of excessive sun.

Oral: Wider practice of early detection measures.

Basic: Regular physical examination for all adults.

DIABETES

Diabetes mellitus, referred to nonprofessionally as "sugar diabetes," is a disorder of carbohydrate metabolism due to a deficiency in insulin utilization or production. Possibly 5 percent of the population are now diabetic, and diabetes is on the increase. Diabetes is among the top ten causes of death. Symptoms become apparent most often in the forty-year-old overweight female who is related to a diabetic. When the onset is in childhood or adolescence, it may begin quite abruptly and requires stringent treatment. In adults, like many other chronic illnesses, the signs begin insidiously and are so mild that the victim frequently fails to seek medical advice early. Too often this disorder is detected in the late stages as a result of examinations for some other condition. Very early diagnosis, long before the symptoms of thirst, itching, hunger, weakness, weight loss, and frequent urination (polyuria) appear, can markedly alter the course, treatment, and outcome of diabetes.

Glucose is necessary for cell metabolism, and usable insulin must be present for this simple sugar to pass through the cell membrane. In the past, the belief was that the islets of Langerhans in the pancreas did not secrete sufficient insulin. Current research indicates that in the early stages of the disease, sufficient insulin is present but so is an antagonist in the body that prevents utilization. The condition causes the pancreas to increase insulin production, which results in a wearing out of the Langerhans cells and then eventually a decreased secretion of insulin. Such wearing out occurs within a few months to several years in the very young, but adults may never completely lose the ability to produce insulin.

A strong hereditary predisposition is a factor in the acquisition of diabetes mellitus, though probably what is inherited is the tendency to produce large amounts of insulin antagonists, of which there are several. The exact cause and mechanism of this disorder is not fully understood. What is known are these characteristics of *potential diabetics.*

1. A family history of blood relatives with diabetes. (This risk is greater if the disease is present on both sides of the family; the incidence is $2^1/_2$ percent greater.)
2. Obesity. (This risk precedes diabetes in 85 percent of the cases; the incidence is $1^1/_2$ to 4 times greater among the overweight. Mortality rates from diabetes are greatly increased among men 20 percent overweight and women 15 percent overweight.)
3. Gestational diabetes (during pregnancy) and giving birth to babies nine pounds or more in weight.
4. Subclinical or chemical diabetes wherein there are positive laboratory findings without other clinical evidence especially during times of severe emotional or physical stress.
5. Over forty years of age.

Treatment consists of a balanced regimen of medication, diet, and exercise. Diabetes that develops late in life can sometimes be controlled by diet and exercise alone. The obese and overweight will have difficulty in maintaining control. Some patients are able to take medicine by mouth to lower blood sugar levels (oral hypoglycemic compounds), but the severe form of the disease requires insulin by injection. Some oral medications appear to increase cardiovascular complications so should not be used by those who can control diabetes by diet alone. Contraceptive pills may also precipitate symptoms in some prediabetic women.

Diabetics have greatly increased life spans today and can lead almost normal lives and follow almost all types of occupations. The primary danger in diabetes is the early development of vascular changes, particularly in the kidneys and the eyes. Even these can be minimized by early detection and treatment. Maintenance of normal weight is presumed to reduce the danger and effect of diabetes. People who are potential diabetics should receive careful periodic examinations, including a blood test for sugar taken one to two hours after ingesting 50 to 100 grams of carbohydrate.

HYPOGLYCEMIA

Hypoglycemia, or *hyperinsulinism,* which is evidenced by abnormally low blood sugar levels, is being diagnosed more frequently. Seventy percent of the time it is functional in origin. It is thought to be the result of oversecretion of insulin by islet cells of Langerhans due to an excessive response to glucose absorption. Organic causes precipitate low blood sugar in the remaining 30 percent. These causes include a number of conditions such as tumors, glandular disorders, and infections. Attacks occur after the patient has gone several hours without food. The first symptoms may include sweating, flushing, chilliness, trembling, weakness, hunger, headache, apprehensiveness, and fainting. Diagnosis is confirmed by a glucose tolerance test. Treatment of the symptoms is dietary—a high protein, high fat, and low carbohydrate diet given in frequent, small feedings including a snack on waking and another before going to bed. Since emotional disturbances are background features of functional hypoglycemia, psychotherapy may be necessary.

CIRRHOSIS OF THE LIVER

Mortality from cirrhosis of the liver has been increasing steadily the last few years, and this cause of death is now among the top ten. Part of the steady rise might be attributed to improved diagnostic techniques such as liver function tests and liver biopsy procedures. The rates are appreciably higher among men than women. Currently, about a third of the deaths are certified as alcoholic. However, alcohol as a primary cause of mortality is notoriously underreported because of the social stigma attached to this disorder. When alcoholism is treated early, irreversible damage such as occurs in cirrhosis can be prevented.

The etiology is unknown or obscure in many cases. The disease process is characterized by decreasing liver function and increasing pressure in the portal venous system. Dietary deficiencies, diseases of the bile duct, chemical toxins, and infections are considered to be contributory factors, but alcoholism is thought to be the major one. The exact relationship of alcoholism to cirrhosis has not been definitely determined even though alcohol has a direct toxic effect on the liver. The incidence of alcoholism is high among those who have cirrhosis, but most alcoholics do not develop this disease. Possibly, genetic factors are involved.[23]

Moderate cirrhosis may be asymptomatic; the onset of liver failure is gradual with ill defined symptoms. Gastrointestinal upsets are frequent and consist of anorexia, flatulence, nausea, vomiting, and abdominal pain. Advanced cases have a slight fever, are emaciated, may be jaundiced, have distended abdominal veins and enlarged esophageal blood vessels (which may hemorrhage), and have vascular "Spiders" over the face, neck, arms, and upper trunk. Ultimately, swelling, accumulation of fluid in the tissues (edema and ascites), and mental torpor develop. Active treatment can retard and may cure early cases.

CHRONIC RESPIRATORY DISEASE

Chronic respiratory diseases affect the lungs in numerous ways. They can attack at any age, and the incidence of these is increasing. Respiratory conditions account for 55 percent of all acute medical conditions, and those that are chronic, cause major limitations of activity in two and one-half million people.[24]

Up to the age of eight years the lung is still growing and is quite susceptible to permanent injury caused by infections such as whooping cough. The American Lung Association says, "There is a growing recognition that the quality of medical care given to someone with chronic respiratory disease is not only important, it can be crucial. In some cases, the kind of care given can mean the difference between years of health and years of disability—particularly in pediatric care."[25] The person with chronic RD needs an efficient muscular engine so that he can use energy more efficiently and does not need so much oxygen. He will not have to work so hard in breathing.

The Respiratory System

Respiration occurs in all living things, both plants and animals and is directly related to exercise. Proper functioning of this system is perhaps the single most important factor in the sustaining of life. Respiration consists of those processes by which the body cells and tissues make use of oxygen and by which carbon dioxide or the waste products of respiration are removed.

Inhaled air contains about 20 percent oxygen and 4/100 of 1 percent carbon dioxide. Exhaled air consists of approximately 16 percent oxygen and 4 percent carbon dioxide. Nitrogen, which makes up about 79 percent of the atmosphere, is not involved in the breathing process. When air is inhaled into the lungs, a portion of the oxygen passes into the blood and is circulated through the body. At the same time, carbon dioxide is diffused out of the blood into the lungs and exhaled.

Air is breathed through either the mouth or nose into the oral cavity, or *pharynx*. It then passes through the *larynx* into the *trachea*. The trachea ultimately divides into two smaller tubes called *bronchi,* one going to each lung. The bronchi in turn divide into tiny passageways called *bronchioles* that lead to minute air sacs, or *alveoli*. The exchange of gases is effected through the membranous walls of the alveoli.

Mechanisms in the upper respiratory tract serve to filter, humidify, and warm the air in its journey to the alveoli. The hairs, or cilia, in the passages partially filter out dust particles as does the sticky mucus that is produced by mucous cells lining the nasal passages, pharynx, trachea, bronchi, and bronchioles. Figure 12.12 illustrates the respiratory system.

Two kinds of potentially injurious materials can enter the lung—tiny particles and toxic gases. Tiny particles of air pollutants, dust, or other materials when breathed in can travel rapidly down through the respiratory system. Larger particles are screened out by the nose. Medium-sized ones —five to ten microns in size—continue on. In a healthy lung the particles drop out of the air stream onto the surface of the bronchial tree where they are trapped in mucus and are removed back up the passageways by the muco-ciliary cleaning system. Very small particles—one to five microns in size—may penetrate deeply into the lung as far as the alveoli. Here, *dust cells* may ingest them. Sometimes the particles are sufficiently irritating that they cause direct injury to alveolar cells.[26]

The lung not only has a capacity to clean out particles, but it can absorb tremendous amounts of toxic gases. These can cause significant damage to the respiratory mechanism and tissues. Much of irritating gases are absorbed by the upper respiratory tract and may never reach the alveoli. When they are inhaled with particles, particularly moist particles, they are distributed deep into the lungs where they may be extremely injurious.[27]

FOUNDATIONS OF HEALTH SCIENCE

Figure 12.12 Respiratory System. (From *American Lung Association Bulletin*, April, 1974, p. 5. Illustration copyright 1974, American Lung Association. Reproduced with permission.)

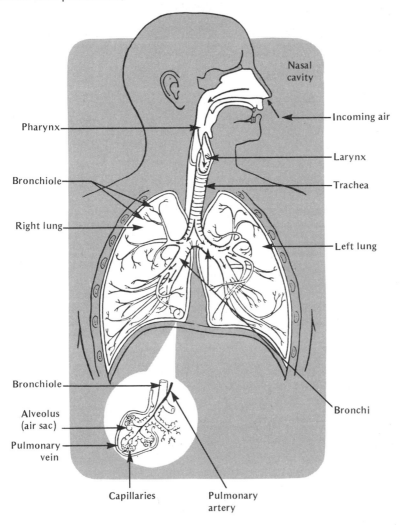

EMPHYSEMA

Emphysema is a disease that was relatively unheard of by the average person before 1950, but today it is the fourth leading cause of permanent and total disability in the United States compensated by governmental agencies in amounts over one billion dollars a year.[28]

As the disease progresses, the patient has greater and greater difficulty in meeting the demands of endurance, speed of work, and travel required by his vocation. His attendance at work may be irregular, and he may have to abandon his occupation. Ultimately, he may even reach a point where he is unable to attend to his own personal daily activities without help. Generally, the crippling stage is reached in the late forties, and to blacken the picture, the medical profession today knows of no cure for this chronic and progressive disease.[29]

Nature of Emphysema

Emphysema is a disease or group of diseases in which the alveoli or lung sacs are permanently damaged. The walls of the alveoli become stretched, thin, and lose their elasticity. This condition reduces the extent of the capillary bed for oxygenation of the blood and the excretion of waste products (see Figure 12.13). Eventually the supporting structures of the bronchi and bronchioles constrict and collapse. The lungs gradually become distended with air, which the victim is unable to exhale. As the patient reaches the limits of physical distention of his lungs his blood will contain too much carbon dioxide and too little oxygen, so he will no longer be able to function. The heart attempts to compensate by working harder and harder, but it reaches its limits of endurance and eventually becomes malfunctioning and fails. This type of heart disease is called *cor pulmonale.*

Emphysema begins insidiously. The first warnings are usually a persistent cough producing sputum for months at a time and a prolonged recovery from mild infections. The victim refers to himself as having bronchial trouble or a cigarette cough. After a period of years, he will notice a shortness of breath out of all proportion to activity. Slowly, breathing becomes more and more difficult and the coughing attacks more frequent. As oxygen decompensation increases, the fingers will develop a club-like appearance; the chest becomes barrel shaped; the shoulders are rounded; the veins in the shoulder, neck, and head are distended; and the lips blue and pursed-looking.

Emphysema appears to have several underlying causes. Patients with emphysema give histories of recurrent infections, with several bouts of pneumonia requiring hospitalization, and have frequent attacks of influenza. Nine-tenths of the victims smoke more than one package of cigarettes per day. The incidence is also much greater in areas of heavy air pollution, and in occupations requiring exposure to dusts such as in mining, foundry work, sugar fields, welding, plastics grinding, and even paint spraying. This disease has some tendency to be familial. The child who suffers severe asthma is much more likely to develop emphysema.

464   FOUNDATIONS OF HEALTH SCIENCE

Figure 12.13 Emphysema. (1) Healthy: The alveoli expand for intake—snap back for exhalation. (2) Diseased: Air enters a diseased alveolus but is poorly expelled owing to a saggy-balloon effect and tube collapse. (From *Today's Health,* 47:30, September, 1969, published by the American Medical Association.)

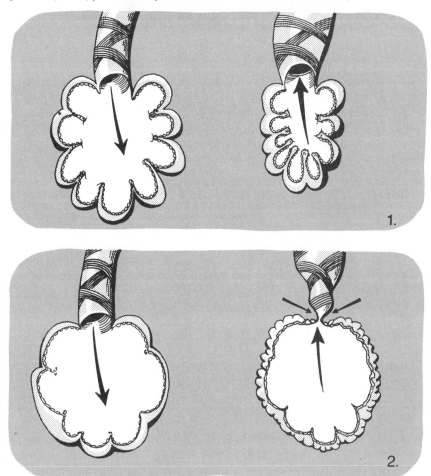

Treatment

Treatment is palliative, but much can be done to retard progressive lung destruction once the diagnosis is made. Therapy assists the patient in using his remaining respiratory potentials more efficiently. The physician will prescribe medications that relax the bronchi and bronchioles and that liquify mucus so it can be more easily coughed up. Aggravating conditions such as recurring infections, allergies, and other disorders are prevented if possible. Breathing exercises to expel collections of mucus are a most important phase of therapy. The victim must avoid respiratory irritants such as smoking, dusts, or other air pollutants.

Detection and Prevention

No completely satisfactory method of detecting emphysema early is known. The inability to expel the air in the lungs rapidly is a valid measure of obstructive lung disease. Checks of forced expirations and of vital capacity pulmonary function tests, should be included in routine medical examinations. Chest X-rays do not show emphysematous changes until rather late in the course of the disease.

ARTHRITIS

Arthritis is a term used for a group of over one hundred related diseases involving the joints and supporting structures. The results are inflammation, swelling, pain, and sometimes deformity. The two most prevalent types are *osteoarthritis* and *rheumatoid arthritis*. These account for 70 percent of this group of disorders. Two other common types are *gout* and *rheumatism* (involvement of tendons and ligaments around the joints).

All arthritic disorders have certain factors in common: Etiology in most instances is unknown; they are all characterized by chronicity and by periods of exacerbation and remission; and, with the exception of a few, no one course of treatment works. However, proper medical care can prevent most of the crippling if it is started early and used conscientiously. About 90 percent of the population has some degree of arthritis by the time they are sixty, but of those "crippled," half are under forty-five years of age.

Osteoarthritis

Osteoarthritis is by far the most common type of arthritis, but it receives less attention than the other forms. In most patients, it involves only a few joints and is relatively mild. Secondly, most people view osteoarthritis, which develops slowly, as an inevitable accompaniment of aging. This presumes that joint cartilage, which acts as a shock absorber for the joint, wears out in time and permits the two bones in the joint to come

466   FOUNDATIONS OF HEALTH SCIENCE

into direct contact with each other. "While it is true that osteoarthritis is progressively more common as people get older, evidence is accumulating to suggest that it is not an inevitable occurrence. The term wear and tear arthritis, which is frequently used synonymously with osteoarthritis, may not be correct."[30]

Osteoarthritis most commonly occurs in people past forty, but many middle-aged women who have not done strenuous physical work demonstrate osteoarthritic changes in the distal small joints of their fingers. This instance appears to be one of familial predisposition. Changes are most often present in the weight-bearing joints such as the hips, knees, and spine, as well as in the fingers. Less than 10 percent of those afflicted have disabling pain and crippling. People who engage in hard physical work and the obese seem to be more susceptible. Although this condition is annoying and sometimes painful, rarely are its victims immobilized or deformed. Poor posture and overweight aggravate wear and tear on joints. Exercises help keep such people more limber, and the physician will probably prescribe aspirin, heat, and massage during periods of especial discomfort.

Rheumatoid Arthritis

The second most prevalent of these disorders is rheumatoid arthritis. It is crippling as well as painful and strikes the younger age group, including children under five. It is nearly always a slowly progressing disease that involves the whole body. During periods of exacerbation, the victim may have fever, general weakness, and weight loss. Sometimes the eyes, heart, muscles, and glands are affected, and the joints may become rigid. It is three times more prevalent in women than in men. Again, three-fourths of severe crippling can be retarded by prescribed medication, physical therapy, and rest. The drug of choice is aspirin, which in addition to relieving pain decreases swelling and inflammation. No other medicine equals aspirin in the treatment of rheumatoid arthritis. Others that produce a modicum of success in some patients are ACTH, cortisone, other steroids, and gold injections. All of these have dangerous toxic effects, and many people cannot tolerate them. Figure 12.14 illustrates a woman with rheumatoid arthritis.

More economical than elaborate treatments of whirlpool baths, short wave, and other forms of diathermy, and just as effective for either rheumatoid or osteoarthritis, are the simple measures of hot tub baths, hot moist towel packs, an electric blanket, and prescribed exercises. Vitamins, patented medicines, vaccines from bee and snake venom, linaments, and special dietary regimens are nearly always useless.

The causes of rheumatoid arthritis and osteoarthritis are still unknown,

Figure 12.14 Arthritis. (Courtesy of the National Arthritis Foundation.)

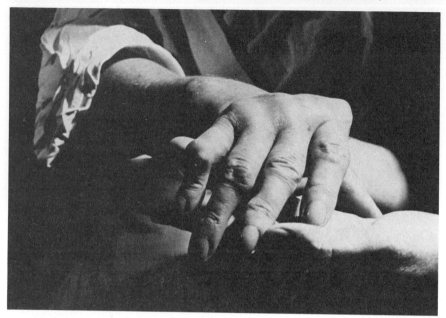

but much research is being done. Virus-like organisms are suspected, and heredity and emotions seem to be common denominators in some cases. Also under investigation is the role of allergies and hypersensitive reactions. The blood of rheumatoid patients contains a special kind of protein called the *rheumatoid factor,* but its significance is not known. As yet, no test has been devised that accurately diagnoses rheumatoid arthritis in the early stages, when treatment might be more successful in preventing crippling. Even the severely handicapped, though, can benefit from rehabilitation, and surgery can make a deformed joint more functional. Research is being done on surgically replacing the hip by cementing an artificial joint to the pelvis. This prosthesis has relieved pain, restored mobility, and resulted in a rapid return to weight-bearing ability in a number of people. Artificial finger joints are another new device.

Gout

Gout probably accounts for at least 5 percent of all patients suffering from arthritis. (Ninety-five percent of those with gout are males.) It customarily attacks the metatarsal joint of the big toe, the ankle, and knee, but may affect other joints. This condition is not related necessarily to "high

FOUNDATIONS OF HEALTH SCIENCE

living" or rich foods. Emotional upsets, drugs, and infections may precipitate an attack in the gout-prone individual. This condition is a metabolic disorder in which uric acid builds up in the blood and results in deposits of sodium urate crystals that cause inflammation of the lining of joints. The pain is excruciating during an attack, which lasts for several days. Treatment with regular doses of colchicine and other medications to reduce the uric acid level is very effective. A balance between work and recreation, sufficient sleep, reduction in tension-producing activities, regular exercise, and adequate nutrition are advocated to reduce attacks. Special diets are prescribed by some physicians. (Gout, or low-purine, diets are limited in meats, high-fat foods, lentils, cereals, and alcoholic beverages.) If gout is allowed to go untreated, it will become progressively worse and result in permanent deformities and eventually kidney disease. Aspirin can produce hyperuricemia and precipitate an acute attack.

Rheumatism

In popular usage, the term *rheumatism* means aches and pains in the joints and muscles. More specifically, this term applies to conditions affecting the supporting structures of the joints—tendons, ligaments, and bursae. Ligaments and tendons become less elastic with age, and any sudden strain on a joint or unaccustomed activity may irritate, producing quite sudden pain. People seem to be susceptible to recurrent attacks. Usually aspirin and heat help, but cortisone, other steroids, or novocaine may be injected locally to reduce inflammation and muscle spasm. Following the remission of symptoms, the physician will prescribe exercises to help strengthen the joint against future strain.

The Arthritis Foundation recommends that the following warnings may come and go, but if neglected, may recur with sudden violence. People should not delay in seeing a physician when these sign of arthritis occur or persist:

1. Persistent pain and stiffness upon arising
2. Pain or tenderness in one or more joints
3. Swelling in one or more joints
4. Recurrence of these symptoms, particularly involving more than one joint
5. Noticeable pain and stiffness in lower back, knees, and other joints
6. Tingling sensation in fingertips, hands and feet
7. Unexplained weight loss, fever, weakness, and fatigue.

Decker, of the National Institute of Arthritis, Metabolism, and Digestive Diseases reports that "We can diagnose" [arthritis] very early. . . . We can't stop it, but with consistent and careful management, we can do much to prevent the difficulties it causes."[31] Charles Sisk, of the Arthritis Foundation, says:

> "If left untreated, arthritis can lead to death. . . . We say that 5,000 to 10,000 people die every year from the arthritic diseases, but this is an underestimation." Arthritis can lower a person's resistance—according to the doctor—making him more susceptible to other diseases, such as pneumonia . . . . arthritis does reduce the victim's life span.[32]

ALLERGIES

About one-sixth of all people suffer from an annoying allergy of one kind or another. They have hives, rashes, itches, twitches, runny noses, and watery eyes; they cough, sneeze and wheeze; and some have digestive upsets and headaches. All in all, people with allergies have an unhappy lot.

Nature of Allergies

Allergy is in part an undesirable immunological response of the body. A person may be hypersensitive to certain proteins and polysaccharides; when exposed, he develops antibodies. Future contact then results in an antigenic reaction, which produces the symptoms described above.

Research shows that allergy is characterized by two features: heredity and the demonstration of reaginic antibodies or reagins in the patient. Seventy-five percent of allergic people have an immediate member of their family who is allergic. The term "atopy" implies that the allergy is inherited. What is inherited is the tendency or capacity to become sensitive or allergic. Parents sensitive to pollen may have children who are sensitive to eggs, but not to pollen. An asthmatic may have children who have hives, but who never develop asthma. The capacity to be allergic is general and does not specify the body organ that will be affected or the allergens that will cause the symptoms.

Factors that may trigger, but do not *cause*, allergic reactions include: changes in the weather, air pollution, fatigue, chilling, and emotional upsets if the individual is simultaneously exposed to the allergen to which he is sensitive. A person who is allergic is usually sensitive to more than one allergen (antigen). Allergens fall into the following groups:

1. *Inhalants* are the most common allergens and cause respiratory symptoms. They include pollens, fungi, all kinds of dusts, animal dander,

vapors, smokes, cosmetics, perfumes, and many compounds causing strong odors.

2. *Foods* are quite frequently antigenic and may also be offenders in one allergic to inhalants. The most common are wheat, eggs, milk, fish, nuts, chocolate, pork, and strawberries.

3. *Contactants* cause dermatitis when they come in direct contact with the skin or mucous membranes. This group includes plants (such as poison oak and sumac), flowers, dyes, rubber, metals, plastics, synthetic fabrics, cosmetics, furs, leather, and insecticides.

4. *Drugs, medicines, pathogens, and physical agents* such as heat, cold, pressure, and radiation also produce allergic manifestations in the hypersensitive person.

Allergic Rhinitis

Allergic Rhinitis may be called "hay fever," but this is a misnomer because hay and fever have nothing to do with allergic rhinitis. Although no one knows the exact number that are afflicted, experts say that probably 20 percent of the population is a conservative estimate. Sneezing, nasal obstruction, watery discharge, tearing of the eyes, and itching or pruritus are typical symptoms of allergic rhinitis. If either the mother or father have had allergic rhinitis, asthma, or atopic dermatitis, their children have approximately a 50 percent chance of developing one of these disorders in their lifetimes. If both parents have had one of these disorders, their children have an almost 100 percent chance of having some type of allergy. It is a myth that allergies are outgrown.[33] Control of symptoms is aided by antihistamines, decongestants, and a change of environment for several weeks. If symptoms are prolonged, a trial of hyposensitization (allergy shots), may be helpful. Children between the ages of three and eight who have chronic allergic rhinitis may experience involvement of the middle ear, such as otitis media, which can cause impairment of hearing.

Asthma

In terms of consequences, bronchial asthma is the most dangerous of the allergies. In bronchial asthma, the bronchi becomes narrowed and plugged with mucus. The patient has difficulty breathing and makes a typical wheezing sound when exhaling. About half the cases are due to allergies and the other half to infection. The symptoms may come on quite slowly or very suddenly. In the asthmatic, emotional stress frequently triggers an attack. The acute state always entails the danger of suffocation, but chronic asthma eventually can produce the changes leading to emphysema and heart disease.

Treatment

The basis of all treatment is avoidance of the allergen when it is possible: change of diet; removal of the offending substance from the environment in the case of clothes, cosmetics, and pets; and change of geographic and occupational environment when the allergen is pollen, dust, or any other inhalant.

Desensitization may be used when reactions are severe and it is impossible to eliminate the allergen. Antihistamines and steroids such as cortisone can help alleviate the symptoms. Since emotional stress precipitates symptoms, tension-producing situations should be minimized. A combined program of avoidance, desensitization, alleviation of symptoms, and reduction of stress will bring about improvement 80 percent of the time. Detection of specific allergens usually requires the skill of an allergist, a medical specialist.

VASCULAR AND TENSION HEADACHES

Probably 70 percent of the population have had a headache at one time or another. About 10 percent of this group have such severe pain that they seek medical attention. Among this 10 percent, 90 percent have vascular headaches, muscle contraction or tension headaches, or a combination of the two. People with recurring headaches should have general physical, neurological, and laboratory tests to rule out organic causes such as trauma, tumors, or hemorrhages. Once these causes are eliminated, the process of identifying the triggering factors of the headache and the effective methods of treatment can begin. This process is time consuming and not always successful.

Either vascular or tension headaches may be called migraine. Migraine sufferers are often characterized as being perfectionistic, rigid, compulsive, extremely sensitive, and conscientious. They may be ambitious, hard-driving people who work themselves to exhaustion and then develop a headache that allows them to relax and rebuild their energy. They frequently come from families that do not express their emotions and that set high standards. They tend to repress hostility and anger.[34] Understanding the characteristics of headaches can give clues as to preventive measures, or at least techniques for ameliorating their severity.

FOUNDATIONS OF HEALTH SCIENCE

Vascular Type Headache

These headaches are usually generalized, but may be unilateral, throbbing, or begin in and about the eye and spread to involve one or both sides of the head. They may be accompanied by nausea and vomiting; they are periodic and recurrent. The *classic migraine* lasts about four to six hours and is severe. Its onset tends to be unilateral, frontal, and temporal. The *common migraine* can persist for several days. It often starts slowly and builds up to severe throbbing. Victims may awaken with it. It, too, may begin on one side, but then may spread. This type frequently occurs on weekends, Mondays, premenstrual days, and when relaxing. It is correlated with "let down" activities.

Vascular migraines have a high incidence of occurrence among other members of the family. Attacks are often preceded by physical and emotional signs, which might include changes in mood, anorexia, and transient visual aberrations. They may begin at any age, usually during adolescence.

Muscle Contraction or Tension Headache

No family history is involved in this type of headache. Although episodic, the onset is gradual, and without treatment, the headache can become constant. The pain is usually dull, nonthrobbing, and varies in intensity. The neck, shoulders, and head muscles may also be tense and/or painful. An individual can suffer from both vascular and tension types of migraines.

NEUROLOGICAL DISEASES

A number of diseases in which the nervous system is affected leave the patient with some kind of physical handicap. Although these are not as prevalent as the disorders just described, we are becoming more aware of and concerned about them because of the severe degree of disability they cause.

The Nervous System

The nervous system, which does much to control and integrate bodily processes, is one of the most complex mechanisms of the human organism. Physiologists have differentiated this system into three parts, each of which is very closely interrelated with the others. The *central nervous system* is composed of the brain and the spinal cord. The *peripheral nervous system* includes the nerves that connect with the various parts of the body, such as the glands, muscles, and sense organs. The *autonomic nervous system,* sometimes considered a part of the peripheral system, helps to regulate the automatically performed fundamental physiological processes, such as circulation, digestion, excretion, and respiration.

The brain is a delicate structure protected by bones of the skull, or *cranium.* The uppermost portion consists of two hemispheres and is called the *cerebrum.* Centers in the cerebral cortex control such bodily activities as voluntary movements and sensations of various kinds. Thinking, memory, and emotions are also functions of the cerebral cortex but do not seem to be localized in any special center. The *cerebellum,* which lies just below the posterior portion of the cerebrum, apparently assists in the coordination of voluntary muscular responses. The *midbrain* connects the cerebrum and the cerebellum. Control of certain automatic activities, such as breathing, sweating, heartbeat, and swallowing, is located in the *medulla,* which is a continuation of the upper part of the spinal cord. Twelve major pairs of nerves emanate from the brain.

The *spinal cord* emerges from the brain at its upper end and extends downward inside the vertebral column. It is bathed, as is the brain, by the *cerebrospinal fluid.* Thirty-one pairs of nerves originate from the spinal cord, each pair extending out between adjacent vertebrae to all parts of the body. These serve as pathways or tracts for the transmission of impulses to and away from the brain.

The unit of structure of the nervous system is known as a *neuron.* It is composed of a central part called the cell body and fibers that extend outward from it. Most neurons possess one long fiber and several shorter ones. Nerves consist of many long fibers bound together into ropelike structures that connect parts of the body with the brain and spinal cord. Groups of cell bodies of neurons, known as *ganglia,* are located in the brain and spinal cord.

Impulses travel along the nerve fiber, which can transmit only in a single direction. Impulses moving toward the brain or spinal cord are known as *afferent,* or sensory, impulses; those traveling away are called *efferent,* or motor, impulses. A synapse is the juncture between two neurons.

Figures 12.15 and 12.16 illustrate the human brain and nervous system, respectively.

Epilepsy or Seizures

Epilepsy, seizure, or convulsion state is a group of symptoms. So-called "epilepsy" in itself does not result in mental retardation, psycho-

Figure 12.15 The Brain. (Adapted from Hollis F. Fait, *Health and Fitness for Modern Living* [Boston: Allyn and Bacon, 1967].)

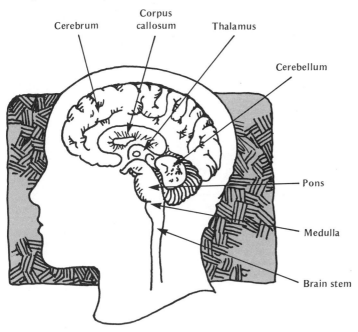

logical disturbances, impairment in function, or degeneration. Some of the causes of this syndrome (anoxia during birth, infectious disease, tumors, circulatory defects, injury) may produce these undesirable consequences. In only 25 percent of the victims is the cause or etiology known. The remaining 75 percent are of "unknown origin."

This disorder is characterized by:

> . . . periodic transient episodes in which one or more of the following phenomena occur: alteration in the state of consciousness, convulsive movements, disturbances in feeling or behavior . . . a wide variety of clinical manifestations are encountered . . . certain features based on the site and nature of brain involvement allow for a grouping into categories that serve as a guide in evaluation and treatment. . . .[35]

Exactly what happens neurologically to produce the seizure is not known. In normal persons, these symptoms can be precipitated by convulsant agents such as drugs and electric shock, and by photic and auditory stimuli. As soon as the effects of such stimuli wear off, the brain in these normals returns to a seizure-free state. The electroencephalograms of patients with convulsive disorders are abnormal even during symptom-free periods. Organic lesions produce a high incidence of seizures, but

Figure 12.16 The Nervous System. The nervous system regulates the activities of all other systems of the body. It is generally divided into three related systems of specialized function. The *central nervous system* includes the brain and spinal cord. The nerves that extend outward from the base of the brain and the spinal cord are called the *peripheral nervous system*. The third division is known as the *autonomic nervous system*. The central and the peripheral nervous systems are primarily concerned with conscious activities and sensations of the body. The autonomic system controls the slowing down or speeding up of the involuntary functions of the body, such as digestion, heartbeat, perspiring, and adrenal secretion. (From *Instructoscope*. Copyright © 1964 by Scott Foresman and Company. Reprinted by permission of the publisher.)

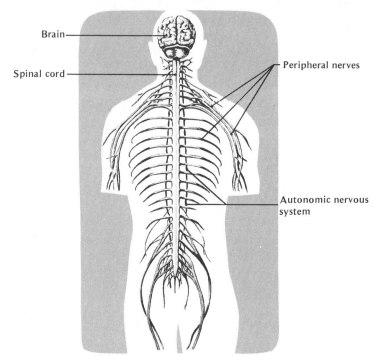

many convulsives demonstrate no such physiological change. One hypothesis is that disturbances in enzyme systems may be responsible. A tendency to this disorder is transmitted genetically, but a precipitating factor is required for the disease to occur.

Seizures are of five types or categories. The first and most frequent of these is the dramatic *grand mal*. Grand mal attacks may be preceded by an aura or warning and consist of: unconsciousness, intermittent muscle contractions or spasms, tongue biting, difficulty in breathing, and incontinence. These attacks may last from a few seconds to as long as ten minutes. The victim may be sleepy and confused and have headaches or gastric upsets for several hours following such a seizure. Grand mal epi-

FOUNDATIONS OF HEALTH SCIENCE

sodes might occur more than once in a day or be as much as a year or more apart.

The *petit mal* is a different type of seizure. It is not just a mild grand mal. This type more commonly occurs in children and disappears during the teens. The episode lasts only a few seconds and consists of a brief loss of consciousness, sometimes minor movement of the eyes, head, and extremities, staggering, and once in a while, incontinence. The victim is alert immediately afterwards.

Psychomotor attacks are episodes in which there is alteration in behavior and perception. The victim may become confused and do such things as clap his hands or run aimlessly and then not remember what has happened (amnesia). Sometimes he behaves aggressively but rarely is he violent. The seizure may last for two or three minutes, following which the victim may be confused.

In a *focal seizure,* the area in the brain that is disturbed can be pinpointed; the symptoms correspond to the functions controlled by that area. The fifth type is *minor motor*.

Treatment of the underlying cause in the 25 percent of patients in which the etiology is known can reduce or eliminate some of the seizures. The remaining cases can be partially or completely controlled by such therapy as anticonvulsant drugs and regimens for maintaining physical and emotional health. Because of the social stigma still attached to this disorder, psychological counseling for both the patient and his family may be required.

Public education programs are doing much to dispel the erroneous beliefs that people with convulsive disorders cannot be gainfully employed, need to be institutionalized, are dangerous, or cannot be helped medically. The incidence of this disorder is greater than most people realize—approximately 10 percent of the population have this condition in either a latent or symptomatic stage. At present, either complete control or a marked reduction in symptoms is obtained in over 75 percent of the cases; the greatest success is in the grand and petit mal types. The life span is not necessarily shortened by epilepsy.

Muscular Dystrophy

Muscular dystrophy is a chronic disease in which there is a gradual wasting away of muscle tissue. Most of the victims are children between the ages of three and thirteen years. Almost all of them will die before reaching adulthood. In children, the muscles of the legs and lower back are affected first. The victim initially becomes clumsy, later is unable to walk, gets weak, and eventually is helpless. When this condition develops in adults, muscles of the pelvic and shoulder girdle become involved; if the facial muscles are affected, the patient loses the ability to smile, scowl, or grimace.

Muscular dystrophy is considered an inherited disorder, but it does appear without any family history. Apparently, it is the result of a mutation, and such mutations are then transmitted to any offspring. The actual incidence is unknown, but some estimates indicate possibly one in five hundred.

No cure is known, but supportive care aids the patient to live more comfortably. Since the respiratory muscles will eventually be affected, prevention and treatment of infection is necessary. Physical therapy can reduce the effects of disability, and helping the child to live as normal a life as possible lessens emotional problems. The Muscular Dystrophy Association of America, Incorporated, provides funds for diagnostic examinations, for wheel chairs and other equipment, and for research.

Multiple Sclerosis

Multiple sclerosis is a chronic, usually progressive, neurological disease that affects persons between twenty and forty years of age. It is one of the most common disorders of the nervous system, and fortunately is rarely fatal. It is characterized by periods of exacerbation and remission and may cause prolonged disability.

The symptoms are loss of muscular coordination and strength, inability to maintain balance, trembling, paralysis, visual and speech disturbances, and impaired bowel and bladder control. Sometimes patients become severely emotionally depressed. The symptoms may come and go, but in time recovery becomes less and less. In multiple sclerosis, the myelin sheaths covering the nerve fibers in the brain and spinal cord dissolve or disintegrate and are replaced by scar tissue. As long as only the sheath is affected, nerve impulses can still be transmitted. Ultimately the scar tissue will impinge upon the nerve itself. Many with mild or even moderately severe symptoms are able to work for many years.

The cause is unknown, but the condition is more common in cold, damp climates. Adequate rest and proper nutrition are prescribed, but no particular diet, vitamin supplements, or other regimen is of special value. Physical therapy can relieve spastic muscles and increase coordination. In cases of spasticity, muscle-relaxing drugs may be used.

Parkinson's Disease

Parkinson's disease, or "shaking palsy," cause unknown, is not a disease entity but a syndrome associated with dysfunction of the basal ganglia

FOUNDATIONS OF HEALTH SCIENCE

in the nervous system. It is present in approximately 2 percent of the population over sixty years of age. The first symptom is a tremor or shaking in one of the limbs. At first the tremor is rhythmic and slight, but gradually it increases in intensity and may become widespread. Soon muscular rigidity appears, there is loss of equilibrium, the face becomes masklike, and the gait is rapid and shuffling. These symptoms develop more slowly in some cases than others, but they gradually increase in severity.

Various drugs are used to reduce the symptoms of rigidity and tremors. Physical therapy is most effective in relaxing rigid muscles, but neither drugs nor physical therapy can restore automatic movements and correct weakness. In a few instances, neurosurgery is helpful to reduce tremors and rigidity. Helplessness can be postponed, in some cases indefinitely, by the patient who follows a program of medication, special exercises, and healthful habits.

The patient with Parkinson's disease usually can do only one thing at a time. For example, he cannot turn pages in a book and reach for a light switch simultaneously. This disability means that his schedule must be altered considerably. He is accident-prone because of his clumsy, stiff movements, so his environment should be organized to reduce the danger of stumbling and falls. Handrails throughout the home will give him needed support, and furniture that is high will make it easier for him to get up or down.

Cerebral Palsy

Cerebral palsy is a rather general term used to describe a group of disabilities resulting from damage to the developing brain that occurred before, during, or after birth. It is the primary cause of handicaps in children. The child has some loss or impairment of control over voluntary muscles. The condition may be severe or mild, with just a few or many muscles affected. Lack of control may be in the arms, legs, tongue, speech mechanism, eyes, or movements. Those afflicted have awkward or involuntary movements, lack balance, have an irregular gait and guttural speech, and frequently grimace and drool. Other types of defects are present and frequently include mental retardation, convulsions, and impairment of sight and hearing.

Modern medical treatment has greatly expanded the life expectancy of the cerebral palsied as well as all other handicapped persons, but it is not yet able to repair damaged brain tissue. These victims must live within the limits of their handicaps. Present techniques of habilitation have markedly increased these limits, however. About 20 percent of those afflicted can become self-sufficient, another 20 percent partially self-sufficient, and the remaining three-fifths will need partial or complete care throughout life.

Prevention is accomplished by improved prenatal care to reduce the effects of viral infections, syphilis, radiation, toxemia of pregnancy, injury, blood incompatibilities, medicines that interfere with embryonic development or oxygenation of the fetus, and by improved obstetrical care. The greatest number of cerebral palsies have their cause in abnormalities occurring during birth because of interference in the oxygen supply to the fetus. Infections and injuries after birth also may result in cerebral palsy.

IN CONCLUSION

Cardiovascular diseases and cancer are the major killers in the United States. Emphysema is rapidly increasing, and deaths from all types of chronic respiratory disorders combined are now among the top ten killers. Arthritis and other rheumatic conditions cause most of the disabling, and allergies annoy or temporarily incapacitate approximately one-sixth of the population. In addition to these, a number of neurological disorders and birth defects severely handicap many children and adults. Research is slowly disclosing the "know-how" to aid in preventing, controlling, and treating the chronic and degenerative diseases that cause so much suffering, loss of productive years, and needless premature deaths.

We can do a number of things personally to reduce the ravages of many of these conditions. One, *we must keep informed!* As consumers of medical services we need to know what constitutes "good" care. We must be constantly alert to the "pitch" of the huckster who offers panaceas of little or no value. Second, we must know and practice techniques of self-examination such as those described to detect possible disorders of the breast and testes. Third, we must be aware of the early danger signals of disease in order to obtain medical attention early when treatment may have the best chance of ameliorating symptoms or of curing. Fourth, we must follow our health advisor's recommendations! This may be the only way some diseases can be controlled—diabetes and hypertension, for example. And last, we must apply the proper health maintenance procedures outlined in preceding chapters.

Notes

1. "Focus on the News," *Medical World News,* 15:4, April 9, 1974.
2. "Alerting Public to Heart Attack Signs—Without a Stampede," *Medical World News,* 14:18, March 9, 1973.

FOUNDATIONS OF HEALTH SCIENCE

3. "Survival Among Metropolitan Employees with Coronary Heart Disease," *Statistical Bulletin,* 54:7, August, 1973.

4. Ibid.

5. "Type A Theory: Only an E for Effort?" *Medical World News,* 15:52, May 17, 1974.

6. Ibid.

7. Margaret R. Keller and B. Lionel Truscott, "Transient Ischemic Attacks," *American Journal of Nursing,* 73:1330, 1973.

8. Ibid.

9. Keller and Truscott, "Transient Ischemic Attacks."

10. Alice D. Chenoweth, "High Blood Pressure: A National Concern," *The Journal of School Health,* 43:307, 1973.

11. Ibid., p. 308.

12. "Reduced Mortality from Hypertension," *Statistical Bulletin,* 53:6–7, May, 1972.

13. *High Blood Pressure, Facts on Disease of Some 23 Million Americans,* pamphlet (Merck Sharp and Dohme, 1974), pp. 2–10; William B. Kannel and Thomas S. Dawber, "Framingham Revisited" *Medical World News,* 17:11–14, April 26, 1976.

14. "Trends in Cancer—1974," *1976 Cancer Facts and Figures* (New York: American Cancer Society, 1976), p. 6.

15. "Cancer Survival Among Women," *Statistical Bulletin,* 55:4, June, 1974.

16. "Recent Mortality from Hodgkin's Disease and Leukemia," *Statistical Bulletin,* 54:6, March, 1973.

17. "75 Years of Pioneering Cancer Research," *Medical World News,* 14:101, September 7, 1973.

18. "Setting Safer Limits On Mammography," *Medical World News,* 16:23, 24, August 11, 1975.

19. "Two Attacks Against Testicular Cancer," *Medical World News,* 16:58, June 30, 1975.

20. Ibid.

21. Ibid.

22. "Better Ways of Examining the Bowel," *Medical World News,* 14:61, October 19, 1974.

23. "Mortality from Cirrhosis of the Liver—United States, Canada, and Western Europe," *Statistical Bulletin,* 54:8, October, 1973.

24. Alan K. Pierce, "The Shortage of Trained Chest Specialists," *American Lung Association Bulletin,* 59:14, October, 1973.

25. "Improving Medical Care for People with Chronic Lung Disease," *American Lung Association Bulletin,* 60:14, April, 1974.

26. "An Odyssey to the Depths of the Lung," *American Lung Association Bulletin,* 60:5, April, 1974.

27. Ibid.

28. Pierce, "The Shortage of Trained Chest Specialists."

29. "Reported Frequency of Chronic Respiratory Diseases as Causes of Death: Age Variations," *Statistical Bulletin,* 46:6, August, 1965.

30. Edward S. Mongan, "Osteoarthritis—Most Common," *Headlines from The Arthritis Foundation,* February, 1974.

31. "What Doctors Can Do for Today's Arthritis Victims," *Today's Health,* 51:35, October, 1973.

32. Ibid.

33. "Overcoming Seasonal Allergies," *Medical World News,* 15:39, August 9, 1974.

34. Lois M. Hoskins, "Vascular and Tension Headaches," *American Journal of Nursing,* 74:848, 1974.

35. Paul Beeson and Walsh McDermott, *Cecil-Loeb Textbook of Medicine* (Philadelphia: W. B. Saunders, 1963), p. 1553.

INFECTIOUS DISEASES

chapter thirteen

The infectious diseases account for many premature deaths, many days of suffering, many hours of heartache for loved ones, and many millions of dollars of economic loss. These diseases may produce symptoms that range from mild and transitory to severe, debilitating, and persistent. Some infections that were problems in the early nineteen hundreds are now controlled, and some that were rare, unknown, or undiagnosed fifty years ago, such as Asian flu, hepatitis, and mononucleosis, are matters of current concern. With the emphasis on chronic and degenerative illnesses in the United States, we are prone to forget about infections, many of which are contagious. The war against these invaders is not won, and constant vigilance must be maintained. The destruction of some of them enables others to live and become threats to life. Increasing mobility of the world population is introducing new problems of control. Participants in this never ending battle are not just "government" or "someone else," they are all of us.

To appreciate and understand how to maintain the vigilance that promotes good health requires knowledge of the nature of infections, how they can be prevented, how they can be controlled, and the characteristics of some of the more prevalent diseases.

THE NATURE OF INFECTION

Of the millions of microorganisms that inhabit the universe, only a few are harmful to man. The average size of microbes is about 1/15,000 of an inch long. It would take about two trillion to weigh one gram (one-quarter teaspoon). Each of these minutes forms of life has the ability to reproduce, grow, and effect changes in its immediate environment.

Classification of Microorganisms

Many of the organisms that cause disease are members of the plant kingdom, others belong to the animal kingdom, and viruses are intermediate between plants and animals. An organism that lives off the body of another plant or animal (host) is known as a parasite. Parasites, such as the protozoa, obtain food by ingesting and then digesting solid particles of food, or as in the case of bacteria, they absorb organic molecules through their cell membranes. We do not know whether viruses obtain nourishment. They divert host cells to carry on functions for them. The parasites that produce disease in man are called *pathogens* (*path* means suffering or disease).

Specific parasites are usually found in only few kinds of hosts and often in only one kind. Most of those that live off man cannot live off other forms of life. They require specific environments with limited variations in temperature, moisture, sugars, amino acids, vitamins, and minerals. A few can survive and multiply only within the living cells of the host. Some parasites have the ability to withstand adverse conditions, such as drying or

This is responsible behavior showing concern for others as well as for self.

The last time I was really sick enough to have it interfere with anything was when I had the flu. I had just gotten a new job, as a waitress, and now I was too sick to go to work. Even if I had felt well enough to move around that much, sneezing and sniffling around all that food is very bad for business. So I kept calling in sick, and I felt terrible. I was so powerless. I kept thinking that I should be able to control it, that I couldn't really be all that sick, that I should be able to live with it and go about my business. But even if I had tried that, I would have infected half the population of the city after a couple nights work, so I stayed home. I felt guilty and helpless and altogether awful.

FOUNDATIONS OF HEALTH SCIENCE

wide variations in temperature. A few, such as tetanus bacilli, develop spores in which the cell itself shrinks and a thick membrane grows inside the original wall. In this form, a bacterium may live many years until it accidentally is placed in a suitable host. Table 13.1 describes the different pathogens, some of their characteristics, and examples of diseases they can cause.

Ecological studies provide information that enables man to control the growth of microorganisms and therefore prevent many parasitic diseases. Those that are spread through poor sanitation and by insects are controlled best in the United States. In most of the world the situation is entirely different, since the majority of people live in overcrowded areas characterized by little or no safe water for drinking or bathing, few or no sanitary facilities, and an abundance of insects and vermin. Intestinal parasites are still determining much of man's destiny.

How Pathogens Cause Disease

Microbes multiply so quickly that within a few hours one organism can produce billions of its kind. They produce toxins that interfere with the functions of the host's cells. Endotoxin is a poison elaborated within a microorganism that is liberated only upon destruction of the organism. Exotoxin is a poison produced by an organism without its destruction.

In people, these toxins may affect any cell in the body or just particular kinds of cells, such as nervous tissue, connective tissue, or blood. When particular sets of cells or organs are affected, characteristic symptoms develop. Pathogens can be classified by the toxicity of the poisons they produce as well as by the ease by which they can invade the body. We are fortunate that the most poisonous are not always the most invasive.

Pathogens invade the host through several different systems. A common portal of entry in persons in the United States is through the respiratory system. Microorganisms that are "breathed in" and "breathed out" usually settle in the throat, nose, and respiratory tract. Colds and influenza, the most common of all respiratory disorders, may primarily weaken tissues, which enables other less invasive organisms to infect secondarily

This is irresponsible behavior to self and others.

The last time I had the flu I hated being sick so consequently I did not rest and it took me twice as long to recover. I hate to be sick and when I am I try to ignore the sickness.

Table 13.1 Classification of Pathogenic Microorganisms

Pathogenic Microorganism	Characteristics
Viruses: myxovirus, adenovirus, enterovirus, reovirus	The virus is possibly the smallest parasite. It grows only in living cells and must utilize the protoplasm of other cells to multiply and live. The virus usually becomes an integral part of the cell that it invades and diverts the nucleic acids of the host cell to making new viruses. When the host cell becomes full it bursts and disseminates the new viruses to invade other cells. Some viruses grow on cell walls. Chemotherapy is rarely effective against viruses which are the most virulent of all pathogens. The cell in which they multiply must be destroyed. Viruses are very antigenic. Unrelated viruses may cause the same symptoms and the same virus may cause different symptoms. Viruses are spread by direct contact. They cause such diseases as colds, influenza, mumps, smallpox, poliomyelitis, enteritis, hepatitis, rabies, and lymphogranuloma venereum.
Rickettsiae	These grow only in living cells, unlike viruses they are a complete cell unit and can reproduce themselves and carry out life functions. They are intermediate in size and biological activity between viruses and bacteria. They are arthropod-borne and must spend time in an arthropod host. They are transmitted to man through bites and it is probably only accidental that man becomes infected. Rickettsiae cause such diseases as typhus, Rocky Mountain fever, and Q fever.
Bacteria: 1. Cocci (round shaped) diplococci in pairs streptococci in chains staphylococci in clusters 2. Spirochetes (spiral shaped) 3. Bacilli (rod shaped) 4. Actinomycetes (tree shaped)	Bacteria are one-celled; some have flagella and are motile. Some are encapsulated with a shell-like covering that prevents them from drying out. Others have a spore form that can withstand quite adverse conditions. Certain bacteria multiply only in the presence of free oxygen (aerobic), and others multiply deep in tissues using oxygen compounds (anaerobic). They tend to exist extracellularly. Bacteria produce exotoxins and endotoxins. The latter are released only when the bacteria die and disintegrate. Antibiotics are effective against many of the bacteria. Typical diseases include: pneumonia and gonorrhea from diplococci; boils and other common skin infections from staphylococcus; scarlet fever, impetigo, and strep throat from streptococcus; syphilis and yaws from spirochetes; tuberculosis and tetanus from bacilli; and actinomycosis from actinomycetes.
Protozoa: Trypanosoma, Leishmania, Giardia, Amoeba, Trichomonas, and Plasmodia	These are the largest and most complex of the microbes. They are unicellular and many are motile. They react to many stimuli and ingest, digest, and store food. Some live on human tissue. Drugs of different kinds may prevent the growth of various protozoans. Some diseases caused by these microbes are malaria, amoebic dysentery, sleeping sickness, Chagas disease, and trichomoniasis.

Table 13.1 *(Continued)*

Pathogenic Microorganism	Characteristics
Molds and Fungi (yeasts)	These are multicellular plants. The difference between molds and fungi is more a matter of structure than composition. Fungi are usually single-celled and molds have a branching formation.
	Some of these affect skin, nails, and hair, while others produce systemic symptoms. Antibiotics of the broad spectrum type control some, particularly those producing local rather than systemic symptoms.
	Molds and fungi are the causes of such conditions as: ringworm or tinea, histoplasmosis, coccidioidomycosis, candidiasis or thrush, blastomycosis, cryptococcosis, and athlete's foot.

the lungs and airways, thereby causing pneumonia and bronchitis. The pathogens that enter through the mouth invade the digestive tract and cause symptoms of gastrointestinal disturbances and then are excreted in the feces. Organisms that invade the skin and mucous membranes are most often spread through direct contact with an infected person, animal, or insect.

Characteristic of some infectious agents is their ability to spread easily and rapidly from one host to another. The body has several mechanisms by which it can prevent microorganisms from invading and taking over.

DEFENSE AGAINST INFECTION

Man's constant battle against parasites is in his favor. Once a pathogen enters the human body, the body has deterrents to its growth: general body defenses and antigenic responses. When these are insufficient, chemotherapy may retard growth or destroy the parasite.

General Body Defenses

We have what is known as species immunity against many organisms. Man is not susceptible to most of the parasites infecting other animals and plants. Differences in degree of susceptibility to infection also appear among people. Geneticists have demonstrated that there seem to be hereditary factors predisposing people to such diseases as tuberculosis, leprosy, diphtheria, and scarlet fever. The genes influence resistance through the enzyme systems that affect the biochemistry of the host, which is well demonstrated in breeding specific strains of plants and animals that are resistant to parasites. The parasites may in turn become resistant to chemicals that man devises to destroy them.

Barriers to entry. Several mechanisms of the body prevent organisms from becoming established and multiplying. Many parasites cannot penetrate skin, especially when it is unbroken. The secretions on the skin, which are acid, are not conducive to most microbial growth. The various body orifices also have protective barriers. The epithelial tissue lining these openings secretes mucus, which entraps organisms. In the nose and mouth, these secretions are swallowed and any remaining viable agents are acted upon by gastric secretions. The cilia, or fine hairs, that are in the trachea and bronchi return the parasites up the respiratory passages to be swallowed. The tears that constantly bathe the eyes wash any matter through the lacrimal duct into the nose. Both tears and saliva are antibiotic. In the ears, wax provides protection. Urine is not only bacteriostatic but mechanically washes out pathogens. The normal bacterial content of the bowel and vagina appear to inhibit the growth of some pathogens.

Barriers to internal growth. Several kinds of connective tissue cells function to destroy foreign agents that manage to gain entry. These cells fall into two groups: those that stay in one area and those that move about freely in the blood or lymph systems. The so-called *fixed cells* move about only in a more or less circumscribed area and are named *endothelial, fibroblastic,* and *macrophagic.* Endothelial cells are flat and line the inside of the body cavities and the interior of all blood vessels. They repair blood vessels that become damaged by infection. Fibroblasts are scattered throughout the connective tissue. They form scar tissue and wall off or encapsulate parasites and other foreign material. The macrophages actually ingest foreign material. They are quite large cells and are numerous in all connective tissue. Many organs that have passageways or sinuses have macrophages present in their linings—sinuses of bone, lymph glands, spleen and liver, and alveoli of the lungs.

Although these fixed cells do move about to some extent, the free cells are much more mobile and are found in the blood and lymph. When they leave the freely moving circulatory systems, they can travel over other cells in the tissue by an amoeboid or slithering motion. These free cells are known as *leukocytes,* or white blood cells. They are of two types: the monocytes with one nucleus, and the polymorphonuclear cells or granulocytes with more than one nucleus. Granulocytes act by walling off and occasionally digesting foreign material. The monocytes are quite large and not only ingest and digest pathogens and other debris associated with infection but also ingest other leukocytes that have become weak and ineffectual.

FOUNDATIONS OF HEALTH SCIENCE

A defense that aids in protecting against viral infections is a substance called *interferon*. Viruses have the ability to interfere with the growth of each other. One kind of virus present in the intestinal tract can stimulate host cells to produce interferon, a protein than can prevent a new or different virus from multiplying in the cell. Research may enable man to use this substance to protect against pathogenic viruses.

Systemic internal defenses. There are also systemic defense mechanisms. Elevated body temperature or fever increases such cellular activities as phagocytosis and antibody formation. The chills and shaking that may accompany fevers are thought by some to be a physiological attempt to maintain the fever. Chills are much like shivering, which is an involuntary reaction to increase body temperature when the environment carries away too much heat. Fever is also presumed to deter the multiplication of infectious organisms. Consequently, a slight increase in body temperature of two to three degrees Fahrenheit during infection may be desirable.

Antigenic Responses

Through its antigenic responses, the body can protect itself against specific pathogens. Antigenic response is the production of antibodies. Antibodies are globulins created in the body when specific foreign substances called *antigens* are introduced. Antigens may be proteins, some complex carbohydrates, toxins, or microorganisms. The major globulin in antibody formation is the gamma fraction. Certain nonantigenic substances (adjuvants), such as calcium phosphate, when mixed with an antigen, increase antibody production as well as does the manner in which the antigen enters the body. The spleen, lymph nodes, and lungs are most active in producing antibodies, but other tissues have this capacity, too. In general, each antigen produces its own specific antibody. Antibodies fight infection by actually destroying the pathogens or by causing them to clump together or agglutinate so that the white cells can destroy them.

Whether or not antigenic substances produce antibodies and how successful these antibodies are in combatting the effects of the antigen depends on many factors: the nutritional level of the host; age, since the very young and the aged produce fewer antibodies; the extent of exposure to the antigen; and the nature of the antigen, since it may vary in virulence and in ability to stimulate antibody formation. Antibodies themselves can differ in their protective capacities. The reasons for this difference are currently being investigated. Due to slight variations in their structure, a few people lack the ability to produce antibodies, a condition called agammaglobulinemia. They have little or no gamma globulin. All pathogens do not stimulate antibody production, and in some infections the antibodies produced last such a short time that little protection is provided against future infections. The level of antibodies or degree of protection against future infections as well as the length of time that protection lasts varies with each pathogen and with the way a pathogen stimulates the production of antibodies.

Active immunity. Active immunity occurs when an individual makes his own antibodies as the result of antigenic stimulation. This process takes anywhere from a few days to many months to develop, but such immunity lasts for months, years, or even a lifetime depending on the specific antigen and the nature of exposure to it. Antibodies may result from an acute infection, from an atypical or missed infection in which the symptoms of disease may not be apparent, and from oral or parenteral (injection) administration of a modified form of the pathogen in controlled doses. Administering doses of the modified pathogen, called *artificial immunization*, stimulates antibody formation but causes few or no symptoms of disease.

In some acute infections when the victim has a frank (obvious) case, the resulting immunity is so great that protection may last a lifetime. Of the common childhood diseases, such as measles, chickenpox, and mumps, second infections are rare because of high immunity. Protection resulting from an atypical case is also high, but whether or not it exists is difficult to determine. Immunity obtained from atypical infections is one reason why adults who apparently have never had mumps, or any of the other so-called "childhood diseases," still may not become infected when exposed to such illnesses.

Immunizing by artificial techniques does not produce as effective protection as do either frank or inapparent infections. Vaccinations must be periodically repeated or "boosted." However, such repetition is preferable to coming down with a disease that may result in serious after-effects or even death. Skin tests and laboratory examinations may or may not indicate whether or not a person is immune to certain pathogens.

Passive immunity. Sometimes a person who has no antibodies after he has been exposed to an infectious agent can be protected by injecting him with already prepared antibodies. This process is called *passive immunization*. It provides immediate protection but lasts only a few weeks. The active immunity process may not produce antibodies quickly enough to give protection to someone exposed to the pathogen. Antibodies that are used in passive immunizations are obtained from "blood products" of other human beings or animals such as horses. Some people are quite sensitive to a foreign serum (horse serum), and may develop a severe,

FOUNDATIONS OF HEALTH SCIENCE

possibly fatal allergic reaction. The modified pathogen used in active immunity rarely causes dangerous side effects. Therefore, it is better to be actively immunized.

Human blood, particularly from adults, contains a mixture of different antibodies, and when it is given prophylactically, it can provide the recipient with some protection against infections. Newborn infants have passive immunity against those diseases to which the mother is immune, since maternal antibodies can filter through the placenta into the fetus. Consequently, for the first several months of life, infants may have some protection against the different types of measles, chickenpox, whooping cough, and so forth. In all probability, infants will not be as well protected by placental transfer when they are born to mothers who have never had these diseases because of controlled artificial immunizations.

Laboratories combine many pints of blood and extract such products as gamma globulin and immune serum globulin, which contain antibodies. These are used to protect unimmunized people who have been exposed to regular measles and poliomyelitis. This protection is about 50 percent effective in preventing infection and reduces the severity of disease in another 30 percent.

Chemotherapy

Chemotherapy is the use of chemicals to treat disease. A desirable chemical or drug is one that destroys the parasite without doing too much damage to the host. It must have high toxicity for the one and low toxicity for the other. The two major groups of antibacterials are the sulfonamides and the antibiotics. The sulfonamides are made synthetically and the antibiotics are usually obtained from living organisms. Each group contains a variety of compounds, some of which are more effective for one kind of pathogen than for another.

Physicians may use "sulfa" drugs and antibodies together. The sulfonamide drugs are used in the treatment of infections caused by different cocci: meningococcus; which causes meningitis, and the streptococcus and staphylococcus, which cause many infections of the respiratory and urinary systems as well as of the skin. These pathogens frequently invade tissues that are weakened by viruses, thus producing secondary infections that can leave the patient with permanent damage to such organs as the brain, middle ear, heart, and lungs. The modern application of antibiotics began with the use of penicillin. Dozens of similar products are available today to retard the growth of many different pathogens.

Both sulfonamides and antibiotics must be used with caution. They do not work against all infectious agents. Most viruses are not susceptible to their action, including those viruses that cause the common cold and influenza. Indiscriminate use can be dangerous. Over a period of years, some of the pathogens have become resistant to these drugs. Resistance has become a serious problem in the control of tuberculosis, gonorrhea, and certain strains of staphylococci. The patient also may become highly allergic to antibiotics. As consumers of health products, laymen should not demand or use these products promiscuously.

PREVENTION OF COMMUNICABLE DISEASES

Communicable diseases are always caused by infectious agents or their toxins. These agents are transmitted from one host to another, either directly or indirectly. Although many microorganisms can be communicated from one host to another, the term *communicable*, or contagious, is usually reserved for infections that are fairly easily transmitted or spread. Epidemiology is a study of how disease spreads. It requires a knowledge of the source or reservoir for the pathogen, how it lives and is transmitted, and the nature of the susceptible host. Actions that render the pathogen noninfectious, prevent its spread, or make the potential or susceptible host resistant are based on the science of epidemiology. Spread of infection from the obviously ill person can be prevented, but less apparent sources of communicable disease are carriers and those so recently infected that they are still asymptomatic.

A *carrier* is a person who harbors a specific infectious agent in the absence of discernible clinical disease. The host and the pathogen have established a symbiotic relationship in which neither appears to suffer. Carriers are potential reservoirs of infection. The carrier state may last only a short time or, as in typhoid, it may extend over periods of months and years. Curing a person who is a carrier can be very difficult. He may be excluded from certain occupations, as are carriers of typhoid or other salmonella organisms, who should not work in any kind of food handling jobs, or carriers of hemolytic streptococcus, who should not work with newborn infants or with obstetrical patients.

The incubation period of a disease is that time between the entrance of the infectious organism into a new host and the appearance of symptoms. The new host is particularly a source of trouble during the prodromal stage—the period from the appearance of nonspecific symptoms until the symptoms typical of that infection appear. Many upper respiratory illnesses begin with a sore throat or a runny nose, a prodrome of

492

what is to come. In several hours to several days, additional signs develop that indicate more clearly the nature of the particular disease. During the prodromal period the infected person can spread a communicable disease, before anyone knows that the illness is contagious.

Spread of Infection

The causative agent is spread from the reservoir of infection to a new host by several means. These include contact, vector, and air.

Contact. Infections spread through contact may be directly or indirectly transmitted. Direct transmission occurs when there is body contact between the infected and the susceptible host or when the infected person sneezes, coughs, or talks within a radius of several feet of the susceptible host. In the latter instance, the germs are carried from one person to another in droplets of moisture. Respiratory infections are spread primarily through droplets. Contact can also take place indirectly when droplets or body secretions are deposited on articles (fomites) that are then handled by a susceptible host. When the pathogen is short-lived, the fomite must be something used immediately, such as eating utensils, clothing, cosmetics, bedding, or towels. These intermediate objects are said to be *contaminated*.

Vector. Vector spread of disease demands the presence of a so-called "third party," frequently an insect or rodent. The pathogen may be mechanically carried on the body of the vector, such as on the feet or mouth parts of flies and roaches; or it may actually infect the vector. Infection in the vector may be of two types: accidental or required. Some pathogens, such as protozoa and worms, grow and develop in different stages. Each stage in their life cycle may need to take place in a different species. The mosquito is a required vector for the protozoa causing malaria, as is the snail for the fluke in schistosomiasis, or bilharziasis, and beef, pork, or fish for tapeworms.

Air. Organisms may drop toward the ground and become attached to particles of dust. Stirring the dust can disseminate the microbe through the air. This particulate mode of transmission is usually short-lived, since many germs can stay alive outside the host for only a few days. Some pathogens, though, can attach themselves to molecules in the air, live long periods of time, and, because of wind currents, spread over a wide area.

Inhibiting the Growth of Microorganisms

The most effective method of destroying pathogens is by using moist heat, which coagulates cellular proteins. Boiling (at sea level) for fifteen to twenty minutes is usually sufficient to destroy germs and is reliable and economical. Steam under pressure is more efficient than boiling since in a short period of time the heat penetrates through the material being disinfected. Either procedure is practical to use in the home for small articles of clothing and eating utensils. Bedding and other similar large items as a rule can be cared for safely by washing in hot water and soap and then drying in the sun. Exposing nonwashable mattresses and pillows to air and sunlight for several days is usually sufficient. Expendable items, especially those soiled by any body secretions, should be flushed down the toilet, or wrapped well in paper and burned.

Chemical disinfectants are well known. Some are bacteriostatic and others are bacteriocidal. No one compound affects all pathogens, nor is any one compound "safe" to use on all things. Disinfectants are dangerous if used improperly: They can poison if taken internally, they can burn if they come in contact with the skin, and some can be absorbed in lethal amounts through the skin. Soap is the commonest and probably the safest disinfectant available for home use. The value of soap lies in its mechanical action rather than its bacteriocidal affect, though some soaps contain a phenol derivative that is particularly good in reducing the number of microbes on the skin.

Immunization and Chemotherapy

Good levels of health probably make people less susceptible to infection, but the most satisfactory protection is provided by immunizations and chemotherapy. The fact that immunization is available does not always mean that it will or should be used. Public health personnel and physicians consider a number of variables before deciding whether or not to vaccinate. These include the chance of becoming infected; effectiveness of treatment; fatality rate; aftereffects of the infection; efficiency of the vaccine; and complications from the vaccine.

Because of the availability of the sulfonamides in the 1930s, penicillin a decade later, and the broad-spectrum antibiotics in the 1950s, doctors can prevent many infections and treat successfully many others for which there are no vaccines. Such chemotherapy can render a contact noncommunicable in a short period of time even if it does not prevent illness. Chemotherapy and chemoprophylaxis are occasionally considered preferable to incurring the slight risk involved in using some vaccines, especially those that are not very efficient.

Everyone in the United States should be immunized against some of the more dangerous communicable diseases. Specific immunizations are different for children and adults. Children, starting two months after birth, should be vaccinated against: diphtheria, tetanus, pertussis (DPT), poliomyelitis, regular measles, rubella, and mumps.

Adults should maintain immunity against tetanus, and poliomyelitis. Several months before traveling to foreign countries, travelers should check with their physician or health department to find out what additional immunizations they need. Among the more commonly recommended are smallpox, typhoid, yellow fever, and cholera. Chemoprophylaxis is recommended against malaria in tropical regions.

Tables 13.2 and 13.3 show the communicable diseases that the United States Public Health Service recommends individuals be immunized against.

RESPIRATORY DISEASES

The most prevalent and some of the most annoying illnesses plaguing mankind are the respiratory infections. Some are acute, some are chronic, many are minor, and a few are serious. Most of these infections are caused by viruses, which are responsible for colds, influenza, and sometimes pneumonia. A few infections lead to prolonged disability and sometimes death. Bacteria and fungi also precipitate both acute and chronic respiratory disease. More frequently, the bacteria invade tissues already weakened by viruses, to produce complications and sometimes permanent tissue damage. Despite the fact that viruses are rarely affected by chemotherapy, people spend millions of dollars yearly on worthless remedies imputed to "cure." Much can be done to alleviate symptoms and make the patient more comfortable, but this is palliative therapy, not curative treatment.

The Common Cold

Colds are differentiated by their predominate symptoms and may be labeled accordingly: head colds—rhinitis; sore throat—pharyngitis; and chest cold—tracheobronchitis. More than one hundred viruses cause colds, and these pathogens are not only widespread but can be recovered from the noses and throats of many apparently healthy persons. Exactly how colds are spread is not known. Logically, they seem to be spread from person to person through droplets sprayed into the air when talking, coughing, sneezing, and by using or touching articles contaminated by

Table 13.2 Commonly Recommended Immunizations for Children

Disease	Prevalence	Immunization	Who Needs	Dosage	Booster
Poliomyelitis	Among those with low immunization rates. Vaccines have almost eliminated disease.	Live, modified polio virus vaccine (TOPV), by mouth.	Children, 6–12 wks. old. Infants usually get at same time as DPT.	3-dose series: 6–8 wks. apart.	Single dose at 18 mo. and again 4–6 yrs.
Diphtheria-* Tetanus- Pertussis (whooping cough)	Localized outbreaks. Incidence has declined with routine immunization.	Combined toxoids and vaccine. DPT (3-in-1 shot) injected into muscle.	Children, 2 mos.–6 yrs. Ideally given at usual 6-wk. checkup.	3 doses at 4–6 wk. intervals. Booster 1 yr. later.	Children, 3–6 yrs. preferably at time of school entrance.
Measles†	Among unvaccinated children. Occurs in epidemics.	Live, modified, measles-virus vaccine injected under skin.	Children over 1 yr. especially those with chronic illness.	Single shot.	None needed.
Rubella†	Among school children, especially in winter and spring. Mild in children but can damage fetus of women infected early in pregnancy.	Live, modified rubella-virus vaccine injected under skin.	Children 1 yr. to puberty. Top priority for kindergartners and early graders.	Single shot.	None needed.
Mumps†	Among young school children. Highly communicable.	Live, modified mumps-virus vaccine injected under skin.	Children over 1 yr. (especially those nearing puberty), adolescents, and men.	Single shot.	None needed.

*DT: diphtheria-tetanus toxoids, adult type, should be given ten years after the last DPT and every ten years thereafter. For a contaminated wound, a tetanus booster is needed if five years since last booster.

†May be given as measles-rubella or measles, mumps, rubella combined vaccines.

Table 13.3 Commonly Recommended Immunizations for Adults and Travelers

Disease	Prevalence	Immunization	Who Needs	Dosage	Booster
Smallpox	Endemic, though decreasing, in Asia, Africa, South America. Routine vaccination has virtually eliminated disease in U.S.	Pressed into outer skin layer with needle or injected into skin.	Travelers to some countries.	Single dose.	Revaccination every 10 yrs; every 3 yrs. for international travel to some countries.
Influenza	Epidemics in two- to three-year cycles.	Combined Hong Kong and Type B vaccine injected under skin.	Older persons; people with chronic debilitating conditions. Not for those hypersensitive to eggs.	2 doses, 6–8 wks. apart.	Single doses for high-risk persons who regularly get flu vaccines.
Typhoid	Endemic in poorly sanitized areas. Fewer than 400 cases annually in U.S.	Vaccine injected under skin.	Travelers to typhoid areas; persons exposed to known carrier or regional outbreak.	2 shots 4 wks. apart.	For continued or repeated exposure every 3 yrs.
Yellow Fever	Africa and South America.	Live, modified vaccine (17D) injected under skin.	Travelers to yellow-fever areas. Single shot. Must be given at Public Health Service vaccination center.	Single shot.	Revaccination every 10 yrs.
Cholera	South and Southeast Asia, Middle East. Occurs in endemic (native to region) and epidemic form.	Vaccine injected under skin or into muscle.	Persons traveling to or from cholera countries (list available from U.S. Public Health Service).	Single shot. 2 doses a month or more apart for extended travel in cholera areas.	Every 6 mos. when likelihood of exposure exists.
Typhus	Primitive mountainous area with cold climate. No U.S. epidemic since 1922.	Vaccine injected under skin.	Special-risk groups only. Not required as condition of entry by any country.	2 shots, 4 wks. apart.	Single shot every 6–12 mos. if exposure persists.
Plague	Parts of Asia, Africa, South America. Occasionally in western U.S. Vietnam now peak plague area.	Vaccine injected into muscle.	Persons traveling to Vietnam, Cambodia, Laos or who have contact with wild rodents in other plague areas.	3 shots about 4 wks. apart. Same for children under 10 but smaller doses.	Every 6–12 mos. when risk of exposure persists.

these droplets. The incubation period is quite short, anywhere from one to three days. Communicability apparently starts with the beginning symptoms and lasts for several days. The development of a cold seems to require several predisposing factors: fatigue, nervous tension, poor nutrition, and chilling. Some individuals seem to be more susceptible than others, and colds occur more frequently in children. As we get older, we can expect fewer colds but may have more serious complications from them.

Colds in themselves are rarely a life-and-death matter. Occasionally, a cold may involve such complications as bacterial pneumonia, tracheo-bronchitis, laryngitis, sinusitis, or ear infection. Whenever a cold is accompanied by pain in the chest and ears, extreme tenderness over the sinus areas, and an elevation of temperature, such as 102°F. or 103°F., complications should be suspected and medical advice sought. Chemotherapy at this point may be prescribed.

We should re-emphasize here that treatments of colds relieve symptoms but do not cure the infection, and antibiotics are of no value against the pathogens causing colds. Ideally, of course, the cold victim would benefit from a day or two in bed, and in bed he probably would not communicate his affliction to others. A variety of cold medications are available at pharmacies. The bases of most such medicines are aspirin to relieve pain; a stimulant, such as caffeine, to reduce the feeling of depression; and decongestants to shrink mucous membranes and reduce secretions. These are usually quite safe when self-prescribed as long as the directions on the label are followed closely as to dose, length of time they should be used, and contraindications. Their purpose is to alleviate discomfort during the acute phase only. Continued use can produce problems more serious than the original condition. Prolonged use of decongestants can weaken normal protective mechanisms so that secondary infections may develop. Nose drops themselves may irritate, may spread the infection, and, if they have an oil base, may cause pneumonia.

Other effective palliative measures include a light diet with plenty of fluids; maintenance of a constant temperature that is warm and draft free; increasing the humidity by using a vaporizer or a pan of water on a hot plate; and keeping comfortably warm. Sweating out a cold by taking hot baths, exercising, or using alcoholic beverages, instead of helping, may weaken body resistance and make the victim more susceptible to secondary infections. We have no statistical evidence that massive doses of vitamins and antihistamines prevent such infections, nor in the foreseeable future are we likely to have efficient medicines to cure or vaccines to prevent colds.

People believe in numerous myths about colds. The following examples contain little or no truth:

FOUNDATIONS OF HEALTH SCIENCE

1. Cold vaccines are quite effective. No, many viruses causing cold symptoms are still unidentified.
2. Use of antibiotics immediately will stop the cold before it gets a hold. No, antibiotics have no affect on these rhinoviruses.
3. Vitamins help prevent and/or cure colds. No scientific evidence is available to back this myth up, even relative to Vitamin C. Most physicians do not object, but they do not recommend massive doses of C; people with gout or renal stones, for example, should not take large doses of C.
4. Alcohol will help sweat out a cold. No, alcohol decreases mobilization of white cells and resistance is lowered. Some doctors believe judicious use may have a psychic effect on the depression and malaise accompanying such infection.
5. Herbal teas and mustard plasters are good adjunctive therapy. No, but their value is in "doing something," which people feel is necessary when they are ill. They certainly do no harm.
6. Chilling and wet weather contribute to colds. This is a moot point; some researchers think it does, some do not.

Influenza

Influenza is an acute respiratory disease caused by four groups of viruses: A, B, C, and D. These are spread by droplets, intimate contact, and recently contaminated towels, dishes, or other objects, and are probably also airborne. The incubation period is quite short—one to two days. The surfaces of all the air passages are inflamed and the lining becomes thickened, necrotic (the cells die), and sloughs off. The symptoms are systemic. They begin suddenly and include: marked malaise, chilliness, headache, and muscular aches in the back and limbs; a sharp elevation of temperature; a flushed face; red throat; inflamed eyelids; a watery nasal discharge and usually a dry hacking cough. Two or three days of these symptoms can leave the patient exhausted and in a run-down condition for some time. Frequently, secondary infection follows, but most people recover without permanent effects.

Influenza tends to occur in epidemics every two to three years, and an epidemic plus the symptoms described above are sufficient for diagnosis. During the "flu season" microscopic examinations are made of a sample of the population to determine the specific virus involved This information is used to prepare appropriate vaccines. About 50 percent of those immunized are protected. High-risk groups should be vaccinated annually starting September 1 so that by December, when the "flu season" begins, effective immunity is attained. The Public Health Service especially recommends that these high-risk people be immunized: those with a chronic or debilitating disease, older age groups, pregnant women, and patients in nursing homes or chronic disease hospitals. During an epidemic, as many as 40 percent of the population may be ill.

Avoiding infection is most difficult, but staying out of crowds during an epidemic may help. The antimicrobial drugs are ineffective and treatment is palliative. Bedrest in a warm room, lots of fluids such as high caloric fruit juices, and aspirin will reduce discomfort. Staying away from others may prevent complications due to additional infections. Physicians should be consulted when there is a high fever, a rapid pulse, difficulty in breathing, or any symptoms lasting more than several days.

Bronchitis

What is commonly called "bronchitis" is really tracheobronchitis, since both the trachea and bronchi are inflamed. This condition is a complication of acute viral respiratory infections. Several days after the beginning of such illnesses as colds or influenza, a mild fever will develop and coughing will be severe and produce thick purulent sputum. Acute bronchitis seldom results in serious complications even though sinusitis and laryngitis may be present.

Chronic bronchitis tends to recur each year. The periods of expectoration and coughing last several months at a time. The etiology of this condition appears to vary but can be recurrent acute upper respiratory infections; air pollution; heavy smoking; or prolonged dust inhalation usually associated with such occupations as mining and quarrying. Over long periods of exposure in such occupations, the bronchi are continuously irritated, which causes the membranous lining to thicken and become more susceptible to infection. Changes in the epithelium result in inflammation and increased mucus, which at times plugs up the small bronchioles. The symptoms last for longer and longer periods until they are continuous, month after month. The typical patient raises more than an ounce of sputum daily, and has a loose cough that is more severe in the morning and evening and worse in damp, cold weather. After a prolonged siege of coughing, the sputum may contain streaks of blood. Eventually, shortness of breath occurs and emphysema may develop.

Most people are not aware of the prevalence of this chronic condition, which is one of the major causes of disability in the United States. The incidence is increasing, and the ultimate result can be irreversible emphysema, which is discussed in the previous chapter. Those who are subject to bronchitis should be particularly conscientious about obtaining immunizations against influenza.

FOUNDATIONS OF HEALTH SCIENCE

Pneumonias

Pneumonia is an inflammation of the lungs and a filling of the air sacs with fluid or pus. It has a number of causes. Viruses are more frequently the culprits in young adults, while in infants and the aged the causes are bacteria. Aspiration of chemicals and other irritants may also result in pneumonia.

In about 80 percent of the cases the first symptom is a severe, shaking chill, and 70 percent of the victims have severe chest pain that is of a "stabbing" nature. A high fever is followed soon by a cough, and three out of four of the victims produce bloody sputum. When antibiotics are administered, a crisis (rapid drop in temperature) occurs in approximately twenty-four hours. Although serious complications may develop, more than 95 percent of all patients recover from bacterial pneumonia when treated properly. Vaccines are being developed to prevent certain of the bacterial pneumonias.

Tuberculosis

Tuberculosis is still a serious respiratory infection in the United States. Estimates indicate that possibly 10 percent of the population are infected with the tubercle bacilli and that one out of twenty people so infected will have clinical tuberculosis. Over three-fourths of the newly discovered cases of the disease tuberculosis are in an advanced stage, when it is most contagious. Only one out of five is found at an early stage, when treatment and recovery is apt to be the most successful.

The only cause of tuberculosis is the tubercle bacillus, but several factors may determine whether or not one becomes infected upon exposure. Sex, age, race, and body build appear to affect chances of infection, and people who are more susceptible are referred to as high-risk groups. In the United States, males are twice as likely as females to develop the disease, tuberculosis, and they are twice as likely to die from the disease. Almost one-half of the male victims are over forty-five years of age. Non-Caucasian races are thought to be more susceptible, but separating the influence of living conditions from race is difficult. Poverty, with its low levels of nutrition, lack of facilities for personal hygiene, and crowded conditions provides the environment in which the tuberculosis bacillus spreads most easily.

In the United States, the bacillus is nearly always spread through direct contact with someone who has clinical disease. Infection seldom results from ingesting contaminated milk, since dairy herds are screened for bovine tuberculosis and pasteurization of milk destroys this pathogen, or from contaminated objects.

A few weeks after the initial invasion, all the cells in the body have become allergic to the bacillus or its proteins (tuberculins) and the victim will demonstrate a positive skin test. Several months or more elapse before change is apparent at the usual site of invasion, the alveoli of the lungs or the surrounding lymph nodes. White blood cells and other cells surround the bacilli to form a tubercle. As the healing process continues, lime is deposited around the lesion and it eventually becomes calcified. If this calcification is complete, the pathogens will be walled inside, some of them continuing to live in a dormant stage. If the process is imperfect, the germs multiply and leave to set up new infections in other areas. If the victim's health declines, the calcified lesion can break down and the dormant bacilli become active and spread. In either case, the final effect is cavities or scars in the lungs that can be seen in an X-ray several months after infection. (See Figure 13.1.)

In open cavities bacteria continue to multiply and may be discharged for many years. As long as the bacilli multiply and spread throughout the body, continue to destroy body tissue, and are disseminated into the environment, the patient is considered to have clinical disease. The course of this disease is insidious. Without treatment, 70 percent of those afflicted will die in ten years, 5 percent continue to be chronically ill, and 25 percent have no symptoms. Modern chemotherapy gives the patient a twenty-to-one chance of living a productive life without being chronically ill. The earlier the disease is detected, the more quickly it can be controlled. But if a person waits until symptoms are pronounced enough to require medical attention, the odds are four to one that his illness will be widespread before it is diagnosed.

Chest X-rays are one screening technique used for detecting pulmonary tuberculosis. The screenee is informed, however, of *any* abnormal findings disclosed by the X-ray that require further medical evaluation. Skin tests are another valuable adjunct to screening and diagnosis. These tests detect whether or not the screenee has been infected with the tubercle bacillus. The most valid and widely accepted skin test is the Mantoux. This consists of injecting a small amount of tuberculin between the layers of the skin (intradermally). If the screenee is infected, a red wheal or raised spot will develop. Skin tests and X-rays discover only those persons who require further study. Diagnosis of clinical disease requires a series of X-rays showing changing pathology and laboratory examinations demonstrating live tubercle bacilli.

The control and eradication of this scourge is case-finding and treatment. Starting during the first year of life, people should have periodic examinations for tuberculosis infection. The examinations are accomplished by skin testing. Should skin tests be positive, follow-up by X-ray is necessary. When a person who has skin tested negatively suddenly

FOUNDATIONS OF HEALTH SCIENCE

Figure 13.1 Pulmonary Tuberculosis. Diagrammatic drawing of lungs shows progressive stages of pulmonary TB: (1) Healed and calcified complex of primary infection—primary focus and tributary lymph glands at base of right lung. (2) Healed lesion in left lung apex. (3) TB disease with cavity formation in right lung subapical region. (4) Disease spreads to opposite lower lobe through bronchial channels. (From *Introduction to Lung Diseases* [New York: American Lung Association, 1975], p. 35.)

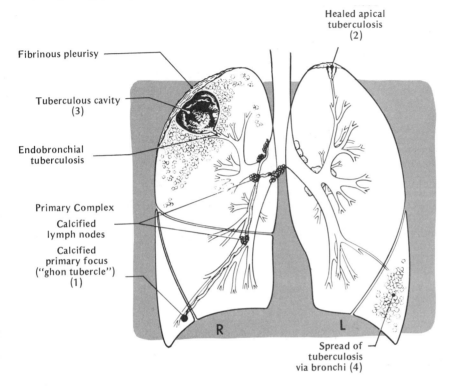

Healed apical
tuberculosis
(2)

Fibrinous pleurisy

Tuberculous cavity
(3)

Endobronchial
tuberculosis

Primary Complex

Calcified
lymph nodes

Calcified
primary focus
("ghon tubercle")
(1)

R

L

Spread of
tuberculosis
via bronchi (4)

becomes positive—is a recent converter—(1) his associates should be examined for infection and for clinical disease, and (2) he should be given antitubercular drugs. With chemotherapy, plus rest and proper nutrition, the time needed to control the disease and to render the patient non-infectious has been reduced from years to a few months. And in increasing cases, the patient is cured.

The development of efficient chemotherapy has made the general hospital inpatient and outpatient facilities a primary source for treatment. Drugs have not only shortened the period of infectiousness, but also the length of time necessary for hospitalization. The American Hospital Association no longer emphasizes that all tuberculosis patients need to be hospitalized—only those who are symptomatically ill or those with major complications.[1] Tuberculosis patients under certain conditions, even though still harboring viable bacilli, present very little hazard of spreading infection to others in the community, and in these instances, their activities are not limited or confined: (1) had one month of continuous chemotherapy, (2) have responded to treatment clinically and radiologically and are asymptomatic, (3) are and can be expected to remain under medical supervision, (4) have a suitable home situation and are cooperative, (5) understand the nature of their disease, and (6) have negative sputum cultures.[2] In addition, lifetime follow-up by health departments of ex-TB patients who have successfully completed their drug treatment is not considered necessary by medical experts.[3]

Immunization is available against tuberculosis but it is not widely used in the United States. The vaccine, BCG (Bacillus Calmette-Guerin), is safe and about 85 percent effective in preventing infection for a period of six to seven years. Authorities do not completely agree on the best technique of administering the vaccine or on how potent it should be. Anyone who has received BCG may have a positive skin test, so it would not be possible to detect and treat new early infection. The American Thoracic Society and the Surgeon General's Committee recommend BCG be given to those who must be exposed, such as nurses, physicians, or infants in households with tuberculous patients. Some health departments are making it available to people who live in areas where the incidence of tuberculosis is high.

Hemolytic Streptococcus

The hemolytic streptococcus is responsible for a variety of infections. Many streptococci are normal inhabitants of the body and rarely precipitate disease; group A causes most of the trouble. This group is nearly always spread through direct contact with someone who is ill or with a healthy carrier. Occasionally outbreaks have been the result of contaminated food, particularly milk.

The unusual characteristic of this pathogen is that the same serological type can produce sore throat, scarlet fever, erysipelas, cellulitis, impetigo (may be caused by staphylococcus, too), or puerperal fever. It may or may not cause a rash and symptomatology may depend upon the age of the victim.

The term *strep throat* is used to describe several different forms of nonpneumonic infections. People with a rash (scarlet fever) are more ill than those with acute tonsillitis and pharyngitis. In either form of streptococcus infection, the onset is quite abrupt, with chills, headache, a high fever, and frequently nausea and vomiting. Particularly in adults, the severity of the illness, fever, and very sore throat differentiate this infection from the common cold. In many instances, a physician will treat the patient with antibiotics on a presumptive basis, but a differential diagnosis requires laboratory examinations.

Scarlet fever and strep throat are by far the most prevalent streptococcal illnesses. They occur most frequently in children from five to fifteen years of age even though other age groups are susceptible. The most serious complication is rheumatic fever. The nature of the relationship between streptococcal infection and rheumatic fever is not clearly understood. Familial tendencies and poor living conditions appear to be factors. Once invaded by "strep" the victim is prone to repeated infections and additional damage.

Rheumatic fever can be prevented by prompt attention to any streptococcus infection. A throat culture is necessary to confirm the actual presence of the pathogen. Some health departments provide throat swab sets that a parent can use and then mail into the department laboratory for examination. Chemotherapy does control recurring infections, thus preventing cumulative cardiac damage, and surgery can restore the functioning of many rheumatic hearts.

Measles

Measles (red measles, regular measles, rubeolla) is an extremely contagious disease. It can attack anyone who is susceptible regardless of age. In itself it is rarely fatal, but complications do cause the death of a number of children each year—needless deaths. The complications from measles are most often due to secondary bacterial infections, usually pneumococcus, which causes pneumonia, and streptococcus, which causes middle-ear infection. A fraction of 1 percent develop encephalomyelitis, which results in death or permanent brain damage. Highly efficient vaccines are available.

Rubella

Rubella (German measles, three-day measles) is an infection that occurs in late childhood and adolescence. It seldom causes severe symptoms or any complications unless acquired during pregnancy. Immunization affords 96 percent protection against this viral disease. Public health physicians recommend that it be administered between one and twelve years of age to boys and girls. It should not be given to pregnant women or women likely to become pregnant. Protecting the majority of youths will result in limited foci of infection to endanger the pregnant woman, which is the only way to prevent rubella-induced congenital defects including blindness, deafness, missing limbs, and mental retardation. Some states are requiring that women be tested premaritally to see whether they are susceptible to rubella. If they are, immunization could be considered. Figure 13.2 is an illustration of a child with the rubella syndrome.

Mumps

Mumps, or epidemic parotitis, is a viral infection usually found in childhood, but because of its consequences of potential sterility, it is of concern to adults. Laterally, it has been one of the five most common communicable diseases among children. While mumps is generally harmless, the serious complications that occur with enough frequency to be of concern are: meningoencephalitis, nerve deafness, pancreatitis, orchitis (inflammation of the testes), impairments of vision, myocarditis, and mastitis, especially in women. Out of every one hundred adult males with mumps, less than 2 percent, if untreated, may become sterile. Vaccination is 95 percent effective.

Infectious Mononucleosis

Infectious mononucleosis is called the "kissing disease," or glandular fever, by many college students. It is spread by close contact and is fairly common in the age group between fifteen and thirty years. It is particularly prevalent around examination time when students are fatigued and under increased emotional stress. The specific cause is a virus-like organism. It is not known how it is spread. Attempts to reproduce this infection by using preparations from blood, nasopharyngeal washings, stool, or material from excised lymph nodes have been unsuccessful.

Mononucleosis is widespread and is more prevalent among males. Although epidemics have been reported among children, most cases are sporadic. The sporadic form, which college students contract, is not considered especially contagious since roommates, families, or other close contacts do not become infected. Isolating the patient is not necessary.

This disease has a wide variety of symptoms, which are usually quite mild. The initial symptoms of a general nature are malaise, fever of 100° to 103°F., sore throat, and a headache, which can be severe. These are followed by the typical signs of swollen lymph glands, particularly the nasopharyngeal tissues; sometimes the spleen becomes swollen and tender, the liver enlarges, and the patient has jaundice or a yellowing of the skin and a mild rash. The typical signs tend to appear by the fourth or fifth day of illness and last two to eight weeks. The physician makes his diagnosis based on characteristic symptoms plus a blood test.

Figure 13.2 Rubella (German Measles) Syndrome. (Courtesy of the National Foundation–March of Dimes.)

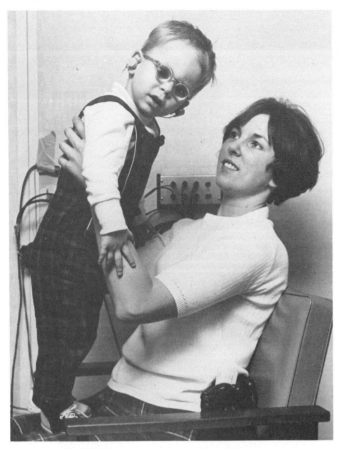

The disease itself has no specific treatment. The patient must rest in bed for a few days to several weeks and medication may be prescribed to ease the discomfort from fever, sore throat, or headache. The course of the illness is usually quite mild. Those with more severe discomfort will be ill longer. Occasionally they may have a relapse. Complications are very rare, and recovery is usually complete.

GASTROINTESTINAL DISEASES

Infections of the intestinal tract can range from mild disorders with transient symptoms of nausea to severe pain, persistent vomiting, and diarrhea. Etiological agents may be viruses and bacteria, one-celled organisms such as the protozoa, and multicelled animals such as tapeworms, pinworms, and roundworms. Some of these are found throughout the world; others are more prevalent in warm and tropical climates. The incidence of human infection by any of these is directly correlated with the level of sanitation and habits of personal cleanliness found in the community.

Viral Infections

Viral enteritis. Viral enteritis is an acute infection of the intestinal tract with symptoms of nausea, vomiting, and fever accompanied by diarrhea. In cases where the body temperature remains normal, the victim has no diarrhea. This disease is probably almost as prevalent as respiratory infections. It is spread by fecal contamination of the hands, and children are frequently carriers of the viruses. The incubation period is from one to five days, and the afebrile type frequently occurs in epidemic form. It is very contagious and usually spreads through the whole family. Treatment other than maintaining body fluid is not necessary. Prevention is accomplished by thorough handwashing after defecation.

Hepatitis A. One of the serious, presumedly viral, diseases is infectious hepatitis. It has no specific treatment, and the convalescent period may be quite prolonged. Occasionally, the condition becomes chronic and causes repeated injury to the liver. One of the typical symptoms is jaundice. The initial discomforts, about five days prior to jaundice, include malaise, loss of appetite, nausea and vomiting, and tenderness over the liver area. Diarrhea, headache, and fever may develop. Most people (over 90 percent) get well without complications in about three months. Hepatitis A is usually spread by food and water contaminated by feces, and infections can occur in epidemics.

Hepatitis B. Another similar disease is serum hepatitis, or Hepatitis B, which is spread usually by the administration of blood or blood products that have been prepared from someone who has had the disease. Possibly 2 percent of the population are carriers of the antigen, which contains virus-like particles.

The control and prevention of Hepatitis B is proper sterilization of surgical instruments, syringes, and hypodermic needles, and not using sera from donors that give a history of jaundice or of recent potential exposure to the virus. For example, a narcotic addict taking drugs by injection or someone who has been tatooed within the last six months could be infected. Hepatitis B or serum hepatitis is considered an occupational disease along laboratory workers and other medical personnel working with equipment that might be contaminated with infected blood or sera. A laboratory test can confirm the presence of the hepatitis B antigen, which is associated with the disease. The organism causing Hepatitis B is also present in semen and saliva. It can be infectious if ingested through kissing or oral sex.

The Committee on Viral Hepatitis of the National Academy of Science –National Research Council recommends:

1. Persons found to have a positive antigen test be considered infectious and control measures be taken with respect to potentially infectious materials such as blood and blood-contaminated secretions.
2. Women found to have hepatitis during pregnancy or during the first two months postpartum be tested for hepatitis B antigen and their infants tested at monthly intervals for at least six months.
3. Testing for hepatitis B antigen be required of all blood donors.
4. Standard Human Immune Serum Globulin is of no demonstrable value in the treatment of carriers.[4]

The incidence of both types of hepatitis is increasing markedly. In some areas there is more than a 100 percent rise in number of cases diagnosed. The people commonly hit are in the age bracket fifteen to twenty-four years, and more than two-thirds of these are males. The clinical symptoms in each disease are somewhat different. Immunity in infectious hepatitis, hepatitis A, appears to last longer than in hepatitis B and the outlook for type A is also much better.

Bacterial Infections

In the United States, bacterial infections of the intestinal tract are commonly caused by organisms belonging to the genus of *Salmonella* or *Shigella*. In other areas of the world, such as sections of the Orient, the pathogen causing cholera is a dangerous health problem.

Typhoid fever. Typhoid fever is an acute illness that lasts several weeks. The causative agent is *Salmonella typhosa,* which is excreted in the feces. Where sanitation is poor, the pathogen may live several months in the soil. Flies may be vectors under these circumstances. This disease can also spread through fecally contaminated water. In areas where sanitation is good, the disease is usually transmitted directly by chronic carriers. If such persons work in food handling occupations, they readily transmit this infection.

The symptoms include continued fever, bronchitis, enlarged spleen, rose spots on the trunk of the body, and constipation followed by diarrhea. With modern chemotherapy, few people die, but a very small percentage of those infected become chronic carriers and may excrete the germ in their feces for years. Although drugs are used to remedy the carrier state, surgery is nearly always necessary. The typhoid bacilli literally "hole-up" in the gall bladder and removal of this organ to eliminate them is successful 90 percent of the time. Immunization is effective.

Salmonellosis or paratyphoid. Infections with other salmonella organisms are usually known as salmonellosis. They are most commonly acquired from infected animals and animal products, particularly poultry products. In meat processing plants, the pathogens from an infected animal can contaminate the whole plant. Some surveys have indicated that anywhere from 1 to 58 percent of the raw meat in the market is contaminated. The usual home cooking temperatures do not kill salmonella, and boiled or fried eggs may contain viable bacteria.

Because of the prevalence of this organism, we are fortunate that man is not very susceptible to infection by it. Several studies indicate that human beings must ingest a large number of salmonella before symptoms develop. Good general health seems to reduce the chance of symptomatic infection. Normal body defenses, such as gastric juices, destroy the bacteria. Immunization against paratyphoid is not always accepted as being of great value, but it is probably desirable if one is exposed in his occupation or is traveling where sanitation is poor.

DISEASES ACQUIRED THROUGH THE SKIN

Microorganisms enter the body through the skin in several ways. Some potential pathogens are normally found on the skin, in the soil, or on objects, but they gain entry into the body only when there is a break in the skin due to some kind of trauma such as scratches, cuts, abrasions, burns, insect bites, or dermatitis. Other groups of pathogens are found in an intermediate host or vector and are introduced into the body by bites or stings. The third group is able to penetrate healthy skin when there is direct contact between host and susceptible. Regardless of the manner by which these germs enter, some of the infections they produce are seldom if ever contagious, some are contagious only under special environmental conditions, and some are readily communicated from one person to another. Certain of these organisms, such as hookworm, are mainly nuisances and rarely result in serious illness; others, such as syphilis, can produce severe damage that may permanently handicap their victim; and one, rabies, nearly always causes death. Of the four diseases discussed in this chapter, two—rabies and tetanus—are ever-present threats to life, and two—syphilis and gonorrhea, the venereal diseases—account for most of the reportable contagious diseases.

Tetanus

Tetanus, or lockjaw, claims several hundred lives each year in the United States. About 35 percent of those diagnosed will die. These deaths are needless since immunization is so very effective. The infectious agent, *Clostridium tetani,* can enter the body through any break in the skin regardless how trivial. The general populace erroneously associates danger of infection with a deep puncture wound made by a rusty nail. Although a puncture wound is more conducive to invasions, any object may cause tetanus whether or not it is rusty—a nail, gravel, twigs, thorns, burns, insects, a sewing needle, or even a hypodermic needle. Either the object causing the wound or the injured skin could be contaminated.

Clostridium tetani is widely present in the soil and in spore form can survive many years. Man and other mammals, such as cows and horses, carry the germ in their intestinal tracts. Human carriers are more prevalent in rural areas, but the pathogens have been recovered from urban house dust and even from operating rooms.

Tissue that is devitalized by injury enables the organism to grow. The infection remains localized but the toxins produced are extremely potent. How these toxins spread and act is not known. The clinical manifestations are usually restlessness, difficulty in swallowing, spasm of the muscles controlling the opening of the jaws (hence the name "lockjaw"), and spasms of the muscles of the neck, face, back, abdomen, and extremities. These spasms interfere with respirations. Death is probably the result of lack of oxygen, exhaustion, shock, and electrolyte imbalance.

Practical and effective prevention consists of routine immunizations beginning the first year of life. The duration of immunity is quite long-lasting, from three to ten or more years. If the initial series of injections with toxoid was completed and a year has elapsed since the last injection, a booster shot at the time of injury affords almost 100 percent protection.

Cleaning wounds is presumed to be of some value, and surgical removal of dirt and damaged tissue helps. Laboratory studies show that antiseptics have little effect on these pathogens. Passive immunization or the administration of antitoxin after injury is not always effective. Prolonged antibiotic treatment may be used.

Rabies

Rabies is an ever-present threat to mankind. The disease is endemic among warm-blooded animals in many areas, and the incidence among wild life seems to be increasing in the United States. The rabies virus appears to be of two types: the sylvatic type found primarily among foxes, coyotes, skunks, raccoons, and bats; and the domestic type most commonly infecting dogs, but occasionally present in cows and cats.

The rabies virus affects the central nervous system and is transmitted by the saliva of an infected host from bites or licking. Whether or not the disease develops following exposure depends to some degree upon the location and severity of the wounds. The most dangerous are bites about the face and neck. Children are more susceptible than adults. The usual incubation period in human beings is from ten days to several months, possibly as long as a year. There is a correlation between the length of incubation and the amount of virus in the saliva of the biting animal as well as the severity of the wounds.

Dogs are infectious several days prior to the appearance of symptoms. The animal can be restless, agitated, erratic, and aggressive, growling and biting at any object or other animal, or it may be dumb and paralyzed, and display little restlessness and agitation. Sometimes dogs will not have apparent signs of illness. Death usually takes place in ten to fourteen days.

In people, the beginning symptoms are fever, loss of appetite, headache, nausea, sore throat, and pain or burning around the wound. Soon muscle spasms develop and convulsions occur. The afflicted may become maniacal. Eventually paralysis results.

No drugs or chemical agents can combat this infection once symptoms appear. However, the use of vaccine and antiserum *after exposure, before symptomatology,* is most effective. In areas where the disease is endemic among the animal population, every animal biting a human being should be suspected. These steps should be taken:

1. All bites or scratches and abrasions exposed to licks of animals must be washed well with soap and rinsed or flushed thoroughly.
2. Severe lacerations should be cleaned out surgically and if possible not sutured for several days.
3. Severely exposed victims should have antiserum injected into the bite or lacerated area.
4. Administration of rabies vaccine and antirabies serum is recommended following severe exposure or if bitten by a wild animal. (The development of antibodies resulting from the vaccine alone may be too slow to provide sufficient protection.)

FOUNDATIONS OF HEALTH SCIENCE

In recent years, vaccines have been developed that produce fewer undesirable reactions. They are now being used prophylactically for veterinarians, laboratory workers, animal handlers, personnel stationed overseas in endemic rabies areas, and others in high-risk occupations.

Wildlife, particularly skunks, bats, and raccoons are the major source of endemic infection to domestic animals and to man. Vaccination of dogs and cats protects them against infection and indirectly protects us. All states have laws regarding dog vaccination programs and programs to control stray dogs.

THE SEXUALLY
TRANSMITTED DISEASES

A number of diseases are transmitted sexually. Some are primarily nuisances, but many have serious consequences to the one initially infected, the sex partner, and/or to a child before birth or as a consequence of birth. Certain of these diseases may be increasing because of changing sexual mores. Birth control pills can alter the vaginal environment enabling some pathogens to produce symptoms or to be more readily transmitted to the sex partner. Both the pill and IUD usage have resulted in less use of condoms, which prevent the spread of several sexually transmitted infections. The consensus of opinion seems to be that, today, people have greater numbers of sexual partners and that relationships are of a more casual nature. Greater numbers of partners certainly increase chance of exposure, and casualness may include less concern for the well-being of the sexual partner as well as knowledge about the partner's behavior and values. More people seem to be resorting to a greater variety of behaviors to satisfy sexual needs. Oral-genital sex and anal intercourse enable the spread of some infections that might otherwise not occur. Since it is becoming more and more acceptable to discuss sexual matters, more people are requesting diagnosis and treatment for symptoms of sexually transmitted infections. In addition, physicians are beginning to screen routinely those who are in the most sexually active years regardless of age, marital status, or their opinion about the person's possible sexual behavior (an opinion that higher socioeconomic groups have less sexually transmitted infections than lower groups, for example). Among the sexually transmitted diseases are those commonly called the venereal diseases (VD). The most important of these in the United States are gonorrhea and syphilis. Laws in all states require that these two infections be reported to the health department. This is not true for most of the other sexually transmitted infections.

Various studies have revealed that in order of frequency, among those going for treatment of inflammation of the urethra the major infectious cause is *Chlamydia trachomatis; Herpes virus hominis Type II* is second; and in third place is *Neisseria gonorrhea*.

Chlamydia Trachomatis

Chlamydia trachomatis causes infections known frequently as Chlamydia or trachomatis when the organism affects the genito-urinary system and trachoma when it invades the conjunctiva of the eyes. It is the major cause of inflammation of male and female genital structures in the sexually active. In one study of those who had nongonococcal urethritis, 36 percent were infected with *Chlamydia;* when only those with a urethral discharge were counted, 57 percent were infected with *Chlamydia*. In women with inflammation of the cervix, 37 percent demonstrated this same pathogen.[5]

Transmission. Trachomatis is spread by contact with one who is infected. Sexual transmission is the most common since the organism requires the warm moist environment found in the genital tract to survive successfully. The newborn may become infected while passing through the birth canal. The consequence is conjunctivitis or opthalmia neonatorum, which, if untreated, causes blindness.

Pathogenesis. The incubation period is from seven to fourteen days. This infection is often asymptomatic. It can produce urethritis, cervical lesions, and sometimes, pelvic inflammation (PID). A small percentage of males develop prostatitis.

Diagnosis. An antigen test and cell cultures can confirm the diagnosis. Current recommendations are to treat those with symptoms of nongonococcal urethritis (NGU) and their sexual partners without waiting for laboratory confirmation.

Treatment. Treatment with antibiotics, usually sulfa drugs or tetracycline is effective. Sometimes in well-established or long-time infections treatment is not successful.

Herpes Virus Hominis Type II

Herpes belongs to a family of viruses that causes many persistent skin problems ranging from fever blisters and cold sores to shingles.

FOUNDATIONS OF HEALTH SCIENCE

When these infections appear above the waist they are generally due to herpes simplex Type I virus; below the waist, they are usually due to herpes virus Type II. Each type can occur outside its customary territory, though.

Herpes virus Type II infections seem to be exploding through the nation. Estimates are that there were a million cases in 1975. The explosion is presumed to be the result of increased numbers of casual sexual encounters and more oral-genital sex. Herpes increases the number of miscarriages; and one-half the children born to infected mothers develop this disease. If the child has skin manifestations only, the prognosis is good. If other organs are involved, permanent brain damage usually results, and the child has a 75–100 percent chance of death. Six percent of women with genital herpes will develop cervical cancer in five years.[6]

Transmission. Herpes genitalis is highly contagious and is readily spread to sex partners. For a pregnant woman with the disease, a cesarean section to deliver the child is desirable since the infant may become infected while passing through the vaginal canal. The Type I virus usually invades and produces symptoms above the waist. However, as a result of oral-genital sex, it too can invade the genital area. Tight-fitting clothing such as panty hose appears to favor a recurrence of symptoms. Pills and IUDs seem to contribute to the transmission to male sex partners since these birth control procedures cause an increase in vaginal secretions that apparently favor spread of the pathogen. Use of the condom can reduce chances of becoming infected.

Pathogenesis. The incubation period is from two to twenty days following exposure, but usually six days suffices for symptoms to appear: sores like fever blisters; single or multiple raised painful lesions; fever, headache, malaise; tender, swollen lymph nodes; and dysuria (painful urination). The symptoms last two to three weeks. The disease has a high rate of recurrence, as much as four to five times the first year of infection, followed by two or three attacks in each succeeding year. Symptoms may also go unnoticed.

Diagnosis. During the symptomatic stage, diagnosis is easy. The lesions are characteristic and a Pap smear will show multinucleated giant cells. Between recurrence of symptoms, herpes cannot be detected.

Treatment. We have no well-established cure for vaginal herpes. Several things are being tried experimentally but the rate of success is low. Dye and light therapy is not too effective and has produced cancer in experimental animals. Prevention is the only means of control; limiting sexual partners and using a condom provide some protection. A vaccine is being used experimentally in Germany. Some physicians find they can forestall recurrences by using repeated smallpox and TB vaccinations.

Trichomoniasis

Trichomoniasas is caused by a protozoa. Some physicians estimate that one-half their female patients who have vaginal infections suffer from this disease. Approximately one-half their sexual partners will also be infected. The trichomonad may migrate to the prostrate, enter the semen, and thus be spread to females during intercourse.

Pathogenesis. Men are usually asymptomatic, but women usually suffer from vaginal irritation, discharge, and intense itching (the discharge is frothy, odorous, and a greenish-yellow color). They may have pain or difficulty when urinating. Chronic inflammation of various glands, the reproductive organs, and urinary system may be complicating consequences. The incubation period is four to twenty-eight days, and trichomonas may be spread by sexual contact. Controversy surrounds the question of whether or not the use of birth control pills contributes to infection, but intercourse without using a condom increases likelihood of spread. Long term infections injure the cervix and therefore increase chance of cancer.

Diagnosis. A cervical smear examined microscopically, is diagnostically accurate. Routine Pap tests can uncover such infections.

Treatment. Flagyl (metronidazole) is most effective. *All male sexual partners should be treated concurrently.* Treatment with the above medicine should not be given during the first trimester of pregnancy because of possible teratogenicity. Vaginal suppositories containing metronidazole are available for pregnant and nursing women.

Gonorrhea

A report to the recent International Venereal Disease Symposium indicates:

A real epidemic of gonorrhea is prevalent throughout the country.
People between the ages of 15 and 19 account for 80 percent of the reported cases of gonorrhea and 65 percent of the reported cases of primary and secondary syphilis .... Geographically the rates of venereal disease in

FOUNDATIONS OF HEALTH SCIENCE

large cities are five to ten times those of smaller cities, and the rates among central city population are as much as ten times higher than among other groups. . . .[7]

Reported cases are only indications of the magnitude of the problem. Several surveys reveal that most cases of gonorrhea and syphilis are treated by the private physician who may report as few as 10 percent of these to the health department.

Transmission. Gonorrhea (GC) is almost wholly transmitted in children, adolescents, and adults through sexual intercourse. The gonococcus re-

Sounds like "True Confessions," but sexual relations can be complicated.

After graduating from a southern college, Maureen spent one year in the Peace Corps. She then "did her thing" on the West Coast, but moved back East to "settle down" for her career. Even though she was a college graduate and had job experience, she could not find a job in her major (history) so in the meantime she took a secretarial job at a university.

She dated around, but then became serious about Bob. However, as she made more definite plans for their life together, he became more evasive. Finally, the whole relationship fell apart. Maureen was heartbroken, but with the help of friends began to pull her life back together. After a few months she noticed that one of the real nice young professors, Scott, had become part of her circle of friends. Although it wasn't intentional on her part, she began spending a lot of time with him— not really dating, but doing a lot of things together. One thing led to another, and Maureen began spending more nights and weekends at Scott's townhouse apartment.

One night Maureen developed severe abdominal pains. The gynecologist at the hospital explained that the pain was from an ectopic pregnancy and scheduled immediate surgery. During surgery it was discovered that it was not an ectopic pregnancy but severely inflamed Fallopian tubes caused by gonorrhea. Maureen blamed Scott who said he never had any signs of gonorrhea or any other venereal disease.

The doctor told Maureen she would never be able to have children. Scott said he wanted to marry her anyway and they could adopt children if they wanted to have a family. Maureen continued to accuse Scott of giving her VD and ruining her life. After a couple of weeks Scott told Maureen that OK, he would get out of her life forever if that's what she wanted.

Maureen went back to Atlanta to live with her parents. She refused to talk to Scott when he called, so he stopped calling.

quires moisture and warmth to exist, and these conditions are found in the tissues of the generative organs. It can live outside the body for only a minute or two and can attack the mucous membranes in the mouth and cause symptoms of a sore throat. A person who has cunnilingus with an infected female has a 5 to 10 percent chance of such infection, and following fellatio with an infected person, the chance is 20 to 30 percent of becoming diseased.[8] Nonsexual infection of the cunjuctiva of the eyes may occur at the time of birth. If the cervix of the mother is infected, the pathogen can get into the eyes of the fetus. The ensuing infection is a congenital ophthalmia neonatorium, and the consequences can be permanent blindness. State laws require prophylactic treatment in the eyes of all newborn to prevent this. Adults can acquire gonorrheal conjunctivitis by infecting themselves with contaminated hands.

Pathogenesis. The course of gonorrhea is different in males than in females. In some three to nine days after exposure, the male usually has severe discomfort from burning when he urinates. Severe inflammation in the urethra may cause thick, yellow, creamy pus that drips from the end of the penis. In fact, one of the slang expressions for this infection is "the drip." If the male remains untreated, the immediate symptoms will abate but the gonococcus may slowly spread up the urethra into the bladder and ureters, or it may spread into the prostate gland, up the vas deferens, through the epididymes and down into the testes. In chronic inflammation of the epididymes, the tubes will eventually be blocked with scar tissue. Sterility results in approximately 5 percent of such cases. Chronic bladder and ureteral irritation can cause urinary obstruction. Possibly 10 percent of males are asymptomatic.

In the female, the disease is primarily one of the reproductive system rather than the urinary system. Women are frequently asymptomatic. Not only are they carriers, but they are reservoirs of infection. The gonococcus prefers to live in the cervix. Since there is little sensation in the cervix, the woman does not realize that she is infected. She may have some discharge, but she usually has discharges and does not recognize this as being abnormal. In 15 percent of women with gonorrhea, the organism infects the urethra, bladder, anus and rectum, uterus, and Fallopian tubes, respectively. Scarring in the tubes causes obstruction and sterility. Gonorrhea may also cause arthritis and heart disease in either male or female.

The effects of gonorrhea are more serious than many realize. One of five women infected with GC develops pelvic inflammatory disease, and over half of these women must be hospitalized. Of those hospitalized, 50 percent are so severely ill that they require radical pelvic surgery.[9] The pill contributes to adverse effects. Clinical evidence indicates that women

FOUNDATIONS OF HEALTH SCIENCE

on the Pill "tend to suffer gonorrhea complications including pelvic in-flammatory diseases, skin lesions and arthritis at almost twice the rate of those not taking oral contraceptives."[10]

Diagnosis. The diagnosis of gonorrhea is difficult, and clinical laboratory examinations may not reveal its presence. The laboratory tests consist of microscopic examinations of smears and of cultures. The microscopic exam is inaccurate 40 to 50 percent of the time; the culture is much more accurate with a rate of 80 to 90 percent, but this type of test takes forty-eight hours to do. One out of three cases in males and three out of four cases in females will be missed on initial examination. In addition, since about 80 percent of the females and 10 to 15 percent of males show no symptoms and may remain asymptomatic for long periods of time, they not only continue spreading the infection, but are more apt to develop serious complications since they usually go untreated.[11]

Treatment. Although the *Neisseria gonococcus* is becoming resistant to penicillin, large doses in one or two injections cure about 85 percent of the infections. Cases that do not respond are treated with one of the other antibiotics. A follow-up examination after treatment is necessary to be sure that antibiotic therapy was effective. Any irritant to the urinary system, such as alcohol, sexual relations, or menstruation during the infectious stage interferes with cure and recovery.

Syphilis

Syphilis is the most serious of all the venereal diseases because of its severe effects. It is known as the great masquerader since not only can it destroy any tissue in the body but its symptoms can mimic those of many other diseases.

Transmission. Syphilis is caused by a spirochete, the *Treponema pallidum*. A treponema can exist only where it is warm and moist, inside or on the surface of the human body. It lives only a few seconds away from the body, since it is so sensitive to drying and changes in temperature. Consequently, with few exceptions, it is spread only by the prolonged close body contact found in sexual relationships, and the act of sexual inter-course is the method by which it is most frequently transmitted from one person to another. However, this disease can spread from other types of contact when lesions containing the spirochete are present on the skin or mucous membranes. This condition can be acquired from kissing dur-ing the infectious stage if mouth lesions are present. It is not contracted from such objects as contaminated dishes, toilet seats, or linens. Approximately 50 percent of those exposed will become infected.

Pathogenesis. The infection is systemic in that it spreads throughout the body. The infectious process takes place in four stages: primary, secondary, early latent, and late latent syphilis. After the organism invades the body, a period of incubation usually lasts from two to twelve weeks. Then at the site of the original inoculation a nonpainful sore appears, called a *chancre*. This chancre is apparent to a male if it is on the external genitalia and if he *happens* to notice it. If it should be in or about the rectum, it may not be seen. The female is not as fortunate since the lesion is most apt to be inside the vaginal tract and not observable to her. Should it be on the external genitalia, she most likely will not see it either, since it gives no discomfort. Treponemas are present in these lesions, and they can be spread to a sexual partner through heterosexual or homosexual relationships. In the primary stage, diagnosis is made only by microscopic examination. The blood is not yet reactive. This sore disappears without treatment. Infection without a chancre is fairly frequent.

The secondary stage appears two to ten weeks later. By this time, the infection is systemic so the symptoms may be widespread, and the blood is becoming reactive and may be tested. Signs can include a rash, mucous patches or whitish areas in the mouth, a sore throat, low fever, and some loss of hair. These, too, go away without treatment but the disease is contagious since pathogens are present in the skin and mouth lesions. Since they are also in the blood, an infected hypodermic needle could spread the infection. These symptoms, like the chancre, can be overlooked. If the victim is undergoing treatment for another condition with antibiotics, these symptoms may be so aborted that they are not evident. *Forty to 60 percent of the patients are unaware of having the disease.*

During the secondary stage, the body marshals its defenses to fight the organism. Antibodies begin to develop plus an antibody-like substance called *reagin*. These are demonstrable in the blood. Sometimes a spontaneous recovery is apparent, but most often relapses occur, some as long as thirteen years after the first invasion. Susceptibility is universal since the body has no natural immunity. The antibodies that do develop can easily be overcome by large reinfecting doses or they may fail to develop because of early treatment.

Between ten and thirty years after the first invasion by this spirochete, thirty to forty out of each one hundred untreated cases will develop severe cardiovascular and nervous system dysfunctions. Some 90 percent of the time private physicians fail to recognize that syphilis is involved in a "heart case." Figure 13.3 shows what happens during the different stages.

FOUNDATIONS OF HEALTH SCIENCE

Figure 13.3 Pathogenesis of Syphilis. (From G. Edward Maxwell, "Why the Rise in Teen-Age Venereal Disease?" *Today's Health,* 43:21, September, 1965, published by the American Medical Association.)

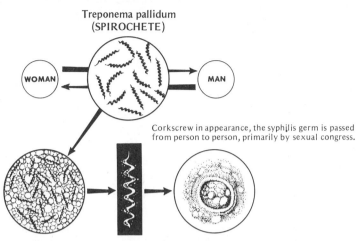

Treponema pallidum
(SPIROCHETE)

WOMAN   MAN

Corkscrew in appearance, the syphilis germ is passed from person to person, primarily by sexual congress.

Burrowing into tissues at entry site, spirochetes may give no indication of their presence from 14 to 90 days. During all this time (the incubation period) they increase in number.

As time of migration to all parts of the body approaches, tempo of spirochete activity increases. Tissues around invasion site become irritated, sometimes giving rise to "soreless" sore—a primary, or **hard** chancre.

Specific Antibodies: Alerted to spirochetes' presence (about 14 days after their invasion), the body builds up its own defenses. Some specific antibodies, capable of killing spirochetes, are produced but in insufficient numbers and potency to annihilate all the hostile invaders.

Reagin, an antibody–like substance, is also produced. More bacteriostatic than bactericidal, reagin inhibits the growth and mobility of the spirochetes rather than kills them.

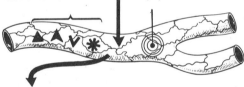

Secondary Stage of Untreated Syphilis

Breaking through every body defense, the spirochetes migrate to all parts of the body, the defensive reagin and antibodies follow in pursuit. Sometimes evidence of the many skirmishes which ensue shows up in intermittent rashes on the body.

Terminal Stage

Rather than wander aimlessly around in the blood the poisonous spirochetes choose to "occupy" body tissues in such choice locations as the heart, liver, and the brain. Eventually, these vital organs become so badly damaged that the patient dies from syphilis.

Latent or Dormant Stage

After two years or thereabouts, the spirochetes seemingly call a truce for five, 10, 15, or even 20 years. During all this time they may give no sign of their presence. But they can and will come out fighting at any time.

The Role of Penicillin

The body never idly accepts the infiltration of any germ. Still, in the case of syphilis, it can only marshal a sluggish — if stubborn — defense. What the body desperately needs is a potent ally capable of annihilating on contact the great hordes of poisonous spirochetes. This it has in penicillin.

Diagnosis. The diagnosis is made by both clinical and laboratory examinations. During the primary stage, spirochetes can be scraped from skin lesions and seen by a microscopic darkfield process. A diagnosis can be missed at this time since the spirochetes may not be visible if the lesions are unclean, have been treated with antiseptics, or if the patient has taken antibiotics. About four to five weeks after the infection has become systemic, the blood test can be used for diagnosis. Occasionally, the tests show false positives because of similar reactive changes in the blood resulting from pregnancy; chronic diseases such as tuberculosis, malaria, and diabetes; hepatitis; narcotic addiction; recent blood transfusion; a new smallpox vaccination; or some acute infections.

Treatment. Curing syphilis today takes the same amount of penicillin as it did twenty years ago. Physicians prefer to give a series of intramuscular injections over several weeks. If they believe the patient is not likely to complete the series, the total dose can be administered at one time. Oral antibiotics, such as tetracycline, kill the treponema and are used in penicillin-sensitive patients. Twenty-four hours after commencing antibiotic therapy, the patient is usually noninfectious. When treatment is started during the latent stages, it may not be effective in halting cellular destruction. Once tissue is destroyed, the resultant defects are seldom correctable. A baby who acquires congenital syphilis from its mother and is born with physical handicaps and is mentally retarded will live his life through with these handicaps. The patient who becomes psychotic or in whom there is extensive neural damage or paresis will always be symptomatic.

Moniliasis or Candidiasis

Moniliasis or Candidiasis is caused by the fungus, *Candida* or *Monilia albicans*. This organism is commonly present in the vaginal tract and large intestine of men and women. Symptoms may be precipitated by pregnancy, diabetes, birth control pills, antibiotic treatment, and lowered resistance.

Pathogenesis. The organism is commonly present in the vaginal tract and may be spread through sexual contact; it can be acquired by infants during birth. The symptoms include intense genital itching, an inflamed, dry vaginal tract, and a thick curd-like white discharge, all of which frequently recur. Infected males are usually asymptomatic.

Diagnosis. The *Candida* can be detected by special smears and cultures.

Treatment. Treatment is effective: Miconazole nitrate (Monistat Cream) and Nystatin tablets used vaginally.

Condylomata Acuminata— Venereal Warts

Condylomata acuminata, or venereal warts, are caused by a Papova Group virus. Physicians are seeing more and more of these infections, too. Depending on their location, these warts may be subject to chronic irritation and secondary infection. If they are in the rectum or urethra, they may obstruct urination and defecation; such obstructions can be very painful. The presence of genital warts can be disfiguring, to say the least; they may occur around the anus, scrotum, and on the penis and labia. They may recur and ultimately become malignant.

Pathogenesis. The incubation period is from one to three months. The appearance of Condylomata is similar to common skin warts. They may be single or multiple growths, may be pink colored, indented and moist with a cauliflower-like texture, or be hard and yellow-gray. They are usually transmitted by sexual intercourse, and the probability of infection after intercourse with an infected partner is 60 to 70 percent. Circumsized males are much less frequently afflicted.[12]

Diagnosis. Simple observation is sufficient for diagnosis.

Treatment. Chemotherapy such as Podophyllin is effective. Keeping the genital area clean and dry and using a condom may be of value in preventing infection.

Nongonococcal Urethritis (NGU)

Nongonococcal urethritis, or NGU, is any inflammation of the urethra that is not caused by gonorrhea infection. This disease may also be diagnosed as nonspecific urethritis, or NSU. NGU is as common as gonorrhea in males and seems to be increasing. Such infections are not known to occur in females.

The causes include mycoplasmas that are something like viruses, chlamydia, allergies, trichomonads, and chemical irritations. Infection appears to be transmitted sexually in that males who have not had intercourse do not contract this disease. Their sexual partner may not be infected, though.

Pathogenesis. The symptoms usually include usually a clear discharge from the penis, especially noticeable before urinating in the morning (sometimes the discharge is thick and white) as well as mild to moderate pain when voiding (while in gonorrhea the pain is nearly always severe).

Diagnosis. The diagnosis may be missed if the physician suspects all discharges to be gonorrheal. Men should refuse to accept treatment until a sample of the discharge is taken for laboratory testing. Relapses occur when the victim becomes tired, has poor body resistance, and is emotionally upset. Gonorrhea increases susceptibility to such infections.

Treatment. Symptoms may disappear in two weeks without treatment. However, antibiotics, namely tetracycline, is the drug of choice.

Vaginitis and Cystitis

Vaginitis may also be labeled NSV or NGV—nonspecific vaginitis or nongonorrheal vaginitis. As in treating males, physicians do not always utilize laboratory procedures to identify the specific cause.

Pathogenesis. In vaginitis the symptoms are the same when caused by one of several microorganisms: inflammation, severe genital itching, and vaginal discharge. The most common urinary tract disorder is cystitis, or inflammation of the bladder. This condition occurs almost exclusively in women between puberty and age forty-five. In cystitis, too, several different pathogens could be responsible. Symptoms include burning and frequency of urination, blood-tinged urine, low back pain, and fever. Untreated cystitis can result in kidney infection.

Diagnosis. In the case of either vaginitis or cystitis, diagnosis must include laboratory testing and a microscopic examination.

Treatment. Depending on the cause, sulfa drugs and antibiotics are successful in curing most such infections.

MEASURES TO CONTROL SEXUALLY TRANSMITTED DISEASES

Public health personnel consider that we are in the midst of an epidemic of sexually transmitted diseases. The accuracy of any data is questionable, of course, since physicians do not report all the cases they treat and reporting depends on such variables as the use of private versus public medical facilities and the reactions of a physician to a young patient with a sexually contracted disease, to disease acquired through either extramarital or variant sexual behavior, and the success of public health authorities in getting physicians to comply with reporting regulations.

Education of physicians has improved their rate of reporting. The physician does not have the time or facilities to track down sexual contacts, examine them for infection, and treat them when necessary, but a number of states have laws and regulations that require doctors, in addition to reporting suspected and diagnosed cases to health authorities, to instruct their patients in the seriousness and prevention of the disease:

> It shall be the duty of the physician in attendance on a person having a venereal disease, or suspected of having a venereal disease, to instruct such patient in precautionary measures for preventing the spread of the disease, the seriousness of the disease, and the necessity for treatment and prolonged medical supervision, and the physician shall, in addition, furnish approved literature on these subjects.[13]

Since diagnosing gonorrhea in the female is difficult, women should be treated presumptively on the basis of infected contact rather than waiting for medical confirmation of disease. Diagnosing and treating a patient without examining the sexual partner is also foolish, for in all likelihood one has infected the other.

The responsibility for case finding is legally delegated to the public health department. The health officers or investigators are invested with full powers of inspection, examination, and isolation of all persons known to be infected with venereal disease in an infective stage. Health departments also provide clinics in which anyone can be examined and in many instances treated free of charge. In many states, this service is available without parental consent to minors. The law in California is quoted here:

> Notwithstanding any other provision of law, a minor 12 years of age or older who may have come into contact with any infectious, contagious, or communicable disease may give consent to the furnishing of hospital, medical and surgical care related to the diagnosis or treatment of such disease, if the disease or condition is one which is required by law or regulation adopted pursuant to law to be reported to the local health officer. Such consent shall not be subject to disaffirmance because of minority. The consent of the parent, parents, or legal guardian of such minor shall not be necessary to authorize hospital, medical and surgical care related to such disease and such parent, parents, or legal guardian shall not be liable for payment for any care rendered pursuant to this section.[14]

Gonorrheal case finding is difficult not only because of the numbers infected but because the period of communicability occurs within several days of infection. In addition, no highly efficient techniques for rapid diagnosis are available. On the other hand, in syphilis, the long incubation period enables the finding of sexual contacts before they become contagious, and we do have reliable laboratory procedures for making a diagnosis.

Many of these sexual-related infections in the United States are contracted primarily through so-called free promiscuous homosexual or heterosexual relationships, not from the male or female prostitute or professional purveyor of sex, which makes public health procedures of control extremely difficult. In the promiscuous, nonprostitute relationship the sources of infection cannot be easily tracked down. The name of the sexual partner may not be known, and people are frequently untruthful about such behavior.

These personal prophylactic measures can reduce to some extent the chance of infection:

1. Use of a mechanical contraceptive such as the condom
2. Urinating immediately after intercourse by males
3. Douching immediately after intercourse by females
4. Washing genital area with soap and water
5. Physician treatment with antibiotics: (a) after sexual relationships with a potentially infected partner, or (b) treatment of suspicious symptoms prior to obtaining laboratory confirmation of disease.

In the United States, premarital and prenatal blood tests have almost eradicated congenital syphilis, and the installation of silver nitrate or penicillin into the eyes of all newborn has practically obliterated blindness due to gonorrheal ophthalmia neonatorum.

Control of the epidemic of sexual-related diseases requires that those infected be found and treated; physicians be educated about the problem so that they have a higher index of suspicion when examining patients and that they report infections to health departments so that sexual contacts can be traced; parents be sufficiently educated so that they can teach their children; and, since the general public is uninformed, teachers be prepared to provide for education about sexually transmitted diseases in the schools, not by waiting until college and senior high school, but starting in the fifth, sixth, seventh, and eighth grades, where the infection rate is increasing so rapidly.

IN CONCLUSION

Myriad microorganisms cause all kinds of infection in man. These gain entry into the body through the respiratory system, intestinal tract, and the skin. While the body has physiological defenses that protect against onslaughts of germs, some survive and produce disease. We can do much, communally and personally, to reduce the ravages and deaths caused by these organisms.

The best way to prevent many infections, of course, is to avoid becoming infected. Knowing how they are transmitted gives us a basis for taking measures to reduce exposure. Immunizations and chemoprophylaxis are available for some of these communicable disease. But, they are of little value when not utilized. Recognizing symptoms of such diseases in the beginning stages enables us to obtain prompt treatment. The control of contagious conditions requires case finding and treatment. Personally, periodic examinations are one way case finding is done. On a communitywide basis, we must support detection programs.

Notes

1. Madison B. Brown, "The American Hospital Association Spells Out the Reasons Why," *American Lung Association Bulletin,* 58:16, July–August, 1972.

2. Betsy B. MacCracken, "Tuberculosis Control-Changing Scene," *Morbidity and Mortality Reportable Diseases,* County of Los Angeles, March, 1974.

3. Helen Jones, "Lifetime Followup No Longer Recommended," *American Lung Association Bulletin,* 60:7, July–August, 1974.

4. Ralph R. Sachs, "The Public Health Implications of Hepatitis B Antigen in Human Blood," *Morbidity and Mortality Reportable Diseases,* County of Los Angeles, June, 1974.

5. "More Kinds and Cases of VD," *Medical World News,* 16:44, July 28, 1975.

6. Genell Subak-Sharpe, "The Venereal Disease of the New Morality," *Today's Health,* 53:42, March, 1975.

7. Betty S. Baker, "International Venereal Disease Symposium: A Report," *The Journal of School Health,* 44:5, January, 1974.

8. "More Kinds and Cases of VD," p. 43.

9. Baker, "International Venereal Disease Symposium."

10. Charles and Bonnie Remsberg, "The Shocking Facts about Gonorrhea," *Good Housekeeping,* 174:140, February, 1972.

11. Baker, "International Venereal Disease Symposium."

12. *VD Handbook* (Montreal: Montreal Health Press, Inc., 1972), p. 42.

13. *Control of Communicable Diseases,* California State Department of Public Health, 1966, p. 329.

14. *California Civil Code.* Stats. 1968, c. 417, p. 859, para. 1.

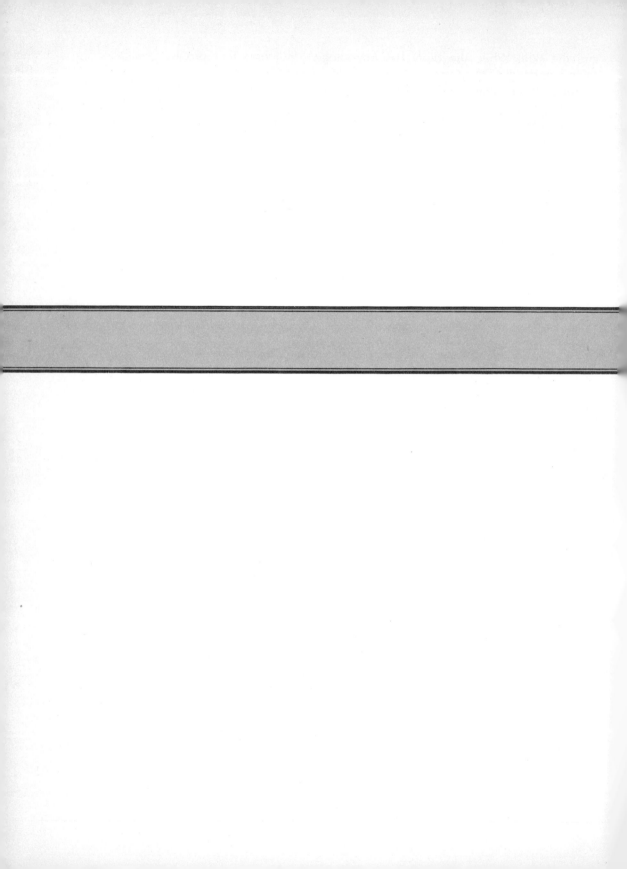

SAFETY AND ACCIDENT PREVENTION

chapter fourteen

Living safely in our times is a challenge that might be considered more difficult to meet than fighting Indians in the old frontier days or conquering space tomorrow. Living safely is a challenge to learn not only what to do and what not to do, but "why we *do or do not.*" Attitudes and emotions about safe living direct behavior.

THE ACCIDENT PROBLEM

If this is a normal "safe" week, 2012 Americans alive this morning will be dead from accidents seven days from now. They will die in mishaps, most of which are avoidable. During this average week, some of the deaths include the 48 people who either will kill themselves by careless handling of their guns or be shot to death by companions who mistake them for four-footed game; 9 firearm deaths will include children between five and fourteen years of age. Among the 22 killed by electricity will be the do-it-yourself handymen who forgot to turn off the current while doing repair jobs. Approximately 314 persons, most of whom are sixty-five and older, will suffer fatal falls in such situations as on slippery pavements, in bathtubs, and on highly polished floors. Fires will claim another 119 lives, and many victims will be smokers who lit their last cigarette in bed just before falling asleep. About 106 people will die from leaking gas or poisons taken by mistake. The leading accident killer, motor vehicles, will claim about 892 persons and motorcycles, another 54 people. Drownings, responsible for about 7876 deaths each year, will account for 151 fatalities during this average week. *Automobile accidents are the leading cause of death for college-age men and women!* The annual accident toll, which varies only slightly from year to year, amounts to approximately 105,000 fatalities and 11 million injuries, 380,000 of which result in permanent disability.[1] Types of accidents listed in descending order of frequency by age group are given in Table 14.1.

Table 14.1 Order of Type of Accidents Causing Death

All Ages	Under 1 Year	Under 5 Years
Motor vehicle	Ingestion of food, object	Motor vehicle
Falls	Mechanical suffocation	Drowning
Drowning	Motor vehicle	Fires, burns
Fires, burns	Fires, burns	Ingestion of food, object
Other	Falls	Falls

5 to 14 Years	15 to 24 Years	25 to 44 Years
Motor vehicle	Motor vehicle	Motor vehicle
Drowning	Drowning	Drowning
Fires, burns	Poison (solid, liquid)	Poison (solid, liquid)
Other	Firearms	Falls
	Other	Other

45 to 64 Years	65 to 74 Years	75 Years and Over
Motor vehicle	Motor vehicle	Falls
Falls	Falls	Motor vehicle
Fires, burns	Fires, burns	Surgical complications
Drowning	Surgical complications	Fires, burns
Other	Other	**Ingestion of food, object**

Source: *Accidental Facts* (Chicago: National Safety Council, 1976), p. 8.

The death rate from accidents for those between the ages fifteen and twenty-four has dropped 2 percent during the years 1965 to 1975. However in 1974 61 percent of all accidental deaths in the age range of fifteen to twenty-four years was due to automobile accidents.[2] It is hoped that as

FOUNDATIONS OF HEALTH SCIENCE

more and more adolescents participate in driver education courses, this increase will be reversed. Statistics show that both the accident rate and the incidence of traffic violations are lower among students who have taken such courses than among other drivers of the same age. On a proportionate basis, five times more infractions are committed by the untrained driver than by the trained driver.

Why Safety Today?

Safety problems of today, as contrasted with the past, are as different as the modes of living then and now. At one time, security of life depended upon man's versatility in a mainly physical setting. Today we must depend more upon our versatility in a social setting wherein elements of intelligence, tolerance, courtesy, judgment, and emotional stability have become all important. An imposing list of new hazards has been added to our lives due to unique and rapid scientific and technological advances. Among the factors that have stimulated new safety problems are the growth of large cities and suburbs, giant strides in industrial development, increasing population, new implements and machines, and high-speed vehicles.

What Is An Accident?

"An *accident* may be thought of as *an unplanned act or event resulting in injury or death to persons or damage to property*," according to Marland Strasser a professor of Safety and Driver Education.[3] Obviously, not all injuries or fatalities are accidental. The differentiating key is intent.

Accidents don't just happen, they are caused by carelessness—someone did not mark the glass door!

I was running to catch someone and ran through a glass door. Fortunately, I was not seriously injured but suffered lacerations of the hands, arms and hip. It required sixty-five stitches, I was operated on by a plastic surgeon. The most distressing part of this experience was the time I spent in the emergency room. I found the hospital staff to be most insensitive. I felt relieved that with therapy, I was able to regain full use of my hands.

An accident often is without apparent cause. It is an occurrence that is unpremeditated, unintentional, and unforeseen.

Only in recent years has the accident situation begun to be studied in behavioral terms. The *true* cause of most accidents has been masked. For example, let us look at a hypothetical case: Professor Hazard, on his way to work by automobile, struck John Frosh who was at the time riding a bicycle. Subsequent investigation resulted in a citation being issued to the Professor for "running a red light." But was this the *true* cause of the accident? In actuality, the underlying reason could have been a bee or wasp in the car, a dropped lighted cigarette, a late appointment with the college president, a fight with his wife before leaving home, a "distracting" coed walking down the sidewalk, a tardy class, or any of a number of other factors. Much accident research is presently focusing in on such aspects of human behavior and activity.

Causes of Accidents

Accidents have no single cause, nor a single cure. Mechanical and personal failures, environmental hazards, inadequate knowledge, insufficient skill, and improper attitudes and habits are all factors. Of all accidents in recent years, 85 percent could have been prevented if the victims had reacted properly to their environment. People have not learned to live safely with the powerful forces at their disposal. They drink before or while driving; they recklessly speed to and from work or vacation; they fish indifferently in a deep lake without knowing how to swim well; they hunt without exercising proper precaution; and they carelessly throw away their lighted cigarettes. Furthermore, they do not take preventive measures to protect the elderly people in their homes from falling.

Many persons have not learned common safety practices. Accidents may be caused by people who attempt to perform feats beyond their ability, who are emotionally disturbed or intoxicated, who have faulty vision or hearing, and who are fatigued. Faulty or negative attitudes, procrastination, and lack of supervision all add to the death toll. Many of these factors are interrelated, and in many cases, faulty attitudes relate to lack of knowledge. (See Table 14.2.)

Attitudes and Emotions

When a new situation develops, a person with the "safe attitude" reacts in a manner that will avoid or decrease the possibility of an accident. A readiness or predisposition to react safely controls and directs his or her behavior. The way attitudes influence behavior is very complex and a

FOUNDATIONS OF HEALTH SCIENCE

Table 14.2 Safety Quiz. What Is Your Safety I.Q.?

	True	False	Sometimes true
1. The best way to assist a drowning person is to jump in after him.	___	___	___
2. Be sure you know how to swim well if you go in alone.	___	___	___
3. If nothing else is available, water will put out oil and grease fires.	___	___	___
4. Bullets require a gun to explode.	___	___	___
5. If you clothing gets on fire get water quickly to put it out.	___	___	___
6. Bicyclists and equestrians should ride on the left hand side of the road.	___	___	___
7. Persons come up to the top of the water three times before drowning.	___	___	___
8. Oil or gasoline is safe to start a fire if it is poured from a safety container.	___	___	___
9. It is a fallacy that electric razors or telephones should not be used while bathing.	___	___	___
10. It is discretionary to run from a dog that is acting peculiarly.	___	___	___
11. More accidents occur at home than at work.	___	___	___
12. It is impossible for a person with cramps to swim.	___	___	___
13. Running stream water is safe to drink.	___	___	___
14. More fatal accidents occur on the highway than at work or at home.	___	___	___
15. Friday the Thirteenth is an unlucky day.	___	___	___

Statements 11 and 14 are the only ones that are true.
Adapted from: Joseph G. Dzenowagis, "What's Your Safety I.Q.?" *Safety Education* (November, 1956), a reprint. Courtesy National Safety Council.

one-to-one relationship rarely exists. Rather, each situation brings together many conflicting as well as supporting attitudes and values that interact to determine the behavior response.

Research studies show that emotional patterns of behavior play an important role in accident causation. In a comparison study of sixteen-year-old traffic violators and nonviolators, Beamish and Malfetti point out that "members of the violator group rated (significantly) lower in emotional stability, conformity, objectivity and mood."[4] Under conditions of emotional stress, even an ordinarily safety-conscious person may temporarily behave dangerously.

Habitual emotional patterns of handling problems and frustration are evident in safety behavior. The different ways of responding to stress are described in the chapter on mental health. The immature person uses many of the maladjustive types of behavior to reduce his frustrations and meet the needs of living. For example, the adjustive mechanism of regression relative to driving practices might manifest itself as an infantile disregard for the rights of others, road hogging, beating the lights, demanding the right of way, or speeding.

Attempts have been made to single out the characteristics that separate those who are susceptible to accidents from those who are not. Such attempts are motivated by the need to identify the group that might profit most from the efforts of safety education. This group has been labeled *accident-prone*. The theories about accident-proneness have been numerous, varied, and often contradictory. In a study of personality characteristics of youthful accident-repeating drivers, Rommell points out:

> ... individuals who have had the following experiences have a tendency to manifest accident-producing behavior: (1) a desire to leave home, (2) an urge to do something harmful or shocking, (3) a tendency to be influenced by people about them, (4) association with peers to whom parents object, (5) a desire to frighten other individuals for the fun of it, (6) a tendency to become readily impatient with people, (7) a tendency to be somewhat suspicious of overly friendly people, and (8) a possibility of having been in trouble with the law.[5]

Effect of Alcohol on Physical Abilities

The relationship between alcoholic beverages and accidents probably has received more publicity than any other facet of accident prevention, and rightly so! Alcohol is involved in at least one-third of all motor vehicle fatalities. Research has repeatedly demonstrated that alcohol reduces a person's ability to reason, evaluate, and determine action—all of which are needed for safe living. In addition, alcohol slows down all physical capabilities. Reaction speed, distance judgment, and visual skills decrease in proportion to the amount of alcohol in the blood. This reduction in physical proficiency plus the decreased psychophysical skills can easily result in an accident.

MOTOR VEHICLE SAFETY

Accidents on the public highways have killed more Americans since the advent of the automobile than were killed in all the past wars of our country. Year after year, more than 55,000 Americans die from motor vehicle accidents.

College-age Drivers

We know from accident statistics that the college-age driver is involved in more accidents and has a higher fatality rate than those who are older. Over eighteen thousand persons in this age range are killed in motoring accidents each year. Drivers under twenty have an accident rate of two and one-half times that of all other drivers, and those twenty to twenty-four, nearly twice that of other drivers. Insuring the young drivers is so expensive that insurance companies have had to increase their rates on cars driven by people under age twenty-five. Exceptions to this increase are young men and women who have had a course in driver education and driver training (usually a 10–15 percent discount) and young married couples because of their lower accident rates.

Driving is a privilege granted by the state. Once a license is granted, the driver must demonstrate with every mile driven that he is entitled to this privilege. The driver's ability to obey the state's safety rules and laws is called *driver responsibility*. Parents must assume financial responsibility for any damages minors may cause; for married people, this type of economic loss affects their spouses and children. Each driver, then, assumes what is called *family responsibility*. Few motorists expect to be involved in a collision or to hit a pedestrian or cyclist, yet every day thousands are injured or killed in these ways. A car is more than just a means of transportation. On crowded streets, it has become a deadly weapon. The driver's concern for the safety of others is called *social responsibility*.

Young drivers, because of their age, have special strengths and special weaknesses. Their strengths are their physical characteristics. Their weaknesses are lack of knowledge and inappropriate attitudes. Reaction time, manual dexterity, and alertness are near peak levels in the teen and early adult years. Young drivers get a great deal of pleasure out of using these skills. As a result, they often attempt maneuvers that test the limits of these skills, and occasionally they go too far and experience accidents. Also, in their concentration on their display of skill, they neglect to consider what some other driver might do, and so are easily caught in a hazardous situation.

Drugs and Driving

An estimated twenty million or more American motorists are taking some kind of prescribed medication, and many do not realize that the drugs can affect their ability to drive safely. Many drugs slow reaction time, and at the high speeds driven today, fast reactions are needed.

Drugs affect people differently. For some, an antibiotic prescribed by a physician may have the desired therapeutic result with no undesirable side effects. For others, the same drug may produce drowsiness that can make it dangerous to drive a car. Every motorist should be alerted to this possibility when taking any drug, and he should be even more concerned about the likely possibility of a dangerous reaction when drugs are combined with alcoholic beverages. Drugs and alcohol can have a synergistic action, whereby the total effect is greater than the sum of the two taken independently.

The wise approach is to find out beforehand how any medication, either prescribed or acquired over the counter, may affect driving. The physician or the pharmacist can tell how it may affect vision, coordination, or alertness; whether it can have side effects when combined with other prescribed medicine or with alcohol; and how long the effects will last. The driver who takes a nonprescription drug should read the label carefully, particularly any warnings in fine print.

Causes of Motor Vehicle Accidents

The need for safer automobiles has received widespread publicity. Legislative committees conduct hearings, and laws regulating safety standards for automobiles are continually reviewed. Two comprehensive references on the general subject of car safety were written by lawyers who had been alarmed for many years at the built-in hazards of automobiles. Both *Unsafe at Any Speed* by Nader[6] and *Safety Last* by O'Connell[7] concluded that while research is needed on many aspects of auto safety, present knowledge and technology, if applied, could provide us with vehicles far more crashworthy than anything available today. Both books have a common theme: that the manufacturers for over five decades have shown little regard for safety-oriented automotive design. Consequently, the authors advised that the federal government should regulate safety requirements for this industry just as it has done for aviation, railroads, and other means of public transportation.

A number of techniques are used to increase the safety of the automobile by protecting occupants from the effects of collision. Unrestrained occupants of crash-involved cars may be injured when they strike interior surfaces or when they are thrown out of the vehicle.

The most widely used method of attenuating the energy of vehicle occupants in crashes is to restrain their movement by safety belts.[8] Safety belts require the active cooperation of vehicle occupants. The *National Traffic and Motor Vehicle Safety Act of 1966* required lap belts and shoulder harnesses in the frontal outboard seating positions and lap belts in other positions in all automobiles manufactured after January, 1968. However, a 1970 survey revealed that lap belts were used by less than one in four and shoulder harnesses by less than one in twenty.[9]

Waller and Barry report that 23 percent of persons observed not wearing belts in their home town said in a follow-up questionnaire that they wore them always on short trips. Over 50 percent of those observed not wearing belts some distance from their homes, said they always used them on long trips.[10]

Since the active participation of motor vehicle occupants to protect themselves by using either lap belts or harnesses is inefficient, the federal government as of August, 1973, required a belt system on all new cars that allows the automobile to start only under certain conditions. These include the buzzer-light system in which the buzzer-light operates until the belt or shoulder harness is fastened (occupants of front outboard seats). A second device is the interlock system that prevents starting a vehicle unless the driver and front seat passenger are belted. Unfortunately, both these devices can be circumvented.

In a study of 1974 vehicles compared by type of belt-wearing inducement system, 59 percent of the occupants used belts with the interlock devices and 28 percent used belts with the buzzer-light devices. However, as a result of strong negative public reaction to the interlock devices, federal law has now banned the interlock.[11] No laws in the United States require that occupants of motor vehicles *use* seat belts. In Victoria, Australia, where such laws are in effect, urban use reportedly exceeded 70 percent, rural use 60 percent, and significant drops in morbidity and mortality followed.[12]

Since "active" protective devices are not giving adequate protection, what about passive devices? Some of the passive means of reducing hazards include steering assemblies that yield at a controlled rate in a collision and windshields that reduce energy. These two protective devices have been required by federal standard for machines sold since 1968.[13]

Modification of the automobile by air cushions requires no "action" on the part of the driver or passenger either. Air cushions that inflate in a crash have tested out to be most efficient, but only a few vehicles are so equipped. The air bag systems have had more than one hundred million miles of successful performance in the United States. "These air bags respond in a few milliseconds to crash onsets, inflating between vehicle occupants and structures on which they would otherwise impact."[14] These devices cost approximately $75 more to install than belt-buzzer-light or interlock devices. Why haven't the executive and judicial branches of government taken the necessary steps to mandate additional measures to reduce injuries to more than 10,000 people daily from motor vehicle crashes and deaths to tens of thousands yearly?[15]

Law Enforcement

In those states where the motor vehicle accident rate is decreasing, officials point to the rigid enforcement of the following safety measures:

1. Increased police patrols on highways (this has top priority in most states)
2. New laws—or rigid enforcement of existing laws—calling for suspension of licenses and/or fines and imprisonment for motorists convicted of drunk driving, "chronic" negligence, and speeding
3. More strict examinations for vehicle licenses and mandatory automobile inspection programs
4. Use of special forces to reinforce regular highway police during peak travel periods, such as holiday weekends
5. Periodic roadblocks to check on licenses, intoxication, and vehicle condition
6. Expansion of the use of radar devices in apprehending speeders
7. Establishing state speed limits where they are not already in force and reducing maximum speed limits to lower levels such as 55 miles per hour
8. Designing and manufacturing cars with more effective safety features.

Connecticut is an example of a state that found the key to its safety program in the rigid enforcement of speed laws. The most potent weapon in that program is suspending the licenses of convicted speeders for a period of thirty days. The experiment has proved that people will slow down to save their drivers' licenses, if not their lives. Former Governor Ribicoff of Connecticut insisted that a good traffic safety program should include in addition to those points just mentioned: strict control of drivers through good examination and licensing as well as fearless use of suspension and revocation, and proper education and training of all drivers to develop knowledge, attitudes, and skills.

The Human Factor

The human aspect of traffic accidents, although it constitutes the chief causative factor, has not been given the attention that has been afforded to the design of the vehicle, the design of the roadway, or traffic flow. Motor vehicle administrators are required by law to prohibit drivers who are mentally or physically unfit from driving motor vehicles. They are seeking aid from the medical profession through health departments for establishing standards for this purpose. One of every thirteen drivers involved in fatal accidents has a physical condition that could have been a contributing factor: fatigue or lack of sleep is the condition in two-thirds of the cases; defective eyesight, illness, and defective hearing rank next in order.

Certain physical disabilities should motivate the conscientious person to stop driving. Many, certainly not all, persons with heart disease, diabetes, epilepsy, and other disabling illnesses should put themselves in the nondriver category. Vision problems are obviously a handicap, but not always obviously considered to be. A high degree of nearsightedness, night blindness, glaucoma, or tunnel vision are particularly dangerous. Persons with sight in only one eye often have difficulty judging distance and getting a clear perspective. Yet only a few states(including California, Michigan, Iowa, and Colorado) require eye tests for drivers' license renewals. Most states appear to ignore the fact that good vision at seventeen years of age does not assure good vision at sixty-five.

Age itself is not necessarily a ban to driving, since a fortunate few retain alert senses and good muscular coordination up to the age of seventy. However, giving up the wheel at that age is good advice. Some states require stringent and more frequent testing for license renewals for those over seventy years of age.

In Pennsylvania's required medical examinations, ten conditions of severe medical or physical impairments are cause for refusal to issue or renew a driver's license. All new licensees are examined. The program is automated so that individuals may be examined every ten years on the anniversary of their original licensing date. Of the several million persons examined so far, 1.7 percent did not receive their licenses or have them renewed. Most of these voluntarily withdrew their request for license or renewal when they learned an examination was required.[16]

An examination system such as this one by no means solves all the human factors involved in the causation of accidents. Perhaps the largest group of persons who should give serious consideration to whether or not they are fit to drive is that group with recognized emotional instability. The excitable, the quick-tempered, the absent-minded, the "touchy," and the easily upset person becomes a serious threat behind the wheels of a fast-moving vehicle.

Fatigue

Fatigue is more of a major cause of traffic accidents than most people realize. So important is it in traffic safety that the Interstate Commerce Commission regulates the number of hours that truck and bus drivers can drive. Fatigue and sleepiness are usually the result of long and continuous driving hours, failure to get adequate rest each night while on a trip, and trying to cover an excessive number of miles in a few hours. Shorter driving hours, frequent rest stops, adequate sleep each night, and sharing the driving will help eliminate accidents caused by fatigue and sleepiness.

Is falling asleep at the wheel careless driving? The Courts have ruled yes. Some may argue that falling asleep was not careless driving because there was no proof of willful intent. This is not so, since we do have prior warnings of fatigue and drowsiness. Because of these warnings, it is inferred that falling asleep at the wheel is negligent behavior. College students as well as other drivers should keep in mind that the penalty may be a serious accident as well as an arrest.

ACCIDENT AND LIABILITY INSURANCE

Although the aim of safety education is to prevent or reduce accidents, wise drivers should be prepared for an accident's happening and should be protected against possible liability action resulting from the accident. This protection can be gained by carrying liability insurance. In view of the fact that the highest accident rate is in the fifteen-to-twenty-four-year-old age group, this group should carry liability and accident insurance even though the premium rates are high. This age group, or those financially responsible for them, usually could not afford the financial burden involved in a court suit, and the price of the insurance premium, which covers many benefits in case of an accident, is indeed small by comparison.

Liability is based on negligence, and negligence is the absence of prudent action. A person who successfully appraises dangers inherent in an anticipated act and uses precautionary measures to avoid a possible accident is acting prudently. The circumstances of an automobile accident determine whether or not the driver has been negligent.

THE SAFE DRIVER

Perhaps the largest group of persons who should give serious consideration to whether or not they are fit to drive is that group with recognized emotional instability. As we have said before, excitable, quick-tempered, absent-minded, "touchy," and easily upset persons become serious threats behind the wheels of fast-moving vehicles. On days when you are in one of the above moods, why not let someone else do the driving?

The Kemper Insurance Companies list the following habits as dangerous:

Unreasonable speed (high)

Driving in spurts, slow, then fast, then slow, and so forth

Frequent lane changing with excessive speed

Improper passing with insufficient clearance, also taking too long or swerving too much in overtaking and passing (i.e., overcontrol)

Overshooting or disregarding traffic control signals

Approaching signals unreasonably fast or slow and stopping or attempting to stop with uneven motion

Driving at night without lights; delay in turning lights on when starting from a parked position

Failure to dim lights to oncoming traffic

Driving in lower gears without apparent reason, or repeatedly clashing gears

Jerky starting or stopping

Driving unreasonably slow

Driving too close to shoulders or curbs, or appearing to hog the edge of the road or continually straddling the centerline

Driving with windows down in cold weather

Driving or riding with head partly or completely out of the window.

The character of the good, safe driver is comprised of these six qualities:

1. Through experience under instruction, he has developed mechanical and technical skill in controlling his car.
2. He knows what to expect of his car under both favorable and adverse driving conditions.
3. He avoids taking foolish chances; he never overdrives the danger zone projecting ahead of his car.
4. He has a courteous and sportsmanlike regard for the rights of all other users of the public highway, including pedestrians, bicyclists, motorcyclists, and other motorists.
5. He signals his intentions to all persons who may be affected by the course of the car of which he is the brain; he does not expect other people to be mind readers.
6. He is alert for the mistakes of these people, and he does what he can to compensate for them; he does not demand the right-of-way to his own or anyone else's hurt.[17]

MOTORCYCLE ACCIDENTS

Recent years have witnessed a tremendous growth in motorcycle use in the United States. Between 1961 and 1973, the number of motorcycle registrations jumped over 600 percent totalling over a million.[18] Some of the factors that contribute to this growing popularity include: an improved public image of the riders, symbolic of the "Pepsi generation"; economical as a means of travel; more disposable income and time for recreation; and motorcycling is fun.[19]

Unfortunately, accidents involving motorcycles have reached epidemic proportions. Speca and Cowell predict that during the summer months, alone, approximately 10,000 injuries severe enough to require medical attention will occur to users of minibikes and motorcycles. As a result of these accidents, some one thousand young persons will suffer lifelong disabilities.[20] Studies conducted in a number of states reveal that more than 90 percent of motorcycle accidents result in death or injury. For motor vehicles, the percent is only eight.[21]

Most of the fatalities occur when the cycle collides with another vehicle, usually a car. The blame is not necessarily that of the cyclist since between 60 and 70 percent of such accidents are the fault of the automobile driver.[22] Frequently, the automobile driver does not see the cyclist.

Persons connected with motorcycle associations, insurance companies, and highway traffic safety state that the major cause of accidents appears to be inexperience; 25 percent of such accidents involve cyclists with less than six months' experience.[23]

Some safety experts are recommending the incorporation of motorcycle driving instruction in driver education courses. Special attention is also being given to making the vehicle itself safer, and laws are being enacted and enforced to bring about more responsible use.[24]

I wonder what "safety" precautions this cyclist used?

Two years ago I was in a motorcycle accident. I hit a car broadside who had cut across the road I was traveling. I blacked out completely not remembering anything until waking in the hospital. My body was shaking pretty heavily. I had multiple contusions and also a concussion. I had dizzy spells for about a week, but was fine after that except for many lacerations.

FOUNDATIONS OF HEALTH SCIENCE

Despite the hazards of serious injury and the chance of death, if you decide to cycle, you should remember that these behaviors can reduce the chances of trouble:

1. *Wear a helmet.* Head injuries are the cause of death in two-thirds of cycle fatalities.
2. Wear heavy clothing and boots.
3. Protect your eyes with glasses, goggles, or a face shield. You may be easily blinded by glaring light, wind, or rain.
4. Wear bright colored clothing and helmet to make yourself more visible.
5. Use your lights, even during the day, to increase your visibility.
6. The best safety device is experience. Do not drive on highways or well-traveled roads until you have had some five hundred miles driving experience—says Buchanan of the National Highway Traffic Safety Administration, a specialist in motorcycle highway safety.[25]

HOME SAFETY

Home accidents account for approximately 27,000 deaths each year. Falls and fire burns cause more than 60 percent of these fatalities. Most of the falls occur in the bedroom and involve aged persons. Home fire deaths occur most frequently to helpless infants and aged persons who become trapped. The fires are primarily due to smoking and faulty electrical equipment.

Accidental Poisoning in Children

One of the most important and increasingly common causes of childhood accidents is poisoning. A lengthening list of deodorants, depilatories, detergents, herbicides, insecticides, rodenticides, petroleum products, stimulants, sedatives, and analgesics contribute to the magnitude of the problem. Recent cumulative studies indicate that the major toxic agents responsible for poisoning cases are aspirin, sleeping pills, and birth control medications. The kitchen, bedroom, and bathroom contain many poison hazards.

Poison control centers have been established to help cope with this problem. These centers maintain 24-hour telephone service and offer immediate information to the attending physician concerning the contents, toxicity, and means of combating the poison. A public health nurse may later visit the family at home to try to determine the cause of the accident and suggest ways to remove hazards and prevent future accidents.

The first poison control center was organized in Chicago in 1953 by the American Academy of Pediatrics, the Chicago Board of Health, the Illinois State Toxicology Laboratory, the University of Illinois, and six major teaching hospitals. Since then, several hundred centers have been established throughout the country. These centers provide a long-term study of frequency and causes of poisoning as they occur, so that better methods of prevention can be devised.

Although manufacturers have devised hard-to-open safety closures for containers in an effort to protect small children against potentially harmful compounds, parents do not realize how dangerous substances commonly found in the kitchen can be. For example, solvents such as kerosine can cause fatal pulmonary damage if swallowed. Adults as well as children may accidentally become poisoned. The following procedures are recommended to prevent such accidents:

1. Keep all drugs, poisonous substances, and household chemicals out of the reach of children, the senile, and the severely emotionally disturbed.
2. Do not store nonedible products on shelves used for storing food.
3. Do not transfer poisonous substances to unlabeled containers.
4. Never re-use containers of chemical substances.
5. Do not leave discarded medicines where children or pets might get at them.
6. Never tell children you are giving them candy when you are actually giving them medicine.
7. Read labels before using chemical products.
8. Never give or take medicines in the dark.

RECREATION SAFETY

The primary problem in recreation safety is drowning. Each year, almost 9,000 people lose their lives in rivers, lakes, streams, pools, and oceans. Many were good swimmers. In fact, half of all drownings are within twenty feet of safety. Numerous drownings occur at supervised beaches and pools where the personnel on duty attempt rescue procedures that prove to be inadequate. Generally, these victims were believed to have been beyond the point of a successful rescue, and no

544   FOUNDATIONS OF HEALTH SCIENCE

questions were asked about the methods used or whether additional steps could have been taken to revive the victims.

Within the past few years various research articles have appeared in the *Journal of the American Medical Association* dealing with the physiology of drowning and the rescue procedures that should be used on the drowning victim. These indicate that a number of fatality victims might have been revived through intelligent and efficient action. Many drownings could be avoided if individuals would adhere to a few basic rules while swimming or engaging in water sports. Some of these include:

1. Learn to swim and relax in the water.
2. Never swim alone.
3. Do not swim when overly tired or when the water is extremely cold.
4. Do not overestimate ability and endurance.
5. Swim at protected pools or beaches under the supervision of a trained lifeguard.
6. If a boat overturns, stay with it and don't try to swim a long distance to shore.
7. Never dive into unknown water.
8. Try new activities only after learning the skills from qualified instructors.
9. Know how to float.

Figures 14.1 and 14.2 illustrate water safety techniques that can help you to save your own or another person's life.

Some times emergency measures require more than pulmonary resuscitation. The heart may not be beating adequately. This is determined by checking the carotid artery for presence of a pulse as shown in Figure 14.3. If no pulsation in the artery is felt, then cardiac resuscitation is imperative. Figure 14.3 illustrates the procedures recommended by the American Heart Association to begin artificial circulation.

The number of private pools is increasing rapidly in the United States. Those who have a private pool, or use a neighbor's, should observe these fundamentals of safety. Make certain the pool is kept clean and the water chemically purified. Walk, don't run, about the pool; horseplay should be forbidden. Fence the pool and keep the gate locked to keep out small children. Keep hand rescue equipment, such as long poles and ring buoys, readily available. Keep bottles and glasses away from the concrete or metal pool decks. Be sure that phone numbers of fire department and ambulance service are readily available. Be sure that someone who can give artificial respiration is always present.

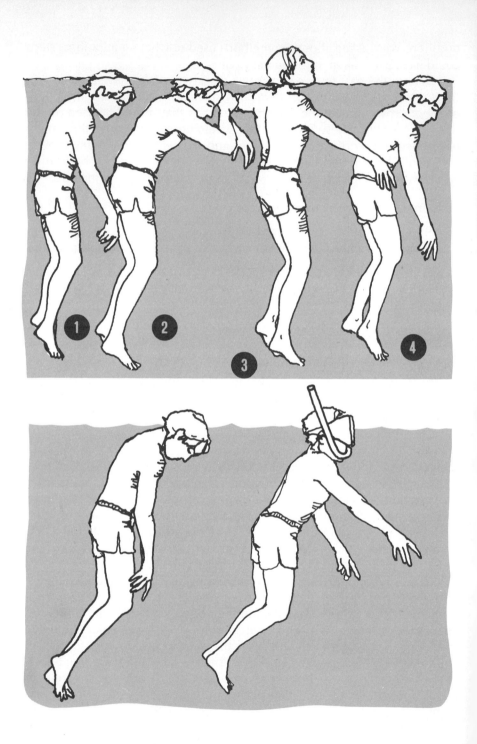

FOUNDATIONS OF HEALTH SCIENCE

Approximately one-quarter million Americans have nonvisible medical problems that can interfere with emergency treatment. Over two hundred conditions are of the type that should require a person to carry emergency medical identification to ensure correct first aid. For example, many diabetics and epileptics are jailed as drunks when they are ill. One in every ten thousand Caucasian males is a hemophiliac who may bleed to death with the slightest cut. Persons who are allergic to penicillin, tetanus antitoxin, aspirin, codeine, novocaine, and sulfa might be given treatment that does more harm than good.

A person who does not speak English or the deaf and mute need to carry instructions about any special health problem, as do people who wear contact lenses, because if these are left on an unconscious accident victim for twenty-four hours or more they may "chew up" the cornea of the eye and impair vision or cause blindness. Alcoholics who take antabuse need protection because they will become violently ill if they are given drugs dissolved in alcohol. Cardiovascular and some radical surgery patients also need special recognition.

Medical I.D. Tags

In 1963 the nation's doctors, working through the American Medical Association, recommended use of a universal symbol, Medic-Alert (shown in Figure 14.4), which tells first-aid workers at a glance that its wearer has a condition requiring special attention. It may be displayed on a wrist, an anklet, a medallion, or a card. Usually the condition requiring urgent attention can be imprinted upon the anklet, bracelet, or medallion. The symbol also is a sign that there are vital medical facts on a card in the person's purse or wallet. Since its existence, Medic-Alert has saved

◀ **Figure 14.1** Float to Safety, the Lanoue Style. Work only enough to bring your mouth above the surface to inhale, then sink down again into the natural floating position to rest. Exhale under water. The lazier you are the better. The basic floating technique: (1) Rest just below surface, letting arms and legs hang limp. (2) Slowly raise arms as if to fend off a blow to forehead. (3) Extend arms and float to surface. When mask and snorkel is not used, this is the time to take breath, having expelled the last breath through the nose under water. (4) After rising for breath, rest by hanging limp under water.

Only back of head is above water as man floats Fred R. Lanoue style in fresh water. When learning to float, it might be helpful if the student starts off with the face mask and snorkel. (From W. S. Kals, "Float to Safety," *Today's Health,* 47:47, June, 1969.)

Figure 14.2 Mouth-To-Mouth Ventilation. (From *First Aid Manual*, Copyright 1971, American Medical Association. Courtesy of the American Medical Association.)

MOUTH–TO–MOUTH RESUSCITATION FOR INFANTS AND SMALL CHILDREN

Put child in a face-up position. Tilt child's head backward.

Lift child's lower jaw with fingers of both hands so that it juts out. Keep child in this position so that the tongue will not fall back to block the air passage.

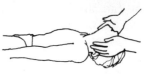

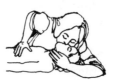

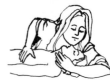

Take a deep breath and place your mouth over the child's MOUTH AND NOSE. Blow your breath gently into the child's mouth and nose until you see the chest rise and you feel the lungs expand. The air you blow into the child's lungs has enough oxygen to save his life.

Remove your mouth and let the child exhale. As soon as you hear the child breathe out, replace your mouth over his mouth and nose and repeat procedure. Repeat 20 times per minute. When possible, place your hand over the child's stomach. Use moderate pressure to keep the stomach from becoming inflated.

REPEAT STEPS ONE AND TWO 20 TIMES PER MINUTE

MOUTH–TO–MOUTH RESUSCITATION FOR ADULTS

Place victim on his back.

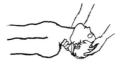

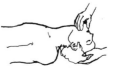

Lift victim's neck with one hand and tilt his head back by holding the top of his head with your other hand.

Pull the victim's chin up with the hand that was lifting the neck so that the tongue does not fall back to block the air passage.

PLACE YOUR MOUTH OVER VICTIM'S NOSE OR MOUTH

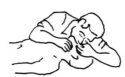

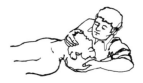

Take a deep breath and place your mouth over the victim's nose or mouth, making a leak–proof seal. Blow your breath into the victim's mouth or nose until you see the chest rise. The air you blow into the victim's lungs has enough oxygen to save his life.

Remove your mouth and let the victim exhale while you take another deep breath. As soon as you hear the victim breathe out, replace your mouth over his mouth or nose and repeat procedure.

REPEAT CYCLE 12 TIMES PER MINUTE

Start immediately. Seconds count.

Check mouth and throat for obstructions.

Place victim in position and begin artificial respiration.

Maintain steady rhythm of 12 breaths per minute.

Remain in position. After the victim revives, be ready to resume artificial ventilation if necessary.

Call a physician.

Do not move the victim unless absolutely necessary to remove from danger.

Do not wait or look for help.

Do not stop to loosen clothing or warm the victim.

Do not give up.

Figure 14.3 Cardiopulmonary Resuscitation. (© American Heart Association. Reprinted with permission.)

EMERGENCY MEASURES IN CARDIOPULMONARY RESUSCITATION

Place Victim Flat On His Back On A Hard Surface

IF UNCONSCIOUS, OPEN AIRWAY

    LIFT UP NECK
    PUSH FOREHEAD BACK
    CLEAR OUT MOUTH IF NECESSARY

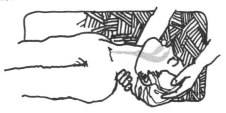

IF NOT BREATHING, BEGIN ARTIFICIAL BREATHING

    CONTINUE AT A RATE OF
    12 INFLATIONS PER MINUTE

CHECK CAROTID PULSE

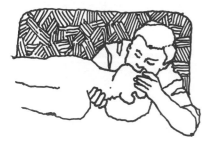

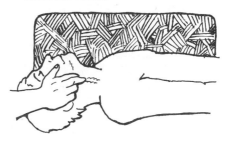

IF PULSE ABSENT, BEGIN ARTIFICIAL CIRCULATION

LOCATE PRESSURE POINT

DEPRESS STERNUM 1½" TO 2"
60 TO 80 TIMES PER MINUTE

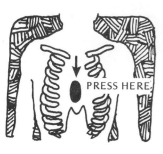

ONE RESCUER
15 compressions
2 quick inflations

TWO RESCUERS
5 compressions
1 inflation

PRESS HERE

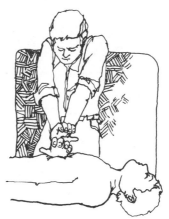

Figure 14.4 Medic Alert. Example of Medic Alert wallet card (top) and Typical Medic Alert emblem (bottom). (Courtesy of Medic Alert Foundation International.)

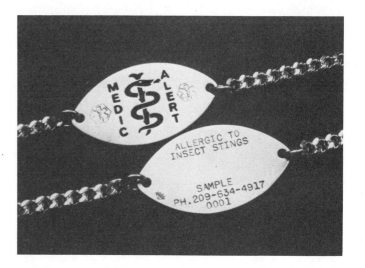

```
MEDIC ALERT MEMBER INFORMATION        MEMBER NUMBER
SMITH, MARY JANE                         6548369
7605 PARK AVE
NEW YORK, NY  11554
                                     (212)634-1987
             IN AN EMERGENCY CALL
DR THOMAS JOHNSON                    (212)687-1492
GERALD SMITH                        (212)634-1987
             MY MEDICAL PROBLEM IS

DIABETES
HEART CONDITION
WEARING CONTACT LENSES
)TAKES NPH U100 INSULIN, DIGOXIN

DATE ISSUED 6/10/76
IN AN EMERGENCY CALL COLLECT (209) 634-4917
```

hundreds of lives. Medic-Alert's founder, Marion C. Collins, M.D., a Turlock, California, practitioner, relates that more lives could be saved with Medic-Alert than can be saved in the operating room.

Emergency Care of the Sick and Injured

Personal bodily injury or sudden illness requires emergency care in the form of first aid. First aid, defined as the immediate and temporary care offered to the stricken victim until the services of a physician can be obtained, minimizes the aggravation of injury and enhances the earliest possible return of the person to peak performance. Since this may mean life or death, procedures used in emergency care situations must be applied intelligently by a competent first aider. The control of bleeding, promotion of breathing, removal of the object choking a hapless victim, cardiac resuscitation, and reduction of shock are immediate life control measures that require special training. Such training is available to all of us through first aid courses taught in all communities.

The appendix contains instructions for giving basic first aid.

IN CONCLUSION

Reducing accidents requires that society be made aware of the complexity of the accident problem as well as being made aware of its extent. The principal method of creating this awareness is an organized program of safety education. Each of us must assume responsibility for our own actions. We must develop the skills necessary for living safely in our time and behave in such a manner that we promote our own safety as well as the safety of those around us.

Notes

1. *Accident Facts* (Chicago: National Safety Council, 1976), pp. 3, 12, 14, 56.

2. Ibid., p. 14.

3. Marland K. Strasser et al., *Fundamentals of Safety Education* (New York: Macmillan, 1973), p. 4.

4. Jerome J. Beamish and James L. Malfetti, "A Psychological Comparison of Violator and Non-Violator Automobile Drivers in the 16th and 19th Year Age Group," *Traffic Safety Research Review,* 8:13, March, 1962.

5. Quoted by M. K. Strasser et al., *Fundamentals of Safety Education,* p. 100.

6. Ralph Nader. *Unsafe at Any Speed: The Designed-in Dangers of the American Automobile* (New York: Grossman Publishers, 1965).

7. J. O'Connell and A. Myers. *Safety Last: An Indictment of the Auto Industry* (New York: Random House, 1966).

8. Leon S. Robertson. "Safety Belt Use in Automobiles with Starter-Interlock and Buzzer-Light Reminder Systems," *American Journal of Public Health,* 65:1319, December, 1975.

9. L. S. Robertson, B. O'Neill, and C. W. Wixom. "Factors Associated with Observed Safety Belt Use," *Journal of Health and Social Behavior,* 13:18–24, 1972.

10. P. F. Waller and P. Z. Barry. "Seat Belts: A Comparison of Observed and Reported Use," *University of North Carolina Highway Research Center,* Chapel Hill, 1969.

11. Robertson, "Safety Belt Use in Automobiles with Starter-Interlock and Buzzer-Light Systems," p. 1324.

12. William Haddon, "Perspective on a Current Public Health Controversy," *American Journal of Public Health,* 65:1343, December, 1975.

13. Robertson, "Safety Belt Use in Automobiles with Starter-Interlock and Buzzer-Light Systems," p. 1319.

14. Haddon, "Perspective on a Current Public Health Controversy," p. 1343.

15. Ibid., p. 1344.

16. Charles L. Wilbar, Jr., "Health Aspects of the Driver Licensure Program of Pennsylvania," *American Journal of Public Health,* 55:1811–1812, November, 1965.

17. Justus J. Schifferes, *Healthier Living* (New York: John Wiley & Sons, 1965), p. 361.

18. Laurie Cray Sadler, "Motorcycling: A Hazardous Two-Wheel Ride," *Today's Health,* 53:28, July–August, 1975.

19. Ibid., p. 29.

20. John M. Speca and Henry R. Cowell, "Minibike and Motorcycle Accidents in Adolescents," *Journal of the American Medical Association,* 232:55–56, April 7, 1975.

21. Sadler, "Motorcycling," p. 28.

22. Ibid., p. 29.

23. Ibid.

24. "Motorcycle Accident Fatalities," *Statistical Bulletin,* 54:9–11, August, 1973.

25. Sadler, "Motorcycling," p. 29.

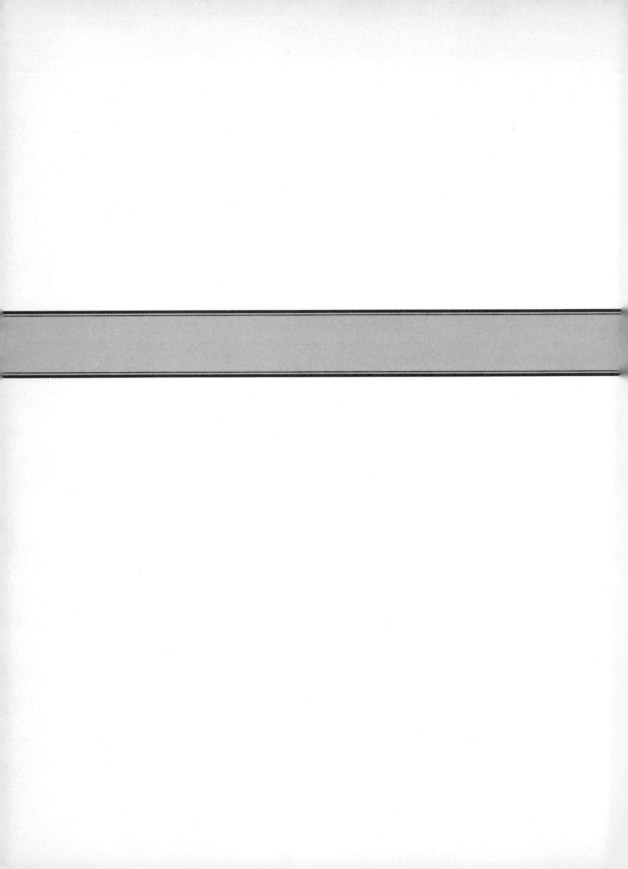

COMMUNITY HEALTH IN ECOLOGICAL PERSPECTIVE

chapter fifteen

For every American, environmental decay has become a personal experience—a glass of water bitter with impurities, a mountain view obscured by haze, an acrid smell of industrial smoke or automobile exhaust, and earpiercing noises from the boom of jets or rumbles of trucks. Every nation, large and small, is confronted with environmental hazards.

From his earliest beginnings, man has sought ways to manipulate and control his environment and to create favorable conditions for his activities. Through the years, the inventions of man have created many sources of pollution. The new, more subtle, insidious contaminants are the undesirable byproducts of technological progress. Ubiquitous and rapidly increasing numbers of chemicals, drugs, and other pollutants are finding their way into the air people breathe, the water they drink, and the food they eat.

Although the problem is enormously complicated and difficult, the gap between technology and biology must be closed quickly. In the last analysis, though, progress depends upon the attitudes and values of the community. Our industrial, mobile public, made more aware by increased education and mass communication, is demanding a higher living standard and a better environment. This awareness is reflected by some citizens' demanding "reasonably clean air and water at reasonable costs"; and other citizens' demanding "clean air and water at all costs." In either extreme, everyone must realize that control programs for water, air, and food sanitation can respect no city or state boundary. Cooperation, co-ordination, and support at the local, state, and national levels are necessary to further the growth, development, and health of the nation.

Although we have many answers, we need to know a lot more about pollutants, their combined effects, and what they can do to man. Ecologists, students of natural resources, physicians, and public health officers have long recognized that technological innovations create dangers for human health. The problem is not to protect man from exposure to a few poisonous substances but rather to consider, as a whole, the dangers to health that are created by the innumerable products and processes of modern technology. Dubos stimulates our thinking in this area by saying:

> For the time being, we must accept as a fact that it is impossible to detect beforehand all the potential dangers of new technological developments. No legislation or administrative regulation can cope with this problem because the scientific background is far too inadequate. It must be recognized, furthermore, that to exact a certificate of absolute safety before licensing a new process or a new product would completely paralyze technological progress.
>
> It is almost certain that any substance possessing biological activity will also prove to have some toxic properties. Each one of the drugs introduced into the practice of medicine during the past twenty years—from penicillin to cortisone or the tranquilizers—is now known to be capable of causing severe toxic reactions under certain circumstances; this is true even of acetylsalicylic acid (aspirin). . . .
>
> All technological innovations, whether concerned with industrial, agricultural, or medical practices, are bound to upset the balance of nature. In fact, to achieve mastery over nature is synonymous with disturbing the order of nature. Technological progress necessarily involves dangers, and these cannot always be foreseen.[1]

Ehrlich is not quite as soft spoken as Dubos, since he believes:

> There are no simple answers to . . . threats, no technological panaceas for the complex of problems comprising the population-food-environment crisis. Of course, technology, properly applied in such areas as pollution abatement, communications, and fertility control, can provide valuable assistance. But the essential solutions entail dramatic and rapid changes in human *attitudes*, especially those relating to reproductive behavior, economic growth, technology, the environment, and resolution of conflicts.[2]

Johns, Sutton, and Cooley have spelled out these attitudes and behaviors that promote continuing abuse of our environment:

> . . . economic growth remains our highest national priority, with everything else—including environmental quality—subservient to that end

556   FOUNDATIONS OF HEALTH SCIENCE

... loopholes in environmental protection laws are not plugged

... exemptions and variances from the law are granted whenever the economic pinch is felt

... local, state and federal supervisory, regulatory, and planning agencies are underfinanced and understaffed

... major industrial polluters found in violation of the law are assessed fines of no economic consequence

... we retain our national pride in technological achievement for its own sake, with little or no thought to the long-range environmental consequences of such achievement

... major industrial polluters spend more money on public relations programs designed to whitewash their activities in the eyes of the public than on research and development programs to combat pollution

... transportation cost differentials encourage the use of raw materials in the production of consumer goods rather than the recovery of used materials for recycling

... we value personal gain and private rights to the exclusion of concern for the public good

... our individual appetites for "the latest model," "the newest gimmick," "the easiest," "the most convenient," feed the fires of higher and higher levels of production of consumer goods to embellish unnecessarily an already high standard of living.[3]

We now see that if we are to have a suitable environment, we must be concerned with the total management of the natural resources of air, water, food, land, and space. This goal means that federal, state, and local governments must develop organizational patterns and tools, in an effort to promote the fullest possible coordination and cooperation with all agencies that have programs with significant implications for public health.

THE SCIENCE OF ECOLOGY

The word "ecology" derives from the Greek *oikos*, meaning "house." Ecology, therefore, is translated as the study of houses, or in a broader sense, environments. The science of ecology examines the precarious relationships between living things and their surroundings.

To understand ecology—and the present dilemma that we have created for ourselves—we must first understand the concept of "ecosystem." An ecosystem is the sum total of all of the living and nonliving parts that support a chain of life within a selected area. These are the four primary links in the chain:

Nonliving matter: sunlight, water, oxygen, carbon dioxide, organic compounds and other nutrients used by plants for their growth.

Plants: ranging in size from the microscopic phytoplankton in water up through grass and shrubs to trees. These organisms convert carbon dioxide and water, in a process called *photosynthesis,* into carbohydrates required both by themselves and other organisms in the ecosystem.

Consumers: those higher organisms that feed on the producers. Herbivores, such as cows and sheep, are primary consumers. Carnivorous man and such animals as the wolf feed upon the herbivores and are secondary consumers.

Decomposers: those tiny creatures—bacteria, fungi, and insects—that close the circle of the ecosystem when they break down the dead producers and consumers and return their chemical compounds to the ecosystem for reuse by the plants.

Although growth and decay are going on simultaneously and continuously in an ecosystem, they tend to balance each other over the long run

What are you doing?

It's a bunch of garbage! I *do* care about the oil spills in the ocean. I do care about the beer cans on the highways. But does it really matter what I think or even what I do. I don't feel I can have any real impact on the problem. I don't even tell my friends, but I'm worried and I'm trying to do my thing. I gave up my electric hot lather machine and replaced it with the old-fashioned non-aerosal shaving lather. I also gave up my spray deodorant and replaced it with a stick deodorant. My aerosol hair spray has been replaced by a liquid hair spray. I'm not a fanatic about pollution but I'm afraid to just sit by and let it all happen. The hardest thing for me to believe is that what I am doing, no matter how small it is, is really worthwhile. I want someone to say it really doesn't matter. I want someone to say that even though I don't carry banners or write my congressman, that I'm making a dent in the pollution problem. I'm doing all I can. Let the others with their free time and money carry on the cause. I dare them to say I'm not doing enough. I'm doing more than others are. They laugh at me—I laugh at them. If everyone thought as they do, that they, as only one person couldn't make a dent in the pollution problem, where would we be? I refuse to admit that I carry the cause too far. My overreaction perhaps will make up for my friends' lack of reaction.

I save newspapers and cans, I wash dishes once a day to save hot water, i.e. fuel. I use one light for reading and turn it off when I leave the room. I use tobacco juice from my neighbors cigarettes as a garden duster and bug repellent. I am trying in my own small way to prevent the disaster that is going to occur. Laugh at me if you will, but I'm trying. What are you doing?

FOUNDATIONS OF HEALTH SCIENCE

—and thus the chain is said to be in equilibrium. Nonhuman environments have a remarkable resiliency; as many as 25 to 60 percent of a certain fish or rodent population might be lost in a habitat during a plague or disaster, yet the species will recover its original strength within one or two years. Manmade interference can profoundly disturb the ecosystem and its equilibrium. One type of interference is pollution.

For example, in the shallow waters of the Pacific Ocean, sea urchins—a small sea animal—are enjoying a population boom, thanks to the organic materials in sewage being washed out to sea. Normally, the sea urchins' population levels are tied to the quantity of kelp on the ocean bottoms; the animals die off when they have eaten all the kelp, thus allowing new crops of the seaweed to grow. But now that sewage is available to nourish the sea urchins they don't die off and the kelp beds do not get a chance to recover. In many places the kelp, for which man has found hundreds of uses, has disappeared altogether.

We have no way of calculating the precise effects of the loss of kelp on its particular ecosystem. This inability has been one of the failings in the science of ecology; precious few quantitative measurements are available to support the ecologists' empirical observations. But this fact is rapidly changing. At scores of universities across the nation, projects are under way to determine just what happens, for example, in a fresh-water ecosystem or a coastal estuary. Perhaps the most comprehensive and exhaustive of these projects is the International Biological Program, a cooperative effort to study distinctly different environments such as grasslands, types of forests, deserts, arctic tundra, and the life web of each. The scientists, working at instrumented field sites, are not only trying to determine who eats what and with what effect, but also attempting to measure the total energy flow starting with the sunlight and rain falling on the designated site and ending with the total amounts of herbiage and animal weight growth. In the United States, ecologists are conducting a series of studies of environmental programs that focus on man—Eskimos, migrant people, American Indians—and nutritional adaptations to specific climatic zones.

Highly technological societies, such as this nation is, call upon new technology to cure the ills wrought by the old. Scientists are hopeful of finding technical solutions for many pollution problems; cleaner fuels for automobiles, for example, with more efficient engines to make up for the loss in volatility, and recycling systems to make use of the wastes that are currently pumped into streams or spewed into the air. These attempts can be dangerous, though, since often the technological solutions have a way of creating new environmental problems of their own. Nuclear power plants avoid smoke pollution but introduce heat pollution (temperature rises that upset the balance of life) in the rivers they use for coolants; and detergents used to disperse oil slicks do more damage to marine life than the oil itself. For this reason, a number of today's environmental reformers conclude that mankind's main hope lies not in technology but in abstinence—fewer births and less gadgetry.

Ecological Balance

Clear Lake, California, is a shallow, forty-thousand-acre body of fresh water that lies about one hundred miles north of San Francisco. For centuries, it was home for a large colony of Western grebes, lovely birds that swim with the stately grace of swans and dive as skillfully as loons. But some years ago, in an environmental tragedy unwittingly perpetrated by man, large numbers of grebes began dying off, and the once-clear waters of the lake turned murky and green. Now, by introducing a new ecological cycle, scientists have saved Clear Lake's grebes and even clarified its water.

The grebe's problems began in the late '40s when the local mosquito abatement district sprayed thousands of pounds of DDD, a chlorinated hydrocarbon pesticide, on Clear Lake to rid the area of swarms of buzzing black gnats. The chemical, a close cousin of DDT, worked so well that people previously repelled by the gnats began building houses around the lake.

Unhappily, after an absence of several years, the gnats returned. In 1954 and again in 1957, stronger doses of DDD eliminated them. About the same time, the lake's population of grebes began to decrease, dropping from one thousand pairs to only twenty within one year. The baffling change was explained in 1962 by Rachel Carson, in *Silent Spring*. Grebes, she wrote, feed mainly on fish. The fish, in turn, eat insect larvae and zooplankton, and these foods had become saturated with the DDD dumped into Clear Lake. Thus, over a long period, the grebes accumulated lethal amounts of the long-lasting pesticide in their tissues and died by the hundreds. Even worse, because of the DDD in their eggs, thousands of grebes never hatched. Between 1958 and 1963 only one young bird was seen at Clear Lake.

Meanwhile, the proliferation of residential areas around the lake was having another, equally unforeseen effect. Household wastes, laden with nutrients, seeped into the water and promoted the growth of algae. By 1961, the lake and its beaches were covered with algae, a green slime.

What could be done to solve the problem. The mosquito abatement district switched from the persistent DDD to methyl parathion, a chemical that is effective against gnats but that deteriorates and becomes harmless in a short time. At the same time, the district hired a team of scientists

FOUNDATIONS OF HEALTH SCIENCE

from the University of California at Davis to find a way to control the gnats biologically. The team decided that a small fresh-water smelt, the Mississippi silverside, might find the gnats appetizing. In 1967 they "planted" 3,000 fingerlings in the lake.

The silversides have multiplied prodigiously. They not only eat the gnats but also compete for the nutrients that stimulate algae growth. As a result, the algae are disappearing, and the lake has regained 80 percent of its original clarity. No longer troubled by DDD, the grebes are returning. But an ecological balance is not easily restored; large game fish now have to be imported to feed on the wildly proliferating silversides. Nevertheless, at least one balance has been restored.

AIR POLLUTION

Over ten thousand communities in the United States have some kind of serious air pollution problem, and each year keeping the air supply fresh and healthful becomes more difficult. The past tendency to associate the smoking industrial stack with prosperity has consistently deterred community rebellion, but today people are not so accepting of wealth first, health second. Throughout the industrialized world, men are awakening to the air pollution hazard.

Smog and other forms of contaminated air, previously considered a local annoyance, are now recognized as a national problem in America and a menace to the future health of this country. Evidence from disastrous occurrences and from ongoing studies, though limited, indicates that air pollution poses a significant threat to wellness. Furthermore, investigation reveals that air pollution is injurious to agricultural crops, livestock, and to air and ground transportation.

Air and Health

Accumulating evidence indicates that pollutants in the air produce harmful effects in humans. Many studies plus common sense show that air pollution may cause reduced visibility, eye irritation, and respiratory irritation. Medical research links air quality with lung cancer, emphysema, heart disease, and allergies.

The severity of symptoms of illness increases proportionately with concentration of pollutants in the air. The first effects are likely to lead to annoying discomfort though not necessarily serious disease. These effects include eye irritation, rasping sensation in the throat, or headaches. At this pollution level, vegetation is damaged, visibility is reduced, and property damage is of sufficient magnitude to cause significant economic loss. At a higher level of pollution, insidious or chronic disease, or significant alteration of physiological functions, may occur in "sensitive groups" such as the aged or sufferers from chronic respiratory and heart disease. Pollution would not necessarily be a risk for persons without a health problem. Under conditions of very heavy pollution this "sensitive group" might die.

Three episodes of acute air pollution have been characterized by sudden death. These tragedies occurred in Belgium's Meuse Valley in 1930, in Donora, Pennsylvania, in 1948, and London in 1952. In each case a heavy fog settled over the area and did not lift; in each case the phenomenon was produced by a temperature inversion, or a layer of warm air over a layer of cold air; and in each case a heavy concentration of smoke and pollutants covered the area. During these periods, sixty-three deaths in Meuse Valley, twenty deaths in Donora, and three thousand deaths in London were attributed to air pollution. Most of those who died were elderly people already suffering from diseases of the respiratory or circulatory systems. In any large metropolis, periods of heavy air pollution are accompanied by increased deaths from respiratory illness.

Of the various constituents of air pollution some have been investigated in controlled studies. Continued, prolonged exposure to ozone produces loss of alveolar walls and damaged bronchiole walls that causes emphysema. Pulmonary artery walls thicken and the artery becomes narrowed. This condition can lead to an inadequate supply of oxygen in the blood, increased activity by the heart in an attempt to increase the supply, and thence to cor pulmonale—pulmonary heart disease.[4]

Another study showed that emphysema is related to air pollution as demonstrated by postmortem examination of the lungs of three hundred adults who had resided in St. Louis, Missouri, and a like number who had lived in Winnipeg, Canada. St. Louis, at the time of the study, was heavily polluted, with thirteen times as much sulfur oxide, seven times as much hydrocarbon, and twice as much particulate pollution as Winnipeg had. The subjects whose lungs were examined were matched by sex, occupation, socioeconomic status, length of residence, smoking habits, and age at death. The investigators found that the contribution of air pollution to emphysema was in addition to that of smoking—the latter, though, was a much greater factor. Four times as much severe emphysema was found among cigarette smokers from St. Louis as among cigarette smokers from Winnipeg. No severe emphysema was found in the lungs of nonsmokers who had lived in either city, but three times as much mild to moderate emphysema was found among nonsmoking St. Louis inhabitants as among nonsmokers from Winnipeg. In general, emphysema appears to be more

562

prevalent in St. Louis than in Winnipeg, to develop much earlier, and to progress more rapidly.[5] Figure 15.1 illustrates the findings of this study.

Stomach cancer appears to be associated with suspended particulate pollution. Mortality rates for gastric cancer in white men and women fifty to sixty-nine years of age are almost twice as high in areas of high suspended particulate air pollution as in areas of low pollution.[6] Childhood allergic disease rates are greater as air pollution levels rise. In a comparison of hospitalized cases of childhood eczema, the difference between eczema incidence at low and high levels of pollution was threefold (300 percent). This figure does not consider the effect of pollution on asthma patients and the vast majority of eczema patients who never require hospitalization.[7]

Kinds of Air Pollution

Three general types of substances are known to pollute the atmospheres of all industrial environments: chemical, radioactive, and biological. Chemical pollutants are the major concern because of expanding industrial, automotive, and domestic wastes. However, radioactive pollutants add to the total radiation exposure in both urban and rural air. Biological dusts and pollens likewise may cause harmful effects, especially in persons who react to them with hay fever, asthma, and other allergies.

The accidental industrial fumigation of the Mexican town, Poza Rica, during a temperature inversion in 1950, poisoned 329 persons and killed 22 in the immediate vicinity of an oil refinery. This catastrophe showed that hydrogen sulfide can diffuse through the air in concentrations sufficient to kill individuals in normal health. Other lethal concentrations can also occur to a degree far above tolerance levels.

Industry. Two major causes of chemical air pollution are the steady, rapid industrialization that has come with urbanization and meteorological factors. More than forty damaging substances have been identified in the atmosphere of coastal cities. These include *hydrocarbons* from motor vehicle exhausts, petroleum refinery processes, and the storage and marketing of petroleum products; *nitrogen oxides* from auto exhausts, household and industrial fuels, and oil and gas burners; *smoke* from domestic incinerators and fuel oil burners; *dust and fumes* from mineral and earth processes, metal industries, grain and feed processes, and a wide variety of chemical industries; and *sulfur oxides* emitted from fuel oil burners, petroleum processes and chemical processes.

A study made in Louisville, Kentucky, revealed that a daily average of 440 tons of manmade substances are thrown into the air over the city's

Figure 15.1 Prevalence of Emphysema in Two Cities with Contrasting Levels of Air Pollution. Prevalence of emphysema, as found in a 1960–66 postmortem examination of the lungs of 300 residents of heavily industrialized St. Louis, Missouri, and an equal number from relatively unpolluted Winnipeg, Canada. The subjects were well matched by sex, occupation, socioeconomic status, length of residence, smoking habits, and age at death. The findings clearly suggest a link between air pollution and pulmonary emphysema. (Courtesy of National Tuberculosis and Respiratory Disease Association, *Pollution Primer*, 1969, p. 73.)

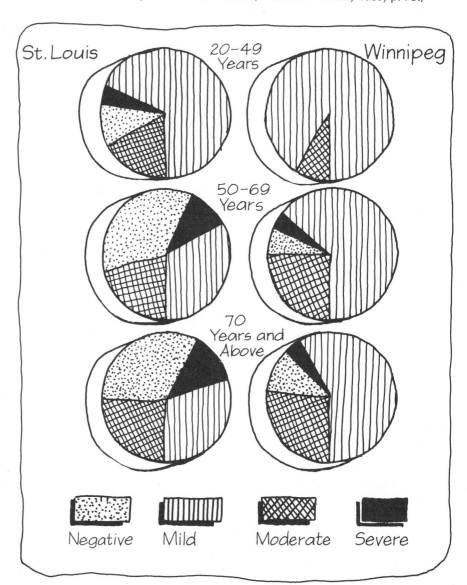

FOUNDATIONS OF HEALTH SCIENCE

main industrial section. In Seattle, Washington, autos and trucks alone were found to be putting 100 tons of hydrocarbons, 20 to 80 tons of nitrogen dioxide, and 4 tons of sulfur dioxide into the city's air each day. In Chicago, the Illinois Institute of Technology found that each month dust fall, a measure of air contamination, was averaging 52.9 tons per square mile, compared with 71 tons in the same period when industrial activity was significantly higher.

The automobile. The major source of air pollution is the automobile. As Ayres says in the *Lung Association Bulletin*:

> A list of the air pollutants produced by the internal combustion engine resembles an alchemist's collection of mysterious potions. Unburned gasoline appears in the exhaust as hydrocarbons; partially burned gasoline forms formaldehyde, acrolein, and other irritant substances. While complete combustion of petroleum hydrocarbons produces carbon dioxide and water . . . incomplete combustion due to high fuel-air ratios produces carbon monoxide . . . . The high temperatures produced within the engine chemically unite oxygen and the ordinarily inert nitrogen, liberating nitric oxide . . . and nitrogen dioxide . . . .[8]

Ayres, a specialist in cardiopulmonary disease is most concerned about the effects of carbon monoxide and the nitrous oxides. Carbon monoxide causes headache, nausea, vomiting, dizziness, palpitations, and death. Hemoglobin has a greater affinity for carbon monoxide than for carbon dioxide, and it also holds on to CO for several hours even after the person leaves the polluted area. An hour in congested traffic can raise the carboxyhemoglobin levels for four to five hours. The average urban dweller has about 2 percent of his blood combined with carbon monoxide. As little as 3 percent of the total body hemoglobin combined with CO interferes with body function. Low levels of CO can critically endanger people with coronary artery disease and emphysema. A 50 percent concentration causes death, but 5 to 10 percent may initiate events leading to death.[9] Figure 15.2 illustrates auto pollution.

Nitrogen dioxide and photochemical oxidants are irritant pollutants that damage the nose, throat, and lungs. In addition, they decrease physical performance. Studies of people have demonstrated that higher concentrations of these substances cause long-lasting damage to airways and lungs.

The pollution problems are not the only ecological effects of the automobile. It shapes our cities and the way we live:

> The impact of the auto on the physique of the city has been as pervasive as its consequences for urban people. The major physical effect has been to rend apart the structure of the compact city. Separation and distance are

Figure 15.2 Illustration of Auto Pollution, Contributing to Smog. (Photo by Norman Wexler, courtesy Los Angeles County.)

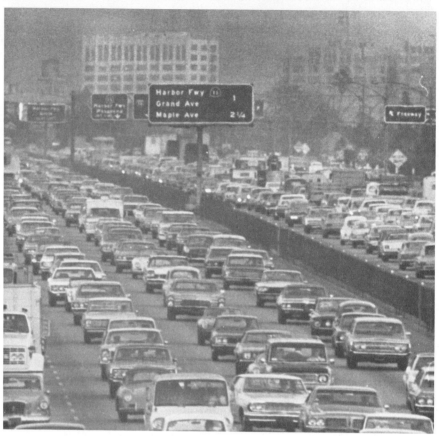

now the rule—houses from jobs, production from consumption, schools from pupils, doctors from hospitals, and both from patients . . . . The automobile requires space—lots of it. As much as 60 percent of the area of our metropolis is given over to serving it—roads, highways, and freeways; parking lots; garages; driveways.

. . . the close-in older suburbs, are now stained permanently by the twice-a-day roar of commuter traffic in and out of the central city. How such areas shall be rescued from a downward spiral of blight and decay due to being corridors between old city and new suburb is a major problem.[10]

Meteorological factors. The virulence of Los Angeles' smog stems from the very meteorological factors that give Southern California its superb mild climate. Warm air, trapped in the basin bounded on three sides by

FOUNDATIONS OF HEALTH SCIENCE

mountains, often hangs over the city. When the upper-level air is warmer than the air at ground level (a condition known as *thermal inversion*), the resulting stagnant air mass becomes a transparent lid, preventing the rise and dispersion of the contaminants. Sunlight then "cooks" the hydrocarbon by-products of incomplete combustion and converts them into noxious polluting gases and vapors that sting eyes, hamper breathing, scorch vegetables, and embrittle rubber. Low-altitude temperature inversions, common throughout the United States, create this photochemical smog in at least nineteen states plus the District of Columbia. Los Angeles' smog differs more in frequency than in severity from that of most large United States cities. Photochemical smog contains ozone and aldehyde derivatives.

Rural pollution. Many rural areas are now engulfed by air pollution. Unlike cities, though, rural areas and their problems differ greatly in character from place to place. They reflect the nature of localized agricultural and industrial activities. Principal rural air pollution problems include: dust storms; smoke and charred sawdust from sawdust burners; dust clouds in delta lands; dust from cement plants; smoke; irritating vapors from hot road mix plants; odors from faulty disposal or organic industrial waste; toxic aerosols from the use of insecticides; and smoke from orchard smudge pots.

The Cost of Air Pollution

City officials and businessmen have learned how expensive air pollution can be. They count the billions of dollars worth of damage from smog in cleaning bills, corrosion, crop losses, and lowered property values. Economic damage alone is estimated at billions per year. This figure can be expected to increase if the levels of toxic substances in the air are allowed to rise. The use of devices designed to "launder" the air used in manufacturing and utility plants have doubled in the last several years at the cost of about $600 million per year. Private industry is now spending more than a billion dollars per year on air pollution control work, and much more will be spent in the future. Figure 15.3 depicts the economics of air pollution.

Prevention and Control

Present control programs are aimed at reducing the quantity of waste materials disposed into the air, because no other method of improving air

Figure 15.3 The Economics of Polluted Air. (Courtesy of National Tuberculosis and Respiratory Disease Association, *Pollution Primer*, 1969, p. 85.)

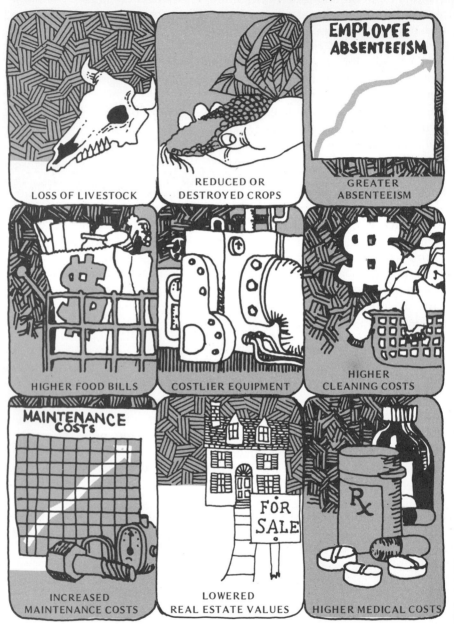

FOUNDATIONS OF HEALTH SCIENCE

quality has yet been developed. Before a community can intelligently plan an air pollution control program, it must have an understanding of the quantity of air available, a knowledge of the kind and amount of pollutants, and an understanding of the reactions that take place in the atmosphere.

To narrow the gap between the known and unknown factors in the air pollution problem, investigations are being carried on by many groups. Effective control of smog is not possible because of a lack of fundamental information. The Public Health Service's National Air Sampling Network, which gathers scientific data on air pollution throughout the country, currently has several hundred individual air sampling stations, located in every state, the District of Columbia, and Puerto Rico. The network samples suspended particulates—smoke, dust, and other such solid contaminants—that are emitted into the atmosphere from a variety of sources and that remain suspended for varying periods of time.

No simple, inexpensive solution is at hand, but all groups involved in air pollution are working toward some solution and realize that they must: extend scientific studies to determine the nature of reactions taking place in the atmosphere, the substances entering into these reactions, and the compounds formed; learn more about the adverse effects of air pollution on human beings and identify the specific substances responsible; develop additional knowledge so that standards for air quality can be established and hazards to health and damage to vegetation can be prevented; devise reliable and practical means for continuously measuring air quality; and develop practical and effective means of controlling certain emissions (particularly hydrocarbons from motor vehicles).

WATER POLLUTION

Water pollution is perhaps an even greater hazard to our health, threat to our economic growth, menace to recreation, and disgrace to the American people than air pollution. Millions of fish are killed in coastal waters and rivers each year. Radioactive wastes, detergents, pesticides, and other chemicals are found in numerous rivers and streams, and unsewered septic tanks drain into underground waters. In many cities drinking water is becoming less and less palatable because of pollutants. In addition, demands upon available municipal water have multiplied because of a large population, concentrations of people in large urban areas, higher standards of living, growing industry, increased agriculture, and the production of new chemical substances requiring water in the manufacturing process.

A study made by the Department of Health, Education and Welfare in the early 1970s disclosed that as many "as eight million people could be served water that is potentially dangerous. Physical facilities supplying drinking water were poorly constructed, unqualified operators were staffing water treatment plants, and state inspections were insufficient if not lacking."[11] In addition, in 1974 potentially dangerous organic chemicals, which could form compounds suspected to be carcinogenic, were discovered in the drinking water of New Orleans and Cincinnati.[12] We do not have the "pure" drinking water that most citizens believe!

If water and people were uniformly distributed throughout the country, water pollution problems would be lessened. However, most of the population of the United States now live on less than 10 percent of the land. The unequal distribution of mist, rain, and snow over the country and variability in "wet and dry" periods aggravate the situation.

Virtually all water supply has its origin in rainfall. When society was predominantly rural, rain fell on soil, through which it percolated down to underground rivers and lakes. Increased suburbanization, with larger and larger houses, two-car garages, supermarkets, and drive-in movies, prevents underground accumulation. Now rain hits the top of the ranch house, carport, driveway, or shopping area parking lot and runs quickly off to a storm drain and thence to a river channel, sometimes in a flood, rather than becoming part of the underground water reservoir. In the United States, by 1980, requirements for water will have risen to 600 billion gallons and by 2000, to 1,000 billion gallons per day. Yet the most that the United States can ever hope to have available from present resources will be about 650 billion gallons each day.

Water is not limitless; the supply is relatively fixed. The increasing use of water already has resulted in its re-use. As water is used or re-used, it becomes contaminated or polluted in many ways. Before each re-use it must be cleaned, which poses economic and technical problems of considerable magnitude. The concept of water re-use is not new. Researchers have computed that for some years now the water in the Ohio River is used 3.7 times before it reaches the Mississippi, and some water in almost every stream is used one or more times.

In light of the best available information on population increase, industrial and general economic expansions, and water use, the nation must do these things: as rapidly as possible complete the works necessary to capture the available 650 billion gallons of water per day; reduce water pollution; and treat the water to make each gallon usable at least twice.

Increase Water Supplies

The following techniques of augmenting water resources were described in a report to the Select Committee on National Water Sources of the United States Senate: improved planning and design and better construction and operation of multipurpose water systems; weather modification; exploration of underground aquifers; evaporation suppression; recycling of used water; water conserving agronomy; forest and range management to improve water yield; and, the treatment and use of water having very poor quality such as waste and sea water. These sophisticated operations, after considerable expenditure, can yield a marginal increase in water supply.

Prevention of Pollution

Waters generally are classified as surface waters and ground waters. Surface waters are lakes, reservoirs, interstate and intrastate streams, and the coastal waters of twenty-three states. Generally, treating polluted surface waters is somewhat simpler than eliminating pollution from ground waters, where the pollution can travel rapidly or slowly depending on the nature of the ground strata through which the supply moves and on the nature of the pollution itself. Pollution of ground waters by septic-tank effluents in suburban and rural areas is frequent. Ground waters also may be polluted from waste lagoons or oxidation ponds, by oil field brines, and, in some coastal areas, by salt-water intrusion.

Types of pollution. Water pollutants are classified as follows:

1. Organic wastes from domestic sewage and industrial discharges of plant and animal origin, which remove oxygen from the water through decomposition
2. Infectious agents contributed by domestic sewage and by some kinds of industrial wastes, which may transmit disease
3. Plant nutrients, which promote nuisance growths of aquatic plant life such as algae and water weeds
4. Synthetic-organic chemicals such as pesticides and detergents resulting from the constantly changing chemical technology, which may be toxic to aquatic life and human beings (Some of these are carcinogenic.)
5. Inorganic chemicals and mineral substances from mining, manufacturing processes, petroleum plants, and agricultural industry, which interfere with natural stream purification, destroy fish and other aquatic life, cause excessive hardness in water supplies, produce corrosive damage, and in general add to costs of water treatment
6. Sediments, which fill stream channels, reservoirs, harbors; erode hydroelectric power and pumping equipment; affect fish and shellfish by blanketing fish nests, spawns, and food supplies; and increase costs of water treatment

7. Radioactive pollution from mining and processing of radioactive ores, from use of refined radioactive material, and from fallout following nuclear testing

8. Excessive temperatures (heat) from use of water for cooling purposes and from impoundment of water in reservoirs, which may result in harmful effects on fish and aquatic life and may reduce the capacity of the receiving water to assimilate wastes.

Detection of contaminants. Government agencies are responsible for detecting contaminants in water supplies. Contaminated water may carry infection from human or animal waste, or it may be rendered unwholesome by poisonous chemical compounds. This contamination can be easily checked by field or laboratory analysis. One danger is pollution from the discharges from the human body; there is very little danger of infection from lower animals or from the organic matter of plant life. Organisms discharged from human beings are grouped as "colon bacilli" and are called the "coliforms." These are always present in human intestines and feces, and their presence indicates water contamination.

In December, 1974, the *Safe Drinking Water Act* was finally made law, after nearly four years in the making! This law requires the Environmental Protection Agency to identify contaminants in public drinking water that could constitute health hazards and to establish minimum standards and regulations that will limit such contaminants to safe levels. Regulations of underground injection of wastes to prevent contamination of ground waters—a source of many communities' drinking water—is also controlled by this law. Exemptions from the standards will not be allowed if they will result in unreasonable health hazards (the states can grant public water systems variances and exemptions from standards up to seven years).[13]

Sewage treatment. Today, disposal of sewage into the waterways is considered a privilege rather than a right. Nevertheless, raw sewage is drained into many rivers and bays throughout the country, and many treatment plants are inadequate and ineffective in coping with the increased wastes, chemicals, and detergents. Sewage treatment plants should at least provide primary and secondary treatment in larger communities.

Primary sewage treatment processes the solid matter in waste. Screening first removes large objects. Next, sedimentation or settling out of the remaining solids takes place in settling tanks. These solids, called sludge, are then transported to the digestion tank, where anaerobic bacteria initiate biochemical oxidation. The end product is transported to open-air drying beds, and the residue is then buried, burned, dumped, or sold for fertilizer.

Secondary treatment processes the liquid portion from the settling

FOUNDATIONS OF HEALTH SCIENCE

tank in such a device as the open-air trickling filter. The liquid is sprayed on top of a large, deep open bed of coarse stones, and the droplets trickle from stone to stone to the bottom of the bed, where they collect and flow into an underground drainage system; the cycle is then repeated. This system utilizes aerobic bacteria, air, water, and sunlight to help oxidize and purify the liquid portion of the sewage. It is then chlorinated to reduce bacterial content and odor and transported to the river or bay.

Facilities for the treatment of sewage are inadequate. First, we do not have enough of them. Many of our municipalities still discharge their wastes into the most convenient stream without giving them any treatment. Some provide only primary treatment. Second, our waste treatment plants are not efficient enough. Primary treatment at best removes 35 percent of the organic wastes (of animal or vegetable origin) and secondary treatment removes up to 90 percent. (In terms of total wastes, organic plus inorganic, the plants remove much less than this.) As a result of the size of cities and industries today, an enormous amount of pollution is being expelled into our rivers and streams. The pollution load in rivers is already six times as much as it was sixty years ago. Third, the procedures of waste treatment plants are based mainly on bacterial action, which is inefficient in removing many of the pollutants resulting from the use or manufacture of such new substances as plastics, detergents, nylon and similar fibers, pesticides, herbicides, medicines, and salt. These procedures are also inefficient against other mineral and chemical substances such as acids produced by mine drainage, radioactive substances, and heat, which harms aquatic life by affecting the metabolism of fish and lowering the water's ability to hold oxygen.

Even if secondary treatment by conventional methods is provided at greatly accelerated rates of construction for all the population using present sewage systems, by 1980 the amount of municipal pollution reaching watercourses will be substantially the same as today. Another fact is that if the present rate of municipal treatment plant construction is not accelerated, given the projected urban growth for 1980, the municipal sewage discharge in that year will be 52 percent greater than the pollutant load from the same source in 1960.

Industry is becoming more aware of its responsibility for controlling the waste materials it discards. Today many manufacturers are cooperating, but a large number are still discharging untreated wastes directly into the community streams. One way in which industries can help clean up the water supply is to build treatment plants. They can also recover valuable natural resources from wastes rather than dispose of them in the waterways—for example, the steel industry recently introduced a process for recovery of valuable chemicals from waste liquids.

Although most states have enacted antipollution legislation, many communities have refused to finance the construction of sewage treatment plants. The *Federal Water Pollution Control Act of 1956* for the first time permitted the federal government to join with local governments in financing sewage treatment facilities. This act, adopted in January, 1965, established a national policy for prevention, control, and abatement of water pollution by setting water quality standards for the rivers, by funding research grants, and by increasing federal authorizations for the construction of sewage treatment works.

Water Renovation

Intensive and increased research is needed to discover better and more efficient techniques for treating water. One promising search for new methods of removing wastes is the Advanced Waste Treatment Research Program of the Public Health Service. Scientists in universities and research laboratories are studying a very wide range of renovation techniques. Among them are absorption by carbon or other absorptive filters, distillation, foaming, freezing, ion exchange, solvent extraction, electrodialysis, and even electrolysis. The problem is how to make the application of such techniques to huge volumes of wastes economically feasible.

PESTICIDES

Pesticides contribute to health and welfare by augmenting the production of food and fiber and by helping in the control of vector-borne diseases. Concurrently, the application of pesticides has resulted in human health and environmental contamination problems. The problems are technically complex, cause scientific controversy, and promote public apprehension and confusion:

> Insects and other arthropods are all around us: they live in our houses, puncture our skin, and consume our food and clothing. There is scarcely a place on the planet that is not home to at least one insect . . . . Different species are adapted for life in the air, on land, in soil, and in fresh water, brackish water, or salt water . . . . Wherever they live, they seem indestructible.[14]

Before chemical insecticides were available, millions of people died each year from a number of insect-borne diseases; malaria, typhus, plague, yellow fever, and encephalitis are a few of the more widely known. The use of pesticides and herbicides not only increases the yield of food crops per acre, but it also enhances quality. With more and more people to feed, and less arable land to use, time-consuming methods of weed control and loss of foods because of insect devastation cannot be tolerated.

FOUNDATIONS OF HEALTH SCIENCE

The chemicals used to improve agricultural production act in different ways. Some are ingested by the insects and are suitable for biting or sucking species of pests; some are contact poisons that enter the covering or skin of the insect; others, such as fumigants, are breathed in through the insects' respiratory system. Pesticides can be classified according to their composition:

1. Naturally occurring plant products, such as pyrethrin I and II, rotenone, nicotine
2. Inorganic products containing such metals as copper, arsenic, lead, mercury
3. Chlorinated organic products, such as DDT, benzene hexachloride, methoxychlor, dieldrin, chlordane
4. Organic phosphorus products, such as of parathion, malathion, diazinon
5. Petroleum oil fractions (used as larvicides).

All chemicals have a potential for harming humans, and people vary with respect to their sensitivity to them. A danger of great concern to the general public has been the fact that some of these can accumulate in our tissues, which happened in the case of DDT. Although we have no evidence of untoward effects up to this time, the use of DDT is greatly restricted in the United States. Many people believe that the accumulation of pesticides in the environment causes actual and potential harm in the form of residues ingested in food and water. We do not have evidence that such is true, but continuing studies are being made of the long-term effects of these chemicals on mankind.

We do know some of the effects on insects, which have a fantastic ability to reproduce and to develop resistance to insecticides. We have had to constantly increase dosages to maintain the same levels of control. At times, some desirable insects are sufficiently destroyed that other problems of pest control develop: "This pattern has repeated itself many times. Man would use a chemical to kill insect A and accidently kill insect B, which had been controlling insect C. Often C would prove to be a greater pest than A had been . . . ."[15]

Some pesticides, when incorrectly used, are severely toxic. Children may ingest them accidently, and they pose an occupational hazard to the people working with them. For example, the following types of situations occur every year:

Case 1.
A young sprayer was found dead in the field in the tractor that had been pulling his spray-rig. He had been working alone, pouring and mixing parathion concentrate into the spray-rig tank. In the process of mixing the concentrate, the worker contaminated his gloves inside and out. He rested

his gloved hands on his trousers as he pulled the rig to apply the spray. Parathion was absorbed through the skin of his hands and thighs. He began to vomit, an early symptom of parathion poisoning. He could not remove his respirator and he aspirated the vomitus and choked. The diagnosis of poisoning was confirmed by postmortem cholinesterase tests.

Case 2.

A young man came to work as a swamper for an agricultural aircraft operator. On the first day, he was put to work steam cleaning and washing a crop dusting aircraft. It was reported that he was not informed of any hazard, nor was he given any protective clothing or equipment. His clothing was observed to have been thoroughly wet while he was working. In the early afternoon, he complained of not feeling well. His employer gave him two atropine tablets and the swamper returned to work. Not long afterwards, he was found unconscious. He was admitted to the hospital and died several hours later. Apparently, the aircraft he was cleaning had been used to make several applications of demeton. The diagnosis of phosphate ester pesticide poisoning was confirmed by postmortem cholinesterase tests.[16]

The controversy over how to control insect pests has led to an interest in biological methods: "It is the natural order of life that nature provides for the survival of both beneficial and destructive insects."[17] (In utilizing this attribute, we must be careful, though, that a predator introduced to check a specific pest population will not itself become a pest.)

The attack occurred at a laboratory in Tifton, Georgia. An entomologist placed a single corn earworm in a plastic pan containing several dozen assassin bugs. At first nothing happened and the corn earworm crawled calmly along.

Then one assassin bug sensed a victim and began to stalk it. For a moment the bug glided sideways in step with the worm, like a basketball player guarding his man one-on-one. Suddenly the corn earworm jumped as though jolted by electricity. The assassin bug had stabbed it, injecting a paralyzing venom. The attacker waited for his victim's writhing to subside, then began sucking its body fluids.[18]

Biological control is based on the use of predators, pathogens, or parasites. The predator quickly kills his prey as the assassin bug did the corn earworm. Pathogens, of course, produce a disease that is specific to certain classes of crop-damaging pests, but has no affect on man. Parasites comprise the most successful biological control programs. The pest insect becomes host for the growth and development of its enemies. In the process, it is destroyed. Rarely does a single parasite species provide complete pest control; it must be used in combination with predators and pathogens, chemicals, and cultural practices.

FOUNDATIONS OF HEALTH SCIENCE

Application of cultural practices requires knowledge of how pests like to live and eat. For example, the cereal leaf beetle prefers to eat oats, but if necessary, it can survive on wheat. The farmer will plant a plot of oats amongst the wheat to attract the beetle who then does little damage to the wheat. One acre of oats amidst fifty acres of winter wheat can save most of the wheat from damage.

Successful pest management depends on the use of all weapons. All must be used with forethought rather than hindsight, though, for we do not know the ultimate result of each method.

NOISE POLLUTION

Noise is taking its place with air and water pollution as a major and growing concern to the American public. Actually, men differ from women in their tolerance to "sound pollution." Males endure lower frequency sounds while women tolerate higher frequency sounds better. With a substantial body of medical opinion now agreeing that too much noise is not good for people, many communities and some states are beginning to do more than just "sympathize." Heavy industry—especially drop forging, steel pouring, metal cutting, riveting, drilling, air blasting, sawing, and high-speed paper shredding—has deafened countless people over the years. Not much was done about this problem until 1948 when the New York Court of Appeals awarded $1,661.25 in compensation to a partially deafened drop-forge worker. As a result, companies engaged in noisy work have taken noise-abatement measures, and they conduct regular tests of workers' hearing. States have legal limits to industrial noise. For instance, ear protection devices must be issued if the noise level reaches 95 to 110 decibels depending on frequency and duration of the sound.

Variations in air pressure cause the eardrum to vibrate. These vibrations in turn are processed through the ear to the brain where they are interpreted as sound. The quality of loudness is due to the magnitude of these variations, and pitch is due to the frequency with which these variations occur. Human sensitivity to sound is a function of these two qualities plus duration. Loudness is expressed in decibels, frequency in cycles per second (pitch), and duration in seconds.

If we define noise pollution as being sound that is annoying, then other attributes of sound are of consideration. The more annoying sounds are those of high frequency, those that are intermittent rather than steady, those that vary in level and are of high intensity, those that are of unfamiliar content, and those that are unexpected.

Effects of Noise

Evidence indicates that levels of noise below 75 decibels are not dangerous. Above 80 to 85 decibels, levels in the frequency range of 1,200 to 4,800 cycles per second seem to be unsafe. In noise-induced deafness, the ability to hear high-pitched sounds of speech is lost first, and the victims complain of inability to understand what other people say.[19] Figure 15.4 illustrates the effects of comparative intensities of sound.

Some of the possible physical effects of noise pollution are aggravation of disease, impairment of function, and interference with activities. These effects may be in addition to feelings of annoyance.[20] Peterson and Gross report that people working or living in a moderately noisy environment (above 70 decibels) may experience physiological changes in their body resulting in disease of the circulatory system, nervousness, hypertension, or heart disease. High noise exposure over a long time span will manifest temporary or permanent hearing loss.[21] Goldsmith and Jonsson have summarized the effects of such exposure, as shown in Table 15.1.

"Noise pollution is unwanted sound which produces unwanted effects."[22] The goal in programs to control this aspect of community health should be ". . . the achievement of a desirable environment in which noise levels do not interfere with the health and well-being of man or adversely affect other values which he regards highly."[23]

THE ENVIRONMENTAL PROTECTION AGENCY (EPA)

Control of the environment has customarily been a responsibility of the states. However, environmental hazards are not contained within geographic and/or political boundaries. Consequently, in 1970 the forma-

Table 15.1 Noise and Health

1. Symptoms of aggravation or disease	headache, muscle tension, anxiety, insomnia, fatigue
2. Impairment of function	impairment of hearing including temporary threshold shifts and presbycusis
3. Interference with activities	relaxation, rest, communication such as conversation and listening to TV or radio
4. Feelings of annoyance	fear, resentment, distraction, need to concentrate

Source: Adapted from, John R. Goldsmith and Erland Jonsson, "Health Effects of Community Noise," *American Journal of Public Health,* 63:787, September, 1973.

FOUNDATIONS OF HEALTH SCIENCE

Figure 15.4   Comparative Intensities

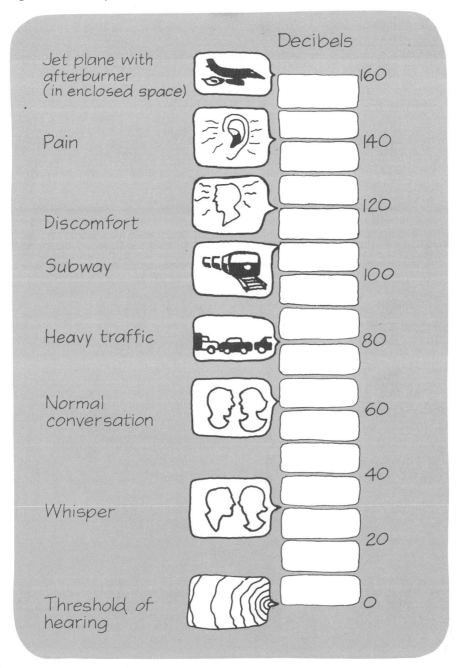

tion of the Environmental Protection Agency, the EPA, combined units from a number of other federal agencies who had been dealing with pollution of the air and water, regulating pesticides, atomic radiation, and waste control.

The EPA conducts research and demonstration projects, establishes and enforces environmental standards, monitors pollution, and assists state and local governments in combating pollution. As stated in the *U.S. Government Organizational Manual 1973/1974*:

> The Environmental Protection Agency was created to permit coordinated and effective governmental action on behalf of the environment. EPA endeavors to abate and control pollution systematically, by proper integration of a variety of research, monitoring, standard setting, and enforcement activities. As a complement to its other activities, EPA coordinates and supports research and antipollution activities by State and local governments, private and public groups, individuals, and educational institutions. EPA also reinforces efforts among other Federal agencies with respect to the impact of their operations on the environment, and it is specifically charged with making public its written comments on environmental impact statements and with publishing its determinations when those hold that a proposal is unsatisfactory from the standpoint of public health or welfare or environmental quality. In all, EPA is designed to serve as the public's advocate for a livable environment.[24]

Environmental Impact Statements

All federal agencies must file an analysis of the environmental impact of any proposed major environmental action. Such statements must include long-term as well as short-term effects of such changes and direct and indirect consequences on ecological systems as well as alternatives to the proposed action that might reduce adverse effects. Impact statements have been broadened to include effects on mental and social well-being as well as physical well-being.

COMMUNITY HEALTH PROGRAMS

Many of the problems stemming from our environment and from our living so closely together require public measures that are called community health programs. Community health is achieved through the organized efforts of groups of people whose aim is to promote and maintain the physical, emotional, and social health of the people. Their efforts are directed toward programs of education, prevention and treatment of disease and infirmities, rehabilitation of the handicapped, and research.

A number of agencies are devoted to community health. They can be classified in three general categories: (1) government, official, or public agencies having the legal responsibility for fulfilling specific obligations; (2) private, nonofficial, or voluntarily organized groups that have assumed certain responsibilities; and (3) both public and private agencies in which health programs are but one of several functions.

Workers in community health have witnessed rapidly growing health organizations striving to keep pace with rapidly growing societies. Public financial support has been increasing steadily as citizens realize more fully how health services, such as those provided by a public health department, prevent misery and death as well as save taxpayers' money. Unfortunately, many areas still lack the services of a health department. While health departments have responsibility for enforcing a great many laws and regulations, compulsion has never been their most important method of protecting the health of the public. Education and persuasion are the keys to community wellness. The ultimate responsibility for community health, therefore, rests with interested people who live in

1. a community composed of individuals motivated to observe the personal practices conducive to physical, mental, and emotional health
2. a community that accepts responsibility for solving its health problems
3. a community that is informed of its health status because it knows:
   a. the nature and extent of prevailing health problems
   b. the measures for preventing and controlling problems as individuals and as community members
   c. the resources or community facilities and services for prevention and control
   d. the program and services of the health department
4. a community that participates in coordinated planning and programing in these ways:
   a. appraising present facilities and services
   b. examining ways by which present facilities and services could be used more efficiently and then acting upon the findings
   c. obtaining facilities and services that are needed.

The Public Health Department

The protection of the public health is primarily an obligation of the governments of the individual states. To fulfill this obligation, each state has created a state department of public health, which sees that the mandates established by the legislators are carried out. To meet local needs, city and county governments have enacted additional ordinances and regulations. The local ordinances and regulations as well as most of the state mandates are effected by the city or county health department.

Many people are poorly informed about public health agencies and activities. The programs of the local health department are varied and interrelated. They include the following broad categories: (1) health education, (2) environmental health, (3) disease control, (4) maternal and child health, (5) vital and health statistics, (6) laboratory services, and (7) comprehensive health planning. Under the impact of expanding health and health-related problems—such as water and air pollution, radiological hazards, mental illness including alcoholism and drug dependency, accidents, chronic disease, nutritional deficiencies, and many others—programs are being continually evaluated and slowly adapted to changing needs.

The public health department staff in general consists of medical and allied health personnel who, preferably, have academic preparation in the field of public health in addition to specific professional education. For example, the health officer and other physicians in the department should, and many do, have a Master's in Public Health (MPH) in addition to a medical degree. Two professional positions requisite to any public health program are the public health nurse and the sanitarian (or environmental health specialist), both of which require a minimum of a bachelor's degree. Also required are laboratory technicians, health educators, medical social workers, nutritionists, epidemiologists, statisticians, industrial hygienists, dentists, dental hygienists, and veterinarians. Professional preparation with advanced degrees is available primarily in schools of public health associated with universities.

Health education. Health education in the public health department is the nucleus or core of all other activities; it permeates each program. Every member of the public health team is first and foremost a teacher: Only by creating attitudes favorable to healthful behavior can the staff assure that practices promoting good health are carried out. However, some functions of the public health department staff are designated as *health education services*.

Health educators provide educational materials, disseminate reliable health information to the public through newspapers, radio, and television, advise on the use of educational methods pertinent to public health, and assist in community health education programs sponsored by the department or other community agencies. Educational materials not available from other sources are prepared or assembled in the health education workshop. These include films, slides, exhibits, pamphlets, posters, and other teaching aids for use in conjunction with the educational programs carried out in schools, homes, industries, communities, and professional groups.

FOUNDATIONS OF HEALTH SCIENCE

Health workers know that solving community health problems is more than providing adequate facilities and services. People must be persuaded to use what is available. Public health educators are concerned with motivating people to take advantage of the resources in the community. The lower socioeconomic or disadvantaged groups in society have more of the major public health problems. They tend to wait until a condition is serious before seeking medical aid (this waiting can be due to ignorance, apathy, suspiciousness, inconvenience, or values). They are, so to speak, more concerned with immediate problems than with the prevention of some possible future illness. Therefore, many programs are provided for people who are not basically interested in prevention. Attitudes of disinterest pose special problems for all public health workers, problems for which few satisfactory answers have as yet been found.

Another responsibility of the health educator is assisting the community to organize for solving its own health problems. Community leaders must be made aware of health needs and how they can be met. This task is difficult. Community members may resist the inception of new programs and effectively oppose a public health measure despite the endorsement of professional public health, dental, and medical associations.

Environmental health. The activities of the environmental health division include such things as provisions for the safety of public water, air, and milk supplies; supervision of safe and adequate disposal of wastes; supervision and assistance to food establishments; study of health factors in new subdivision proposals and community developments; mosquito, vector, and rodent control services; auto court, motel, and trailer camp sanitation; consultation to schools for sanitation and safety; recreational sanitation; investigation of citizens' complaints; abatement of public health nuisances, and occupational health.

Prevention of the spread of water-borne diseases necessitates inspection and survey of water systems and collection of water samples for analysis in the public health laboratory. Periodic inspection of swimming pools ensures both water purity and pool safety, thereby protecting swimmers from disease and injury. Plans for proposed new public pools must have health department approval prior to construction.

Sanitarians supervise dairies, creameries, and milk distribution plants to ensure clean, pure milk and milk products. Consultant service is provided to milk producers and processors. Food processing plants are supervised.

Animal disease control services include the inspection of livestock to prevent the transmission of tuberculosis, undulant fever (brucellosis), and other diseases to human beings. The rabies control program is maintained primarily to avoid the possibility of human beings' becoming infected with this disease and to protect dogs and cats from the threat of rabies. Rabies control is accomplished by vaccination and licensing of dogs and cats, control of stray animals, investigation of animal bite cases, and the isolation of known or suspected rabid animals to minimize the dangers of rabies outbreaks. The health department may provide all animal control services, or some services may be delegated to another governmental agency such as the city pound or animal shelter.

The ultimate goal of a sewage disposal program is the complete sewering of urbanized residential areas. The sanitation division assists as a consultant in the promotion and construction of sanitary sewers. It establishes standards for the construction of septic tank sewage disposal systems for use in areas where sewers are not available. The rapid population increase and growth of new residential areas require the study of each proposed subdivision to ensure adequate supplies of potable water, the safe disposal of sewage and other wastes, and protection from such nuisance or disease carriers as flies, mosquitoes, and rodents. Builders of new residences are required to obtain approval for underground disposal of sewage. Sanitarians aid the builder by performing scientifically engineered soil studies and advising on desirable construction.

The objective of the vector control program is to reduce and eliminate sources of insects and rodents on private and public premises. This goal is accomplished by education, persuasion, and cooperation. Spraying and elimination of breeding places are routinely conducted.

Disease control. Disease control as a department function has been traditionally concerned with communicable diseases. The major health problems in the United States, as far as premature deaths and degree of disability are concerned, are the chronic and degenerative disorders and mental illness, including alcohol and drug dependency. The current trend is for the department to engage in activities to prevent these conditions through education and early detection. All departments do not provide the same services. Some have diagnostic clinics, others sponsor mass surveys, and all provide immunizations, chemotherapy, and chemoprophylaxis to select groups, particularly children. Nearly all have outpatient clinics to treat patients with tuberculosis and the sexually transmitted diseases; many have rehabilitation clinics for those dependent on alcohol and dangerous drugs. Large departments may provide youth clinics where the adolescent may obtain health advice and care.

Maternal and child health. Maternal and child health services are predicated on the premise that healthy mothers and babies lead to healthy citizens. Care of the child starts long before birth when the mother may be examined during the period of gestation. Frequently, obstetricians are employed to give prenatal examinations; public health nurses, nurse-

FOUNDATIONS OF HEALTH SCIENCE

practitioners, and nutritionists help the mother plan for a safe and satisfying pregnancy; and many departments sponsor classes in expectant parenthood to which both of the parents-to-be are invited. Nearly all departments have financial eligibility requirements for persons who receive prenatal care.

The department refers the mother to a hospital for the birth of the baby, but after delivery, she may return for a postnatal medical check. The public health nurse by this time may have visited the mother at home to advise her about infant care.

Well-child conferences are another service of the public health department. Usually any mother is eligible for these, but those who can afford private care are encouraged to obtain such. A pediatrician or a pediatric nurse-practitioner routinely examines children in these conferences that commence when a baby is four to six weeks old and continue until the child is of school age. The physician, nurses, and nutritionist advise mothers on such matters as normal growth and development of children and how to feed and care for them and meet their emotional needs. Immunizations are administered to the children, and those who are acutely ill are referred to another agency such as a clinic for treatment. Some departments provide special services for the physically and developmentally disabled (mentally handicapped) child, and a public health dentist or hygienist may give prophylactic dental examinations and treatment.

When the child starts school, his health may still be partially supervised by health department personnel. Although many large school districts employ their own school health staff, some schools rely on the public health physician and nurse for such services as giving the children screening examination for conditions that might interfere with their education, counseling the parents or the child about health status, referring a child with a problem to the appropriate community resource for treatment or rehabilitation, offering immunizations at school, and aiding the school faculty and staff in planning the overall school health program including health instruction.

Consultation about family planning is available in nearly all public health departments. The mother and father may be advised about eugenics, receive information about the desirability of child spacing, and obtain birth control devices. Figure 15.5 shows a waiting room in a maternity clinic.

Vital and health statistics. The major responsibility of the health department in this area is to compile data about births, deaths, and diseases. Personnel may register and issue certificates of birth and death and must maintain records of the incidence of reportable diseases (primarily com-

Figure 15.5 Maternity Clinic. (Courtesy of the National Foundation–March of Dimes.)

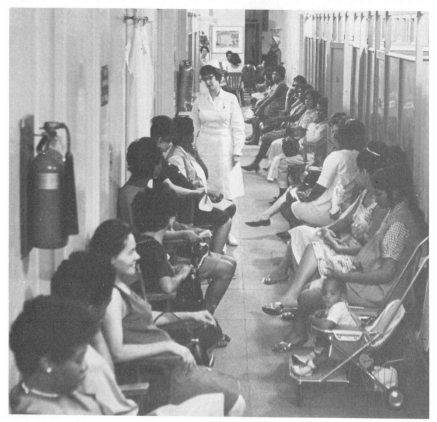

municable). All these data are tabulated, analyzed, and then used to determine health needs, plan programs, detect changes and trends in health levels, and evaluate progress.

Laboratory services. The facilities of the public health laboratory are used by private physicians and health department personnel for diagnosing, treating, and controlling communicable disease in particular. Examinations performed in the laboratory each year, for example, include serological tests for syphilis; bacteriological examinations for typhoid, paratyphoid, diphtheria, streptococcal infections, TB, bacillary dysentery, gonorrhea, parasitic infections, and ringworm, analysis of water samples taken by the health department sanitarians; and testing of milk samples for total bacterial count, amount of butter fat and nonfat solids, presence of coliform organisms, and the completion of pasteurization.

FOUNDATIONS OF HEALTH SCIENCE

Occupational health. The division of occupational health is designed to conserve and promote the health of employed persons, to prevent the occurrence of disease or injury from occupational sources through control over the industrial environment, and to restore health and earning capacity to injured or ill workers. The team of occupational health workers includes radiological inspectors, safety engineers, health physicists, dentists, chemists, industrial hygienists, and the regular staff of public health doctors and nurses. The team provides consultations, surveys, investigations, analyses of health hazards, and educational programs in industries with or without established health programs.

The World Health Organization

The creation of the World Health Organization, WHO, in 1948 was the culmination of a long series of efforts made for several centuries to prevent the spread of disease from one continent to another and to achieve international cooperation for better health throughout the world. The organization occupies the status of a specialized agency in the framework of the United Nations. However, a country does not need to be a member of the United Nations in order to be a member of WHO.

Central technical services. Central technical services form the basis of international health activities, and all countries benefit from them. The International Sanitary Regulations, an important accomplishment of WHO, apply to land, sea, and air traffic throughout the world. They provide for maximal protection against epidemics with minimal interference in international transport and travel. Governments voluntarily adhere to these standards. The Epidemiological Intelligence Service collects information about the occurrence of disease throughout the world, and broadcasts information daily over an international radio network to health authorities, ports, airports, and ships at sea.

An international disease classification system provides for uniform health statistics about diseases and causes of death, thereby making it possible to evaluate health problems more accurately and to adopt more effective public health measures. The list established by WHO comprises approximately one thousand categories of diseases, injuries, and causes of death.

WHO published the first International Pharmacopoeia, which contains recommended specifications for use of drugs in all countries. WHO participates in international efforts for the control of drug dependency and studies new synthetic drugs suspected of causing dependency.

The World Health Organization has been instructed by its member states to study the health problems that arise from the use of atomic energy. Although the peaceful application of atomic energy can improve living conditions, its use is always a threat to the health of workers in atomic establishments and the general public. The amount of background radiation in the atmosphere increases with the development of atomic energy plants and industrial uses of radiation. Radioactive wastes, if not carefully disposed of, can pollute the air, soil, and water. In order to provide protection against these dangers, WHO, in cooperation with the atomic energy industry, has been requested to collect information and to advise governments and public health agencies regarding this hazard.

The Pan American Health Organization, with offices in Washington, D.C., is the regional representative of WHO in the Americas.

VOLUNTARY HEALTH AND WELFARE AGENCIES

The voluntary health and welfare movement is peculiar to the United States. We value individual initiative, being able to look after ourselves and solve our own problems, private ownership, and helping our fellow man in time of adversity. These values together with an increasing amount of personal wealth and leisure time, contributed to the growth of the voluntary agency movement at the turn of the century. Presently over two thousand agencies or chapters of agencies are carrying out health programs. Their work is funded by donations, bequests, fees, profits, and investments. Their support is voluntarily subscribed rather than subsidized by tax funds, though some are given federal funds to support demonstration projects.

The major contributions of the voluntary health and welfare agencies are:

1. Stimulation of the public's interest in health problems
2. Education of the public about the need for specific programs
3. Research and demonstration of improved methods for maintaining the health of the individual and of the community
4. Guarding the public's interests in matters pertaining to health
5. Promotion of efficient health legislation
6. Prodding of governmental agencies to assume those functions that logically appear to be theirs
7. Supplementing programs of the official agencies
8. Meeting the needs of select groups of people.

The voluntary health agencies can be classified as giving direct or indirect services. The direct service agencies do something personal for the individual recipient by offering such things as classes in first aid, water safety, and expectant parenthood or by providing bandages, friendly home visits, limited aid to needy patients, tumor clinics, chest X-rays, tuberculin testing, counseling, sheltered workshops, rehabilitation clinics, weight-control programs, blood, and transportation.

The indirect service agencies provide for education, research, and demonstration projects. For example, one local lung association—Christmas Seals—uses its budget of one million dollars a year for public and school health education; for research in tuberculin testing and chronic respiratory conditions; and for community surveys of the incidence of chronic respiratory disease in children and adults. This association believes that through education and research it is serving seven million rather than the few people it could help if it used its budget for patient care. Figure 15.6 illustrates the demonstration project—Breathmobil.

The research aspect of the voluntary program is most rewarding and

Figure 15.6 Determining the Incidence of Chronic Respiratory Disease. A voluntary agency project. (Courtesy of Lung Association of Los Angeles County.)

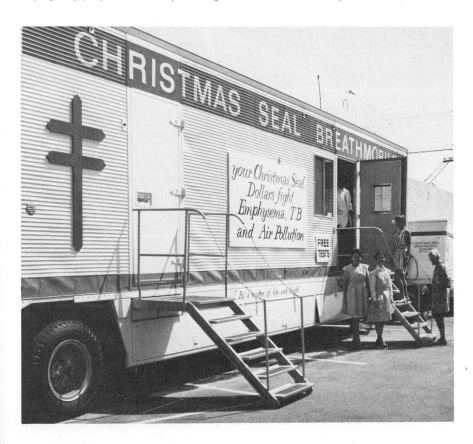

dramatic, as evidenced by the discovery of the Salk poliomyelitis vaccine. Jonas Salk and others worked under research grants sponsored by the National Foundation–March of Dimes. Mass screening for diabetes, glaucoma, and tuberculosis, public health nursing, public health education, cancer detection, heart rehabilitation, and the heart-lung machine are but a few demonstration programs made possible through the auspices of the voluntary health agency.

The American Heart Association, the American Cancer Society, and the National Foundation–March of Dimes, as well as a number of the other voluntary agencies offer undergraduate and graduate scholarships to motivate and encourage students to work in the public health field. Fellowships are available to physicians, nurses, educators, and other related professionals.

Most of the major voluntary health organizations have a national administrative office that is responsible for supervising and guiding activities, functions, responsibilities, programs, and projects. The national office works through the regional or state office. Actual service is rendered at the local level. Large local chapters are usually administered by a salaried executive secretary plus additional professional staff. The board of directors, comprised of volunteer citizens, determines local programs and policies.

Each agency stresses prevention through health education and disseminates health information through films, pamphlets, television, radio, exhibits, and other media. Some have professional public health educators on their staffs who assist individuals, schools, and community agencies and organizations in understanding and adopting preventive health measures.

None of these agencies could function without the volunteer lay worker. Physicians and other professional people also give many hours of their time and support. The volunteer has made the voluntary agency movement a success, and this movement, in turn, has stimulated the growth of many health programs in the United States.

Problems of the Voluntary Agency Movement

Voluntary health organizations have given many people an opportunity to become involved in serving members of their communities. They help the volunteers to keep active and to feel self-satisfied and at the same time stimulate feelings of community spirit and cooperation. Many organizations are responsive to the needs of the community. They have devoted members who participate extensively in the respective programs, who have positions of leadership, and who have a full voice in making

FOUNDATIONS OF HEALTH SCIENCE

policy. Most important, of course, is that this group effort leads to the promotion of health and prevention of disease.

Voluntary health agencies, however, are not without their problems. Voluntary agencies coexist with governmental health agencies and this frequently contributes to competition. A continuing major problem revolves around fund raising. Because of the growth in the number of voluntary agencies, the search for the charity dollar has become extremely competitive. Tax increases and extensive federal appropriations for health research have led many persons to construct impressive theories about the good and evil of organized fund raising. In the interest of protecting the public against never-ending campaigns for funds, consolidated fund raising is now practiced by such organizations as Community Chest and United Federated Funds. People in favor of such consolidated plans argue that the health of a community is essentially a single interest with different aspects. To exalt one agency or aspect of community health is to get it out of focus, they believe, and to encourage one at the expense of other essentials is unscientific, wasteful, and misleading. Further, supporters claim that more money can be raised in consolidated campaigns with less annoyance to the donor.

The attempts at consolidation, though logical, receive considerable opposition and rarely are completely successful. Some agencies prefer to conduct separate fund campaigns and believe that while united drives are a sound process for raising money for some local services, they are not satisfactory for all organizations. Documentary evidence is available to back this belief. Figure 15.7 is an example of one method of fund raising.

Most authorities agree that the voluntary agencies will continue to flourish and offer the public the kind of creative leadership and vital services that have distinguished these agencies for many years. Many also believe that the combined efforts of government and nongovernment organizations, each with their special contributions, are vital to maintaining and promoting the health levels we have today and to improving the levels we expect in the future.

IN CONCLUSION

No matter what the form of life or its habitat, one ecological rule is unchanging, immutable: Populations of animals or plants grow, slowly or rapidly, to some point of equilibrium with their environment. This point of equilibrium is the carrying capacity of the environment. It may be circumscribed by food supply, moisture, nesting sites, competition, or combinations of these; but its capacity is inevitably reached. Man has an edge

Figure 15.7 Fund raising. (Courtesy of the National Foundation–March of Dimes.)

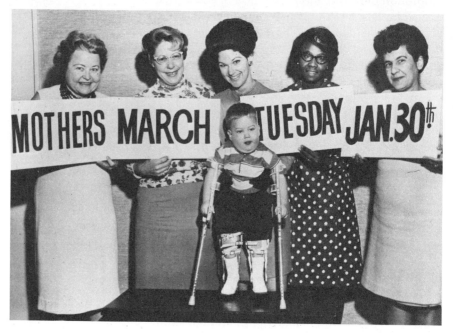

on other forms of life in that he can manipulate his environment. He has done this until now and has reached a dangerous point of disequilibrium. Most of the environmental problems we face today are directly due to overpopulation. We demand more and expend more than the environment can support. In addition, we disrupt the environment with technological innovations and then try to correct the consequences of such disruption by applying more technology. However, Wagner says:

> Clearly technology is not responsible for our current environmental woes any more than a hammer would be for a bruised thumb. The basic cause is man's lack of ecological sensitivity. Until man can become aware of his fellow organisms and the correspondence between their well-being and his, until the environment is regarded as a responsibility rather than an economic opportunity, population control can only partially solve environmental problems.[25]

Programs to develop resources, to prevent pollution, and to reclaim used air and water are costly. These are usually considered to be governmental responsibilities. The federal, state, and local branches of government are working cooperatively, but successful efforts require an educated citizenry who will personally avoid adding unnecessary wastes, who will abide by and support government programs, and who will demand that industry assume its share of responsibility. The level of health in the community is influenced by how well we support health programs through personal concern, understanding, and action, not only financially, but physically by giving time and energy to community activities.

What Can One Person Do?

We can each do a number of things to alleviate environmental decay. Some of them take minimal effort, some take dedicated effort. In your day-to-day, personal activities, you might:

1. Repair leaky faucets.
2. Make a compost pile of lawn clippings and fallen leaves.
3. Avoid persistent and broad spectrum biocides; use natural control of garden pests by encouraging their natural enemies.
4. Keep your automobile tuned up to reduce harmful emissions.
5. Replace a noisy muffler on your car; use the horn only when necessary.
6. Walk whenever you can instead of driving.
7. Use public transportation when possible.
8. Use the litter bag in your car.
9. Use nonleaded gasoline.
10. Turn off air conditioners, furnaces, lights when they are not needed.
11. Avoid eating foods with chemical additives.
12. Don't buy clothing or other items made from endangered species.
13. Be aware of environmental values when buying a house; make your wants known to builders and realtors.
14. Consider safety aspects of purchases as well as luxury aspects.
15. Use returnable bottles.
16. Use biodegradable soaps and cleansing agents.
17. Limit the size of your family; adopt children.[26]

As an informed citizen you might:

18. Insist on good zoning ordinances, balanced community planning, effective conservation agencies, and pollution control measures.
19. Demand attractive communities that have adequate open spaces; playgrounds, parks, and recreation areas; underground utility lines; maintenance of public places; sign and billboard controls.
20. Protect watercourses, natural areas, wildlife.
21. Join groups that work for better environments.
22. Insist on conservation education in the schools.

23. Write your elected representatives about good conservation projects.

24. Support bond issues and tax increases.

As individuals we can do something!

Notes

1. R. Dubos, "The Conflict Between Progress and Safety," *Archives of Environmental Health,* 6:449, April, 1963.

2. Paul R. Ehrlich, Anne H. Ehrlich, and John P. Holdren, *Human Ecology* (San Francisco: W. H. Freeman, 1973), p. 278.

3. Edward B. Johns, Wilfred C. Sutton, and Barbara A. Cooley, *Health for Effective Living* (New York: McGraw-Hill, 1975), p. 138.

4. Alice Y. S. P'an et al., "Ozone-Induced Arterial Lesions," *Archives of Environmental Health,* 24:229–233, April, 1972.

5. S. Ishikawa et al., "The 'Emphysema Profile' in Two Midwestern Cities in North America," *Archives of Environmental Health,* 18:660–667, April, 1969.

6. Warren Winkelstein and Seymour Kantor, "Stomach Cancer," *Archives of Environmental Health,* 18:544–548, April, 1969.

7. Harry A. Sultz et al., "An Effect of Continued Exposure to Air Pollution on the Incidence of Chronic Childhood Allergic Disease," *American Journal of Public Health,* 60:891–901, May, 1970.

8. Stephen M. Ayres, "The Automobile—What a way to go!" *Lung Association Bulletin,* 58:2, June, 1972.

9. Ibid., p. 4.

10. Arthur A. Davis, "Transportation—Shaper of Cities," *Lung Association Bulletin,* 58:8, June, 1972.

11. "Safe Drinking Water Act Passed After States Granted More Power," *"The Nation's Health,* 5:1, January, 1975.

12. Ibid.

13. Ibid.

14. Melvin A. Benarde, *Our Precarious Habitat,* 2nd ed. (New York: W. W. Norton, 1973), pp. 86–87.

15. Hal Higdon, "Bug vs. Bug," *The Kiwanis Magazine,* 58:34, February, 1973.

16. I. West, "Public Health Problems are Created by Pesticides," *California's Health,* 23:11–18, July, 1965.

17. Melvin A. Bernarde, *Our Precarious Habitat,* 1st ed. (New York: W. W. Norton, 1970), p. 98.

18. Higdon, "Bug vs. Bug," p. 33.

19. Bernarde, *Our Precarious Habitat,* 2nd ed., p. 281.

20. John R. Goldsmith and Erland Jonsson, "Health Effects of Community Noise," *American Journal of Public Health,* 63:784, September, 1973.

21. Arnold Peterson and Ervine Gross, *Handbook of Noise Measurement* (Concord, Mass.: General Radio Company, 1972), p. 47.

22. Goldsmith and Jonsson, "Health Effects of Community Noise," p. 782.

23. Ibid.

24. *U.S. Government Organization Manual 1973/74* (Washington, D.C.: U.S. Government Printing Office, 1973), p. 430.

25. Richard H. Wagner, *Environment and Man* (New York: W. W. Norton, 1974), pp. 508, 509.

26. Ibid., pp. 509, 510.

FOUNDATIONS OF HEALTH SCIENCE

THE DISPOSAL OF WASTE IN THE OCEAN

Willard Bascom

current issues

No one would dispute the wisdom of protecting the sea and its life against harm from man's wastes. An argument can be made, however, that some of the laws the U.S. and the coastal states have adopted in recent years to regulate the wastes that can be put into the oceans are based on inadequate knowledge of the sea. It is possible that a great effort will be made to comply with laws that will do little to make the ocean cleaner.

This discussion of waste disposal will be limited to disposal in the ocean; it will not take up disposal in lakes, rivers estuaries, harbors and landlocked bays. Indeed, part of the

Scientific American, 231:16–26, August, 1974. Reprinted with permission. Copyright © 1974 by Scientific American, Inc. All rights reserved.

problem is that insufficient distinction has been drawn between the ocean and the other bodies of water, whose chemistry, circulation, biota and utilization differ from those of the ocean in many ways. It is not sensible to try to write one set of water-quality specifications that will cover all bodies of water. My concern here is only with the quality of ocean water and marine life along the U.S. Atlantic, Gulf, and Pacific coasts. The scientific findings in those areas apply, however, to nearly any other coastal waters that are exposed to ocean waves and currents.

Some of the changes that human activities have wrought in the ocean environment are already irreversible. For example, rivers have been dammed, so that they release much smaller quantities of fresh water and sediment. Ports have been built at the mouth of estuaries, changing patterns of flow and altering habits. On the other hand, certain abuses of the ocean have already been stopped almost completely by the U.S. Nuclear tests are no longer conducted in the atmosphere, so that radioactive material is no longer distributed over the land and the sea; the massive dumping of DDT has been halted, and the reckless development of coastal lands has been restrained by laws calling for detailed consideration of the impact on the environment.

Between these extremes is a broad realm of uncertainty. Exactly how clean should the ocean be? How unchanged should man try to keep an environment that nature is changing anyway? The problem is to decide what is in the best interest of the community and to achieve the objective at some acceptable cost. At the same time it is necessary to guard against the danger that excessive demands made in the name of preserving ecosystems will lead to action that is both useless and expensive.

Waste disposal automatically suggests pollution, which is a highly charged word meaning different things to different people. A definition is needed for evaluating accidental and deliberate inputs into the ocean. Athelstan F. Spilhaus of the National Oceanic and Atmospheric Administration, who has written extensively on pollution, defines it as "anything animate or inanimate that by its excess reduces the quality of living." The key word is excess, because most of the substances that are called pollutants are already in the ocean in vast quantities: sediments, salts, dissolved metals and all kinds of organic

material. The ocean can tolerate more of them; the question is how much more it can tolerate without damage.

One approach to the question was suggested by the National Water Commission in its report of June, 1973, to the President and Congress: "Water is polluted if it is not of sufficiently high quality to be suitable for the highest uses people wish to make of it at present or in the future." What are "the highest uses" that can be foreseen for ocean waters, particularly those near the shore? They are probably water-contact sports, the production of seafood and the preservation of marine life.

Water-contact sports are occasionally inhibited by pollutants on the seacoasts of the U.S. Where such conditions exist they should be corrected at once. Even where coastal waters are clean the community must be alert to keep them so.

To maintain the ocean waters at an acceptable level of quality it is necessary to consider the main inputs of possible pollutants resulting from human activity. One of them is fecal waste (75 grams dry weight of solids per person per day), which after various degrees of treatment ends up in the ocean as "Municipal effluent." Wastes also flow from a host of industrial activities. They are usually processed for the removal of the constituents that are most likely to be harmful, and the remaining effluent is discharged through pipes into the ocean. Dumping from barges into deep water offshore is a means of disposing of dredged materials, sewage sludge and chemical wastes. Thermal wastes include the warmed water from coastal power plants and cooled water from terminals where ships carrying liquid natural gas are

596

berthed. In addition ships heave trash and garbage overboard and pump oily waste from their ballast tanks and bilges.

Such are the intentional discharges, but pollutants reach the ocean in other ways. Aerial fallout brings minute globules of pesticide sprayed on crops, particles of soot from chimneys and the residue of the exhaust of automobiles and airplanes. Painted boat bottoms exude small amounts of toxicants intended to discourage the growth of algae and barnacles. Forest fires put huge amounts of carbon and metallic oxides into the air and thence into the sea. Oil spills from ship collisions and blowouts during underwater drilling operations add an entire class of compounds.

Moreover, natural processes contribute things to the sea that would be called pollutants if man put them there. Streams add fresh water, which is damaging to marine organisms such as coral, and they also bring pollutants washed by rain from trees and land. Volcanic eruptions add large quantities of heavy metals, heat and new rock. Oil has seeped from the bottom since long before man arrived.

Finally, the ocean is neither "pure" nor the same everywhere. It already contains vast amounts of nearly everything, including a substantial burden of metals at low concentration and oxygen at relatively high concentration, plus all kinds of nutrients and chemicals. It has hot and cold layers, well stratified by the thermocline (the boundary between the warm, oxygen-rich upper layer and the cold, oxygen-poor depths). Waves and currents keep the water constantly in motion. It is against this complex background that man must measure the effects of his own discharges.

Even if there were no people living on seacoasts, it would be impossible to predict accurately the kind and quality of marine life because of the natural variability of the ocean. The biota shifts constantly because the temperature and the currents change. Great "blooms" of plankton develop rapidly when conditions have become exactly right and then die off in a few days, depleting the oxygen in the water on both occasions. Within a single year the population of such organisms as salps, copepods and euphausids can change by a factor of 10. When the waters off California become warmer as the current structure shifts, red "crabs" (which look more like small lobsters and are of the genus *Pleuroncodes*) float by in fantastic numbers, followed by large populations of bonito and swordfish. They came in 1973 as they did in 1958 and 1963, but the water soon turned cold again and the fish departed, leaving windrows of dead *Pleuroncodes* along the beaches.

The investigator's problem is to learn enough about the major natural changes so that he can tell whether or not human activities have any effect, either positive or negative. It is a signal-to-noise problem; here the changes one is trying to detect are often only a tenth of the natural biological and oceanic background variations. Both types of variation are hard to quantify.

In the case of the sardine, however, a record of the natural changes has been preserved below the floor of the Santa Barbara Basin off the coast of southern California. The bottom of the basin is anaerobic, that is lacking in oxygen and so supporting little life. The particles that sift down to form sediments are undisturbed by burrowing creatures and therefore remain exactly as they land, in thin strata, layer on layer, one per year. The years can be counted backward, and the count can be confirmed with the lead-210 dating technique.

Some years ago John D. Isaacs of the Scripps Institution of Oceanography, who is also director of the California Marine Life Program, discovered in work with Andrew Soutar that each layer contains identifiable fish scales. Each layer showed a more or less constant number of anchovy and hake scales, but the sardine scales were present erratically, indicating major changes in the population. When the sardines disappeared about 1950, human activities were blamed. The geologic record clearly shows, however, that the sardines had come and gone many times before man arrived. Someday they will return.

It is obvious that some of man's wastes can be damaging to sea life; indeed, products such as DDT, chlorine and ship-bottom paint have been specifically designed to protect man against insects, bacteria and barnacles. Ionic solutions of certain metals are also known to be toxic at some level, as are numerous other substances. The problem is to determine what level is harmful, remembering that some of the substances are actually required for life processes. For example, copper is beneficial or essential for a number of organisms, including crabs, mollusks and oyster larvae. Other marine animals seem to require nickel, cobalt, vanadium and zinc.

Oceanographers would like to be able to demonstrate cause and effect in the ocean, that is, to show that some specific level of a metal does not harm marine life. Proving the absence of damage, however, including long-term and genetic effects, is difficult. Only on fairly rare occasions has it been possible to directly link a specific oceanic pollutant with biological damage. Examples include the finding by Robert Risebrough of the University of California at Berkeley that the decline of the brown pelican off California was attributable to DDT, which inhibits the metabolism of calcium and so makes the shells of the eggs so thin that the mother pelican breaks her own eggs by sitting on them. After patient scientific detective work the source was found to be a single chemical plant in the Los Angeles area. As a result of the work the plant was required to stop discharging DDT wastes into the ocean, and the brown pelican is now returning to California.

From what I have said so far it can be seen that the question of what is a pollutant or what amount of a substance represents pollution is not always easy to answer. Let me now try to put the main kinds of waste in proper perspective.

Municipal sewage containing human fecal material is the type of waste one usually thinks of first. It is certainly a natural substance; indeed, as "night soil" it has long been in demand as a fertilizer in many countries. Since it is not appreciably different from the fecal material discharged by marine animals, is there any reason to think it will be damaging to the ocean, even without treatment? Isaacs has pointed out that the six million metric tons of anchovies off southern California produce as much fecal material as 90 million people, that is, 10 times as much as the population of Los Angeles, and the anchovies of course comprise only one of hundreds of species of marine life.

Two aspects of municipal sewage do require attention. One of them is disease microorganisms. Human waste contains vast numbers of coliform bacteria; they are not themselves harmful, and they die rapidly in seawater (90 percent of them in the first two hours), but they are routinely sampled along public beaches because they indicate the level of disease microorganisms. When there are no endemic diseases in the city discharging the waste (the normal condition in the U.S.), there will be none in the water. It should be noted, however, that the assumption that disease microoganisms die off at the same rate as coliform bacteria is being questioned. It is necessary to guard against the possibility that such organisms will survive in bottom muds long enough to be stirred up by a major storm.

The usual way of reducing the bacterial count is to add chlorine to waste water that is about to be discharged. This approach seems reasonable, since chlorine is commonly added to drinking water and swimming pools to kill bacteria and algae. The trick is to add just the right amount, so that the chlorine exactly neutralizes the bacteria and no excess of either enters the ocean.

The other problem with sewage is one of aesthetics. People do not like to look at discolored water or oily films. A greater effort to reduce effluent "floatables" (tiny particles of plastic, wood, wax and grease) will help to reduce such effects. It will also reduce the number of bacteria reaching the shore, since many of them are attached to the particles.

Petroleum products are perhaps the most controversial marine pollutants. They are seen as small, tar-like lumps far out to sea and on beaches, as great slicks and as brown froth. From two to five million metric tons of oil enter the ocean annually. At least half of it is from land-based sources such as petroleum-refinery wastes and flushings from service stations. Significant quantities of oil enter the marine environment from airborne hydrocarbons. A considerable amount of oil must enter the ocean as natural seepage from the bottom, but it is obviously difficult to estimate how much.

Oil pollution from ships is the most serious problem. Oceangoing vessels shed oil in three ways: by accidents such as collisions; during loading and unloading, and by intentional discharge, which includes the pumping of bilges, the discharge of ballast by tankers and the cleaning of oil tanks by tankers. The ballast component is the worst.

After a tanker unloads its cargo of oil it takes on seawater (about 40 percent of the full load of oil) so that it will not ride too high in the water and be unmanageable. Any oil that remains in the tanks mixes with the water and is discharged with it when the ballast is pumped out in preparation for reloading the vessel with oil. The discharge of oil can be reduced in two ways. One is to wash the tank with water and stow the water aboard in a "slop tank," where the oil slowly separates from it. Then the water is discharged and the next load of oil is put on top of the oil that remains in the slop tank. This practice, which is described as being 80 percent effective, is followed in tankers carrying about 80 percent of the oil now transported at sea. The other stratagem is to build segregated ballast spaces into the double bottoms of new tankers, which reduces the discharge by 95 percent.

A system of international controls could virtually eliminate such discharges. There is an extra incentive for international controls because wherever oil is discharged, and by whatever ship, there is no telling to what shore it will be carried by winds, waves and currents. Substantial progress toward this kind of agreement has been made recently.

Ships are also responsible for most of the littering of the ocean and its shores. Waste consisting of paper, plastics, wood, metal, glass and garbage is customarily thrown overboard. The heavier material sinks quickly, littering the bottom; paper products disintegrate or become waterlogged and sink slowly, and the foods are soon consumed by marine scavengers. The wood, sealed containers and light plastics float ashore.

The estimated yearly litter from ships is about three million metric tons, much of which seems to come from the fishing fleets. The litter that Americans see and are annoyed by comes mostly from the land by way of streams or is thrown into harbors or tossed overboard from pleasure craft. Littering is an aesthetic problem rather than an ecological one, but it certainly reduces the quality of living. It can be curbed by the force of public opinion.

Dumping is a word with a specific meaning; it should not be confused with littering or with discharges from pipes. Dumping means carrying waste out to sea and discharging it at a designated site. Barges carrying solids simply open bottom doors and drop their cargo. Barges carrying liquids generally pump the material out through a submerged pipe into the turbulent wake of the vessel. Still other barges dump wastes enclosed in steel drums or other containers.

Much of the material is dredge spoil sucked up from harbor bottoms by hopper dredges to deepen ship channels. Some 28 million tons of this material were dumped into the Atlantic in 1968. Next in quantity in the New York area is relatively clean material removed from excavations for buildings; then comes sewage sludge, and finally industrial waste such as acids and other chemicals.

The amount of sludge dumped annually into New York Bight is about 4.6 million tons. Much of it is sewage sludge, which is a slurry of solid waste formed by sedimentation in primary sewage treatment or by secondary treatment in the activated-sludge process. For ocean discharge the material is thickened by settling or centrifuging to from 3 to 8 percent solids. Much of the solid material is silt, but complex organic materials and heavy metals are also present.

In some parts of the country the sludge is not dumped but is discharged into the ocean through special pipes. In others it is buried in landfill or spread as fertilizer, although the metals it contains may cause problems later. A broad spectrum of industrial effluents (solvents from pharmaceutical production, waste acid from the titanium-pigment industry, caustic solutions from oil refineries, metallic sodium and calcium, filter cake, salts and chlorinated hydrocarbons) are dumped intermittently at certain sites under Government license.

What damage is done to marine organisms by materials of this kind? The turbidity created by dumping is usually dispersed within a day. Dumped dredge spoil buries bottom-dwelling animals under a thin blanket of sediment, but many of them dig out and the others are replaced by recolonization in about a year. Sewage sludge is high in heavy metals, which may be toxic, particularly when they combine with organic materials to create a reducing (oxygen-poor) environment in which few animals can live. Sludge can also have a high bacterial count. It is clear that much industrial waste could be harmful to marine life and should not be dumped into the sea.

The entire matter of dumping needs more study. With reliable data it will be possible to retain the option of disposal at sea for some materials, such as dredge spoil, and to reject it for others, such as chemicals. Deep-water sites could be set aside for dumping on the same logic that applies to city dumps, namely that it is a suitable use for space of low value where few animals could be harmed.

Thermal waste is discharged into the sea by power plants because the sea is a convenient source of cooling water. The temperature of the water on discharge is typically 10 degrees Celsius higher than it was on intake. The difference is within the range of natural temperature variations and so is not harmful to most adult marine animals. The eggs, larvae, and young animals that live in coastal waters, however, are sucked through the power plant with the cooling water. They are subjected to a sud-den rise in temperature and decrease in pressure that is likely to be fatal. For this reason and others it would seem logical to put new power plants offshore. There they could draw deeper and cooler water from a level that is not rich in living organisms. For a nuclear plant the hazards of a nuclear accident would be reduced; for an oil- or coal-fired plant fuel could be delivered directly by ship, and the shoreline could be reserved for non-industrial purposes.

Some industries discharge substantial quantities of heavy metals and complex organic compounds into municipal waste-water systems whose effluent reaches the ocean. Certain of the metals (mercury, chromium, lead, zinc, cadmium, copper, nickel and silver) are notably toxic and so are subject to stringent regulation. The most dangerous substances, however, are synthetic organic compounds such as DDT and polychlorinated biphenyls. The discharge of these substances as well as the heavy metals must be prevented. The best way to do so is by "source control," meaning the prevention of discharge into the sewer system. Each plant must be held responsible for removing and disposing of its own pollutants.

Other waste substances that generate controversy are those with nutrient value. Since they are decomposed by bacteria, oxygen is required. This biological oxygen demand is commonly measured in units that express how much oxygen (in milligrams per liter) will be required in a five-day period.

There is good reason to restrict the amount of nutrient material that is discharged into lakes and rivers, where oxygen is limited and a reducing environment can be created. The ocean is another matter. It is an essentially unlimited reservoir of dissolved oxygen, which is kept in motion by currents and is constantly being replenished by natural mechanisms.

It is nonetheless possible to overwhelm a local area of the ocean with a huge discharge of nutrient material that may form a deposit on the sea floor if the local conditions are not carefully considered. The materials must be presented to the ocean in the right places and at reasonable rates. Among the ways of achieving that objective are the use of discharge pipes that lead well offshore and have many small diffuser ports and, if the volume of discharge is exceptionally large, the distribution of the effluent through several widely dispersed pipes.

Problems caused by the addition of nitrogen and phosphate to inland waters, which they overfertilize, do not apply to the ocean. There they could be helpful by producing the equivalent of upwelling, the natural process that brings nutrients from deep water to the surface waters where most marine organisms are found. As Isaacs has pointed out, "the sea is *starved* for the basic plant nutrients, and it is a mystery to me why we should be concerned with their thoughtful introduction into coastal seas in any quantity that man can generate in the foreseeable future."

Once possible pollutants reach the ocean it is necessary to keep track of where they go, the extent to which they are altered or diluted and what animals they affect. In order to obtain this information many of the techniques of oceanography are brought into play. Currents are measured above and below the thermocline; other instruments measure the temperature, salinity and dissolved oxygen. Water is sampled at various depths, and so are bottom sediments. It is also useful to directly monitor any changes in plant and animal communities with divers or television cameras.

A good indicator of change is the response of the polychaete worms in the bottom mud. Close to an effluent-discharge point the number of species may be as low as from four to 10 per sample and the total weight of worms as low as 50 grams per square meter. A short distance away the number of species may be 40 or more and the total weight 700 grams per square meter. At greater distances the figures drop off to normal: about 25 species and 300 grams per square meter. This local enrichment shows that worms thrive at some optimum level of organic material. Laboratory tests by Donald Reish and Jack Word of California State University at Long Beach show that worms have a similar optimum for toxic metals such as zinc and copper.

Man must do something with his wastes, and the ocean is a logical place for some of them. No single solution will be sensible for all kinds of waste or all locations, but the following suggestions may help to protect both the land and the sea in the long run. (1) Clearly define what is ocean, separating it from inland freshwaters and from harbors and shallow bays, and make laws that are appropriate for each environment. (2) Avoid the assumption that anything added to the ocean is necessarily harmful and consider instead what substances might cause damage and

FOUNDATIONS OF HEALTH SCIENCE

eliminate excesses of them. (3) Rigorously prohibit the disposal in the ocean of all man-made radioactive materials, halogenated hydrocarbons (such as DDT and polychlorinated biphenyls) and other synthetic organic materials that are toxic and against which marine organisms have no natural defenses. (4) Set standards based on water quality (after reasonable mixing) that are compatible with what is known about the threshold of damage to marine life, providing a safety factor of at least 10. (5) Work to obtain international cooperation in prohibiting ships from disposing of litter or oil and from pumping bilges. (6) Set aside ocean areas of deep water and slow current where certain materials can be dumped with minimal damage. (7) Require each discharger to make studies to demonstrate how his specific effluent will influence the adjacent ocean. (8) Support additional research on the effect of pollutants on the ocean and its life. (9) Anticipate pollutants that may become serious as technology produces new chemical compounds in greater quantities.

A more rational basis is needed for making decisions about how to treat wastes and where to put them. No oceanographer wants damaging waste in the ocean where he works or on land where he lives. Since the waste must go to one place or the other, however, one would prefer the choice to be based on a knowledge of all the factors. Unemotional consideration of which materials can be introduced into the sea without serious damage to marine life will result in both an unpolluted ocean and a large saving of national resources.

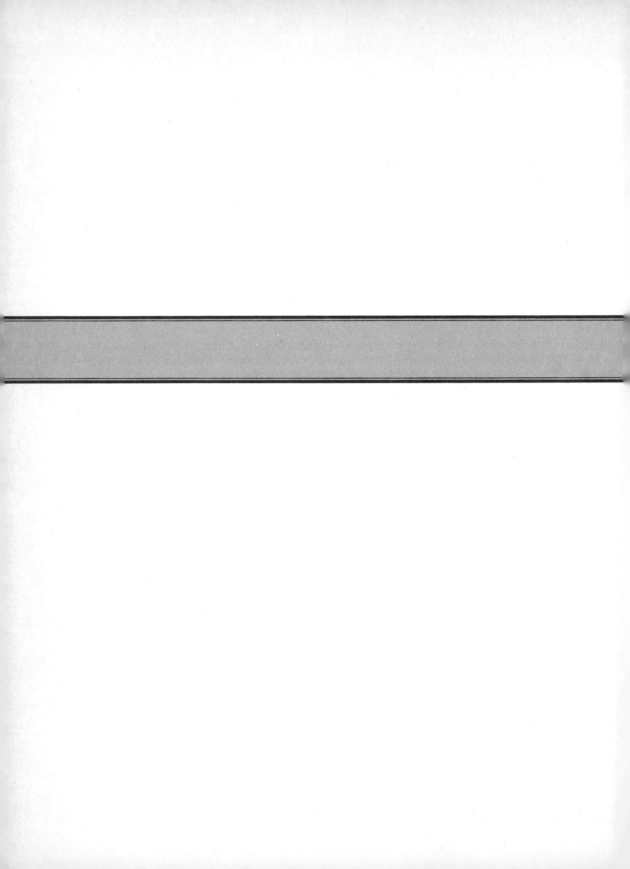

RETROSPECT
AND PROSPECT
IN HEALTH

chapter sixteen

Since the beginning of mankind, health and safety have been considered not only fundamental to survival but also a prime requisite for most effective living. The history of civilizations in certain ways demonstrates a continuing strong concern and deep regard for sound health. An awareness of some of the past practices and the recent rapid increase in knowledge and technological advances contribute to an appreciation of both how much and how little we know.

EARLY IDEAS CONCERNING HEALTH AND DISEASE

The story of health is intrinsically interwoven with stories of the human race and man's struggle from the forest and jungle to the complexities of modern life and the triumphs of present-day science. The very brief historical perspective outlined on the following pages should help to highlight the emergence from mysticism and superstition to the modern scientific approach in man's fight to preserve health and prolong life.

Health in Ancient Civilizations

Although the earliest documents on health and medicine date back only four thousand years, we have evidences that provide information on life before the beginning of recorded history. These clues to early life include bones and teeth, implements and instruments, mummies, and other fossilized remains. The study of such evidences is called *paleontology*. The science concerned with disease relationships in these remains is termed *paleopathology*.

Disease is far older than mankind. Geological formations, for example, have been uncovered that reveal the existence 500 million years ago of fossilized bacteria similar to the micrococci of today. In all likelihood, certain forms of life during this early period suffered from various infectious diseases.[1] Certain other events and circumstances of this early period are set forth in Figure 16.1.

Figure 16.1   Health and Ancient Civilizations

Prehistoric Times:

Age of mystery, superstition and fear; belief in evil spirits and the supernatural. Demons of ill health were combated by magical spells, ritual sacrifices, mystical omens, and magico-religious rites.

Code of Hammurabi (2250 B.C.):

Babylonian set of laws, including individual, family, and community health procedures. "An eye for an eye and a tooth for a tooth" was applied to physicians.

Mosaic Code (1490 B.C.):

Set forth hygienic measures concerned with quarantine and isolation, first aid, medical inspection, cleanliness, safety, chemotherapy, sewage disposal, disease prevention and control, and other factors.

Early Indians in Mexico:

Utilized some 1,200 medicinal plants; practiced surgery, suturing, fumigation, blood-letting, narcotic therapy, and proper bathing and diet.

Peru and India:

Surgery was a highly developed art; successful amputations were not uncommon.

Greece (circa 500 B.C.):

Helped establish principles of scientific rationality. Emphasis was on importance of personal hygiene-nutrition, cleanliness, exercise, and disease control.

Hippocrates:

Father of scientific medicine. Originated the Oath of Hippocrates and established fundamental principles of health observation and treatment.

Rome (circa 200 B.C.):

Refined administrative and engineering accomplishments pertaining to community health; provided aqueducts, paved streets, bathing installations, sewage systems, medical societies and hospitals.

Figure 16.2 Trephining in Ancient Peru. Peru was the center of intensive practice of trephining in the New World. Described as a "surgical operation in life on the head and skull," trephining was used to release the demons associated with headaches, mental illness, and wounds of the head. (Courtesy, Parke, Davis & Company © 1957.)

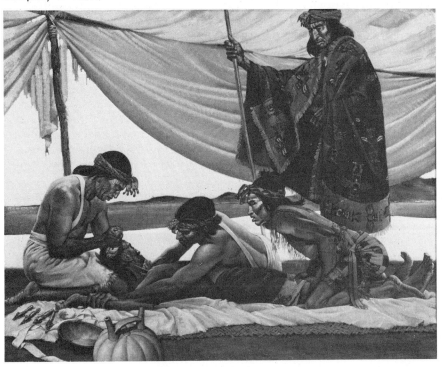

The Middle Ages

The medieval period was a time of great strife, aggression, political upheaval, and social change. The ruthless destruction of centers of learning by conquering barbarians, the domination of life by the church, and waves of epidemic diseases combined to destroy much previously acquired knowledge in Western civilization and to stifle originality of thought and practice with respect to the sciences and other fields. Figure 16.3 describes this period.

The Rebirth of Science

The period immediately following the Middle Ages and extending into the next several centuries brought about a slow emergence from the

Figure 16.3   Health and the Middle Ages

Middle Ages:
    Superstition and witchcraft at their height. Bloodletting, alchemy, astrological healing, quackery, and herb-doctoring were common.
Health Measures:
    Necessary due to widespread epidemics of disease. Quarantine, isolation, and fumigation were initiated.
Hospitals:
    Widespread establishment in France, Italy, England, Spain, and other European countries.

spell of the past. Although medical thought and practice were still associated with lingering superstition and with magical, religious, and supernatural phenomena, significant beginnings were made toward modern scientific ideas.

The Renaissance and Reformation

The discoveries, notable achievements, and rapid progress made in the many areas relating to well-being during the Renaissance and Reformation periods of history can be only briefly sketched. During this era of the fourteenth through seventeenth centuries, the firm foundations of science and medicine were established. The contributions of several famous men of this era are described in Figure 16.4.

Figure 16.4   The Renaissance and Reformation

Leonardo da Vinci:
    Performed physiological experiments and dissections to provide detail to his famous anatomical illustrations.
Paracelsus:
    Father of chemotherapy; was known for his "chemical kitchens."
Andreas Vesalius:
    First man of modern science; based study of anatomy on direct observation.
William Harvey:
    Discovered the circulation of the blood.
Thomas Sydenham:
    Developed the science of internal medicine.
Antony van Leeuwenhoek:
    Invented the microscope and observed bacteria for the first time in 1675.

The Eighteenth and Nineteenth Centuries

The eighteenth and nineteenth centuries were a period of consolidation during which steady progress was made in the health-related sciences. New discoveries, made possible because of the foundations established by previous work, were consolidated with the old to mold the disciplines of physics, chemistry, anatomy, biology, physiology, bacteriology, and other sciences. Great men and some of their contributions are given in Figure 16.5.

Figure 16.5   Health and the Eighteenth and Nineteenth Centuries

Giovanni B. Morgagni:
> First great pathologist; correlated symptoms of disease in the living with anatomical findings at autopsy.

James Lind:
> English naval surgeon; conquered scurvy.

John Hunter:
> Founder of scientific surgery and a great comparative anatomist.

Antoine Lavoisier:
> Provided significant experimental data on oxidation and the respiratory process.

René Laennec:
> Invented the stethoscope.

Edward Jenner:
> Introduced immunology in 1796 with the smallpox vaccine.

Benjamin Rush:
> America's first great physician.

Philippe Pinel:
> Father of psychiatry.

Lemuel Shattuck:
> Published the classic report *Sanitary Survey of the State of Massachusetts* in 1850.

Oliver Wendell Holmes:
> Author and physician; provided insight into modes of disease transmission and prevention.

Ignaz Semmelweis:
> Laid the foundation for cleanliness in obstetrics.

William Morton:
> Successfully demonstrated ether anesthesia in 1846.

Marion Sims:
> Helped establish the first women's hospital in the United States; became a leader in gynecology.

Gregor Mendel:
> Contributed to the science of heredity and genetics.

(Continued on next page)

Figure 16.5 *(Continued)*

Louis Pasteur:

    Originator of the "germ theory" of disease; perfected the immunization against rabies, discovered fermentation and pasteurization, and many other accomplishments.

Florence Nightingale:

    Laid the foundation for modern nursing programs.

Joseph Lister:

    Introduced antiseptic surgery in 1867.

Wilhelm K. Roentgen:

    Discovered the X-ray in 1895.

Sigmund Freud:

    Introduced psychoanalysis and other psychotherapeutic methods.

Figure 16.6 James Lind: Conqueror of Scurvy. In 1747 James Lind, a British naval surgeon, conducted a series of clinical experiments that definitely proved citrus fruits or their juices would cure scurvy. This dread dietary deficiency disease killed a million seamen between 1600 and 1800. (Courtesy, Parke, Davis & Company © 1959.)

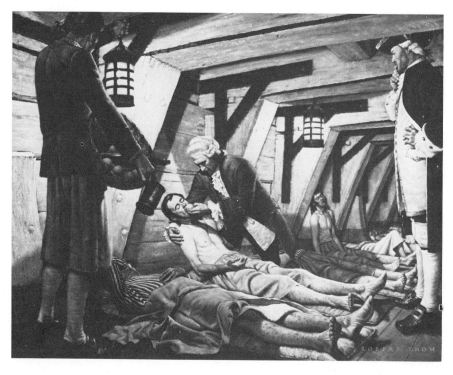

The early twentieth century is noted for the tremendous progress made in scientific knowledge and discovery. Great advances were made in public health organization, preventive medicine, chemotherapy, medical and surgical techniques, nursing and health care, and other activities. Some of the individuals and programs contributing to the accomplishments of the early 1900s are shown in Figure 16.7.

Figure 16.7 The 1900s

Men

Walter Reed:
Helped to prove that yellow fever was transmitted by the mosquito in 1901.
Karl Landsteiner:
Discovered the blood groups.
Paul Ehrlick:
Developed salvarsan, the first effective treatment for syphilis.
Alexander Fleming:
Founder of the modern science of antibiosis with the discovery of penicillin.
Gerhard Domagh:
Introduced sulfanilamide in the mid-thirties.

Programs

Large-scale vaccination programs against the diseases of smallpox, diphtheria, tetanus, poliomyelitis (oral vaccine, 1961), rubella (1969), measles (1963), and mumps.

The introduction of insecticides and pesticides as measures of disease control.

The concept of accessory foodstuffs, the application of knowledge about vitamins and their successful synthesis, and other important discoveries in nutrition.

Successful international campaigns against such problems as yellow fever, hookworm, trachoma, tuberculosis, and malaria.

New discoveries in endocrinology and hormone functions.

Introduction and improved therapeutic uses of radioactive materials and X-rays.

Significant developments in biophysics, such as the medical uses of isotopes and tracer elements.

Remarkable progress in drug research, like the discovery of antihistamines used in the control of allergies and the tranquilizers.

MEDICAL ADVANCES IN THE SECOND HALF OF THIS CENTURY

Laser beams that coagulate tissue are being used to repair tears in the retina, destroy tumors, and seal broken blood vessels. Organs are being successfully transplanted into the human body. Electronic devices such as the mental pacemaker are being implanted that control thought processes.

These devices can also be hooked up to computers that are programed to take orders directly from the subject's thoughts. Artificial parts are increasingly available to replace defective heart valves, diseased joints, such as the hip and knuckles, and within the near future artificial hearts are expected to be a reality. It is now possible to transplant genes (in bacteria), to diagnose congenital disorders prior to birth, to cure some people with leukemia, to use spectrum analysis for diagnosis, and to utilize computers to diagnose and check vital signs. By using biofeedback techniques man can now alter some of the physiological processes in the body that were once considered involuntary—brain wave patterns, heart rate, blood pressure, and circulatory flow. Figure 16.8 shows a modern operating room.

Figure 16.8 Surgery. Notable progress in the field of surgery has greatly contributed to the control and treatment of many dread diseases and disorders. (Photograph courtesy of The National Foundation–March of Dimes.)

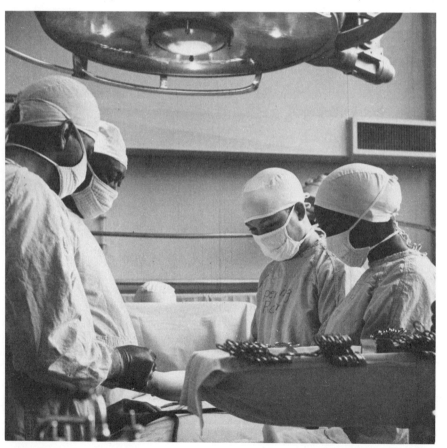

FOUNDATIONS OF HEALTH SCIENCE

On the other hand, increased technology, space travel, traveling faster than sound, automation, urbanization, and advanced educational requirements are creating new problems and intensifying some of the older ones. The high rate of mental illness, alcoholism, drug dependency, juvenile and adult delinquency, and divorce could be the result of the stresses of living in these times. The demands from the aged supersede even present accomplishments produced by technical marvels. People are demanding more of everything, including health services, products and protection.

An Era of Decisions

The public is more aware and informed about health matters and problems now than ever before in history. The more one learns, the more one realizes how little is known and that a little knowledge can be dangerous because of twisted statistics, incomplete, inconclusive, and inaccurate evidence, faulty research, and emotionally influenced controversy. Who should be believed and what is the best thing to do? Even a well-read person with superior intelligence experiences difficulty in evaluating health information.

The Medical Paradox

The spectacular advances in medical science and technology, which have so greatly increased the capacity of medicine as a whole, also have made the physician's job more difficult for him to practice. He cannot begin to keep up with increased medical knowledge, much less become proficient in the skills required to apply new procedures. He is no longer independent. Improved technology has gradually transformed medical care from an individual enterprise into one highly organized and institutionalized. Not only are many specialists required within the medical profession, but the health care of each person requires the cooperative efforts of a multiplicity of health personnel plus the sociologist, anthropologist, geneticist, statistician, health educator, and scientist. All of these factors lead to vastly increased financial costs. The need for highly skilled professionals and technicians is growing faster even than the population explosion.

American medicine has attempted to meet the problems of cost and lack of personnel by taking advantage of technology to increase productivity. More efficient organization, more effective utilization of paramedical personnel, modern diagnostic tools, and chemotherapy have permitted the doctor to see many more patients during a week than he could in the past. But this in itself causes resentment and misunderstanding. Physicians complain that in an institutionally organized program they are tied down by red tape and are restricted in using their individual initiative. Some have made allegations that the ten-minute hasty office call is too impersonal and demoralizing to the patient and that the ill will engendered is contributing to the boom in malpractice suits—and thus they believe in the need for adjustments.

Some may debate whether American medicine is the best in the world or the 16th best in the world, but both of these positions are myths of a sort.

It is hardly edifying to see government officials inflating our infant mortality statistics and medical officials minimizing them, when what they both should be doing is analyzing them together.

What is important is that we all know that American medicine can be improved, and therefore I have been pleased to see the decreased frequency with which the American Medical Association invokes the "sacred doctor-patient relationship," the sanctity of which was often lost upon people who could neither find nor afford a physician when they needed one.

But if organized medicine can lay aside some of its myths, and I think it should and has, then might we ask the same of the planners and academic physicians, and the government officials, because if they cannot, and if we cannot, and if we cannot reach some kind of mutual respect and mutual understanding, if we cannot get some honest research rather than preordained, self-fulfilling "studies," then American medicine is not going to be reformed. It may be changed, but it will not be improved.

The AMA is no longer the medical establishment. It is the sociologists and the economists and the medical academicians who have become that establishment and who have the ear of government agencies and insurance companies and labor unions.

Let us examine some of the myths of these planners.

Take, for example, the almost obscene enthusiasm with which our critics have fastened onto the phrase, "Our non-system of medical care," as if it were the ultimately devastating reply to organized medicine (and "organized medicine" itself is a myth, but a convenient one).

Well, of course we have a non-system of medical care. We also have a non-system of education—big colleges, little colleges, good colleges, bad colleges, private colleges, public colleges, Catholic colleges, Protestant colleges; and we have a non-system of food distribution—little farms, supermarkets, corner groceries, scarcities, surpluses, malnutrition, and obesity; and we have a non-system in this country of everything else except postal service and military service.

The American people and American political theorists, both of the right and of the left, have been properly skeptical about such systems, and everyone knows that "the system" is not a term of endearment among young people today. . . .

Medicine usually depends on mutual trust and respect of two people:

the one seeking help, the other offering it. Medicine starts in that cry and ultimately comes back to it.

We can have a system of mass-production medicine, but I think we do not need and do not want it. . . .

There are many more myths. There is the myth that solo practice is doomed in the large cities, but might just possibly have a chance in small towns, whereas insight and intuition show us that it is just the opposite.

There is that touching solicitude with which economists fret about the solo practitioner, locked up in his little cottage office, isolated from his peers, and unwilling and unable to get intellectual stimulation, a myth which is obvious when one realizes that the enforcement agencies of quality, the hospitals and the speciality boards, are the real agents today in how well medical care is practiced, and that no one practices alone in his office.

I would like to ask why these myths develop. Some are what I call "benevolent myths," designed, perhaps unconsciously, to exaggerate a true social problem and thus force government action. But exaggerated statistics may lead to unrealistic responses.

These benevolent myths may get the government spending millions of dollars, billion of dollars, on attempts to upgrade the poor, or upgrade not only the poor but other people, and then when the expected result does not occur, because I do not think it will, . . . there may be a great disillusionment. . . .

Today's practicing physician knows that the real killers in this nation —depression, alcohol, fast driving, tobacco—are very easy to detect, but very hard to cure, and the practicing physician must know, if he has any insight at all, that the patient's wife may be much more valuable in preventive medicine than he will ever be.

But the men in the Public Health Service are just like most other middle-class Americans. They hope that if you devote a day to a yearly physical examination or blood-screening profile, you can eat, drink, and drive fast the other 364 days of the year and you'll be safe, and it isn't true.

Lastly, what except invincible ignorance of what medicine is all about can lead decent, intelligent men to speak so glibly about efficiency in medical care, applying all the cliches about the value of bigness that marked the Blue Eagle NRA era to a field which is not the same as poultry processing or shoe manufacturing? . . .

No, America is not crippled by presymptomatic gout. It is instead tormented by fear, ambition, and loneliness. We have our triumphs, but we have them at a cost. We move too often. Our parents are in Florida, our children on the Coast. Friends are the people that we graduated with from high school 20 years ago. Neighbors are the people who are going to move next month. The friendly neighborhood cop is a face in a squad car. The neighborhood butcher is a pair of hands wrapping supermarket meat.

But the one person who has kept his links to our personal past, not only into our childhood, but into a long tradition of art and literature and science, is the physician, and physicians can in fact best meet the needs of the future by retaining the cornerstone of the past—care of the patient.

We are not city planners, nor were we meant to be.

But physicians have a privileged place in our society, and can use that well by giving honest, imaginative consultation to those economists and sociologists and government officials who wish to help us in the reform of medicine. We can do a great deal together.[2]

HEALTH PROBLEMS IN THE SEVENTIES

The dominant question of the 1970s will be the quality of human life. The prospect is that man in the next decade will not be crowded into marginal existence by famine. Yet his ability to control depredation of the earth's shrinking resources will remain uncertain, even as it is today.

One dire prediction of the early 1960s was that the world, within a generation, would starve itself to death. Happily, this is not coming true. One of the unexpected and unheralded developments of the decade past was what agriculturists call "the green revolution"—the development of new inexpensive high-yield wheat and rice grains. In the next ten years, the experts predict an extraordinary rise in farm productivity; even India, with its hundreds of millions, may become self-supporting in its food supply. Coupled with the gains from the land, man will have the technical ability to farm the sea instead of simply harvesting it; scientists believe that they will soon be able to breed and control fish and shellfish in large quantities and to cultivate underwater plants.

Nevertheless, America is now aware that malnutrition is here. The existence of hunger, in a society that can afford to abolish it, is morally and economically indefensible. A child who is hungry because his family cannot afford to buy food is living reproof to a wealthy society's claim that it treasures human over financial capital. Neither can a society excuse itself from a charge of harboring hungry people on grounds they are ignorant of proper nutritional practices.

Hunger damages the moral and economic fiber of the nation, no matter what the reason for its existence. Ardor for improvement and change is growing amongst the poor, and we should be considering how these newly acquired energies can be harnessed for the good of the nation as a whole.

The concept of population explosion is and will remain more than a simple phrase. The United States now has 212 million people. By 1990, the Census Bureau estimates, it will have at least 225 million (and perhaps as many as 250 million). If present trends continue, the world population will grow from an estimated 3.6 billion today to at least 4.3 billion ten years from now. Compulsory birth control will not be a political issue for

FOUNDATIONS OF HEALTH SCIENCE

America in the 1970s, but it may well be in other lands. The governments of India and perhaps China and Pakistan, for example, will be under continual pressure to try to change traditional social attitudes that favor large families and stigmatize the single.

In all likelihood, man's biblical lifespan of threescore years and ten, the average in the Western world, will not be extended by more than a month or so during the next decade. Nonetheless, expectably, developments in geriatrics, in improved hospital care, and in partial conquest of such killers as cancer and heart disease, will make life better for the old and will undoubtedly add to population pressures.

Government and business will be forced to spread ever increasing sums to control pollution of air and water and to prevent the destruction of natural beauty. Young adults are protesting about problems of environment and are organizing demonstrations against irrepressible corporations and municipalities. In the next few years, increasing attention will be paid to inadequate municipal development and the infamous urban sprawl; wider recognition will be given to the fact that like most forms of pollution, defiling of the landscape, whether it be with shopping centers or expressways, is hard to reverse. In the interests of preserving open spaces —not to mention domestic tranquility—some nations may bar or limit tourism. International relations will certainly be affected by the cause of conservation, since neither air nor water pollution observes boundaries. Nations will discover that sovereignty can be threatened by pollutants just as much as by invasion.

Much more is involved than putting filters on chimneys and car exhausts and building new sewage plants. As the decade advances, we will come to see clearly that if the ecological effort is to succeed, much of today's existing technology will have to be scrapped and something new developed in its place. The gasoline-powered automobile, at present the chief polluter of the air, will be made clean or it will be banned from many urban areas—a threat that some car manufacturers already recognize. Alternatives are electric or gas-turbine-powered autos. Increasingly, we will see that any kind of mass transportation, however, powered, is more efficient than the family car. Some, however, cynically argue that the revolt against the car may not take place until a thermal inversion, combined with a traffic pile-up, asphyxiates thousands on a freeway to nowhere. In addition, factories will have to be built as "closed systems," operated so that there is no waste; everything, in effect, that goes in one end must come out the other as a usable, nonpolluting product. Man's own body wastes will have to find use as fertilizer—the cheapest and most efficient means of disposal.

Popular though the cause is, the struggle to save the environment will by no means be clearly won. The attitude, central to the modern mind, that all technology is good technology will have to be changed radically. "Our society is trained to accept all new technology as progress, or to look upon it as an aspect of fate," says George Wald, Harvard's Nobel-laureate biologist. "Should one do everything one can? The usual answer is 'Of course'; but the right answer is 'Of course not.' "[3]

The less fortunate people of the world are trapped in a whirlpool from which they find it extremely difficult to escape. Illiteracy and poverty contribute to their inability to improve economically. Low income means not enough money to pay for even a limited education, or, for that matter, to purchase food needed for survival. The improvement of health status is both dependent upon and essential to higher standards of living and universal opportunities for education.

Changes in agricultural methods are proving to be worth over thirteen billion dollars a year to the farmer and consumer. Research has shown farmers how to produce abundantly so that a large variety of wholesome and nutritious food is available all year round. If farmers today used 1940 methods, it would cost an extra thirteen billion dollars a year to produce food and grain for the nation. This extra cost would be passed on to the consumers, adding more than five dollars a week to each family's bill for farm products.

Increasingly, people throughout he world are beginning to recognize the importance of education as an investment in economic growth and well-being. In other words, people are noting the relationship between the amount of money, time, and the effort put into education and the standard of living that an individual person or a nation may have. A growing belief is that conditions in other countries or nations have an affect on us. The United States is expending greater amounts of money and effort to promote educational and technological development in the less-advantaged areas of the world. Poorer nations are beginning to demand their greater shares of the resources and wealth available to but a few nations.

Education for health is one of the areas of learning. Health education becomes increasingly important in promoting the health, welfare, and economy of any country. Medical superstitions, myths, folklore, ignorance, and unsanitary practices prevail throughout much of the world. In Nigeria, for example, which is a country of much sickness and malnutrition, over 250 tribes believe that bananas cause illness and eggs cause lying, or "a false tongue." Likewise, many persons in India go hungry because the cow is sacred. The solution to this problem is twofold: (1) sending education specialists and consultants to help the people help themselves, and (2) training the capable, competent leaders of the less-developed countries so that they may initiate local programs utilizing more modern technology and scientific knowledge.

What about health education here? How smart are we? The National Health Test conducted on television a few years ago disclosed that 75 percent of those taking the test could not name even three of the seven dangers signals of cancer and that 40 percent still clung to the schoolboy belief that they could get venereal disease from toilet seats.

THE CHANGING SCENE

The changing scene has significance in planning for the future. Today's problems stem from a combination of forces. Alcoholism, drug dependency, delinquency, suicide, and accidents are representative of "social deviances" as well as "medical deviances." The health science profession tends to view such problems as these as purely medical, whereas the general public sees them as sociological. In fact, the social stigma attached to sexually transmitted diseases and mental illness creates serious difficulties in case finding. Treatment and prevention in the future is going to require that the health professions and the behavioral science professions work together for each other's mutual advantage as well as that of society's.

The shift from communicable diseases to chronic degenerative diseases as major problems requires new approaches in motivating people to action. People now have to be persuaded, rather than compelled by law, to take advantage of preventive measures. Laws can oblige persons to be vaccinated, isolated, or quarantined. Laws cannot oblige persons to procure cancer detection examinations.

These changes and trends appear to fall into five broad categories.

Changes in the Nature of Disease

As we have brought the acute communicable diseases under control, we have correspondingly emphasized the chronic degenerative diseases. Social factors are now much more important in considering etiology, treatment, and prevention. Specific infectious *agents* are being replaced by social and psychological *processes* as "causes" of disease, while changes in one's way of life become a crucial factor in the treatment of these chronic illnesses.

The age groups in which disease is most evident are changing and the most vulnerable groups are the young and the old. Older children and adolescents have many fewer problems than the middle-aged. Attention to the intrauterine child and the neonate is increasing.

The progression of illness is changing from the sudden and spectacular to the long, drawn-out, and routine. Some chronic diseases develop over many symptomless years and require long periods of continued care. Early detection and rehabilitation are becoming the symbols of modern public health.

Changes in Social and Environmental Conditions

Technological changes have produced new public health problems, such as air pollution, radiation, and food contamination from chemicals. The peaceful use of nuclear energy poses a real hazard, and the automobile is an ever-increasing agent of death and disability.

The stress of modern living and the breakdown of social supports, such as the family, appear to increase mental illness. Alcoholism, drug dependency, and delinquency are consequences of poor levels of mental health if not actually a form of mental illness.

The increased numbers of people both chronically ill and senescent have created new demands for long-term care and special facilities. We have more and more need for extended care facilities and home-care services.

Changes in Medical Care

The greater complexity of medical practice and the rapidity of new medical discoveries have caused increases in the number of specialists, with a corresponding decrease in general practitioners. This change has, in turn, created problems in the integration of medical services and in the continuity of care. Group practice or team medicine is offered as one possible answer to this problem.

The high cost of medical care has led to a rapid expansion of health insurance, both private and government-financed. The rise of medical expenses has been accompanied by the trend toward using the hospital as the nucleus for prevention, diagnosis, treatment, rehabilitation, and research rather than only for the treatment of the acutely ill. Another growing movement is toward using extended care facilities and home programs rather than the hospital unit for custodial care of the debilitated.

Medical welfare services are changing from mere "free public clinics" to an integral part of the organized governmental services provided under public assistance funds. The quality of this care and the need for a more comprehensive approach to the problem are subjects of a great deal of controversy. These services are being expanded to provide for those with minimal economic resources as well as the indigent.

Shortages and/or maldistribution of medical and nursing personnel have created serious problems of providing adequate care, and have encouraged the development of health personnel such as nurse's aids, dental assistants, and physician's assistants as well as the nurse practitioner.

Medical education has become more costly and more complex. Medical schools are not turning out enough physicians to maintain the physician-population ratio, and increasing demands are being made for government support. The teaching of "general medicine" is being developed as an antidote to overspecialization. Courses in the behavioral sciences are gradually being introduced. Experimentation with medical curriculum plans is underway to expedite professional preparation.

Changes in Public Health Practice

The prevention of illness is becoming more a matter of changing the habits and customs of people rather than one of controlling environmental conditions or immunizing populations. New methods of health education are needed to produce changes in the behavior of individual people and customary practices of groups. Cultural differences among subgroups of the population require special attention.

The emphasis of public health upon legal mandate and enforcement is giving way to a greater reliance upon voluntary participation. Many of the current sanitary measures are more of an aesthetic consideration than a disease threat; compliance has become a matter of public education and taste.

The initial emphasis of public health was upon establishing and providing services. Today, with many such services in operation, the problem is becoming one of improving utilization. The public must be motivated to make use of these services.

Changes in Public Opinion and Behavior

Health and happiness are being demanded by the public as a basic right rather than a privilege. People no longer expect and accept illness and early death as "natural." Health care has become a necessity of life and an essential part of any welfare program.

The public is taking more active part in the determination of public health policy. The support of public opinion is becoming necessary both from the point of view of budgetary allocations to health departments and community support of voluntary health programs.

People are showing a greater interest in medical matters, as evidenced by an increase in the number of health articles in lay publications and the growth of voluntary health agencies. The merchandising of drugs has become "big business" and has created many problems of communication both for the public and for the medical profession.

INDIVIDUAL INITIATIVE

Even in this day of the powerful establishments, each person can bring about change. Community interest and support are sometimes stimulated or initiated by one person. Upton Sinclair, Jessica Mitford, and Rachel Carson are only a few of these individuals. Ralph Nader is a current modern self-appointed and unpaid guardian of the interests of 212 million United States consumers. He has championed dozens of causes, prompted much of United States industry to reappraise its responsibilities, and against considerable odds, created a new climate of concern for the consumer among both politicians and businessmen.

Nader was able to force off the market General Motors' Corvair, which was withdrawn from production in 1969. Corvair's sales had plunged by 93 percent after Nader condemned the car as a safety hazard in his bestseller, *Unsafe at Any Speed.*[4] That influential book, and Nader's later speeches, articles, and congressional appearances, also forced the Department of Transportation to impose stricter safety standards on automobile and tire manufacturers.

Advocate and crusader, Nader has also been almost solely responsible for the passage of five major federal laws. They are the *National Traffic and Motor Vehicle Safety Act of 1966;* the *Wholesome Meat Act of 1967;* the *Natural Gas Pipeline Safety Act, The Radiation Control for Health and Safety Act,* and the *Wholesale Poultry Products Act,* all of 1968, and in 1969, the *Federal Coal Mine Health and Safety Act.*

One man was responsible for Louisiana's quiet revolution in family planning. Until the summer of 1965, distributing birth control information anywhere in Louisiana was a felony; today, family-planning clinics are operating in nearly all of the state's sixty-four parishes (counties). By July, 1970, clinics in all parishes were offering free—and legal—services to the entire medically indigent population, an estimated 130,000 women, both black and white. In a Deep South state where more than one-third of the people are Roman Catholics, this change was so astonishing that delegations from all over the world flocked to New Orleans to see how the miracle was accomplished.

FOUNDATIONS OF HEALTH SCIENCE

Invariably, the low-income groups in society produce the most children per family and thus perpetuate a grim cycle of poverty, ignorance, and still more children. Past efforts to bring family-planning information and techniques to such people have had limited success, and from such failures gloomy conclusions have been drawn: that the poor do not want birth control; that they will not accept it even when it is available; that "procreation is the poor man's recreation;" and so on—until the Louisiana program came along to prove, quietly, logically, irrefutably, that such assumptions simply are not true.[5]

IN CONCLUSION

Medical science and technology have made tremendous strides in areas affecting well-being. Noticeable progress has been made in the prevention and treatment of cardiovascular disease, cancer, bacterial and viral infections, kidney disorders, allergies, and other leading causes of death and disability. Improvements also are being made in the methods of coping with such problems as suicide, alcoholism, arthritis and rheumatism, muscular dystrophy, drug dependency, and cerebral palsy. Preventive measures such as water fluoridation to protect against tooth decay, infant and maternal care programs, and slum clearance or urban renewal projects have been promoted through well-organized and well-planned programs of services at local, state, county, national, and international levels. Despite these great advances, however, a myriad of problems affecting health remain and still defy the best scientific thinking.

Research may eventually unlock the secrets of the human cell and mind. Nevertheless, such discoveries would not have to lead to "science over nature" and "chemistry over mind," as Aldous Huxley proposes in *Brave New World*. "We live in a finite world with finite resources. Yet we are endowed with a brain of almost infinite inventiveness and capacity, and if we use it wisely and cooperatively, it can give us all a healthier, happier life."

Notes

1. Erwin H. Ackerknecht, *A Short History of Medicine* (New York: The Ronald Press, 1955), p. 4.
2. Reprinted from Michael J. Halberstam, "Modern Medical Myths," *Today's Health,* published by the American Medical Association. 47:72, 71, July, 1969.
3. "Man and Environment," *Time,* December, 1969, pp. 22, 25.
4. John R. Nader, *Unsafe at Any Speed: The Designed-in Dangers of the American Automobile* (New York: Grossman Publishers, 1965).
5. Arthur Gorden, "Louisiana's Quiet Revolution in Family Planning," *Today's Health,* 48:38–42, January, 1970.

Appendix

PHYSIOLOGY AND ANATOMY IN BRIEF

The human body basically consists of the head, neck, trunk, and the limbs or appendages. It is constructed around the skeleton and maintains its shape by means of the bones, muscles, tissues, and other supporting structures. Located in the head region are some of the most important and vital organs, principally the brain and certain sense organs.

The trunk contains *viscera,* or the soft organs. The interior of the trunk is a great body cavity called the *coelom.* It is afforded protection by the vertebrae, ribs, other bones, and muscles. The *diaphragm* is a large dome-shaped muscle that divides the coelom into two parts. The upper portion is called the *chest cavity,* or *thorax,* and contains principally the heart and lungs. The lower part is known as the *abdominal cavity.* Most of the space in this cavity is occupied by the intestines and other organs related to digestion, such as the liver, stomach, pancreas, and gall bladder. The kidneys, urinary bladder, and reproductive organs are also located in the abdominal region.

The Skeleton

The skeleton basically lends form to the body. Its essential components include the bones, which comprise the hard framework, the *cartilage,* which makes up the connecting and supporting structures, and the ligaments, which serve to bind the bones together. In addition to providing a framework for bodily support and for the various systems, the skeletal bones serve as a reservoir for certain minerals and fats, enclose and protect the vital organs, provide attachments for muscles and other supporting structures facilitating movement and locomotion, and perform the "hemeopoietic" function of manufacturing blood cells.

Bones consist of organic and inorganic materials. Together, these account for the amazing strength and the durability of the structures. Yet bones are pliable and relatively light. The skeleton comprises 206 bones, which form two general divisions. The *axial skeleton,* 80 bones, includes those bones that make up the basic framework of the body—the skull, the vertebrae, and the bones of the thorax. The *appendicular skeleton,* 126 bones, consists of the bones of the upper and lower extremities—the shoulders, arms, hands, pelvic girdle, thighs, knees, legs, and feet. See Figure A.1.

The place where two or more bones meet is called an *articulation* or *joint.* Such junctions are held together by cartilage, ligaments, or fibrous tissue. In certain instances the fittings are lubricated by a secretion called *synovial fluid,* which facilitates movement. In general, the body has two major types of articulations. The first type is known as *synarthrosis* or immovable. It lacks an articular cavity, which thus permits very limited or no movement. Such joints are found at junctions of the cranial bones, between adjoining vertebrae, and between ribs and costal cartilage. *Diathroses,* or movable joints, which are the second type, permit a range of movement from slight to great. These include the ball and socket joints of the shoulder and hip, hinge joints of the elbow and knee, and rotating joints of the arm and elbow.

The Muscles

The muscles constitute what has sometimes been called the "red flesh" of the body and are intimately involved in the maintenance of fitness. They account for approximately 50 percent of the total body weight (slightly more in the average male than the female). Tendons, fasciae, and the various organs themselves depend on the muscular system and the functioning of muscle cells.

The functions performed by muscles may be viewed as of two kinds —*voluntary* and *involuntary*—although no strict dichotomy exists between the two. Certain "voluntary" or consciously controlled functions may also take place "involuntarily" and vice versa. Muscular actions that are primarily voluntary include those that help in posture, balance, leverage, locomotion, food manipulation, vocalization, swallowing, and similar movements. Functions of an involuntary nature are those that principally occur internally, such as the propulsion of food through the digestive tract and blood through the vascular system, the expulsion of excretions from

FOUNDATIONS OF HEALTH SCIENCE

Figure A.1 The Skeletal System. The Skeletal system makes up the strong framework that supports the softer organs of the body and provides a firm attachment for the muscles. Most of the important bones are labeled on the diagram. (From *Instructoscope*. Copyright © 1964 by Scott, Foresman and Company. Reprinted by permission of the publisher.)

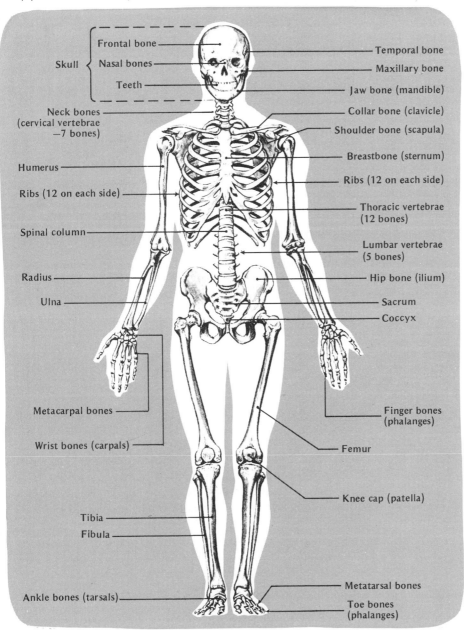

Skull {
Frontal bone
Nasal bones
Teeth

Temporal bone
Maxillary bone
Jaw bone (mandible)
Collar bone (clavicle)
Shoulder bone (scapula)
Breastbone (sternum)

Neck bones (cervical vertebrae —7 bones)
Humerus
Ribs (12 on each side)
Spinal column
Radius
Ulna

Ribs (12 on each side)
Thoracic vertebrae (12 bones)
Lumbar vertebrae (5 bones)
Hip bone (ilium)
Sacrum
Coccyx

Metacarpal bones
Wrist bones (carpals)

Finger bones (phalanges)
Femur
Knee cap (patella)

Tibia
Fibula

Ankle bones (tarsals)

Metatarsal bones
Toe bones (phalanges)

various glands, and the regulation of functions, such as the size of the pupil of the eye. See Figure A.2.

Three types of muscle tissue have been identified and classified on the basis of structure and function. *Smooth* muscle tissue consists of long spindle-shaped cells. Smooth tissue constitutes the visceral or involuntary muscles. *Striated* muscle tissue is made up of large fibers grouped into bundles. This type of tissue is characteristic of the skeletal or voluntary muscles. *Cardiac* muscle tissue is composed of striated cells and is located only in the heart. The four properties of muscle tissue—contractility, extensibility, elasticity, and irritability—permit each specific type to perform its own unique function and are important in exercise.

The Circulatory System

The circulatory system comprises all structures involved in the transportation of body fluids from one region of the body to another. It has two main divisions—the *cardiovascular* system, including the heart and blood vessels, and the *lymphatic* system, composed of vessels that act as a drainage mechanism for specific body fluids.

The center of the circulatory system is the *heart,* a cone-shaped organ slightly larger than the fist, which is located in about the middle of the chest cavity. Its pumping action keeps the blood circulating, thus assuring the distribution of life-giving substances to all parts of the body. It is enclosed in a tough membrane called the *pericardium,* the inside surface of which secretes a fluid that bathes the heart and reduces friction resulting from its movement. Although the heart normally beats from 70 to 80 times a minute, it rests after every contraction. *Diastole* is the term used to describe this relaxation period; *systole* is the period of contraction.

The four chambers making up the interior of the heart are lined with a membrane known as the *endocardium.* Blood is received in the *atria,* two upper chambers, and then passed through *atrioventricular* valves into the thick-walled *ventricles,* from which it is pumped out. Blood returning from the body flows into the right atrium and is pumped into the right ventricle and then into the pulmonary artery to the lungs. The left atrium receives oxygen-laden blood from the lungs through the four *pulmonary veins* and sends it into the left ventricle, which then passes it through the aorta to the general body system. The flow to, through, and from the lungs is called *pulmonary circulation.* The flow throughout all other parts of the body is known as *systemic circulation.* See Figures A.3 and A.4.

The blood is a moving tissue consisting of a fluid called *plasma* and a countless number of floating cells and other substances. The plasma is composed of approximately 90 percent water, in which are found the

628

Figure A.2 The Muscular System. More than 650 muscles surround the internal organs and skeleton of the body. The left half of the diagram shows the outside muscles of the front of the body. The right half shows the outside muscles of the back. (From *Instructoscope*. Copyright © 1964 by Scott, Foresman and Company. Reprinted by permission of the publisher.)

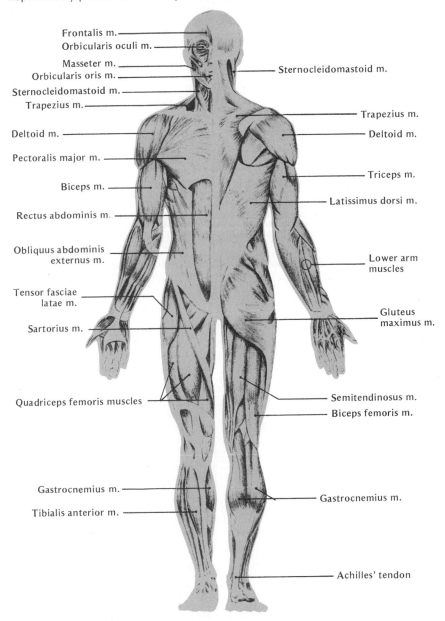

Frontalis m.

Orbicularis oculi m.

Masseter m.

Orbicularis oris m.

Sternocleidomastoid m.

Trapezius m.

Deltoid m.

Pectoralis major m.

Biceps m.

Rectus abdominis m.

Obliquus abdominis externus m.

Tensor fasciae latae m.

Sartorius m.

Quadriceps femoris muscles

Gastrocnemius m.

Tibialis anterior m.

Sternocleidomastoid m.

Trapezius m.

Deltoid m.

Triceps m.

Latissimus dorsi m.

Lower arm muscles

Gluteus maximus m.

Semitendinosus m.

Biceps femoris m.

Gastrocnemius m.

Achilles' tendon

Figure A.3 The Circulatory System. This system carries the blood through the body and is composed of many sizes of the flexible tubes. The diagram shows veins on one side and arteries on the other side. Of course, the body has arteries and veins on both sides. (From *Instructoscope*. Copyright © 1964 by Scott, Foresman and Company. Reprinted by permission of the publisher.)

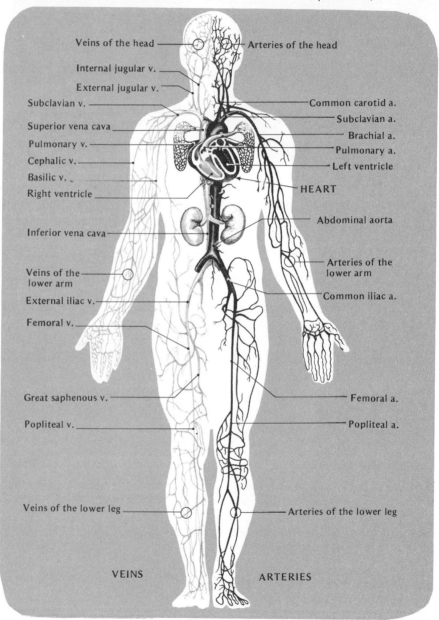

Veins of the head — Arteries of the head

Internal jugular v.

External jugular v.

Subclavian v. — Common carotid a.

Superior vena cava — Subclavian a.

Pulmonary v. — Brachial a.

Cephalic v. — Pulmonary a.

Basilic v. — Left ventricle

Right ventricle — HEART

Inferior vena cava — Abdominal aorta

Veins of the lower arm — Arteries of the lower arm

External iliac v. — Common iliac a.

Femoral v.

Great saphenous v. — Femoral a.

Popliteal v. — Popliteal a.

Veins of the lower leg — Arteries of the lower leg

VEINS   ARTERIES

Figure A.4 The Lymphatic System. The lymphatic system is composed of many thin-walled vessels, some large enough to be called trunks and others no larger than the capillaries of the circulatory system. The lymph is circulated through the system by body action and the squeezing of the muscles. Lymph is formed from blood plasma that diffuses through capillary walls. It nourishes the body cells by carrying food substances to the cells and carries away poisonous substances. The lymph nodes are small clusters of lymph tissue along the lymph vessels, as shown in the diagram above. They contain lymph cells that aid in filtering poisons from the lymph fluid. (From *Instructoscope*. Copyright © 1964 by Scott, Foresman and Company. Reprinted by permission of the publisher.)

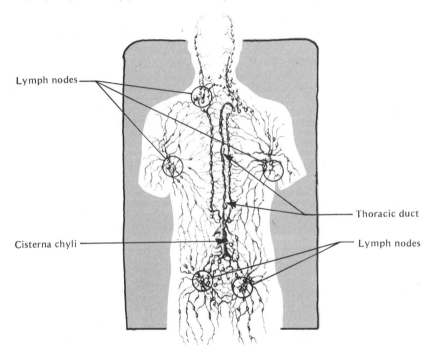

absorbed products of digestion, oxygen, carbon dioxide, antibodies, hormones, and other metabolic waste products. The white blood cells, or *leukocytes*, serve as a circulating defense against disease and infection. The red blood cells, called *erythrocytes*, are the oxygen carriers. Fibrinogen, also carried in the plasma, helps to produce the fibers that function with the platelets to clot the blood when an injury occurs.

Table A.1 Minerals

Nutrient	Best Sources	Function	Deficiency Symptoms

Calcium	Milk
	Cheese
	Vegetables (green)
		Essential for:
		  normal development and
		    maintenance of bones
		    and teeth
		  regulating body
		    processes
		  clotting of the blood
		  normal action of the
		    heart
		  health of the nerves
		  normal activity of the
		    muscles
		  iron utilization
			Retarded growth
			Poor tooth formation
			Rickets
			Slow clotting time of blood
			Porous bones

Phosphorus	Variety meats
	Meat
	Fowl
	Fish
	Soybeans
	Milk
	Cheese
	Legumes
	Eggs
	Whole-grain cereal
	  products
		Essential for:
		  formation of normal
		    bones and teeth
		  cell structure
		  maintenance of normal
		    reaction of the blood
		  output of nervous energy
		  normal activity of the
		    muscles
		  metabolism of
		    carbohydrates and fats
			Retarded growth
			Poor tooth formation
			Rickets
			Porous bones
			Tetany-convulsions

Iron	Variety meats
	Oysters
	Meat
	Vegetables (green)
	Legumes
	Fowl
	Potatoes
	Dried fruits
	Eggs
	Fish
	Whole-grain or enriched
	  cereal products
		Essential for:
		  formation of hemoglobin
			Anemia, characterized by:
			  weakness
			  dizziness
			  loss of weight
			  gastric disturbances
			  pallor

Copper	Oysters
	Liver
	Mushrooms
	Fowl
	Legumes
	Meat
	Fish
	Potatoes
		Essential for:
		  formation of hemoglobin
		  fat metabolism
		  ascorbic acid metabolism
			Anemia (*see* iron)

Iodine	Iodized salt Sea foods	Regulates energy exchange and metabolism	Simple goiter Cretinism (rare in U.S.) Thyroidtoxicosis

Table A.2 Vitamins

Vitamin	Best Sources	Function	Deficiency Symptoms

Vitamin A	Fish liver oils
	Liver and kidney
	Vegetables (green and
	  yellow)
	Fruits (yellow)
	Tomatoes
	Egg yolk
		Essential for:
		  growth
		  health of the eyes
		  structure and functioning
		    of the cells of the skin
		    and mucous
		    membranes
			Retarded growth
			Functional disorders of the
			  eyes (night blindness)
			Increased susceptibility to
			  infections
			Changes in skin and
			  membranes
			Defective tooth formation

Thiamine (B_1)	Pork
	Variety meats
	Meat
	Soybeans
	Oysters
	Potatoes
	Melons
	Milk
	Whole-grain or
	  enriched products
	Vegetables (green)
	Fowl
		Essential for:
		  growth
		  carbohydrate metabolism
		  functioning of the heart,
		    nerves, muscles
			Beriberi (rare in U.S.)
			Enlarged heart
			Irritability
			Retarded growth
			Loss of appetite and weight
			Nerve disorders
			Less resistance to fatigue
			Impairment of digestion
			Emotional instability
			Constipation

Riboflavin (B_2)	Variety meats
	Meat
	Soybeans
	Milk
	Oysters
	Vegetables (green)
	Eggs
	Fowl
		Essential for:
		  growth
		  health of the skin and
		    mouth
		  well-being and vigor
		  functioning of the eyes
		  carbohydrate metabolism
			(Common in U.S.)
			Retarded growth
			Lesions at corners of the
			  mouth
			Dimness of vision
			Cataract-like symptoms
			Intolerance to light
			Inflammation of the tongue
			Premature aging

*Niacin
(Nicotinic
Acid)*
	Variety meats
	Meat
	Fowl
	Fish
	Peanut butter
	Potatoes
	Whole-grain or
	  enriched cereal
	  products
		Essential for:
		  growth
		  carbohydrate metabolism
		  health of the skin
		  functioning of the
		    stomach and
		    intestines
		  functioning of the
		    nervous system
			Pellagra (rare in U.S.)
			Glossitis (smoothness of
			  the tongue)
			Skin eruptions
			Digestive disturbances
			Mental disorders

Pyridoxine (B_6)	Meat (muscle tissue)
	Variety meats
	Fish
	Whole-grain products
	Milk
	Legumes
		Specific function unknown
		Probably essential for:
		  growth
		  health of the skin
		  functioning of the
		    muscles and nervous
		    system
		  protein metabolism
			(Seldom due to poor
			  nutrition)
			Skin eruptions
			Vague symptoms of
			  insomnia, irritability,
			  muscular rigidity

FOUNDATIONS OF HEALTH SCIENCE

Table A.2 *(Continued)*

Vitamin	Best Sources	Function	Deficiency Symptoms
Pantothenic Acid	Liver Meat Milk Whole-grain products Synthesized in body	Specific function unknown Probably essential for: growth health of the skin normal hair production	(Seldom due to poor nutrition) Intestinal disorders Mental disorders Neurological disorders
Vitamin C (Ascorbic Acid)	Citrus fruits Melons Berries Tomatoes Raw cabbage	Essential for: growth cell activity maintaining strength of the blood vessels development of the teeth health of the gums	Scurvy Poor wound healing Sore gums Hemorrhages around the bones Tendency to bruise easily Susceptibility to infections Retardation of growth
Vitamin D	Fish liver oil Fat fish Liver Milk (fortified) Eggs Irradiated foods Sunshine	Essential for: growth regulates calcium and phosphorus metabolism builds and maintains normal bones and teeth	Bowed legs Enlarged joints Soft bones Poor tooth development Dental decay
Vitamin E	Seed germ oils Vegetables (green)	Specific function unknown Probably essential for: growth normal reproduction normal functioning of the muscles and nervous system	Unlikely in humans
Vitamin K	Vegetables (green) Cabbage Cauliflower Soybean oil Tomatoes Orange peel	Essential for: normal clotting of the blood normal liver function	Hemorrhage In liver damage In intestinal disease In antibiotic therapy

Table A.3 Food and Nutrition Board, National Academy of Sciences–National Research Council Recommended Daily Dietary Allowances,[a] Revised 1974.

Designed for the maintenance of good nutrition of practically all healthy people in the U.S.A.

	Age	Weight		Height		Energy	Protein	Fat-Soluble Vitamins			
								Vitamin A Activity		Vitamin D	Vitamin E Activity[e]
	(years)	(kg)	(lbs)	(cm)	(in)	(kcal)[b]	(g)	(RE)[c]	(IU)	(IU)	(IU)
Infants	0.0–0.5	6	14	60	24	kg × 117	kg × 2.2	420[d]	1,400	400	4
	0.5–1.0	9	20	71	28	kg × 108	kg × 2.0	400	2,000	400	5
Children	1–3	13	28	86	34	1,300	23	400	2,000	400	7
	4–6	20	44	110	44	1,800	30	500	2,500	400	9
	7–10	30	66	135	54	2,400	36	700	3,300	400	10
Males	11–14	44	97	158	63	2,800	44	1,000	5,000	400	12
	15–18	61	134	172	69	3,000	54	1,000	5,000	400	15
	19–22	67	147	172	69	3,000	54	1,000	5,000	400	15
	23–50	70	154	172	69	2,700	56	1,000	5,000		15
	51+	70	154	172	69	2,400	56	1,000	5,000		15
Females	11–14	44	97	155	62	2,400	44	800	4,000	400	12
	15–18	54	119	162	65	2,100	48	800	4,000	400	12
	19–22	58	128	162	65	2,100	46	800	4,000	400	12
	23–50	58	128	162	65	2,000	46	800	4,000		12
	51+	58	128	162	65	1,800	46	800	4,000		12
Pregnant						+300	+30	1,000	5,000	400	15
Lactating						+500	+20	1,200	6,000	400	15

[a] The allowances are intended to provide for individual variations among most normal persons as they live in the United States under usual environmental stresses. Diets should be based on a variety of common foods in order to provide other nutrients for which human requirements have been less well defined.

[b] Kilojoules (kJ) = 4.2 × kcal.

[c] Retinol equivalents.

[d] Assumed to be all as retinol in milk during the first six months of life. All subsequent intakes are assumed to be half as retinol and half as β-carotene when calculated from international units. As retinol equivalents, three fourths are as retinol and one fourth as β-carotene.

[e] Total vitamin E activity, estimated to be 80 percent as α-tocopherol and 20 percent other tocopherols.

FOUNDATIONS OF HEALTH SCIENCE

Water-Soluble Vitamins							Minerals					
Ascorbic Acid (mg)	Folacin[f] (µg)	Niacin[g] (mg)	Riboflavin (mg)	Thiamin (mg)	Vitamin B6 (mg)	Vitamin B12 (µg)	Calcium (mg)	Phosphorus (mg)	Iodine (µg)	Iron (mg)	Magnesium (mg)	Zinc (mg)
35	50	5	0.4	0.3	0.3	0.3	360	240	35	10	60	3
35	50	8	0.6	0.5	0.4	0.3	540	400	45	15	70	5
40	100	9	0.8	0.7	0.6	1.0	800	800	60	15	150	10
40	200	12	1.1	0.9	0.9	1.5	800	800	80	10	200	10
40	300	16	1.2	1.2	1.2	2.0	800	800	110	10	250	10
45	400	18	1.5	1.4	1.6	3.0	1,200	1,200	130	18	350	15
45	400	20	1.8	1.5	2.0	3.0	1,200	1,200	150	18	400	15
45	400	20	1.8	1.5	2.0	3.0	800	800	140	10	350	15
45	400	18	1.6	1.4	2.0	3.0	800	800	130	10	350	15
45	400	16	1.5	1.2	2.0	3.0	800	800	110	10	350	15
45	400	16	1.3	1.2	1.6	3.0	1,200	1,200	115	18	300	15
45	400	14	1.4	1.1	2.0	3.0	1,200	1,200	115	18	300	15
45	400	14	1.4	1.1	2.0	3.0	800	800	100	18	300	15
45	400	13	1.2	1.0	2.0	3.0	800	800	100	18	300	15
45	400	12	1.1	1.0	2.0	3.0	800	800	80	10	300	15
60	800	+2	+0.3	+0.3	2.5	4.0	1,200	1,200	125	18+[h]	450	20
80	600	+4	+0.5	+0.3	2.5	4.0	1,200	1,200	150	18	450	25

The folacin allowances refer to dietary sources as determined by **Lactobacillus casei** assay. Pure forms of folacin may be effective in doses less than one fourth of the recommended dietary allowance.

[g] Although allowances are expressed as niacin, it is recognized that on the average 1 mg of niacin is derived from each 60 mg of dietary tryptophan.

[h] This increased requirement cannot be met by ordinary diets; therefore, the use of supplemental iron is recommended.

Source: **Recommended Dietary Allowances,** Eighth Edition, Publication ISBN 0-309-02216-9, Committee on Dietary Allowances, Food and Nutrition Board, National Academy of Sciences–National Research Council, Washington, D.C. 1974.

Table A.4 Common Communicable Diseases

Infection and Symptoms	Etiological Agent and Transmission	Incubation	Com-municability	Immunity or Prophylaxis	Complications
Chickenpox (Varicella): Slight fever followed by rash which looks like small blisters. Blisters keep developing for 3–4 days and leave crusts that fall off in about 14 days.	*Virus* Direct contact and secretions from nose and throat	13–21 days	1 day before rash—2 days after last new lesions appear	Good after infection; no vaccine	Rare fatality; encephalitis; infected lesions
Diphtheria: Sore throat, fever, patches of grayish membrane on tonsils, in nose and throat. Croup in very young children.	*Corynebacterium diphtheriae* Direct contact; secretions nose and throat; skin lesions; carriers; contaminated milk	2–5 days	2–4 weeks after initial symptoms	Effective vaccines; antitoxin for nonimmunized	2–5% fatality though sometimes 10%; cranial nerve palsies; myocarditis
German Measles (Rubella): A rash like that of measles or scarlet fever or both, slight fever, usually swollen glands around the ears, neck and throat.	*Virus* Direct contact; secretions nose and throat; sometimes contaminated articles	14–21 days	4–5 days after first symptoms	Good after infection; vaccine 96% effective	Very rare encephalitis; congenital anomalies in 20–40% of babies of mothers infected prenatally
Hookworm (Anchyostomiasas): Rash and itching where larvae penetrate skin.	*Ancylostoma* Mild climates, rural areas where sanitation poor; penetrates skin, especially soles of feet; spread in feces	6 weeks for eggs to appear in feces	As long as infected	Wearing shoes; sanitation; drug therapy effective; no immunization	Moderate and severe invasions cause anemia, weakness, heart dysfunction, edema

FOUNDATIONS OF HEALTH SCIENCE

		Incubation	Period of communicability	Immunity/prevention	Complications/fatality
Infectious Mononucleosis (Glandular fever): Vague symptoms such as headache, malaise, fatigue, sore throat, swollen glands; rarely a rash or jaundice.	*The Epstein-Barr virus* Unknown how spread; may be direct contact; most often found in children and young adults	Unknown; may be 4–14 days	infection		but may be ruptured spleen, liver involvement, encephalitis, carditis, anemia, pneumonia, or secondary infection of the throat
Malaria: Systemic, sometimes acute, sometimes severe. Begin with malaise and characteristic shaking chill with rapidly rising fever accompanied by headache, nausea, and profuse sweating. The fever, chill, sweating occur in cycles lasting a week or month. Relapse common.	*Plasmodium: a protozoan* Transmitted by the mosquito; no direct contact man to man; can be transmitted by contaminated blood or hypodermic syringes	8–35 days in mosquito then after inoculation into host, another 3–14 days—occasionally 8–10 months	An infected mosquito carries pathogen for life. As long as in blood, humans can infect the mosquito. About 1–3 years	No vaccines; chemo-prophylaxis usually effective	1–10% fatality—treated 1% fatality; mild jaundice; anemia; enlarged spleen; may become chronic
Measles (Rubeola): Sore throat, running nose, inflamed eyes, cough, fever. Rash follows in a few days—blotchy dusky red color starting first on forehead and face.	*Virus* Direct contact; secretions nose and throat; sometimes contaminated articles	7–14 days	4–5 days after rash appears	Good after infection; effective vaccines	Fatality rare, 1%; otitis media; encephalitis 1%; pneumonia and bronchitis
Meningococcus Meningitis: Runny nose, sore throat, headache, fever, pain in neck and back, loss of alertness, sometimes a rash, convulsions, projectile vomiting.	*Neisseria Meningitidis* Direct contact; carriers; secretions nose and throat	1 week	Until no longer found in discharges; with chemo-therapy about 24 hours	Temporary immunity after infection; chemo-prophylaxis	Fatality, 5%; deafness; internal hydrocephalus

(Continued on next page)

Infection and Symptoms	Etiological Agent and Transmission	Incubation	Com- municability	Immunity or Prophylaxis	Complications
Mumps (Infectious parotitis): Fever and swelling of glands at the angles of jaw and in front of ears. The swelling may be painful and may start on one side only, later involve both.	*Virus* Direct contact; mouth secretions and contaminated articles	2–4 weeks, usually 18 days	1 week after exposure until 9 days after symptoms	Good after infection; vaccine 95% effective	Post pubertal males: 2% adult males if untreated will be sterile; 10% CNS involvement
Pink Eye (Acute catarrhal conjunctivitis): Tearing, inflammation, swelling, pus, photophobia, itching, and burning.	*Caused by various bacteria: Haemophilus aegyptius, influenzae, staphylococcus, streptococcus, pneumococcus, and adenoviruses.* Direct contact with discharge from eyes; possible carriers; usually children under 5 years	24–72 hours	During active infection highly contagious— may last 2–4 weeks	No vaccines; immunity following infection is poor	None
Pinworm, Seatworm (Enterobiasis): Pruritis or itching around anus.	*Enterobius vermicularis:* Rural and urban areas; fecal contamination of hands; eggs airborne; ingest eggs	3–6 weeks	All members in family should be suspected; 2–8 weeks unless reinfected	Good hygiene; effective treatment; no immunization	20% of population infected

Signs and Symptoms	Cause/Transmission	Incubation Period	Period of Communicability	Prevention/Control	Complications/Outcome
Usually slight or moderate fever, headache, vomiting, muscular stiffness, soreness, weakness. Flaccid limb paralysis.	Direct contact with infected people; probably through ingestion; discharges from nose, mouth, feces; carriers	...weeks	1 week after symptoms	Effective vaccines	fatality, 4–10%; 25% severe paralysis; 25% mild disabilities; 50% recover with no residuals
Rabies (Hydrophobia): Convulsions, paralysis. Starts with restlessness, malaise, and fever. Excessive salivation. Spasms of pharyngeal and laryngeal muscles.	Virus In saliva of rabid animal; travels up nerve tissue to brain; usually wildlife	10–60 days, sometimes longer—multiple bites, it is shorter	Duration of illness and 3–5 days before symptoms; bats may be carriers; no record of human transmission	Vaccination after contact highly effective; infiltration of area around wound with antiserum	Fatality, 100%
Roundworms (Ascariasis): Vague abdominal pain, hives, edema, loss of weight, nervousness. Signs malnutrition.	Ascaris lumbricoides Usually ingested but may penetrate skin; fecal contamination of foods	2 months	6–12 weeks in humans; months to years in soil	Sanitation; personal hygiene; effective treatment	Possible mental retardation postulated; 3/4 children in U.S. infected
Rubella, see German measles.					
Schistosomiasis: Diarrhea, abdominal pain. Swimmer's itch.	Trematoda Human excreta infects water; snails necessary to life cycle; snails then shed flukes into water and plants; humans ingest plants or swim in infected water	24–48 hours for local irritation	Snails for several months; as long as human sheds eggs	Destruction of snails; sanitation; not too effective treatment	Ulceration of intestines; liver and gall bladder disorders; anemia

(Continued on next page)

Table A.4 *(Continued)*

Infection and Symptoms	Etiological Agent and Transmission	Incubation	Com- municability	Immunity or Prophylaxis	Complications
Smallpox (Variola): Fever, headache, backache. Rash follows —starts on face, arms and wrists. Rash begins as small red spots which fill up with pus. Scabs or pocks form later.	*Virus* Direct contact; contaminated articles; body discharges, exudate from lesions	1–2 weeks	2–3 weeks or from beginning of symptoms until scale and crusts are gone	Effective vaccine	Fatality, 20–40%; sometimes damage to ears and eyes from lesions
Streptococcal sore throat and scarlet fever: Sudden fever, sore throat, swollen glands in the neck. Sometimes vomiting. The same symptoms occur in scarlet fever and are followed by a rash. Strep throat and scarlet fever are the same disease except for the rash.	*Group A hemolytic streptococcus* Direct contact; carriers; contaminated dust, food, and articles; secretion mouth and nose	2–5 days	During incubation and symptoms— about 2 weeks	Chemoprophylaxis, which may prevent or render noncom- municable in 24 hours; vaccines not too effective	Rheumatic fever; glomerulo-nephritis; otitis, broncho- pneumonia; carditis; meningitis
Tapeworm: Vague feelings of discomfort. Segments of worm in stool.	*Cestoda* Improperly cooked infected pork, beef, fish; ingestion of cysts or eggs	2–3 months	As long as infected	Cooking meats well; effective treatment	Anemia; abdominal pain; diarrhea

FOUNDATIONS OF HEALTH SCIENCE

Tetanus: Stiffness of neck muscles, painful spasms of jaw muscles (lockjaw). Rigidity is sometimes limited to the part of the body that is injured.	Clostridium tetani From soil, street dust, manure, articles contaminated by above; injuries indoors and outdoors causing break in skin	4 days to 7 weeks—usually 1–2 weeks	Not communicable from person to person	Effective vaccines; human serum globulin for nonimmunized	Fatality about 35%
Trichinosis: Vague aching in muscles, backache, headache, edema, chills and fever, weakness, prostration.	Trichinella spiralis Infected pork	2–28 days	Animal hosts infective for years	Pasteurization of garbage; cooking pork well; freezing and irradiation of pork, no immunization	Rarely death and that only in very heavy infections; heart failure; 1/8 population infected
Typhoid: Fever, rose spots, enlarged spleen, diarrhea, malaise, headache, constipation, backache, bronchitis, delirium, stupor.	Salmonella typhi Carriers; infected water, food; in feces and urine; direct and indirect contact; flies	1–3 weeks	During symptoms and as long as typhoid bacilli in excreta—10% will discharge bacilli for 3 months, 2–5% become carriers	Effective vaccine	Fatality, 2–3% with treatment; without treatment, 10%; complications in 25–30% of untreated—hemorrhage, intestinal perforation, pneumonia, meningitis, carditis, otitis media, psychoses, arthritis, cholecystitis, nephritis, neuritis

(Continued on next page)

Table A.4 (Continued)

Infection and Symptoms	Etiological Agent and Transmission	Incubation	Com-municability	Immunity or Prophylaxis	Complications
Viral Encephalitis: Abrupt onset with high fever, generalized rigidity, headache, muscle pain, upset stomach and respiratory symptoms. In several days, coma, delirium. May have convulsions.	*Virus* Mosquitoes are vectors; occasionally ticks; man is accidental host	5–15 days	Not spread from man to man—mosquito remains infective for life	Vaccine for high risk groups—usually immune after infection	Fatality range from 5–60%; complications may result in paralysis
Whooping cough (Pertussis): Irritating cough which sometimes becomes worse at night. Some fever. In about two weeks in typical cases the characteristic "whoop," a spasm of coughing, followed by vomiting, usually appears.	*Bordetella pertussis* Direct contact; secretions mouth and nose	7–21 days	From beginning symptoms and lasting about 4 weeks	Effective vaccines	Fatality, 1–2%; pneumonia; CNS involvement; bronchiectasis; spastic paralysis; mental retardation; otitis media
Yellow Fever: Sudden onset, high fever, jaundice, prostration and tendency to hemorrhage. May vomit blood. Nausea and constipation. Delirium, convulsions, coma.	*Virus* Mosquito bite	3–6 days	3–4 days after symptoms the blood is infectious and the pathogen can be transmitted to a mosquito	Effective vaccine	Fatality rate as high as 85%; no aftereffects

LIFE-SAVING MEASURES

Control of Bleeding

Always as a first step, elevate the bleeding part as much as possible.

1. *Direct pressure.* The simplest and often most effective treatment is direct pressure on the bleeding vessel or on the wound. Use a heavy, sterile gauze compress, any clean cloth, or hand and fingers. The danger of infection is minimal.

2. *Use of pressure points.* In the event that a pressure dressing is ineffective, the bleeding can usually be controlled by finger pressure on the main artery supplying the wounded part. Such pressure can be applied most effectively at the pressure points—the points where an artery is relatively near the surface and where it passes close to a bony structure against which it can be compressed. Pressure can be applied wherever a pulse is felt, however. Figure A.5 illustrates the pressure points.

3. *Tourniquets.* If the above measures to control bleeding are not effective, a tourniquet may be used as a last resort. A properly applied tourniquet is safe; improperly applied, it may result in loss of an arm or leg, hand or foot, or life.

   A tourniquet is placed as close to the hemorrhaging wound as possible and is left in place until it is loosened under conditions where immediate, definitive, surgical, supportive measures can be carried out. The two reasons for leaving it in place are: First, frequent loosening of the tourniquet may dislodge clots and result in sufficient bleeding to produce shock or death. Second, the so-called, possibly fatal, "tourniquet shock" is now recognized as a very special type of shock caused from toxins released by the injured tissue. Extensive study has proved that by leaving the tourniquet in place, although more limbs may be lost, more lives will be saved.

   Place the tourniquet as close to the wound as possible, between it and the heart, but not right at the wound edges.

   Tighten it just enough to control bleeding.

   If a regular tourniquet is not available, use some kind of flat article, such as a bandage, stocking, or belt, and be sure to place a pad over the artery to be compressed.

   Remember, note on the victim the time and where the tourniquet was applied.

Figure A.5 Use of Pressure Points. (Courtesy of John Henderson, *Emergency Medical Guide* [New York: McGraw-Hill Book Company, 1963], pp. 94–95.)

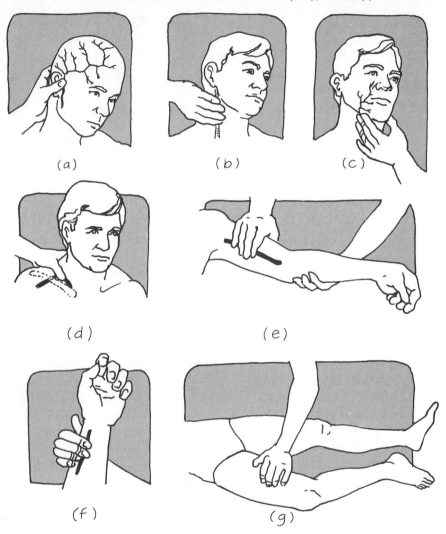

(a)   (b)   (c)

(d)   (e)

(f)   (g)

Reduction of Shock

The term *shock* means a condition in which essential activities of the body are greatly depressed. Shock may be caused by pronounced loss of blood, sera, or by loss of effective circulation. It may occur at times of stress, strong emotion, injury, pain, sudden illness, and accident. If a state

FOUNDATIONS OF HEALTH SCIENCE

of shock continues over a period of only a few hours, it may be fatal or cause permanent damage to essential organs such as the brain.

Shock may begin with a sudden or gradual feeling of unusual weakness or faintness, accompanied by pallor, perspiration, and cold and clammy skin. The pupils of the eyes become noticeably enlarged. The pulse is rapid, weak, and sometimes imperceptible. Shock is also accompanied by changes in the mental state and causes confusion. The shock patient's behavior ranges from a feeling of restlessness at first to a gradual loss of ability to respond to stimulation and finally to stupor and unconsciousness.

In case of shock, the following instructions should be followed:

1. Place the patient on his back or stomach with his head turned gently to one side.
2. Keep the air passages open.
3. Keep the victim warm by coverings underneath as well as over him. Avoid overheating. Shock victims are easily burned by heating pads or heated articles such as water bags or stones.
4. Raise the patient's feet six to twelve inches above the level of his head (in case of head injury, keep victim level).
5. Check for Medic-Alert tag or card.
6. Give conscious victims fluids; burn cases should have salt and soda water; never give alcohol or medicines.
7. Loosen constricting clothing.
8. Place pressure bandages on extensive burns.

FIRST AID FOR COMMONLY OCCURRING INJURIES

Bones and Joints

Fracture: Never move the victim if a fracture of the back, neck, or skull is suspected. If he *can* be moved, carefully splint any possible fracture. Obtain medical care at once.

Dislocation: Support the joint. Apply an ice bag or cold cloths to reduce swelling, and refer the patient to a physician at once.

Bone Bruise: Apply an ice bag or cold cloths and protect the patient from further injury. If the bruise is severe, refer to a physician.

Broken Nose: Apply cold cloths and refer the patient to a physician.

Heat Illnesses

Heat Stroke: Collapse—with *dry,* warm skin—indicates sweating mechanism failure and rising body temperature. This condition is an emergency; *delay could be fatal.* Immediately cool the victim by the most expedient means. Immersion in cool water is best. Obtain medical care at once.

Heat Exhaustion: Weakness—with profuse sweating—indicates a state of shock due to depletion of salt and water. Place the patient in the shade, with head level with or lower than body. Give sips of diluted salt water. Obtain medical care at once.

Sunburn: If severe, apply sterile gauze dressing and refer to a physician.

Impact Blows

Head: If any period of dizziness, headache, incoordination or unconsciousness occurs, disallow any further activity and obtain medical care at once. Keep the victim lying down. If unconscious, give him nothing by mouth.

Teeth: If completely removed from socket, save the tooth. If loosened, do not disturb; cover with a sterile gauze and refer to a dentist at once.

Solar Plexus: Rest the victim on his back and moisten his face with cool water. Loosen clothing around the waist and chest. Do nothing except obtain medical care if needed.

Testicular (Scrotal): Rest the victim on his back and apply an ice bag or cold cloths. Obtain medical care if the pain persists.

Eyes: If vision is impaired, refer to a physician at once. With soft tissue injury, apply an ice bag or cold cloths to reduce swelling.

Muscles and Ligaments

Bruise: Apply an ice bag or cold cloths, and rest the injured muscle. Protect the patient from further aggravation. If severe, refer to a physician.

Cramp: Have the opposite muscles contracted forcefully, using a firm hand pressure on the cramped muscle. If during a hot day, give the patient sips of dilute salt water. If recurring, refer to a physician.

Strain and Sprain: Elevate the injured part and apply an ice bag or cold cloths. Apply a pressure bandage to reduce swelling. Avoid weight bearing and obtain medical care.

Wounds

Heavy Bleeding: Apply sterile pressure bandage; use hand pressure if necessary. Refer to a physician at once.

Cut and Abrasion: Hold briefly under cold water; then cleanse with mild soap and water. Apply a sterile pad firmly until the bleeding stops, then protect with more loosely applied sterile bandage. If extensive, refer to a physician.

Puncture Wound: Handle in the same way as cuts, and refer to a physician.

Nose Bleed: Keep the victim sitting or standing; cover the nose with cold cloths. If bleeding is heavy, pinch the nose and place *small* gauze packs in the nostrils. If bleeding continues, refer the patient to a physician.

Other

Blisters: Keep clean with mild soap and water and protect from aggravation. If already broken, trim ragged edges with sterilized equipment. If extensive or infected, refer to a physician.

Foreign Body in Eye: Do not rub. Gently touch the particle with the point of clean, moist cloth, and wash with cold water. If unsuccessful or if pain persists, refer the patient to a physician.

Burns

Chemical Burns: Wash thoroughly with water. Apply sterile gauze dressing and refer to a physician.

Extensive Thermal Burns: Cover all burned body areas with the cleanest available cloth to exclude air. Have the victim lie down, head and chest slightly lower than the rest of the body. Call a physician.

Small Thermal Burns: Soak a sterile gauze pad in baking soda solution. Place pad on burn and bandage loosely. If the skin is not broken, cold water or clean ice may be applied to relieve pain.

Poisoning

Swallowed Poisons: Call a physician immediately. Begin mouth-to-mouth breathing if victim has difficulty breathing. Give water or milk. If safe, induce vomiting. *Do not* induce vomiting if the victim is unconscious, is in convulsions, has severe pain, or is known to have swallowed acid, strychnine, or a petroleum product.

Inhaled Poisons: Carry or drag the victim to fresh air. Apply artificial respiration if breathing is stopped or irregular. Call a physician. Keep the victim warm and quiet.

Glossary

Abort: (1) To arrest a disease in its earliest stages. (2) To give birth to an embryo or fetus before it is viable.

Abortion: Expulsion of the fetus before it is developed sufficiently to lead an independent existence outside the uterus.

Absorption: Passage of nutrients from the intestine into the blood or lymph.

Acetylcholine: An acid that is presumed to assist in nerve impulses crossing a synapse.

ACTH: A hormone, adrenocorticotropic, secreted by the anterior pituitary.

Active Immunity: The process wherein the body produces specific antibodies or antitoxins, which act to destroy a substance or render it harmless. In infections this is for a particular organism or its toxins.

Acute: Lasting a short period of time; intense (of a disease or condition).

Addiction: An overwhelming desire or need or compulsion to take a drug and to obtain it by any means, with a tendency to increase the dose and with psychological or physiological dependence on the drug.

Adjuvant: Synergist; that which aids or assists; increases the action of.

Adulteration: Addition of an inferior substance or ingredient to a product.

Aerobic: Living in air.

Agape: Brotherly love; love in a nonsexual sense.

Agglutination: A clumping together of blood cells.

Aggression: A disposition to vigorous activity, assertive behavior. Direct attack.

Alcohol Poisoning: A severe or extreme state of alcohol intoxication.

(Alcohol poisoning appears to be distinguished from alcohol intoxication only by the severity of involvement). An extreme state of intoxication, usually at alcohol concentrations in the blood of about 0.4 percent.

Alcohol Tolerance: The capacity to maintain normal function in the presence of a given concentration of alcohol in the tissues.

Alcoholic (noun): A person whose behavior or condition complies with a definition of alcoholism.

Alcoholic Addiction: An uncontrolled use of alcohol.

Alcoholic Beverage: Any beverage containing alcohol, as beer, cider, distilled spirits, wine.

Alcoholism: A chronic disease, or disorder of behavior, characterized by the repeated drinking of alcoholic beverages to an extent that exceeds customary dietary use or ordinary compliance with the social drinking customs of the community, and that interferes with the drinker's health, interpersonal relations, or economic functioning. The alcoholic has lost the ability to control how much he drinks.

Alcometer: An instrument that measures the amount of alcohol in the blood by checking the breath.

Allergen: An agent or substance that produces an allergic reaction.

Alpha Particles (often referred to as "alpha rays"): Positively charged nuclei of certain atoms. They are emitted by radium and other heavy elements and are easily absorbed in a few sheets of paper.

Alveoli: Minute air sacs in the lungs through which respiratory exchanges are made.

Amblyopia: A dimness of vision; partial loss of sight.

Amenorrhea: Absence or abnormal stoppage of the menstrual cycle.

Amino Acid: Organic compound containing both carboxyl (-COOH) and amino ($-NH_2$) groups; it is the fundamental unit in the protein molecule.

Amnesia: Partial or complete inability to recall or recognize past experiences.

Amniocentesis: Aspiration of fluid from the amniotic sac by either abdominal or vaginal route.

Amnion: The membrane surrounding the fetus.

Analgesic: A drug that reduces pain.

Analog: A compound that is almost identical chemically with another, but may have opposite metabolic effects.

Androgen: A testosterone steroid hormone producing masculine characteristics.

Anemia: A deficiency in the hemoglobin or in the number of red blood cells.

Aneurysm: A circumscribed dilation of an artery, or a blood-containing tumor connecting directly with the lumen of an artery.

Angina Pectoris: A characteristic pain produced when oxygen supply to heart muscle is inhibited, as in coronary occlusion.

Anorexia: Loss of appetite.

Anoxia: Lack of oxygen.

Antibiotic: Prejudicial to life.

Antibody: A protein substance formed in the blood in response to an antigen (in the case of infectious disease the organism or its toxin acts as an antigen). Antitoxin is similar to antibody.

Antigen: A substance, commonly protein in nature, that stimulates the production of antibodies upon introduction into the body.

Antiseptic: A substance or compound that prevents the growth of micro-organisms.

Anxiety Neurosis: Syndrome of emotional disorder characterized by anxiety that is not associated with any particular situation.

Apoplexy: Sudden loss of consciousness followed by paralysis, due to cerebral hemorrhage or blocking of an artery of the brain.

Arteriosclerosis: Degeneration of the health status of the artery resulting in loss of elasticity and reduction in lumen size.

Arthropod: Invertebrate animal with jointed limbs. Insect.

Artificial Radioactivity: An element made radioactive by bombardment with nuclear particles. For instance, Iodine-131 is an artificially produced radioactive substance.

Aseptic: Free from pathogenic organisms.

Astigmatism: Unequal curvature of the cornea or lens, which interferes with focusing.

Atherosclerosis: A type of arteriosclerosis in which deposits of calcium or fats (cholesterol) occur in the vessel wall.

Atocia: Sterility in the female.

Attenuation: Weakening of the virulence or toxicity of pathogens.

Autistic: Self-centered; in childhood, an inability to form meaningful interpersonal relationships.

Bactericidal: Causing death of bacteria.

Bacteriostatic: Inhibiting or retarding the growth of bacteria.

B.C.G. (Bacillus Calmette Guerin): A vaccine to protect against tuberculosis.

Benign: Nonmalignant.

Beta Particle (Also called "beta radiation" or "beta ray"): The charged electron emitted from certain radioactive nuclei.

Biological Value: Rating of proteins with respect to their efficiency in maintaining the body in nitrogen equilibrium.

Blackout: Amnesia for the events of any part of a drinking episode, without loss of consciousness. Coma or stupor due to alcohol intoxication.

Blood Lipids: Fats found in the blood.

Blood Serology: Any laboratory examination of the blood. It may be for many different conditions or diseases.

Buerger's Disease (Thromboangiitis obliterans): Disease of the arteries of the extremities causing interference with circulation and producing gangrene.

Calorie: Unit of food energy and of heat. It is the amount of heat required to raise the temperature of 1 kilogram of water 1 degree centigrade (large calorie).

Carbohydrate: Large class of foodstuffs, including the starches and sugars.

Carcinogen: A cancer-producing substance.

Carcinoma: A malignant neoplasm derived from epithelial tissue.

Cardiovascular: Referring to the heart and blood vessels.

Carrier: One who harbors and can transmit pathogens but displays no symptoms of disease.

Castration: Removal of the testicles or ovaries.

Catabolism: Breaking down in the body of chemical compounds into simpler ones.

Cataract: Opacity of the lens of the eye or of its capsule.

Catatonia: Symptoms of negativism, stupor, stereotype, or impulse activity.

Cell: Basic unit of life.

Cellulose: The insoluble and indigestible carbohydrate that forms the fibrous structure of plants.

Cerumen: Waxy substance found in the external canal of the ear.

Chain Reaction: The sequential series of nuclear fissions that maintains itself in a critical assembly of nuclear material.

Chemoprophylaxis: Prevention of disease by the use of chemicals or drugs.

Chemotherapy: Treatment of disease by drugs or chemical reagents.

Chiropractor: One who employs the doctrine and dogma of chiropractic (a philosophic system of mechanical therapeutics that attributes disease to vertebral subluxations; it treats disease with manipulation of the vertebrae in order to relieve pressure on the nerves at the intervertebral foramina). Although he may be privileged to use the term *doctor,* he is limited to the kinds of diagnostic procedures he may use, and he may not prescribe all drugs or use surgery.

Cholesterol: A type of fatty substance found in animal tissues.

Chorea: A disease marked by irregular movements and speech disturbances.

Chromosome: A thread-like body, found in the nucleus of the cell, that contains hereditary traits.

Chronic Alcoholism: Alcoholism with complications; physical or psychological changes due to the prolonged excessive use of alcohol. Alcoholism, alcohol addiction, or repeated drunkenness. Long-lasting inebriety or alcoholic disorder.

Cilia: Hairlike processes of certain cells.

Circumcision: Partial or complete removal of the prepuce or foreskin of the penis, sometimes of the clitoris.

Cirrhosis: A disease of the liver characterized by degeneration and fatty infiltration.

Climacteric: A group of symptoms accompanying the termination of the reproductive period in women; also similar symptoms in the male that accompany the normal diminution of sexual activity.

Climax: The height or acme of sexual feeling; orgasm.

Clinical Diagnosis: Diagnosis of a disease from observing the symptoms and cause of the disease, as distinguished from laboratory diagnosis.

Clinically Active Disease: Disease in the stage when symptoms are evident.

Clitoris: Female homologue of the penis.

Coarctation: Narrowing, compressing.

Coelom: Great body cavity; includes the chest cavity (thorax) and the abdominal cavity, which are divided by the diaphragm.

Coitus: Sexual intercourse, copulation.

Coitus Interruptus: Withdrawal of the penis from the vagina before normal completion of the act of copulation. Onanism.

Collateral Circulation: The enlargement of accessory blood vessels to provide for circulation when the primary vessels are blocked.

College Health Program: Organized set of procedures directed toward the promotion of safe and healthful living for students and staff personnel.

Communicable Disease: A disease that is transmitted from one person to another either directly or indirectly.

Compensation: Overdevelopment of a specific type of behavior to make up for some lack.

Complete Blood Count: A laboratory test in which both red and white blood cells are evaluated as to quantity and quality.

Compulsions: Forced repetitive actions that the performer recognizes to be inappropriate or irrational.

Condom: A thin protective sheath, usually of rubber, worn over the penis to protect against venereal disease or as a contraceptive.

Congenital: Noninherited; present at birth.

Conjunctiva: The mucous membrane covering the anterior surface of the eyeball and lining the lids.

Contagious Disease: A disease that is spread through contact with the sick.

Conversion Reaction: A type of hysteria in which the symptoms are of a physical nature.

Copulation: Sexual intercourse.

Corona Glandis: The rim surrounding the base of the glans penis.

Coronary Occlusion: Blockage of an artery that supplies the heart muscle.

Corpus Luteum: A yellow mass in the ovary formed from the ruptured graafian follicle. Secretes progesterone.

Culture: (1) (verb) To grow organisms on artificial media so that they are sufficient in number to be seen microscopically or be otherwise identified. (2) (noun) Value systems and behavior of a people.

Cunnilingus: Using the tongue or mouth to sexually stimulate the female genitalia.

Curie: A unit used to measure the rate at which radioactive material or a combination of radioactive materials gives off nuclear particles.

CVA: Cerebrovascular accident; stroke.

Cyanosis: A dark bluish coloration of the skin and mucous membrane due to insufficient oxygen.

Cybernetics: The comparative study of the automatic control system formed by the nervous system and brain and by mechanoelectrical communication systems.

Cyst: An abnormal sac containing gas, fluid, or a semisolid material.

Cystocele: Protrusion of the urinary bladder through the fascia of the anterior vaginal wall; a hernia.

Cyte, Cyto: Prefix or suffix meaning *cell*.

Dark Ages: Early part of the medieval period or Middle Ages.

FOUNDATIONS OF HEALTH SCIENCE

Darkfield Microscopy: A type of microscopic examination used to see treponema.

Debility: Weakness, loss of strength.

Decay (also referred to as "disintegration"): The spontaneous nuclear process that may result in the release of energy in the form of alpha, beta, or gamma rays.

Deductible: In major medical insurance, refers to that portion of hospital and medical charges that an insured person must pay before his policy's benefits begin.

Defecate: To excrete feces; move the bowels.

Degenerative Diseases: Diseases occurring as a result of tissue degeneration precipitated by the aging process or prematurely by another disease process.

Delusion: Belief in something that is false.

Demography: The statistical study of populations.

Denial: Inability or refusal to accept and recognize a characteristic, condition, or problem that may be obvious to other people.

Dental Caries: Tooth decay; cavities.

Dental Pulp: The inner soft portion of a tooth where blood vessels and nerves are located. Toothache results when pulp is exposed.

Dentin: The softer bonelike substance under the cementum or enamel portion of a tooth. When dentin is exposed, the tooth may be sensitive to sweets or temperature changes.

Depot Drug (also spelled "depo"): A drug that takes a long time to absorb completely after injection, so that one injection will maintain a curative level of the drug in the blood for three or four days.

Dextrose: Glucose, the sugar of the blood; it is combined in large units to form starch and glycogen.

Dialysis: Separation of substances in a filter-like process; the artificial kidney purifies the blood by such a process.

Diarrhea: Abnormal, frequent, liquid stool.

Diastolic Pressure: The blood pressure during the period in which the heart is at rest.

Digestion: Degradation of food to soluble and absorbable form in the digestive tract.

Diplomate: Holds a certificate from the National Board of Medical Examiners or from one of the American Boards in the specialties.

Dipsomania: Periodic excessive drinking; spree drinking. Craving, or periodic craving, for alcohol.

Direct Contact: Immediate or intimate contact involving physical touching.

Disease: Illness, sickness, abnormal state, interruption or perversion of body function.

Disinfectant: Inhibiting the action of germs or destroying them.

Displaced Aggression: Aggression that is directed toward some source other than that which creates the aggression; frequently known as "scapegoating."

Dissociative Reaction: A type of hysteria characterized by amnesia, fugues, multiple personalities.

Diuretic: A substance that stimulates the excretion of urine.

Doctor: Term used to imply a particular background of advanced study, not necessarily in medicine.

Dropsy: An excessive accumulation of water in tissue or cavities of the body.

Drugs: Any substance used as a medicine in the treatment of disease; term used by some people to mean a narcotic-like medicine.

Dysmenorrhea: Difficult and uncomfortable or even painful menstruation.

Dyspareunia: Painful sexual intercourse.

Dyspepsia: Indigestion or upset stomach.

Dysuria: Difficulty or pain in urination.

Ecology: The study of the interrelationship of organisms and their environment.

Ectomorph: One who has a slender, tall build with small bone structure.

Ectomy: A suffix meaning *to cut out*.

Ectopic Pregnancy: Pregnancy occurring elsewhere than in the cavity of the uterus.

Edema: An abnormal amount of fluid in the tissues causing swelling.

Ego: Usually pertains to the Freudian concept of the conscious, which operates in contact with the external environment on what is called the "Reality Principle."

Ejaculation: The propulsion of the semen from the male urethra normally initiated by the sexual climax or orgasm.

Electrocardiogram (ECG or EKG): A graph of the electrical changes occurring during the contraction of the heart muscle.

Electroencephalogram (EEG): A graph of the electrical impulses in the brain.

Electromyogram (EMG): A graph of the electrical impulses in a muscle.

Electron: A unit of electrical charge, which forms the constituents of the outer part of the atom.

Embolus: A transported blood clot or foreign matter causing a blockage in the circulatory system.

Endemic: Continuously prevalent (said of a disease, as distinguished from an epidemic). Prevailing continuously in a circumscribed area.

Endo: A prefix meaning *within*.

Endocardium: The membrane lining the interior of the heart.

Endocrine: Pertaining to the secretions from the ductless glands.

Endometrium: The tissue lining the uterus.

Endomorph: One who tends to be obese with poor musculature.

Engorged: Filled, distended, congested, hyperemic.

Enzyme: A catalyst; that which promotes chemical change.

Epidemic: A temporary increase in a disease within the community. An increase over the five-year median of a disease within a circumscribed area.

Epidermophytosis: Athlete's foot.

Epididymitis: Inflammation of the epididymis—the excretory duct or canal of the testis.

Epilepsy: A disorder of the nervous system characterized by erratic loss of consciousness, twitching, or convulsions.

Episiotomy: Cutting into the perineum for obstetrical purposes.

Erg: A measure of energy equal to that required for an electron to ionize about 20 billion atoms of air.

Erogenous: Producing sexual excitement.

Erotic: Related to the arousal or stimulation of sexual thoughts or desires.

Erythroblastosis Fetalis: A disorder of the newborn characterized by excessive destruction of red blood cells.

Erythrocytes: Red blood cells that serve as oxygen carriers.

Estrogen: A steroid hormone producing female characteristics.

Etiology: The cause of a disease.

Exacerbation: Increase in the severity of symptoms.

Exercise: Physical activity or exertion that helps keep the body functioning effectively.

Faddist: One who follows a particular course of action with exaggerated zeal and enthusiasm.

Fantasy: Daydreaming or other mental activity that is contrary to the true facts of the situation; a mental make-believe world.

Fatality Rate: The number of deaths due to a particular disease per specified number of cases.

Fatigue: Lessened ability to respond or to react to a given situation due to overstimulation, overexposure, exertion, or other factors.

Fat-soluble: Soluble in fats or fat solvents, such as ether or alcohol.

Fatty Acid: Organic compound containing the carboxyl (-COOH) group that can combine with glycerol to form neutral fat.

Feces: Waste material excreted from the intestinal tract, also referred to as stool, or bowel movement.

Fecundity: Fertility.

Fellatio: The act of taking the penis into the mouth.

Fetishism: Sexual gratification achieved by means of an object, such as an article of clothing, that bears sexual symbolism for the individual.

Fimbria: Finger-like projections from the distal ends of the Fallopian tubes.

Fission: The nuclear process whereby the nucleus of an atom such as uranium is split into two parts. The energy given off during this process is released as heat and radiation.

Fission Products (also called "fission fragments"): Split halves of the uranium or other fissionable atom. They include about 36 different elements and almost 200 different radioactivities.

Flatulence: Excessive amount of gas in the stomach and intestines.

Fourchette: The fold of mucous membrane connecting the labia minora along the posterior wall at the vagina outlet.

Fraud: Intentional perversion of truth to induce another to purchase some product or service.

Frenulum: A small fold of skin retained on the ventral surface of the penis after circumcision.

Frigidity: Sexual indifference or coldness; inability to respond to normal sexual stimuli.

Frustration: A response to the disruption of ongoing behavior.

Fugue: Amnesia in which the individual wanders or runs away.

Functional: Altering the way an organ or system operates without initial demonstrable change. Not caused by an organic defect.

Gamete: A germ cell, whether an ovum or a spermatozoon.

Gamma Ray: A penetrating ray such as is emitted by radium. From a medical standpoint, gamma rays are more penetrating than X-rays, but in a physical sense both are the same in nature. A gamma ray and an X-ray of the same energy are identical.

FOUNDATIONS OF HEALTH SCIENCE

Ganglia: Groups of nerve cells located in the brain and spinal cord.

Genes: The factors located on the chromosome that determine specific characteristics.

Genitalia: Reproductive organs.

Geriatrics: The branch of medicine concerned with the problems of the aged.

Germs: Infectious agents that produce disease.

Gestation: Period from conception to birth; pregnancy.

Gingiva: The gums.

Gingivitis: Inflammation of the gums.

Glans: Cone-shaped body that forms the tip of the penis or clitoris.

Glaucoma: An eye disease characterized by increased pressure, atrophy, and blindness.

Glycogen: The form in which carbohydrate is stored in the body; animal starch.

Gonad: A gland that produces germ cells; the testicle or ovary.

Gynecologist: Specialist in the diseases of women.

Half-life: The length of time required for the decay of one-half of the atoms in a given sample.

Hallucination: A disorder of perception; seeing or hearing things that are not there.

Health (optimal): State of complete physical, mental, and social well-being, not merely the absence of disease or infirmity.

Hebephrenia: Disintegration of the personality accompanied by regression.

Helminth: A parasitic worm such as the tapeworm and hookworm.

Hemiplegia: Paralysis of one side of the body.

Hemoglobin: The compound in red blood cells that has the ability to combine with oxygen.

Hemorrhoids: Enlarged or varicosed veins in the rectum and anal region.

Hermaphrodite: An individual who has generative organs of both sexes or seems to have. True hermaphrodites are extremely rare.

Herpes: An inflammatory reaction of the skin in which small blisters or vessicles appear.

Heterozygous: Dissimilar genetic composition; having unlike genes.

Homeostasis: Maintenance of equilibrium or a steady bodily state.

Homosexuality: The inclination of one sex to the same sex in matters of love and affection, usually with antipathy to such matters with members of the opposite sex.

Homozygous: The same genetic composition; germ cells contain identical genes for a specific character.

Hormone: Chemical substance secreted by an endocrine gland.

Host: An individual or animal or plant that harbors a parasite or pathogen.

Hydrocele: Collection of serous fluid in a cavity, specifically, the tunica vaginalis testis (serous sheath lining testis and epididymis).

Hymen: Membrane fold located at the entrance to the vagina.

Hyperopia: Farsightedness.

Hypertension: Excessive tension; usually means high blood pressure.

Hypochondriasis: A morbid concern about health; exaggerated attention to bodily or mental sensations.

Hypoxia: Low level of oxygen.

Hysterectomy: Partial or total removal of the uterus.

Hysteria: Syndrome of emotional disorder that includes localized sensory and motor symptoms.

Id: The unconscious, which contains all of the primitive urges, emotions, and feelings; operates on the "Pleasure Principle" and is driven by psychic or sexual energy.

Identification: Taking on the characteristics of or acting like an admired individual.

Immunity: Resistance against invading organisms.

Immunology: Bacteriological and chemical science concerned with immunity to disease.

Impotence: Inability of the man to copulate.

Incubation: The development without sign or symptom of an infection from the time it gains entry until the appearance of the first signs or symptoms.

Inebriate: An excessive drinker.

Infarction: Necrotic changes (death of cells) resulting from the obstruction of an end artery.

Infection: Invasion by living pathogenic microorganisms of a part of the body where the conditions are favorable to their growth, and whence their toxins may gain access to, and act injuriously upon, the tissues.

Infectious Disease: A disease that is caused by an invading organism.

Infestation: Invasion by macroparasites, such as worms.

Inflammation: Pain, heat, redness, and swelling of tissues.

Ingestion: Act of taking food into the body by way of the mouth.

Inoculation: The injection of a substance into the body for the purpose of producing immunity.

Insemination: Fertilization of the female by introduction of male sperm.

In Situ: In place or in position.

Insomnia: Inability to fall asleep.

Integration: Organization of experiences, data, and emotional capacities into a unified whole.

Interstitial: Relating to spaces in a structure.

Intractable: Obstinate, resistant to treatment, difficult to control.

Intromission: The entrance of the penis into the vagina.

Invasive: Power to invade.

In Vitro: Within glass; in a test tube or culture dish.

In Vivo: Within the body.

Involutional Melancholia: A depressive form of manic-depressive psychosis occurring during menopause.

Ionization: The process whereby one or more electrons is removed from a neutron by the action of radiation.

Ionizing Radiation: The term applied to electromagnetic radiation, i.e., X-rays or gamma rays, or alpha or beta particles or neutrons, which produce ions as they pass through tissues.

Irradiation: The use of such sources of radiant energy as radioactive, ultraviolet, and infrared rays.

Isometric: Type of muscular contraction that occurs when the ends of the muscle are fixed so that activity is evidenced by increase in tension without change in length. Exercising by tensing a muscle and maintaining the tension (or contraction) beyond the point of comfort (until fatigue occurs). Movement does not take place in this kind of exercise.

Isometrics: Muscular contractions in which the individual exerts force against resistance that does not move.

Isotonic: Pertaining to contraction of a muscle when one end is attached to a light weight, which is lifted when the muscle shortens. Exercising by using weights.

Isotonics: Muscular contractions in which the individual exerts force against resistance that does move.

Isotopes: Atoms of the same element that differ from each other by having different weight. For example, strontium-89 and strontium-90.

Itis: A suffix meaning *inflammation*.

Kwashiorkor: A condition (group of symptoms) resulting from lack of protein.

Kyphosis: Humpback; anterior-posterior anatomical defect of the upper back region.

Labia: Plural for labium, which is a lip-shaped structure.

Larynx: The voice box.

Latent: Not manifest; concealed; a period of incubation of an infectious disease before the appearance of any symptom.

Leukemia: A cancer-like disease of the blood-forming organs.

Leukocytes: White blood cells serving as a body defense against disease and infection.

Leukorrhea: A whitish vaginal discharge.

Libido: Sexual urge or desire.

Licensed Physician: A practitioner of medicine; a medical man; a doctor; a person fitted by knowledge, and licensed by the proper authorities, to examine and care for the sick. He may use any type of therapy including medicines and surgery. He uses the identification "M.D." A minimum of 3 years of college, 4 years of professional school, 1 year of internship, and passing a state examination is required.

Lipids: Fats and oils; comprehensive term including compounds that are insoluble in water but have the capacity to be metabolized by the body.

Local Disease: An infection that is contained within a circumscribed area, or in one part of the body.

Lordosis: Hollow-back; exaggerated forward curvature of the lumbar or lower back region.

Lymphatic System: Drainage mechanism for special body fluids comprised of lymph glands and special vessels.

Macule: A small spot not elevated above the surface of the skin.

Maidenhead: The hymen.

Malaise: A feeling of lethargy and illness.

Malignant: Persistent, unconfined and uncontrolled; severe, unresponsive to treatment, frequently fatal.

Malingering: Conscious feigning of illness.

Malocclusion: Improper or poor contact between maxiliary and mandibular teeth: Abnormal or bad "bite."

Malpractice: Treatment of a medical case by a physician in a manner contrary to accepted procedures and with injurious results.

Mantoux Test: A skin test to detect tuberculosis infection.

Masochism: A sexual deviation in which one derives sexual gratification from having pain inflicted.

Mastectomy: Surgical removal of the breast.

Masturbation: The act of producing sexual orgasm without sexual union, whether by the hand or finger, as the name implies, or by other means.

Medical Specialist: An M.D. who, after licensure or completing basic requirements, obtains additional academic and clinical experiences upon the completion of which he may take oral and written examinations given by a recognized "specialist" in that subject or condition. Upon successful completion of these requirements (2 to 6 years after licensure) he may use the title "certified" or "board man." Examples are surgeons, obstetricians, and pediatricians.

Medicare: Governmental program of medical care for those 65 years of age or over.

Medieval Period: The Middle Ages, from about 500 to 1400 A.D.

Meiosis: Part of the process of maturation of the sex cell in which the paired chromosomes are split and each of the resulting cells contains only 23 rather than 46 chromosomes.

Menarche: Onset of the menstrual period.

Menopause: Cessation of the menses or menstruation.

Menorrhea: Normal menstruation.

Menstruation: The periodic bloody discharge from the uterus.

Mental Retardation: Impaired or inadequate intellectual functioning.

Mesomorph: Of muscular and athletic build.

Metabolism: Bodily transformations of food to produce energy or new tissue.

Metazoa: Multicellular animal in which the cells are differentiated and form tissues.

Metastasis: Spread from one part to another; in neoplasms, appearance of the same, or primary growth in other parts of the body.

Metrorrhagia: Vaginal bleeding unrelated to menstrual bleeding.

Microbe: A minute one-celled form of life either animal or vegetable, a microorganism.

Micturition: Urination.

Millirad: One thousandth (1/1,000) of a rad.

Miscarriage: Expulsion of a fetus from the onset of the fourth to the end of the sixth month of pregnancy.

Mitosis: Cellular division in which the chromosomes duplicate themselves before splitting off into daughter cells each of which will contain the full complement of chromosomes.

Morbidity: A diseased state; ratio of sick to well in a community.

Mores: Customs, established folkways.

Mortality: Death; the death rate.

Mucus: A clear viscid secretion consisting of mucin, epithelial cells, leukocytes, and various inorganic salts suspended in water.

Mutation: A transformation of the gene, which may be induced by radiation and may alter characteristics of the offspring.

Narcissism: Self-love; a state in which the individual regards everything in relation to himself.

Narcotic: A drug that produces stupor, insensibility, or sound sleep; commonly used in reference to opiates and synthetics thereof.

Nematode: A worm, a class in the phylum *Nemathelminthes*.

Neoplasm: Any new growth, particularly that which is unlimited and uncontrolled.

Nephritis: Inflammation of the kidney.

Nephrosis: A noninflammatory disease of the kidney.

Neurasthenic: Syndrome of emotional disorder that includes pathological fatigue, hypochondriasis, and vague aches and pains.

Neurosis: Functional emotional disease of a relatively minor nature characterized by ineffective means of coping with self and environment.

Neutron: A basic constituent of all atomic nuclei that, when released in the fission process, may produce fission in other nuclei or induce radioactivity in them.

Nocturnal Emission: Ejaculation of semen during sleep.

Normal: Common, typical, or standard; like the majority.

Nostrum: Medicine distributed by a quack; generally sold as a cure-all remedy.

Nucleic Acid: Complex compound found in nuclei of cells and composed of phosphoric acid, purines and pyramidines, and sugars. It may serve as template for synthesis of protein from free amino acids.

Nymphomania: Excessive and uncontrollable sexual desire in the female.

Obsessions: Unwanted, irrational, persistent thoughts.

Onanism: A withdrawal of the penis from the vagina before completion of the act of copulation. Coitus interruptus.

Ophthalmologist or Oculist: A licensed physician, M.D., who specializes in medical and surgical treatment of eye disorders and diseases.

Opiate: A drug derived from opium.

Optician: A maker of optical instruments; one who makes and adjusts eyeglasses and spectacles after a formula prescribed by the oculist or optometrist. He may not test for visual defects or prescribe lenses.

Optometrist: A vision specialist who measures the degree of visual acuity and visual functions. In general, he does not have medical training. He may not use medication or surgery. He may use the title of "doctor" or the initials "O.D."

Organic: Characterized by pathological structural change, primarily caused by alteration of the structure of an organ or system.

Organic Disease: A disease that involves some organic impairment to body function. There is alteration in the structure of the organ involved.

Orgasm: The climax of sexual excitement in coitus or sexual intercourse.

Orifice: An opening or aperture.

Orthodontist: A specialist in the field of dentistry who treats irregularities in the position of the teeth.

Os: A mouth or orifice.

Osteopathy: A philosophy of medicine based upon the theory that the normal body, when in correct adjustment, is a vital machine capable of making its own remedies against infections and other toxic conditions. An osteopath may use the title "D.O." or "M.D.," and he can be a licensed physician in the full sense of the word. He completes the same academic and clinical preparation as an M.D., though in a different school.

Otologist: An M.D. specializing in diseases of the ear.

Otomy: A suffix meaning *to cut into.*

Otosclerosis: A formation of spongy bone around the stapes and fenestra vestibuli in the ear resulting in progressively increasing deafness.

Ovary: The female reproductive gland producing the ovum or germinal cell.

Overcompensation: Offsetting some deficiency or a lack in some area to an extreme degree, as in the case of the "obnoxious egotist" who is over-compensating for a gross inferiority complex.

Ovulation: Discharge of an ovum.

Paleopathology: Science dealing with disease relationships evidenced through various remains of life before the beginning of recorded history.

Palliate: To reduce the severity, make more comfortable, or to mitigate.

Pandemic: An epidemic that is worldwide.

"Pap" or Cervical Smear Test: A microscopic examination of cells obtained from secretions found on the cervix (mouth of the uterus).

Papule: A small circumscribed, solid elevation of the skin.

Paranoia: Systematized delusions, frequently of persecution, sometimes of grandeur.

Parasite: A plant or animal that lives off another organism.

Parity: The state of a woman in regard to having children, primiparity is having borne one child.

Parturition: The process of giving birth.

Passive Immunity: Immunity provided by giving antibodies made in the serum of animals or another human.

Pasteurization: Killing of pathogenic bacteria in milk or other liquid by moderate heating (60°C.) for 30 minutes. More intense heat may be applied for a shorter length of time.

Patch Test: A skin test to detect tuberculosis infection.

Patent: Open, expanded.

Patent Medicine: A nonprescription medicine.

Pathogen: Disease-producing agent.

Pathogenesis: The mode of origin and development of a disease.

Pedophilia: Sexual involvement of an adult with a child.

Peri: A prefix meaning *around.*

Pericardium: Tough membranous tissue enclosing the heart.

Perineum: The area between the thighs, extending from the posterior junction of the labia majora to the anus in the female and from the scrotum to the anus in the male.

Periodontitis: Inflammation of the periodontia.

Periodontium: Supporting structure of tooth. Tissue that invests the tooth.

Peristalsis: The rhythmic wave of contractions of the intestinal walls or other tubelike structure.

Peritonitis: Inflammation of the peritoneum, the membrane lining the interior of the abdominal cavity.

Pertussis: Whooping cough.

Phagocyte: A white blood cell.

Phagocytosis: Ingestion by a phagocyte of other cells, bacteria, dead tissue, and foreign particles.

Phallus: The male organ of copulation; the penis.

Phenylketonuria (PKU): An inborn disease of metabolism characterized by mental deficiency and urinary excretion of phenylpyruvic acid.

Phimosis: Excessive tightness of the foreskin of the penis.

Phobia: Morbid or pathological fear.

Physical Fitness: Condition of readiness through which the requirements of daily living can be most effectively met.

Placenta: Organ by which the unborn infant is attached to the inside of the uterus and through which the infant's body needs can be supplied; expelled after birth.

Plaque: A patch, or small differentiated area, on the skin or a mucous surface.

Plasma: Liquid or fluid portion of the blood.

Podiatrist (chiropodist): A specialist in the diagnosis and/or treatment of the diseases, injuries, and defects of the human foot. He is called "doctor," and he may be licensed to use any or all medical and surgical techniques in treating the feet.

Polyunsaturated Fat: A fat with multiple carbon molecules unsaturated. Does not increase the blood level of cholesterol to the same extent as saturated fats.

Posture: Position or bearing of the body.

Potency: Capability or strength. Also the capacity for erection sufficient to engage in sexual intercourse.

Prehistoric: Period of time before written history.

Premature Birth: Birth between the sixth and end of the ninth month.

Premature Ejaculation: Orgasm with loss of semen either before introduction of the penis into the vagina or imediately afterward thus giving the female partner insufficient time to reach a climax.

Prepuce: The foreskin of the penis or clitoris.

Presbyopia: A change in the accommodation power of the eye in aging.

Presumptive: Diagnosis based on medical history and observation without laboratory confirmation.

Prodromal: The initial stage of a disease in which symptoms are general rather than specific to that disease.

Progesterone: A hormone secreted by the corpus luteum. It stimulates growth of the endometrium.

Projection: Seeing in or attributing to others a motive or characteristic of self, frequently of an undesirable nature.

Promiscuity: Indiscriminate sexual relationships.

Proprietary Drugs: Reputable chemicals used by competent physicians in supplement to standard drugs.

Proprietary Hospital: Owned and operated privately for profit.

Prosthesis: An artificial device used to replace a body part.

Prosthodontics: The branch of dentistry pertaining to restoration and maintenance of oral function by replacement of missing teeth and structures by artificial devices.

Protein: Complex foodstuff formed by various combinations of approximately 20 different amino acids. It is essential for growth and maintenance of life.

Pruritus: Itching.

Psychasthenic: Syndrome of emotional disorder that includes severe persistent phobias, obsessions, and compulsions.

Psychic Determinism: The postulate that mental processes and behavior are completely dependent upon and fully explicable in terms of antecedent events, past experiences, and conditions.

Psychoneurosis: Same as neurosis. A personality disorder characterized by the inability to make satisfactory adjustments and to withstand frustrations.

Psychopathic: Having marked deficiency in ethical and moral values plus an inability to follow approved modes of behavior. Also known as sociopathic.

Psychosis: A mental disorder that is so severe that at times the afflicted is incapable of functioning.

Psychosomatic: Having functional emotional causes; particularly referring to dysfunctions of organs controlled by the autonomic nervous system.

Pudenda: The external sex organ.

Pyorrhea: Disease of gums and tissues supporting the teeth in which there is a purulent discharge.

Quack: Fake or incompetent medical practitioner.

Quarantine: The isolation of a person sick with a contagious disease until the period of contagiousness is over. The isolation of all contacts of a person sick with a contagious disease until such time as the period of communicability is passed.

Quiescent: Quiet, without symptoms.

Rad: A unit of absorbed dose, or a measure of radiation exposure, which amounts to 100 ergs of energy imparted to one gram of matter by any ionizing radiation of irradiated material at the place of interest.

Radioactivity: The phenomenon whereby atoms disintegrate and emit radiation.

Rationalization: Developing reasons from some act or thought other than that which may be actually true, such as excuses.

Reagin: A nonspecific tissue antibody that is found circulating in the blood of people who have a collagen disease (diseases or conditions affecting connective tissue, bone, and cartilage).

Rectocele: Protrusion of part of the rectum into the posterior floor of the vagina; herniation of rectum.

Regression: Engaging in behavior that is characteristic of a much younger person.

Remission: An abatement of symptoms or reduction in severity of symptoms.

Renaissance: Transitional period following medieval times; the 14th, 15th, and 16th centuries.

Repression: Blocking from consciousness, or pushing down into unconscious, a feeling or emotion that is completely unacceptable to the individual, hence completely forgotten and very difficult to recall. The severe difficulty in recollection makes repression different from suppression.

Reservoir: Source of infection.

Retrograde: Moving backward or reversing normal growth and development.

Rheumatism: A group of diseases characterized by pains in the muscles, joints, and fibrous tissues.

Rhinitis: An acute inflammation of the mucous membrane of the nose, marked by sneezing, lacrimation, and profuse secretion of watery mucus.

Ribosome: Microscopic body within a cell, the site of protein synthesis.

Sadism: Sexual satisfaction derived from inflicting pain.

Salpingitis: Inflammation of a tube; usually refers to the Fallopian tube.

Sarcoma: Cancer involving connective tissue, e.g., bones and muscles.

Satiety: Feeling of satisfaction and fullness that follows a meal.

Saturated Fat: A fat in which the chemical potential of the carbon molecule is satisfied. Saturated fats are normally solid in form and are found in animal tissue.

Schizophrenia: An emotional illness in which there is a disturbance of one's relationships with people, resulting in withdrawal.

Sclerosis: A word that may be used as a suffix, meaning *hardening*.

Scoliosis: Lateral defect of the spine.

Scrotum: The bag or pouch containing the testicles.

Self-Actualization: A term utilized by Maslow and others, pertaining to the understanding and accepting of oneself; the harmonizing and integrating of one's motives; the state of unity and integration resulting from these processes; the ultimate in self-development and emotional maturation.

Semen: The fluid ejaculated by the male in sexual intercourse.

Semination: Introduction of semen into the vagina.

Seminiferous: Tubules of the testis, carrying or conducting semen.

Sinus: A channel or canal.

Socialized Medicine: Medical care program that is governmentally financed but professionally administered.

Sociopathic: Same as psychopathic.

Somatic: Pertaining to the body in its physical sense.

Sperm: The male germ cell.

Sporadic: Occurring singly, neither epidemic nor endemic.

Spore: The reproductive cell of a sporozoan, a cell of inferior order to an ovum or seed.

State Medicine: Medical care program that is "state" or government-maintained and administered.

Stenosis: A narrowing of any canal; a stricture.

Sterility: Inability to reproduce.

Sterilization: The process of making sterile, usually by operative methods, tying or cutting the vas ductus in the male or the Fallopian tube in the female, though other methods are effective.

Subclinical: Not recognizable by ordinary visual or clinical observations.

Subconscious: Just below the level of consciousness, sometimes used to include the unconscious.

Subcutaneous: Beneath the skin.

Sublimation: The substitution of an unacceptable urge with one that is highly socially approved, as an artist might sublimate unacceptable sexual urges, which are expressed in highly acceptable art forms.

Substitution: Usually relating to a sexual urge that the individual is unable to express in direct form, but which may be expressed in a form of telling dirty stories, or singing risque songs; hence, an expression of the direct urge in a more acceptable fashion.

Superego: A Freudian concept consisting of the ideal self-image—that is, the person one most would like to be; the total sum of the moral values and ideals internalized by the individual.

Suppression: Slightly forgotten material, which may be and usually is unpleasant or unacceptable, and is fairly easily recalled.

Suppuration: The formation of pus.

Susceptibility: Liability to acquire; condition of having little protection against.

Symbiosis: The growth of two or more organisms in mutually satisfying relationship.

FOUNDATIONS OF HEALTH SCIENCE

Synapse: The place where a nerve impulse is transmitted from one neuron to another.

Syncope: Fainting.

Syndrome: An aggregate of symptoms associated with a specific disease.

Synergistic: Working together, cooperation in action.

Systemic Disease: An infection that is widespread throughout the body.

Systole: Contraction of the heart muscle.

Tartar: A brownish or yellow-brown deposit on the teeth.

Teleological: Pertaining to a pulling force in life; concerned with ends, purposes, and goals.

Teratogenic: Producing abnormalities in the embryo and fetus.

Testicle: The male reproductive organ that produces sperm; it also secretes certain hormones related to the sexual activity of the individual.

Testimonial: Statement made by an individual or group attesting to the value or benefits of a particular product or service.

Therapeutic Devices: Machines or instruments promoted by the quack to diagnose and treat disease.

Thrombus: A clot more or less occluding a blood vessel, or a clot in one of the chambers of the heart.

Tissue: Mass or group of cells of a particular type.

Tonometer: An instrument for determining intraocular tension. Used in diagnosing glaucoma.

Toxemia: The clinical symptoms produced by toxins or poisonous substances in the blood.

Toxic: Poisonous.

Toxicity: The degree of being poisonous.

Toxin: Poison.

Toxoid: A toxin that has been treated so as to reduce its poisonous effects but retain its antigenic properties.

T.P.I.: Treponema pallidum immobilization test, a specific antibody test for syphilis used to make a definitive diagnosis. Relatively expensive and not used for screening as a rule.

Trachea: The windpipe.

Trachoma: A specific infection of the lining of the eyelids.

Trauma: Injury; a wound inflicted somewhat suddenly.

Trophoblasts: Cells attaching the fertilized ovum to the uterine wall. These cells contribute to the formation of the placenta.

Tumor: A growth of cells or tissues serving no physiological purpose. Any swelling.

Unconscious: Like the portion of an iceberg below the water's surface, it includes the 90 percent plus of thoughts, feelings, urges, emotions, experiences, and other psychic matter that one is not aware of, or has "forgotten"; sometimes used so as to include the subconscious.

Unsaturated Fat: A fat in which the chemical potential of the carbon molecule is not satisfied. Unsaturated fats are derivatives of vegetable substances. They are normally vegetable oils such as corn oil and tend to be soft or liquid.

Ureter: The tube conducting urine from the kidney to the bladder.

Urethra: A canal leading from the bladder through which urine is discharged.

Uterus: The womb, a hollow pear-shaped organ in which the fertilized ovum develops into a child.

Vaccine: Pathogens treated so as to reduce their disease-producing properties but not their antigenic-producing properties.

Vagina: Literally, a sheath; the female copulative organ.

Varicocele: Hernia varicosa. Varicose enlargement of the veins of the spermatic cord causing boggy tumor of the scrotum.

Vas Deferens: An elongated tube or duct leading from the testicle to the ejaculatory duct.

Vasectomy: Removal of the vas deferens; operation to sterilize the male.

V.D.R.L.: A reagen blood test for syphilis named after the laboratory in which it was developed—Venereal Disease Research Laboratory, Public Health Service Communicable Disease Center, Atlanta, Georgia.

Vector: Animal or insect carrier of disease-producing organisms.

Venereal Disease: Infections relating to or transmitted by sexual intercourse or by prolonged, close, intimate contact of genital organs.

Ventricles: Lower chambers of the heart.

Vertigo: Sensation that the environment is spinning around; a type of dizziness.

Vesicle: A blister; a small circumscribed elevation on the skin containing serum.

Viable: Capable of living.

Vincent's Angina: Trench mouth. Painful bleeding gums and ulcerations of the gums. Not communicable.

FOUNDATIONS OF HEALTH SCIENCE

Virulence: The power of an infectious organism to invade the body and cause disease.

Viscera: The internal organs.

Visual Acuity: Sharpness of vision.

Voyeurism: Peeping Tom. Obtaining sexual gratification by looking at sexual objects or situations.

Vulva: The external genitalia of women.

Wasserman Test: A reagin blood test to determine whether syphilis is present.

Wellness: Sub-health level ranging from low- to high-level wellness.

Zygote: The fertilized ovum; fusion of the nuclei of the sperm and ovum.

BIBLIOGRAPHY AND
SUGGESTED READINGS

Chapter 1. Health Concepts

Abrams, Mark. "The Quality of Life." *World Health,* November, 1974, pp. 4–11.

Asinof, Eliot. "What Doesn't a Campus Doctor Encounter?" *Today's Health,* 50: 35–39, 55–58, January, 1972.

Bardin, John. " 'Must' Books for Every Home Health Library." *Today's Health,* 50: 20–23, 65–66, 71, September, 1972.

Chase, Helen. "The Most Healthful States in the U.S.A." *Today's Health,* 51: 34–37, 67, 70–72, May, 1973.

Dolfman, Michael L. "Toward Operational Definitions of Health." *Journal of School Health,* 44: 206–09, April, 1974.

Douglas, William O. "Toward Greater Vitality." *Today's Health,* 51: 54–57, 72, May, 1973.

Evang, Karl. "Health for Everyone." *World Health,* November, 1973, pp. 2–11.

Halberstam, Michael. "Can You Make Yourself Sick?" *Today's Health,* 50: 24–29, December, 1972.

Hoyman, Howard S. "Rethinking an Ecologic-System Model of Man's Health, Disease, Aging, Death." *The Journal of School Health,* 45: 509–519, November, 1975.

Johnson, Warren R. "Magic, Morals, and Health." *School Health Review,* 1: 5–9, November, 1969.

Koch, Joanne and Lew. "Put a Little More Romance in Your Life." *Today's Health,* 53: 36–39, 52–53, February, 1975.

Matson, Hollis N. "Values: How and From Where?" *School Health Review,* 5: 36–38, January–February, 1974.

Masland, Robert P. "Adolescent Unrest and the Schools—The Impact Upon Health." *J. School Health,* 39: 603–607, November, 1969.

Rennie, Drummond. "What You Can Learn About Health From TV." *Today's Health,* 51: 22–26, January, 1973.

Russell, Robert D. "Toward a Functional Understanding of Ecology for Health Education." *J. School Health,* 39: 702–708, December, 1969.

Smith, G. Kerry (ed.). *Stress and Campus Response.* Washington: American Association for Higher Education, 1968.

"Test Your Health I.Q." *Today's Health,* 52: 36–37, December, 1974.

Tolar, Calvin J. "The Mental Health of Students—Do Teachers Hurt or Help?" *J. School Health,* 45: 71–75, February, 1975.

Wallace, Helen M. "The Training of Adolescent Health Service Personnel." *Journal of School Health,* 45: 535–541, November, 1975.

Werner, Arnold. "Health-Related Concerns of College Students," *Journal of the American College Health Association,* 24: 276–283, June, 1976.

Willgoose, Carl E. "Value Illness," *JOHPER,* 36: 25, 74, March, 1965.

Chapter 2. Health Information: Products and Services

Conniff, James C. "How to Tell a Good Hospital from a Bad One." *Today's Health,* 51: 42–45, 70–71, November, 1973.

Furlong, William B. "You and Your Dangerous Health Practices." *Today's Health,* 50: 54–58, 60, October, 1972.

Holbrook, Stewart H. *The Golden Age of Quackery.* New York: Macmillan, 1969.

Kahn, E. J. "A Stamp of Disapproval for These 'Medical' Malpractitioners." *Today's Health,* 52: 20–23, 67, March, 1974.

Kaplan, Jack. "Frauds Who Prey on Shaky Marriages." *Today's Health,* 47: 16–19, 72, June, 1969.

Linderman, Bard. "What You Can Expect from Cosmetic Surgery." *Today's Health,* 50: 16–19, 56–58, 60, July, 1972.

Littler, Gene. "A Physical Checkup Saved My Life." *Today's Health,* 50: 28–29, November, 1972.

Lu, F. C. "Food Additives: Many Advantages and Some Hazards." *World Health,* February–March, 1974, pp. 34–37.

Masters, William H. "Phoney Sex Clinics—Medicine's Newest Nightmare." *Today's Health,* 52: 22–26, November, 1974.

Rakstis, Ted J. "Sensitivity Training: Fad, Fraud, or New Frontier?" *Today's Health,* 48: 20–25, 86–87, January, 1970.

Rosen, Samuel. "Beware of the 'Quackupuncturist' Who Operates for Profit." *Today's Health,* 52: 6–7, 66–67, August, 1974.

Schultz, Dodi. "When You Should (and Shouldn't) Call the Doctor." *Today's Health,* 50: 20–23, 59–61, August, 1972.

Smith, Ralph L. "Chiropractic: Issues and Answers." *Today's Health,* 48: 64–69, January, 1970.

Squires, Raymond. "A Shut-In's View of Television Commercials." *PTA Magazine,* 63: 32–33, June, 1969.

Chapter 3.   Health Maintenance

Bardin, John. " 'Must' Books for Every Home Health Library." *Today's Health,* 50: 21–24, 65, 66, September, 1972.

Belinsky, Irmgard, Hiromi Shinya, and William I. Wolff. "Colonofibero-scopy: Technique in Colon Examination." *American Journal of Nursing,* 73: 306–309, February, 1973.

Bullough, Bonnie. "The Source of Ambulatory Health Services as It Relates to Preventive Care." *American Journal of Public Health,* 64: 582–589, June, 1974.

"Cancer: Where We Stand Today, Part I." *Medical World News.* 15: 55–64, March 22, 1974.

"Child Immunizing Lag Causes Alarm." *Medical World News,* 15: 49, 48, August 9, 1974.

Donabedian, Avedis. "Issues in National Health Insurance." *American Journal of Public Health,* 66: 345–351, April, 1976.

Eason, Charles F., Barbara G. Brooks. "Should Medical Radiation Exposure Be Recorded?" *American Journal of Public Health,* 62: 1189–1194, September, 1972.

"Early Detection: Reasons To Suspect Colorectal Cancer." *Medical World News,* 14: 49, June 1, 1973.

Egeberg, Roger O. "Fluoridation for All: A National Priority." *Today's Health,* 48:30–32, 58–60, June, 1970.

Evans, Melvin H. "The Politics of Health." *American Lung Association Bulletin,* 60: 3–7, July–August, 1974.

Fishbein, Morris. "The Function of the Pharmacist." *Medical World News,* 14: 116, September 21, 1973.

Fishbein, Morris. "On Seeing the Doctor." *Medical World News,* 13: 68, November 24, 1972.

Fletcher, Joseph. "The Control of Death." *Intellectual Digest,* 4: 82, 83, October, 1973.

Francis, Byron John. "Current Concepts in Immunization." *American Journal of Nursing,* 73: 646–650, April, 1973.

Gieger, H. Jack. "How Acupuncture Anesthetizes: The Chinese Explanation." *Medical World News,* 14:51–62, July 13, 1973.

Gerber, Alex. *The Gerber Report.* New York: David McKay, 1971.

Harrison, Stanley. "The Most Important 30 Minutes of Your Child's Life." *Today's Health,* 54: 42, 45, 67–70, August, 1974.

Halberstam, Michael. "Heart Scares." *Today's Health,* 54: 36–40, April, 1974.

Lander, Louise. *National Health Insurance*. New York: Health/PAC, 1975.

Life and Death and Medicine. San Francisco: W. H. Freeman, 1973.

Lov, Joseph. "Dental Insurance: A Developing Success Story," *Today's Health*, 48: 48, 49, 71, March, 1970.

McTaggart, Aubrey C. *The Health Care Dilemma*. Boston: Holbrook Press, 1976.

"More Kinds and Cases of VD." *Medical World News*, 16: 3747, July 28, 1975.

Mother, Ira. "The Real and Urgent Problems of Science and Ethics, Part 2." *Intellectual Digest*, 4: 66–70, September, 1973.

"Opthalmologist, Oculist, Optometrist, Optician." *Today's Health*, 47: 53–55, March, 1969.

Nolen, William. "Rules to Make You a Better Patient." *Today's Health*, 51: 41, 42, 66, 67, April, 1973.

"Resourceful Ways To Keep Your Medical Bills Down." *Today's Health*, 51: 18–23, 71, 72, October, 1973.

Schultz, Dodi. "When You Should (and Shouldn't) Call the Doctor." *Today's Health*, 50: 21–24, 59, 60, 61, August, 1972.

Soika, Cynthia Vaughan. "Gynecologic Cytology." *American Journal of Nursing*, 73: 2092–2095, December, 1973.

"Vaccines: An Update." *FDA Consumer*, December, 1973/January, 1974, pp. 24–29.

Chapter 4. Physical Fitness

Ashby, Neal. "Togetherness Exercises To Get You in Better Shape." *Today's Health*, 52: 34–37, 60, January, 1974.

Brown, Roscoe C., Jr., and Bryant J. Cratty. *New Perspectives of Man in Action*. Englewood Cliffs, N.J.: Prentice-Hall, 1969.

Cooper, Kenneth H. "The Role of Exercise in Our Contemporary Society." *JOHPER*, 40: 22–25, May, 1969.

Croughan, Jack L. "Insomnia: the Ubiquitous Malady." *Medical World News*, 16: 50, October 27, 1975.

Davis, Flora. "Tick-Tock, The Human Clock." *Family Health*, 7: 26–29, February, 1975.

Devine, Barry. "Run For Your Life," *JOHPER*, 43: 44–46, November–December, 1972.

Edelson, Edward. "The Dream Hunters." *Family Health* 6: 34–37, August, 1974.

Hittleman, Richard. "Give Your Back a Break—Try Yoga." *Family Health*, 6: 44–47, September, 1974.

Hockey, Robert V. *Physical Fitness*, 2nd ed. St. Louis: C. V. Mosby, 1973.

Kock, Joanne and Susan Petrillo. "What You'd Better Know Before Joining a Health Club." *Today's Health*, 50: 16–19, 67–68, February, 1972.

Kretchmar, R. Scott, and William A. Harper. "Why Does Man Play?" *JOHPER*, 40: 57–58, March, 1969.

Lamott, Kenneth. "What to Do When Stress Signs Say You're Killing Yourself." *Today's Health*, 53: 30–33, 59–60, January, 1975.

Maness, Bill. "What Do You Really Know About Exercise?" *Today's Health*, 53: 14–18, 53, November, 1975.

Martin, Alexander Reid. "Idle Hands and Giddy Minds: Our Psychological and Emotional Unpreparedness for Free Time." *Mental Health Digest*, 2: 27–31, February, 1970.

Martin, Mark. "Is There Anything Positive About Negative-Heel Shoes?" *Today's Health*, 53: 36–40, December, 1975.

Morehouse, Laurence E. and Leonard Gross. "Shape Up." *Family Health*, 7: 34–37, 66–67, February, 1975.

Porr, Dennis S. "Male vs. Female." *The Foil*, nv: 9–17, Fall, 1975.

Owens, Jesse. "We're Too Athletic." *Today's Health*, 50: 68–69, January, 1972.

Root, Leon, and Thomas Kiernan. "Positive Advice for Those with Back Miseries." *Today's Health*, 51: 20–23, 68–71, August, 1973.

See, Carolyn. "Ballet: The True Test of Fitness." *Today's Health*, 53: 36–44, March, 1975.

Segal, Julius. "To Sleep: Perchance to Dream." *Today's Health*, 47: 48–51, 86–87, October, 1969.

Selye, Hans. "Stress Without Distress." *World Health*, December, 1974, pp. 2–11.

Shirreffs, Janet H. "Recreational Noise: Implications for Potential Hearing Loss to Participants." *J. School Health*, 44: 548–550, December, 1974.

Tandy, Ruth E., and Joyce Laflin. "Aggression and Sport: Two Theories." *JOHPER*, 44: 19–20, June, 1973.

Taves, Isabella. "Is There a Sleepwalker in the House?" *Today's Health*, 47: 40–41, 76, May, 1969.

Wilkins, Michael H., and Richard L. Ragatz. "Cultural Changes and Leisure Time." *JOHPER*, 43: 35–37, March, 1972.

Wilkinson, Bud. "Our Guide to the Best Sports for Your Health." *Today's Health*, 50: 16–21, 65–67, May, 1972.

Chapter 5.   The Science of Nutrition

Breeling, James L. "Are We Snacking Our Way to Malnutrition." *Today's Health*, 48: 48–51, January, 1970.

Carson, Rachel. *Silent Spring*. Boston: Houghton Mifflin, 1962.

Erhard, Darla. "The New Vegetarians, Part One." *Nutrition Today*, 8: 4–13, November–December, 1973.

Erhard, Darla. "The New Vegetarians, Part Two." *Nutrition Today,* 9: 20–28, January–February, 1974.

"Food Additives: Health Question Awaiting an Answer." *Medical World News,* 14: 7381, September 7, 1973.

"The Food Fad Boom." *FDA Consumer,* December, 1973–January, 1974, pp. 5–13.

Hall, Richard L. "Food Additives." *Nutrition Today,* 8: 20–29, July–August, 1973.

Helzer, John E. "What To Do About Obesity." *Medical World News,* 16: 53, 54, October 27, 1975.

Hicks, Clifford B. " 'Eat!' Says Fat Little Johnny's Mother." *Today's Health,* 48: 48–52, 86–87, February, 1970.

Joseph, Lou. "Foods and Drinks That Will Cause You the Fewest Cavities." *Today's Health,* 51: 41, 42, October, 1973.

Lachance, Paul A. "A Commentary on the New F.D.A. Nutrition Labeling Regulations." *Nutrition Today,* 8: 18–24, January–February, 1973.

The National Nutrition Consortium, Inc. *Nutrition Labeling.* Bethesda, Md.: The National Nutrition Consortium, Inc., 1975.

"The Prudent Diet: Vintage 1973." *Medical World News,* 14: 34, 35, August 10, 1973.

Recommended Dietary Allowances. Washington, D.C.: National Academy of Sciences and the National Research Council, 1974.

Rosenstock, Irwin M. "Psychological Forces, Motivation, and Nutrition Education." *American Journal of Public Health,* 59: 1992–1998, November, 1969.

"Roughage in the Diet." *Medical World News,* 15: 35–43, September 6, 1974.

Schanche, Don A. "Diet Books That Poison Your Mind . . . and Harm Your Body." *Today's Health,* 52: 56–62, April, 1974.

Stare, Fredrick J., and Margaret McWilliams. *Living Nutrition,* New York: John Wiley & Sons, 1973.

"The State of Nutrition Today." *FDA Consumer,* 7: 13–19, November, 1973.

"There's a Fly in the Milk Bottle." *Medical World News,* 15: 30–33, May 17, 1974.

"A Vitamin Answer to Atherosclerosis?" *Medical World News,* 15: 64g–i, September 13, 1974.

"Vitamin E-Miracle or Myth?" *FDA Consumer,* 7: 22–26, July–August, 1973.

"When to Start Dieting? At Birth." *Medical World News,* 14: 31–35, September 7, 1973.

White, Philip L. *Let's Talk About Food.* Chicago: American Medical Association, 1970.

Wilson, Patience. "Iron-Deficiency Anemia." *American Journal of Nursing,* 72: 502–505, March, 1972.

Winick, M. "Childhood Obesity." *Nutrition Today,* 9: 8 May–June, 1974.

Worthington B. S., and L. E. Taylor. "Balanced Low-Calorie vs. High-Protein-Low-Carbohydrate Reducing Diets." *Journal of American Dietetics Association,* 64: 47–52, January, 1974.

Chapter 6. Emotional Health

Breeden, Sue A., and Charles Kondo. "Using Biofeedback to Reduce Tension." *American Journal of Nursing,* 75: 2010–2013, November, 1975.

Curran, W. J. "Policies and Practices Concerning Confidentiality in College Mental Health Services in the United States and Canada." *American Journal of Psychiatry,* 125: 1520–1530, May, 1969.

Harlow, H. F. "The Nature of Love." *American Psychologist,* 13: 673–685, 1958.

Kinsey, A. C., W. B. Pomeroy, and C. E. Martin. *Sexual Behavior in the Human Male.* Philadelphia: W. B. Saunders, 1948.

Kinsey, A. C., W. B. Pomeroy, C. E. Martin, and P. H. Gebhard. *Sexual Behavior in the Human Female.* Philadelphia: W. B. Saunders, 1953.

Korman, A. K. *The Psychology of Motivation.* Englewood Cliffs, N.J.: Prentice-Hall, 1974.

Maslow, A. H. *Motivation and Personality,* 2nd ed. New York: Harper & Row, 1970.

Maslow, A. H. "Self-Actualizing People." In C. E. Moustakas (ed.) *The Self.* New York: Harper & Row, 1956.

Rakstis, T. "Sensitivity Training: Fad, Fraud, or New Frontier." *Today's Health,* 48: 20–25, 86–87, January, 1970.

Rogers, C. R. *On Becoming a Person: A Therapist's View of Psychotherapy.* Boston: Houghton Mifflin, 1961.

Sawrey, James M., and Charles W. Telford. *Personality and Adjustment.* Boston: Allyn and Bacon, 1975.

Chapter 7. People with Psychological Problems

Bandura, Albert. "Behavioral Psychotherapy." *Scientific American,* 216: 78–89, March, 1967.

Chapman, H. H. "The Problem of Prognosis in Psychoneurotic Illness." *American Journal of Psychiatry,* 119: 768–770, 1963.

Coleman, J. C. *Abnormal Psychology and Modern Life,* 4th ed. Fair Lawn, N.J.: Scott, Foresman, 1970.

Goshen, Charles E. "Functional Versus Organic Diagnostic Problems." *Mental Health Digest,* 2: 20–22, January, 1970.

London, P. "The Psychotherapy Boom: From the Long Couch for the Sick to the Push Button for the Bored." *Psychology Today,* 8: 111, 62–68, 1974.

Maris, Ronald W. "The Sociology of Suicide Prevention: Policy Implications of Differences Between Suicidal Patients and Completed Suicides." *Mental Health Digest,* 2: 17–27, February, 1970.

Oswalk, Ian. "Human Brain Protein, Drugs, and Dreams." *Mental Health Digest,* 2: 5–8, January, 1970.

Sawrey, J. M., and C. W. Telford. *Personality and Adjustment.* Boston: Allyn and Bacon, 1975.

Seligman, M. E. P. *Helplessness.* New York: W. H. Freeman, 1974.

Smith, Kathleen, Geoffrey F. Thompson, and Harry D. Koster. "Sweat in Schizophrenic Patients: Identification of the Odorous Substance." *Mental Health Digest,* 2: 19, January, 1970.

Sterman, Lorraine Taylor. "Clinical Biofeedback." *American Journal of Nursing,* 75: 2006–2010, November, 1975.

"Suicide: How to keep patients from killing themselves." *Medical World News,* 17: 86–96, July 12, 1976.

Walker, Robert, William Winick, Earl S. Frost, and J. M. Lieberman. "Social Restoration of Hospitalized Psychiatric Patients Through a Program of Special Employment in Industry." *Mental Health Digest,* 2: 32–34, January, 1970.

Whittington, H. G., and Charles Steenbarger. "Preliminary Evaluation of a Decentralized Community Mental Health Clinic." *American Journal of Public Health,* 60: 64–77, January, 1970.

Williams, Denis, "Neural Factors Related to Habitual Aggression." *Mental Health Digest,* 2: 14–16, January, 1970.

Wilson, G. Terence, and Gerald C. Davison. "A Road to Self-Control." *Psychology Today,* 9: 54–61, October, 1975.

Chapter 8. Alcohol and Tobacco

Berland, Theodore. "Should Children Be Taught to Drink?" *Today's Health,* 47: 46–50, 83–88, February, 1969.

Blue Shield. *The Alcoholic American.* National Association of Blue Shield Plans, 1972.

Cahalan, Don, and Robin Room. "Problem Drinking Among American Men Aged 21–59." *American Journal of Public Health,* 62: 1473–1483, November, 1972.

Carroll, Charles R. *Alcohol: Use, Nonuse and Abuse.* Dubuque, Ia.: Wm. C. Brown, 1970.

Chafetz, Morris E. "New Federal Legislation on Alcoholism—Opportunities and Problems." *American Journal of Public Health,* 63: 206–209, March, 1973.

Chafetz, Morris E. "Problems of Reaching Youth." *Journal of School Health,* 43: 40–45, January, 1973.

The Dangers of Smoking, The Benefits of Quitting. New York: The American Cancer Society, 1972.

Doyle, Nancy C. "The Facts About Second-Hand Cigarette Smoke." *American Lung Association Bulletin,* 60: 13–16, June, 1974.

Globetti, Gerald. "The Use of Beverage Alcohol by Youth in an Abstinence Setting." *Journal of School Health,* 39: 179–183, March, 1969.

Godber, George E. "Smoking Disease: A Self-Inflicted Injury." *American Journal of Public Health,* 60: 235–242, February, 1970.

Goodwin, Donald W. "When is Alcoholism Familial?" *Medical World News,* 16: 52, October 27, 1975.

Health Consequences of Smoking: A Report to the Surgeon General, DHEW Publication No. (HSM) 73–8704. Rockville, Md.: U.S. Department of Health, Education and Welfare, 1973.

Iber, Frank L. "In Alcoholism the Liver Sets the Pace." *Nutrition Today,* 6: 2–10, January–February, 1971.

"The Influence of Alcohol: In Search of Sobriety." *The Kiwanis Magazine,* 59: 24–27, 55, 56, April, 1973.

Lieber, Charles S. "Alcohol and the Liver." *Alcohol Health and Research World,* nv: 23–27, Spring, 1974.

McDonnell, Ashley. "Jellinek Award Winner Concludes: Alcoholism 'Runs in the Family.' " *The Journal,* 4:3, March 1, 1975.

Mueller, John F. "Treatment for the Alcoholic: Cursing or Nursing?" *American Journal of Nursing,* 74: 245–248, February, 1974.

National Institute of Mental Health–National Institute of Alcohol Abuse and Alcoholism. *Alcohol and Alcoholism,* DHEW Publication No. (HSM) 72–9127, Rockville, Md.: U.S. Department of Health, Education and Welfare, 1972.

Neeman, R. L., and M. Neeman. "Complexities of Smoking Education," *Journal of School Health,* 45: 17–24, January, 1975.

Novick, Lloyd, Henry Hudson, and Elaine German. "In-Hospital Detoxification and Rehabilitation of Alcoholics In An Inner City Area." *American Journal of Public Health,* 64: 1089–1095, November, 1974.

Room, Robin. "Minimizing Alcohol Problems." *Alcohol Health and Research World,* nv: 12–18, Fall, 1974.

Steinfeld, Jesse L. "Emphysema." *American Lung Association Bulletin,* 58: 2–7, May, 1972.

Tamerin, John S., and Charles P. Neumann. "Psychological Aspects of Treating Alcoholism." *Alcohol Health and Research World,* Spring, 1974.

Terry, Luther L. "Today's Antismoking Campaign Will Succeed." *Today's Health,* 48: 22, February, 1970.

Tomkins, Silvan S. "Psychological Model for Smoking Behavior." *American Journal of Public Health,* 56: 17–21, Supplement to December, 1966.

"Why Easterners Turn Down Drinks." *Medical World News,* 14: 104, September 21, 1973.

Chapter 9.   Drug Abuse

Adelstein, Michael E., and Jean G. Rival (eds.). *Drugs.* New York: St. Martin's Press, 1972.

Boe, Sue. "Drugs: The Tools of Medical Progress." *American Journal of Public Health,* 40:65–70, February, 1970.

Bowen, Otis R. "The Medico-Legal Conflict in Drug Usage." *Journal of School Health,* 39:165–173, March, 1969.

Brill, Henry. "Drugs and Aggression." *Mental Health Digest,* 2:11–13, January, 1970.

Cohen, Sidney. *The Drug Dilemma.* New York: McGraw-Hill, 1976.

Conrad, Harold T. "New Directions in Treating Narcotic Addicts." *Mental Health Digest,* 2:40–45, February, 1970.

Distasio, Carol, and Marcia Nawrot. "Methaqualone." *American Journal of Nursing,* 73: 1922–1926, November, 1973.

Fort, Joel, and Christopher T. Cory. *American Drugstore.* Boston: Educational Associates, 1975.

Girdano, Daniel A., and Dorothy Dusels Girdano. *Drug Education:* Content *and Methods.* Reading, Mass.: Addison-Wesley, 1972.

Greene, Mark H., and Robert L. Dupont (eds.). "The Epidemiology of Drug Abuse." *American Journal of Public Health,* Vol. 64, December, 1974 Supplement.

Grinspoon, Lester. *Marihuana Reconsidered.* Cambridge, Mass.: Harvard University Press, 1971.

HEW. *Marihuana and Health 2nd Annual Report to Congress.* Washington, D.C.: Superintendent of Documents, 1972.

Jacobson, Leonard D. "Ethanol Education Today." *Journal of School Health,* 43:36–40, January, 1973.

Kaplan, Robert. *Drug Abuse, Perspectives on Drugs.* Dubuque, Ia.: Wm. C. Brown, 1970.

Louria, Donald B. "A Critique of Some Current Approaches to the Problem of Drug Abuse." *American Journal of Public Health,* 65:581–584, June, 1975.

National Commission on Marijuana and Drug Abuse. *Drug Use in America: Problem in Perspective.* Second Report of the National Commission on Marijuana and Drug Abuse, March, 1973. Washington, D.C.: Superintendent of Documents, 1973.

"National Survey of Marijuana Use and Attitudes." *Journal of School Health,* 5:544–546, November, 1975.

Ray, Oakley S. *Drugs, Society and Human Behavior.* St. Louis: C. V. Mosby, 1974.

Taintor, Zebulon. "The 'Why' of Youthful Drug Abuse." *Journal of School Health,* 44:26–30, January, 1974.

Tennant, Forest S., et al. "Effectiveness of Drug Education Classes." *American Journal of Public Health,* 64:422–427, May, 1974.

Thomas, John A., Michael T. Smith, and Glenn R. Knotts. "Current Assessment of Marihuana." *Journal of School Health,* 42:382–385, September, 1972.

Thornburg, Hershel. "The Adolescent and Drugs: An Overview." *Journal of School Health,* 43:640–645, December, 1973.

Weil, Andrew. "Man's Innate Need: Getting High." *Intellectual Digest,* 2:69–73, August, 1972.

Whipple, Dorothy V., and Dodi Schultz. "Answers To the Most Controversial Questions About Drugs." *Today's Health,* 50:1616–1620, 60, 61, March, 1972.

Yankelovich, Daniel. "How Students Control Their Drug Crisis." *Psychology Today,* 9:39–43, October, 1975.

Chapter 10.   Sexuality and Marriage

"Bringing Sex Education for Doctors Up to Date." *Medical World News,* 16:113–129, March 24, 1975.

Brissett, Dennis, and Lionel S. Lewis. "Guidelines for Marital Sex: An Analysis of Fifteen Popular Marriage Manuals." *Mental Health Digest,* 2:10–13, May, 1970.

Cole, J. K., and R. Dienstfier. *Nebraska Symposium on Motivation.* Lincoln: University of Nebraska Press, 1973.

Crase, Dixie R. "Significance of Masculinity and Femininity." *Health Education,* 6:30–36, January–February, 1975.

"The Ethics of Therapist-Patient Sex," *Medical World News,* 17:34–36, July 12, 1976.

Focus: Human Sexuality. An Annual Editions Reader. Guilford, Conn.: The Dushkin Publishing Group, 1976.

Freedman, Mark. "Homosexuals May Be Healthier Than Straights." *Psychology Today,* 8:28–33, March, 1975.

Fulton, G. B. *Sexual Awareness.* Boston: Holbrook Press, 1974.

Gagnon, John. *Human Sexuality—An Aged Ambiguity.* Boston: Little, Brown & Co., 1975.

Gagnon, John H., and William Simon. "They Are Going to Learn in the Street Anyway." *Psychology Today,* 3:48–49, 71, July, 1969.

Goldstein, Bernard. *Human Sexuality*. New York: McGraw-Hill, 1976.

Goodheart, Barbara. "Education on Titillation." *Today's Health*, 48:28–30, 70, February, 1970.

Hall, Mary Harrington. "A Conversation with Masters and Johnson." *Psychology Today*, 3:50–52, 54–58, July, 1969.

Henze, L. F., and J. W. Hudson. "Personal and Family Characteristics of Non-Cohabiting and Cohabiting College Students." *Journal of Marriage and the Family*, 36, No. 4, 1974.

Hettlinger, Richard F. *Human Sexuality: A Psychosocial Perspective*. Belmont, Calif.: Wadsworth Publishing Co., 1975.

Jones, Kenneth L., Louis W. Shainberg, and Curtis O. Byer. *Human Sexuality*, San Francisco: Canfield Press, 1975.

Kaplan, H. S. "No-Nonsense Therapy for Six Sexual Malfunctions." *Psychology Today*, 8(5):76–86, 1974.

Katchadourian, Herant A., and Donald T. Lunde. *Fundamentals of Human Sexuality*. New York: Holt, Rinehart & Winston, 1975.

Kiester, Edwin. "How Divorce Counselors Sweeten the Sour Taste of Separation." *Today's Health*, 53:46–51, November, 1975.

Kinsey, A. C., W. B. Pomeroy, C. E. Martin, and P. H. Gebhard. *Sexual Behavior in the Human Female*. Philadelphia: W. B. Saunders, 1953.

Kogan, B. A. *Human Sexual Expression*. New York: Harcourt, Brace & Jovanovich, 1973.

Masters, William H., and Virginia E. Johnson. *Human Sexual Response*. Boston: Little, Brown & Co., 1966.

Masters, William H., and Virginia E. Johnson. *Human Sexual Inadequacy*. Boston: Little, Brown & Co., 1970.

Michaelson, Mike. "Man in the Middle." *Today's Health*, 48:31–33, 71–73, February, 1970.

Morrison, E. S., and V. Borosage. *Human Sexuality: Contemporary Perspectives*, Palo Alto, Calif.: National Press Books, 1973.

Safran, Claire. "What We're Finding Out About Sexual Stereotypes." *Today's Health*, 53:14–18, October, 1975.

Sawrey, J. M., and C. W. Telford. *Personality and Adjustment*. Boston: Allyn and Bacon, 1975.

Weinberg, Martin S. (ed.). *Sex Research, Studies from the Kinsey Institute*. New York: Oxford University Press, 1976.

"Where Do We Stand—An Editorial." *Today's Health*, 48:30, February, 1970.

Chapter 11.   Reproduction and Family Planning

Ager, Joel, et al. "Vasectomy." *American Journal of Public Health*, 64:680–687, July, 1974.

"Amniocentesis Gets the Green Light." *Medical World News,* 16:17–20, October 20, 1975.

"Aspirin in Pregnancy—Dose of Trouble?" *Medical World News,* 16:81, October 6, 1975.

"Custom-Fitting IUD's with Saline." *Medical World News,* 13:67, June 15, 1973.

Cutright, Phillips. "Illegitimacy: Myths, Causes and Cures." *Family Planning Perspectives,* 3:25–49, January, 1971.

Cutright, Phillips. "The Teenage Sexual Revolution and the Myth of an Abstinent Past." *Family Planning Perspectives,* 4:24–32, January, 1972.

David, Lester. "New Hope for Couples Who Want to Bear Children—and Can't." *Today's Health,* 50:48–54, September, 1972.

Fulton, Gere B. *Sexual Awareness.* Boston: Holbrook Press, 1974.

Goldsmith, Sadja (reviewer). "Birth Planning and Women's Liberation." *Family Planning Perspectives,* 3:1–7, April, 1971.

Goldstein, Phillip, and Gary Stewart. "Trends in Therapeutic Abortion in San Francisco." *American Journal of Public Health,* 62:695–700, May, 1972.

"GP-GYN: What Office Gynecology Should Primary Physicians Do?" *Medical World News,* 14:50–57, December 14, 1973.

Harting, Donald, and Helen J. Hunter. "Abortion Techniques and Services: a Review and Critique." *American Journal of Public Health,* 61:2085–2106, October, 1971.

"Infertility: The Two-sided Puzzle." *Medical World News,* 14:25, 26, 28, 29, 35, 37, January 26, 1973.

"IUDs: the Progress and the Problems." *Medical World News,* 15:55, 56, 58, 60, 61, September 13, 1974.

Kogan, Benjamin A. *Human Sexual Expression.* New York: Harcourt, Brace & Jovanovich, 1973.

Leff, David N. "Boy or Girl: Now Choice, Not Chance." *Medical World News,* 16:45–56, December 1, 1975.

Lincoln, Richard. "Population and the American Future: The Commission's Final Report." *Family Planning Perspectives,* 4:10–23, April, 1972.

Manisoff, Miriam T. "Intrauterine Devices." *American Journal of Nursing,* 73:1188–1193, July, 1973.

Masters, William H., and Virginia E. Johnson. *Human Sexual Response.* Boston: Little, Brown & Co., 1966.

McCary, James Leslie. *Human Sexuality.* New York: D. Van Nostrand, 1973.

McClure, James N. "The Menopause and Psychiatric Symptoms." *Medical World News,* 16:50, 51, October 27, 1975.

Menken, Jane. "The Health and Social Consequences of Teenage Childbearing." *Family Planning Perspectives,* 4:45–54, July, 1972.

Pakter, Jean, et al. "Two Years Experience in New York City With the

Liberalized Abortion Law—Progress and Problems." *American Journal of Public Health,* 63:524–536, June, 1973.

Pengelley, Eric T. *Sex and Human Life.* Menlo Park, Calif.: Addison-Wesley, 1974.

Pilpel, Harriet F., and Nancy F. Wechsler. "Birth Control, Teen-Agers and the Law: A New Look, 1971." *Family Planning Perspectives,* 3:37–48, July, 1971.

"Pitfalls on the Track of Wayward Genes." *Medical World News,* 15:68e–68k, March 8, 1974.

Porter, Cedric W., and Jaroslav F. Hulka. "Female Sterilization in Current Clinical Practice." *Family Planning Perspectives,* 6:30–39, Winter, 1974.

Presser, Harriet B. "Early Motherhood: Ignorance or Bliss?" *Family Planning Perspectives,* 6:8–15, Winter, 1974.

Segal, Sheldon J. "Contraceptive Research: A Male Chauvinist Plot?" *Family Planning Perspectives,* 4:21–26, July, 1972.

Siegler, Alvin M. "Tubal Sterilization." *American Journal of Nursing,* 72:1625–1630, September, 1972.

"Sterilization: Where There's a Will, There Are More and More Ways." *Medical World News,* 14:40, 41, 45, 46, 47, 50, September 21, 1973.

Swanson, Harold D. *Human Reproduction.* New York: Oxford University Press, 1974.

Tietze, Christopher, and Sarah Lewit. "Early Medical Complications of Abortion by Saline: Joint Program for the Study of Abortion (JPSA)." *Studies in Family Planning,* 4:133–139, June, 1973.

"Vasectomy Reversal That Really Works." *Medical World News,* 16:19–22, November 17, 1975.

Wallace, Helen M., et al. "The Maternity Home." *American Journal of Public Health,* 64:568–575, June, 1974.

Westoff, Charles F. "The Modernization of U.S. Contraceptive Practice." *Family Planning Perspectives,* 4:9–13, July, 1972.

Westoff, Leslie Aldridge, and Charles F. Westoff. *From Now to Zero.* Boston: Little, Brown & Co., 1971.

Chapter 12. Debilitators: Chronic and Degenerative Diseases

"Alerting the Public to Heart Attack Signs." *Medical World News,* 14:18, 19, March 9, 1973.

Beeson, Paul B., and Walsh McDermott. *Cecil-Loeb Textbook of Medicine.* Philadelphia: W. B. Saunders, 1970.

"Better Ways of Examining the Bowel." *Medical World News,* 14:61, 62, October 19, 1973.

"Better Screening for Colon Cancer." *Medical World News,* 14:68, May 4, 1973.

"Biofeedback in Action." *Medical World News,* 14:47–52, 57, 60, March 9, 1973.

Cairns, John. "The Cancer Problem." *Scientific American,* 223:64–79, November, 1975.

"Cancer Therapy: How You Can Gauge Adequacy of Treatment." *Medical World News,* 15:38–45, May 17, 1974.

Chenoweth, Alice D. "High Blood Pressure: A National Concern." *Journal of School Health,* 43:307–309, May, 1973.

Cohen, Edward P. "Early Detection is Still Our Best Weapon Against Cancer." *Today's Health,* 53:40–46, December, 1975.

"Co-op Trials: Clinical Key to Advances in Cancer Therapy." *Medical World News,* 14:50f–50j, September 21, 1973.

Cox, Maryann, and Roland F. Wear, Jr. "Campbell Soup's Program to Prevent Atherosclerosis." *American Journal of Nursing,* 72:253–260, February, 1972.

Cushman, Wesley P. *Reducing the Risk of Noncommunicable Diseases.* Dubuque, Ia.: Wm. C. Brown, 1970.

Green, Gareth M. "In Defense of the Lung." *American Lung Association Bulletin,* 60:4–12, April, 1974.

Hoskins, Lois M. "Vascular and Tension Headaches." *American Journal of Nursing,* 74:846–852, May, 1974.

Keller, Margaret R., and B. Lionel Truscott. "Transient Ischemic Attacks." *American Journal of Nursing,* 73:1330–1332, August, 1973.

Kushner, Rose. *Breast Cancer.* New York: Harcourt, Brace, & Jovanovich, 1975.

Lamberg, Lynne. "Diabetes, Researchers Discover some New Links in the Puzzle." *Today's Health,* 53:32–36, 53–56, November, 1975.

"The Lines of Cancer Research." *Medical World News,* 15:31–34, 37, 38, 40, 42, July 12, 1974.

McGovern, John P. "Allergy Problems in School-Aged Children." *Journal of School Health,* 44:260–269, May, 1974.

Milligan, Carol, Dana Cummings, and Virginia Williamson. "Screening for Cervical Cancer." *American Journal of Nursing,* 75:1343–1345, August, 1975.

"New Hope for Diabetics." *U.S. News & World Report, Inc.,* 79:51–55, November 24, 1975.

"Overcoming Seasonal Allergies." *Medical World News,* 15:39–45, August 9, 1974.

"Progress in Cancer Chemotherapy." *Medical World News,* 13:50–60, 63, 65, November 17, 1972.

Rosenman, Ray H., and Meyer Friedman. *Type A Behavior and Your Heart.* New York: Alfred A. Knopf, 1974.

Ross, John, and Robert A. O'Rourke. *Understanding the Heart and Its Diseases.* New York: McGraw-Hill, 1976.
"Setting Safer Limits on Mammography." *Medical World News,* 16:23–25, August 11, 1975.
"74 Years of Pioneering Cancer Research." *Medical World News,* 14:100, 101, 104–107, September 7, 1973.
"Two Attacks Against Testicular Cancer." *Medical World News,* 16:58, June 30, 1975.
" 'Type A' Theory: Only an 'E' for Effort?" *Medical World News,* 15:52, May 17, 1974.
"When the Problem is Neurological." *Medical World News,* 15:39–45, 49, 51, September 20, 1974.

Chapter 13. Infectious Diseases

Baker, Betty S. "International Venereal Disease Symposium: A Report." *Journal of School Health,* 44:5–8, January, 1974.
Beeson, Paul B., and Walsh McDermott (eds.). *Cecil-Loeb Textbook of Medicine.* Philadelphia: W. B. Saunders, 1970.
Blount, Joseph H. "A New Approach for Gonorrhea Epidemiology." *American Journal of Public Health,* 62:710–713, May, 1972.
Holland, John J. "Slow, Inapparent and Recurrent Viruses." *Scientific American,* 230:33–41, February, 1974.
"Mononucleosis: Tender Treatment After Aggressive Diagnosis." *Medical World News,* 14:31, 33, 35, 36, 38, April 6, 1973.
"More Kinds and Cases of VD." *Medical World News,* 16:37–47, July 28, 1975.
"Immunization Levels Inch Up, But 'Conquered Diseases' Remain a Threat." *Medical World News,* 16:86–88, September 22, 1975.
Pariser, Harry, and Harry Wise. "Gonorrhea Epidemiology—Is It Worthwhile?" *American Journal of Public Health,* 62:713, 714, May, 1972.
"Prophylaxis for Rabies With Less Pain, Greater Effect?" *Medical World News,* 14:90e–90h, August 10, 1973.
Reagan, W. Paul. "When the Medical Staff is Convinced, It Can Be Done." *Lung Association Bulletin,* 58:8–16, July–August, 1972.
Remsberg, Charles and Bonnie Remsberg. "The Shocking Facts About Gonorrhea." *Good Housekeeping,* 174:78, 138, 140, 142, February, 1972.
Richards, Robert N. *Venereal Diseases and Their Avoidance.* New York: Holt, Rinehart & Winston, 1974.
Schaefer, Julius, Lavelle Hanna, Edward C. Hill, Susan Massad, Charles W. Sheppard, John E. Conte, Jr., Stephen N. Cohen, and Karl F. Meyer. "Are Chlamydial Infections the Most Prevalent Venereal Disease?"

Journal of American Medical Association, 231:1252–1255, March 24, 1975.

"Treating Colds That Just Won't Quit." *Medical World News,* 15:33–40, March, 1974.

Chapter 14. Safety and Accident Prevention

"Accident Death Toll Drops Sharply in 1974." *Statistical Bulletin,* 56:6–8, January, 1975.

Ashby, Neal. "When You Need to Lift. . . ." *Today's Health,* 50:52–53, 72, March, 1972.

Baker, J. Stannard. "Let's Investigate Serious Accidents." *Analogy,* Autumn, 1969, pp. 10–15.

Howard, Jane. "What Every Woman Should Know About Traveling Alone." *Today's Health,* 52:38–41, 69–70, August, 1974.

Leroux, Susan L. "The Driving Hazard You Inhale." *Concepts,* 7:1–4, Fall–Winter, 1974.

O'Rourke, Thomas W., "The Case for Positive Safety Education." *School Health Review,* 4:35–36, July–August, 1973.

Rushwood, Elizabeth. "Hazards Around Us." *World Health,* May, 1974, pp. 10–13.

Sadler, Laurie Cray. "Motorcycling: A Hazardous Two-Wheel Ride." *Today's Health,* 53:28–30, 50, 51, July–August, 1975.

Strasser, Malaud K., and James E. Aaron, Ralph C. Bohn, and John R. Eales. *Fundamentals of Safety Education.* New York: Macmillan, 1973.

Weaver, Peter. "How Safe Is Your Home?" *Today's Health,* 52:40–43, October, 1974.

White, Carol. "Medical Supplies You Should Always Have on Hand." *Today's Health,* 51:48–51, January, 1973.

Chapter 15. Community Health in Ecological Perspective

American Medical Association. *Physician's Guides to Air Pollution, Water Pollution, Noise Pollution,* and *Odor Pollution.* Chicago, 1973.

Bascom, Willard. "The Disposal of Waste in the Ocean." *Scientific American,* 231:16–26, August, 1974.

Bernarde, Melvin A. *Our Precarious Habitat.* New York: W. W. Norton, 1973.

Burns, Eveline M. *Health Services for Tomorrow.* New York: Dunellen Publishing Co., 1973.

Chanlett, Emil T. *Environmental Protection.* New York: McGraw-Hill, 1973.

Corman, Rena. "Must We Choose Between Energy and Clean Air?" *American Lung Association Bulletin,* 60:2–8, January–February, 1974.

Davis, Arthur A. "Transportation—Shaper of Cities." *American Lung Association Bulletin,* 58:5–10, June, 1972.

Dawson, Barbara, and Charles and Peg Graeff. "Good Volunteers Mind Other People's Business." *Today's Health,* 53:46–51, October, 1975.

Dubos, Rene. *A God Within.* New York: Charles Scribner's Sons, 1972.

Dubos, Rene J. "Humanizing the Earth." *Science,* 179:769–772, February 23, 1973.

Dubos, Rene J. "A Look Into Your Future . . . Ecology." *Today's Health,* 51:50–51, 62–63, April, 1973.

Ehrlich, Paul R., Anne H. Ehrlich, and John P. Holdren. *Human Ecology: Problems and Solution.* San Francisco: W. H. Freeman, 1973.

Glass, David, Sheldon Cohen, and Jerome Singer. "Urban Din Fogs the Brain." *Psychology Today,* 6:94–96, 97–98, May, 1973.

Goldsmith, John R., and Erland Jonsson. "Health Effects of Community Noise." *American Journal of Public Health,* 63:782–791, September, 1973.

Hanlon, John J. *Public Health: Administration and Practice.* St. Louis: C. V. Mosby, 1974.

Henkel, Barbara. *Community Health.* Boston: Allyn and Bacon, 1970.

Higdon, Al. "Bug vs. Bug." *The Kiwanis Magazine,* 58:33–38, 48, February, 1973.

Lehr, Eugene L. "Carbon Monoxide Poisoning: A Preventable Environmental Hazard." *American Journal of Public Health,* 60:289–293, February, 1970.

Longgood, William. *The Darkening Land.* New York: Simon and Schuster, 1972.

Man and His Endangered World: ABC's of Human Ecology. Greenfield, Mass.: Channing L. Bete Co., 1972.

Nader, Ralph, and Donald Ross. *Action for a Change.* New York: Gossman Publishers, 1971.

Nader, Ralph. "Not All of Our Drinking Water Meets Healthful Standards." *Today's Health,* 53:10, 11, 51–56, December, 1975.

"National Wildlife Federation '76 Eq. Index," *National Wildlife,* 14:17–30, February–March, 1976.

"Ozone Alert: Read Before Spraying." *Today's Health,* 53:52–55, October, 1975.

Skalka, Patricia. "Urban Greenery: How Our Cities Can Turn a New Leaf." *Today's Health,* 53:20–24, 53, 54, March, 1975.

Shiffman, Morris A. "The Use of Standards in the Administration of Environmental Pollution Control Programs." *American Journal of Public Health,* 60:255–265, February, 1970.

Smolensky, Jack, and Franklin B. Haar. *Principles of Community Health.* Philadelphia: W. B. Saunders, 1972.

Snow, Donald L. "Standard Needs in Controlling Radiation Exposure of the Public." *American Journal of Public Health,* 60:243–249, February, 1970.

Sultz, Harry A. "An Effect of Continued Exposure to Air Pollution on the Incidence of Chronic Childhood Allergic Disease." *American Journal of Public Health.* 60:891–901, May, 1970.

Task Force on Land Use. *The Use of Land: A Citizens' Policy Guide to Urban Growth,* New York: Thomas Y. Crowell, 1973.

Toffler, Alvin. *Future Shock.* New York: Random House, published by Bantam Books, 1970.

Wagner, Richard H. *Environment and Man.* New York: W. W. Norton, 1974.

Waldbott, George L. *Health Effects of Environmental Pollutants.* St. Louis: C. V. Mosby, 1973.

Walker, Bailus. "Environmental Quality and the Local Health Agency—A Re-examination." *American Journal of Public Health,* 63:352–357, April, 1973.

Chapter 16. Future Prospects in Health

Belson, Abby. "Predictive Medicine." *Family Health,* 7:30–33, January, 1975.

Cross, Farrell. "Sound Waves That Save Lives." *Family Health,* 6:30–33, July, 1974.

Filer, L. J. "The USA Today—Is It Free of Public Health Nutrition Problems?" *American J. of Public Health,* 59:327–328, February, 1969.

Garfield, Sidney R. "The Delivery of Medical Care." *Scientific American,* 222:15–24, April, 1970.

Greenfeld, Josh. "Advances in Genetics That Can Change Your Life." *Today's Health,* 51:20–24, 58, December, 1973.

Gross, Franz. "The Future: Hopes and Fears." *World Health,* April, 1974, pp. 28–32.

Gwynne, Peter. "Acupuncture Update." *Today's Health,* 52:16–19, 66, January, 1974.

Hamburger, Jean. "Physicians, Biologists and the Future of Man." *World Health,* September, 1974, pp. 16–21.

Hickman, James C., and Richard J. Estell. "On The Use of Partial Life Expectancies in Setting Health Goals." *American J. of Public Health,* 59:2243–2251, December, 1969.

Kowet, Don. "Never Say Die." *Today's Health,* 52:20–23, 67–68, July, 1974.

Lambo, T. Adeoye. "The Right to Health." *World Health,* June, 1974, pp. 2–5.

Levin, L. S. "Building Toward the Future: Implications for Health Education." *American J. of Public Health,* 59:1983–1991, November, 1969.

McNerney, Walter J. "Changing the Health Care System." *American J. of Nursing,* 69:2427–2436, November, 1969.

Means, Richard K. *Historical Perspectives in School Health.* Thorofare, N.J.: Charles B. Slack, Inc., 1975.

"Progress, Yesterday, Today, Tomorrow." *Today's Health* (entire issue), 51:1–75, April, 1973.

Robinson, Sharon. "Dial-a-Diagnosis." *Family Health,* 6:41–43, December, 1974.

Schanche, Don A. "Medical Help for Children Who Grow Too Little." *Today's Health,* 53:16–19, 50–51, March, 1975.

Smith, Donald. "Human Experimentation—A Game Without Rules." *Family Health,* 6:24–25, 46–50, June, 1974.

Stewart, Ruth F. and Jo Annalee Irving. "Group Theory Implications for Changing Health Patterns." *American J. of Public Health,* 59:1894–1898, October, 1969.

Terkel, Studs. "Is the Human Spirit Being Snuffed Out in Our Cities?" *Today's Health,* 51:43–47, 72–74, January, 1973.

Train, Russell E. "Prescription for a Planet: The Ninth Bronfman Lecture." *American Journal of Public Health,* 60:433–441, March, 1970.

index

Audiologists, 84
Auricle, the, 85
Automobiles (see Motor
vehicles)
Autonomic nervous system, 474
Autonomy dimension of
adjustment, 176–178
Avoidance-avoidance conflicts,
192–193
Axelrod, Julius, 333–334
Axial skeleton, 626
Ayres, Stephen M., 565

B

Bacilli, 486
Bacteria, 486
fossilized, 606
Bacterial infections, 509–510
paratyphoid, 510
salmonellosis, 510
typhoid fever, 509–510
general data on, 643
immunization against, 495,
497, 510
Bales, R. F., 250
Barbiturates, 309, 311
Barry, P. Z., 537
Bartholin glands, 389
Basal metabolic rate, 133–134
Bascom, Willard, 595–603
Bauer, W. W., 126
Beamish, Jerome, 533
Beaubrun, Michael H., 332
Beck Depression Inventory, 212
Birth of a baby (see Childbirth)
Birth control (see also
Contraception):
compulsory, 616–617
pills, 355, 375, 398–402
Birth defects, 428–431
genetic counseling, 430–431
heredity in, 428–431
Bisexuality, 377
Blacks, Sickle Cell Anemia and,
430
Bleeding:
control of, 645–646
as a symptom requiring
immediate attention, 69
Blisters, first aid for, 649
Blood pressure, 64–65, 446–447
diastolic, 64–65
systolic, 64–65
Bloomquist, E. R., 296, 300
Blue Cross, 97
Blue Shield, 97–98
Body chemistry, effect of

alcohol, 246, 247
Body functions, exercise and,
115
Boggs Act, 318
Bones, first aid for, 647
Bougainville, Louis Antoine de,
16
Bowen, Otis R., 321
Brain, the, 474, 475
effect of alcohol, 248
Brave New World (Huxley), 623
Breasts, examination of, 62,
452–453
Brecher, Edward M., 325–328
Brill, Norman Q., 334
Bromides, misuse of, 289
Bronchi, 462
Bronchial cilia, 268–270
Bronchioles, 462
Bronchitis, 487–500
as a leading cause of death
(current), 11
Brown, Kevin, 117
Bullough, Bonnie, 96
Burns, first aid for, 649

C

Caesarean section, 423–424
Caffeine, 305
Calcium, 633, 637
Caloric needs, 132–134
basal metabolic rate,
133–134
computing daily needs, 134
desirable weights, 134–136
Calories:
defined, 132
expenditure in relation to
activity, 133
Cameron, Charles S., 26
Campbell, A. M. G., 326
Canada, socialized medicine
in, 48, 104
Cancer, 448–458
air pollution and, 563
alcohol and, 90
false cures, 31–32
five-year survival rates, 455
as a leading cause of death
(current), 11, 13
as a leading cause of death
(1900), 11
malignancy detection,
451–455
morbidity, changing patterns
in, 449–451
mortality, changing patterns

in, 449–451
nature of, 448–449
oral, 90–91
prevention of, 457–458
seven warning signals, 452
smoking and, 90, 270–272,
458
treatment of, 456–457
Cancer Quacks, The (Cameron),
26
Candidiasis, 522–523
Carbohydrates (CHO), 136–138
Carbon monoxide, 268, 272
Carcinomas, 449
Cardiac muscles, 628
Cardiologist, description of
specialty, 44
Cardiopulmonary resuscitation,
549
Cardiovascular, definition of
the term, 436
Cardiovascular diseases,
435–448
arteriosclerosis, 436–438
atherosclerosis, 140–141,
438–439
cerebrovascular accidents,
444–446
cholesterol and, 144, 443
congenital heart disease, 444
congestive heart failure,
443–444
coronary artery disease,
439–443
diet and, 161–162
essential hypertension,
446–447
exercise and, 115–116
as a leading cause of death
(current), 11, 435
prevention of, 447–448
primary hypertension,
446–447
smoking and, 439, 443
Carriers, 492
Carson, Rachel, 560, 622
Cartilage, 625
Cataracts, 82, 83
Catatonic schizophrenia, 228
Cecil-Loeb Textbook of
Medicine (eds. Beeson
and McDermott), 255
Central nervous system,
473–474
effect of alcohol, 248
Cerebellum, the, 474
Cerebral palsy, 479–480

Habit patterns (*cont.*)
projection, 201–202
rationalization, 199–200
regression, 199
repression, 200–201
withdrawal, 197–198
Hallucinations, 226
Hammar, Sherrel, 151–152
Hammurabi, Code of, 606
Hangovers, 247
Harlow, H. F., 183
Harmon, Merrill, 8
Harrison Act (1914), 317
Harvey, William, 608
Headaches, 472–473
Health Care Insurance Act, 105
Health concepts, 1–22
ancient civilizations, 606–607
the changing scene, 619–622
environmental conditions, 620
medical care, 620–621
nature of disease, 619–620
public health practice, 621
public opinion and behavior, 621–622
social conditions, 620
college health programs, 9–10
definition of health, 3–4
early ideas of, 605–611
eighteenth century, 609–610
factors determining health, 7
four-step model for making decisions, 8
health instruction, 10
health values and valuing, 7–8
the human body, 5–7
interrelationships of, 6–7
the mind and, 6–7
psychogenic disorders, 7
human ecology, 15–22
adaptation, 17–18
threat of impoverished humanity, 19–22
tolerance, 18–19
individual initiative, 622–623
Middle Ages, 607, 608
the 1900s, 611
in the 1970s, 616–619
nineteenth century, 609–610
optimal health, 5
origin of the word "health," 2
primitive populations, 16–17
rebirth of science, 607–608
the Reformation, 608
the Renaissance, 608

second half of this century, 611–616
as era of decisions, 613
the medical paradox, 613–616
theory and practice, 2–5
the unity of health, 10, 11
well-being, problems affecting, 10–13
Health education in public health departments, 582–583
Health education services, 582
Health history, 61
Health information, 25–56
advertising and, 28, 35–41
appraising, 35–51
criteria for evaluation, 36
sources of health information, 36–41
consumer health protection, 48–54
credentials and testimonials, 41
erroneous beliefs and super-stitions, 37
evaluating health products, 41–42
medical care costs, 46–48
private consumer health protection, 54–55
quackery and fraudulent practice, 26–35
definition of a quack, 26
definition of quackery, 26
modern areas, 28–35
nostrums and drugs, 27
the quack, 26–27
remedies through the ages, 27–28
reliable sources of, 41
selecting health services, 42–46
common medical specialties, list of, 44–45
criteria for selecting advisors, 45–46
Health Institute of St. Louis, 98
Health insurance, 96–107
compulsory, 48
government programs, 100–107
misunderstood facts about, 98–100
voluntary, 97–98
Health maintenance, 59–108

(*see also* Dental health; Health insurance; Hearing; Visual health)
acute symptoms, temporary care for, 71–75
bill of rights for patients, 71, 72–73
cosmetic surgery, 93–94
medical care delivery, 94–96
group practice, 94, 620
Health Maintenance Organization, 95, 107
hospital clinics, 94–95
special clinics, 95–96
periodic medical examinations, 59–66
clinical examination, 61–62
health history, 61
immunizations, 65
laboratory tests, 63
personal medical records, 66, 68–69
radiation exposure, 66
understanding medical findings, 63–65
Professional Standards Review Organizations, 96
rules for being a better patient, 70–71
symptoms requiring imme-diate attention, 67–70
Health Maintenance Organiza-tion (HMO), 95, 107
Health practices, fraudulent, 26–35
definition of a quack, 26
definition of quackery, 26
modern areas of, 28–35
nostrums and drugs, 27
the quack, 26–27
remedies through the ages, 27–28
Health products, evaluating, 41–42
Health protection:
consumer, 48–54
private consumer, 54–55
Health Rights Act, 106
Health Security Act, 105
Health services, selecting, 42–46
common medical specialties, list of, 44–45
criteria for selecting advisors, 45–46
Health statistics, public health departments and, 585–586

Sweeteners, noncaloric, 153
Sydenham, Thomas, 608
Symptoms:
  acute, temporary care for,
    71–75
  requiring immediate attention,
    67–70
Synarthrosis, 626
Synovial fluid, 626
Syphilis, 519–522
Systemic circulation, 628
Systole, 628
Systolic pressure, 64–65
Systolic tension, 64

T
Taintor, Zebulon, 298
Tamerin, John S., 260
Tapeworm, 642
Tay-Sachs Disease, 430
Temperature inversion, 563
Tennant, Forest S., 328
Tension:
  diastolic, 64
  systolic, 64
Tension headaches, 472–473
Testes, 62, 383
  cancer of, 453–454
Testosterone, 383, 385–386
Tetanus, 511
  general data on, 643
  immunization against, 65,
    495, 496, 611
Therapeutic community, the,
  321
Therapeutic devices, fraudulent,
  32–33
Thermal inversion, 567
This Week Magazine, 116
Thomas, John A., 300
Thomburg, Hershel, 297
Thorax, 625
Thorazine, 290, 293
Thornburn, Marigold J., 332
Throat, clinical examination of,
  62
Thrombus, 438
Thwarting, frustration by,
  188–191
Tobacco (see Smoking)
Tolerance, human ecology and,
  18–19
Tompkins, Silvan S., 273–275
Tooth decay (see Dental caries)
Tooth injuries, 91–92
Toxic deliria, 230

Trace nutrient deficiency, 163–
  164
Trachea, the, 462
Tracheobronchitis, 495, 500
Trachoma, 611
Tranquilizers, 237, 611
  misuse of, 290, 293
Transient ischemic attacks (TIA),
  445
Trephining, 607
Treponema pallidum, 519
Trichinosis, 160
  general data on, 643
Trichomonas, 486
Trichomoniasis, 516
Trisomy, 21, 430
Trypanosoma, 486
Tubal ligation, 405, 406, 407
Tuberculosis, 501–504, 611
  immunization against, 504
  as a leading cause of death
    (1900), 11
Tumors, 449
Type A Behavior and Your Heart
  (Friedman and Rosen-
  man), 442–443
Typhoid fever, 509–510
  general data on, 643
  immunization against, 495,
    497, 510
Typhus, 497

U
Underweight, 156–157
Union of Soviet Socialist
  Republics, state
  medicine, 48, 103
United Federated Funds, 591
United Nations, 587
United Nations Educational,
  Scientific, and Cultural
  Organization (UNESCO),
  13
U.S. Census Bureau, 616
U.S. Department of Agriculture,
  49, 52
  description of, 53
U.S. Department of Health,
  Education and Welfare,
  49, 569–570
U.S. Department of Justice, 52
U.S. Government Organizational
  Manual 1973/1974, 580
United States Pharmacopeia, 27
U.S. Postal Service, 52
  description of, 53

U.S. Post Office Department, 41
U.S. Public Health Service, 574
U.S. Recommended Daily
  Allowance, 148, 164, 165
  table of, 636–637
Unsafe at Any Speed (Nader),
  536, 622
Urethra, 384, 431
Urologist, description of
  specialty, 45
Uterus, 62, 387

V
Vaccinations (see Immunization)
Vacuum aspiration, 411–412
Vagina, 387–388
Vaginitis, 524
Valence:
  negative, 192, 193
  positive, 192, 193
Values, 7–8
  clarification process, 8
  defined, 7–8
  prestige, 187–188
Valuing, health, 7–8
Vascular headaches, 472–473
Vas deferens, 383
Vasectomy, 404, 405–406, 408
Vector spread of disease, 493
Vegetarianism, 166–167
Veins, pulmonary, 628
Venereal disease (VD) (see
  Sexual activity, diseases
  transmitted by)
Venereal warts, 523
Ventricles, 628
Vesalius, Andreas, 608
Vibrator chair, 29
Vinci, Leonardo da, 608
Viral enteritis, 508
Viral infections, 508–509
  hepatitis, 508–509
  viral enteritis, 508
Viruses, 486, 489, 499, 501
Viscera, 625
Vision changes, as symptoms
  requiring immediate
  attention, 70
Visual health, maintenance of,
  75–84
  abnormalities, 79–83
  defects, 79–81
  disorders, 79, 81–83
  care of eyes, 76–79
  contact lenses, 83–84
  corneal transplantations, 83